Hepatocellular Carcinoma: Clinical Oncology

Hepatocellular Carcinoma: Clinical Oncology

Editor: Evangeline Hart

FOSTER ACADEMICS
www.fosteracademics.com

www.fosteracademics.com

FOSTER ACADEMICS

Cataloging-in-Publication Data

Hepatocellular carcinoma : clinical oncology / edited by Evangeline Hart.
p. cm.
Includes bibliographical references and index.
ISBN 978-1-63242-895-0
1. Liver--Cancer. 2. Liver--Cancer--Treatment. 3. Oncology. 4. Cancer. I. Hart, Evangeline.
RC280.L5 H47 2020
616.994 36--dc23

Foster Academics,
118-35 Queens Blvd., Suite 400,
Forest Hills, NY 11375, USA

ISBN 978-1-63242-895-0 (Hardback)

Contents

Preface

Hepatocellular carcinoma (HCC) is the most common liver cancer occurring in adults. It is also the leading cause of deaths in patients with liver cirrhosis. Some of the risk factors for this condition are exposure to alcohol or aflatoxin, hepatitis infection, alpha 1-antitrypsin deficiency, hemochromatosis, NASH, metabolic syndrome, etc. HCC may present symptoms such as abdominal swelling due to fluid buildup in the abdominal cavity, yellow skin, loss of appetite, easy bruising, nausea, vomiting, etc. HCC is generally diagnosed at an advanced stage and is thus associated with a high rate of mortality. CT scan, MRI and ultrasound are ideal for liver analysis and detection of HCC. The treatment of HCC is based on a review of the stage of the disease, availability of liver transplant and a person's likelihood of tolerating surgery. Accordingly, a patient may be recommended for a partial hepatectomy, orthotopic liver transplantation, targeted therapies, loco-regional therapy, etc. This book is a valuable compilation of topics, ranging from the basic to the most complex advancements in the field of clinical oncology. It discusses the fundamentals as well as modern approaches in the diagnosis and treatment of this cancer. This book aims to serve as a resource guide for students and experts alike and contribute to the growth of the discipline.

This book is a result of research of several months to collate the most relevant data in the field.

When I was approached with the idea of this book and the proposal to edit it, I was overwhelmed. It gave me an opportunity to reach out to all those who share a common interest with me in this field. I had 3 main parameters for editing this text:

1. Accuracy - The data and information provided in this book should be up-to-date and valuable to the readers.
2. Structure - The data must be presented in a structured format for easy understanding and better grasping of the readers.
3. Universal Approach - This book not only targets students but also experts and innovators in the field, thus my aim was to present topics which are of use to all.

Thus, it took me a couple of months to finish the editing of this book.

I would like to make a special mention of my publisher who considered me worthy of this opportunity and also supported me throughout the editing process. I would also like to thank the editing team at the back-end who extended their help whenever required.

Editor

Glycogen Synthase Kinase-3β is Associated with the Prognosis of Hepatocellular Carcinoma and may Mediate the Influence of Type 2 Diabetes Mellitus on Hepatocellular Carcinoma

Guoliang Qiao[1,9], Yuan Le[2,9], Jun Li[1], Lianghuan Wang[2], Feng Shen[1]*

1 Department of Hepatic Surgery, Eastern Hepatobiliary Surgery Hospital, Second Military Medical University, Shanghai, China, 2 Department of Biochemistry and Molecular Biology, Second Military Medical University, Shanghai, China

Abstract

Background: Although many studies have shown glycogen synthase kinase-3β(GSK-3β) was associated with type 2 diabetes mellitus(T2DM) and implicated with a wide range of cancers, the role of GSK-3β in hepatocellular carcinoma(HCC) and the correlation among GSK-3β, T2DM and HCC remains unclear. Our objectives were to identify the effect of p-Ser9-GSK-3β on the prognosis of patients with HCC and to learn more about the interaction among T2DM, GSK-3β and the prognosis of HCC.

Methods: Firstly we used reverse transcriptase-PCR(RT-PCR) and western blotting to determine the expression levels of GSK-3β and p-Ser9-GSK-3β in human HCC samples. We then used immunohistochemical staining to evaluate the expression pattern of p-Ser9-GSK-3β in 178 patients with HCC after curative partial hepatectomy. Finally we statistically analyzed the association of p-Ser9-GSK-3β and T2DM with the prognosis of patients with HCC.

Results: P-Ser9-GSK-3β was over-expressed in tumor tissues compared with their normal counterparts. Correlation and regression analysis indicated that the over-expression of p-Ser9-GSK-3β was significantly associated with T2DM, and the correlation coefficient was 0.259 ($P = 0.001$). Multivariate analysis showed that the over-expression of p-Ser9-GSK-3β($P < 0.001$) and T2DM($P = 0.008$) were independently associated with poor prognosis of HCC, respectively. Further analysis demonstrated that these two variables are closely related with each other.

Conclusion: The over-expression of p-Ser9-GSK-3β and T2DM are strongly correlated with worse surgical outcome of HCC. P-Ser9-GSK-3β may play a significant role in mediating the influence of T2DM on the prognosis of HCC.

Editor: Xin-Yuan Guan, The University of Hong Kong, China

Funding: The authors have no support or funding to report.

Competing Interests: The authors have declared that no competing interests exist.

* Email: shenfdfgd@163.com

9 These authors contributed equally to this work.

Introduction

Hepatocellular carcinoma(HCC) is the fifth most common malignancy worldwide and the second most frequent cause of cancer-related mortality [1]. Partial hepatectomy remains the standard curative treatment, with a 5-year survival rate of 50%–70% for early HCC [2,3]. Accurately identifying the prognostic factors is important to facilitate screening of high risk patients and make decisions on the adjuvant therapy.

Glycogen synthase kinase 3 (GSK3), a constitutive multi-functional serine threonine kinase, was involved in diversely physiological pathways ranging from insulin signaling pathways which associated with the disease of type 2 diabetes mellitus (T2DM) and Wnt signaling pathways which related to oncogenesis [4–7]. GSK-3β (47 kDa), an isoform of GSK-3, could be inactivated by insulin through phosphorylation of an N-terminal domain serine residue(Ser9 of GSK-3β) [8]. Phosphorylation of Ser9-GSK-3β (p-Ser9-GSK-3β) was associated with the activation of Wnt signaling which could prevent phosphorylation and lead to the stabilization of β-catenin. This mechanism had been reported in a wide range of cancers [9]. However, few researchers reported the significance of GSK-3β or p-Ser9-GSK-3β in the prognostic evaluation of patients with HCC [10].

Currently, epidemiology studies revealed that diabetes mellitus(DM) increased the incidence of HCC [11,12]. Although it remained controversial about the influence of DM on the prognosis of patients with HCC after partial hepatectomy [13,14], accumulating evidence showed that DM was an

Table 1. Correlation between p-Ser9-GSK-3β expression and clinicopathologic features.

Variables		p-Ser9-GSK-3β expression		
		Low(n = 89)	High(n = 89)	*P*
Sex	female	12	14	0.671
	male	77	75	
Age	median	50	49	0.613
	range	15–72	32–74	
AFP level(μg/L)	≤400	53	54	0.878
	>400	36	35	
HBsAg	positive	79	78	0.816
	negative	10	11	
HBeAg	positive	20	13	0.177
	negative	69	76	
Liver cirrhosis	yes	69	75	0.253
	no	20	14	
Edmondson-Steiner grade	I-II	17	20	0.579
	III- IV	72	69	
Diameter(cm)	≤5	52	51	0.879
	>5	37	38	
Encapsulation	complete	32	21	0.071
	no	57	68	
MVI	yes	29	34	0.433
	no	60	55	
Tumor number	single	76	70	0.242
	multiple	13	19	
TBL(umol/l)	median	15.4	16	0.603
	range	4.2-56.7	4.6-64.4	
Alb(g/dl)	median	38.4	40	0.092
	range	24.5–51.4	23.6–53.8	
ALT(U/L)	median	54.9	55.5	0.887
	range	10,6–235.7	8.3–240.3	
WBC	median	5.2	5.1	0.611
	range	2.5–13.7	3.1–14.8	
RBC	median	4.4	4.3	0.348
	range	3.2–5.8	2.8–5.4	
PLT($*10^9$/L)	median	124	122	0.783
	range	22–359	17–367	
INR	median	1.05	1.04	0.308
	range	0.87–1.26	0.89–1.23	
CR	median	70	68	0.454
	range	40–136	38–139	
MELD score	median	7.6	7.5	0.564
	range	6.0–12	6.0–11	
T2DM	yes	6	23	0.001
	no	83	66	

Abbreviations: AFP, alpha-fetoprotein; HBsAg, hepatitis B surface antigen; HBeAg, Hepatitis E antigen; MVI, microvascular invasion; TBIL total bilirubin; ALB, albumin; ALT, alanine; WBC, white blood cell; RBC, red blood cell; PLT, platelet count; INR, international normalized ratio; CR, creatinine; MELD, model for end-stage liver disease; T2DM, type 2 diabetes mellitus.

independent prognostic indicator for patients with HCC after curative resection [15,16]. The purpose of the present study is to identify if the expression level of p-Ser9-GSK-3β is an effective prognostic factor for HCC patients and learn more about the interaction among the T2DM, expression of p-Ser9-GSK-3β and the prognosis of HCC.

Materials and Methods

1. Patients and human HCC specimen

A total of 238 patients with HCC undergoing partial hepatectomy by two independent surgical teams at Eastern Hepatobiliary Surgery Hospital from July 1st, 2003 to May 15th, 2005 were enrolled in this study. The preoperative clinical diagnosis of HCC met the diagnostic criteria of the American Association for the Study of Liver Diseases(AASLD) [17]. Of these surgical HCC specimens, 60 samples which were collected between July 1st and December 15th, 2003, were subjected to RNA and protein extraction that could be done for RT-PCR and western blot analysis. 178 patients collected between December 16th, 2003 and May 15th, 2005 met the following inclusion criteria and then underwent immunohistochemical staining (IHC) and prognostic analyses: had WHO performance status 0-1; did not receive any preoperative anti-cancer therapy; did not have any distant metastasis, image visible ascites, or severe esophageal varices; had the preoperative Child-Pugh class A; received curative hepatectomy; had pathologically proven hepatocellular carcinoma. Patients were excluded from this study if they had a history of other solid tumors, or died from severe postoperative complications. The clinical characteristics of the 178 patients were listed in Table 1.

The definition of curative hepatectomy was described as our previous reports [18]. The histological grade of tumor differentiation was assigned by the Edmondson Steiner grading system [19]. This study was approved by the Institutional Review Board of Eastern Hepatobiliary Surgery Hospital. All patients gave written informed consent to participate. The parents wrote the informed consent on behalf of the patients whose age<18. The ethics committees approved this consent procedure. The data did not contain any information that could identify the patients.

2. Immunohistochemistry and evaluation of immunostaining

Immunohistochemical staining was performed with the Dako Envision Plus System (Dako, Carpinteria, CA) according to the manufacturer's instructions. The primary antibodies were anti-GSK-3β and anti-p-Ser9-GSK-3β (Cell Signaling Technology Inc.,Beverly, MA, 1:50). The tissues were evaluated as positive for GSK-3β and p-Ser9-GSK-3β staining when there were more than 10% of tumor cells demonstrating cytoplasmic and/or nucleus immunoreaction deposits. The sections were scored with a four-tier scale: 0 = negative (0–10%), 1 = weak signal (10–20%), 2 = intermediate signal (20–50%) and 3 = strong signal (> 50%). 0 and 1 were defined as low exprression, while 2 and 3 were defined as over-expression. All sections were scored independently by two observers who did not have any prior knowledge of the clinic-pathologic data. The concordance between scores from different sections of the same tumor was greater than 90%. All discrepancies in scoring were reviewed and a consensus was reached.

3. Western blotting analysis

Fresh surgical specimens were snap frozen in liquid nitrogen and stored in deep freezer. The normal and the tumor tissues were lysed in T-PER Tissue Protein Extraction Reagent(Pierce, Rockford, IL) containing proteinase inhibitors(CalBiochem, San Diego, CA). The extractions were collected and centrifuged at 12,000×g for 5 min. The protein concentrations were determined using the BCA Protein Assay (Pierce) according to the manufacturer's instructions. The following antibodies were used: anti-GSK-3β and anti-p-Ser9-GSK-3β (Cell Signaling Technology Inc., Beverly, MA), we also used β -actin as a loading control.

4. RNA extraction and real-time reverse transcriptase-PCR

Total RNA of tissue samples were isolated using TRIzol (Life Technologies, Inc., Rockville, MD) according to the manufacturer's instructions. cDNA was generated from 1 ug of each RNA sample and a reverse transcribed using a transcription kit (Takara, Kyoto, Japan). Real-time quantitative reverse transcriptase-PCR (RT-PCR) was done in the 7300 Real Time PCR System (Applied Biosystems) to detect GSK-3β gene expression in paired liver samples from 30 HCC patients. The primers were as follows:

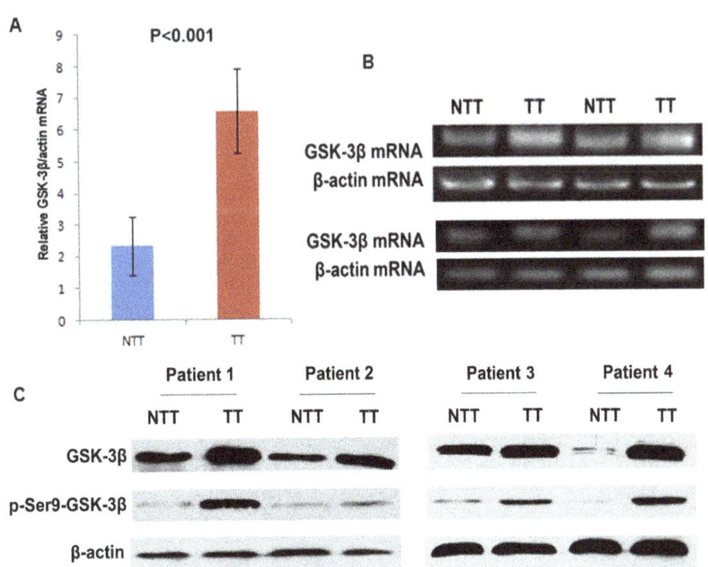

Figure 1. Expression of GSK-3β and p-Ser9-GSK-3β in HCC. (A) Relative expression level of GSK-3β mRNA in 60 tumor tissues(TT) and paired non-tumorous tissues(NTT) by RT-PCR (P<0.001). (B) RT-PCR analysis of GSK-3β mRNA expression. (C) Expressions of p-Ser9-GSK-3β were analyzed by Western Blotting in HCC tumor tissues(TT) and paired non-tumorous tissues(NTT).

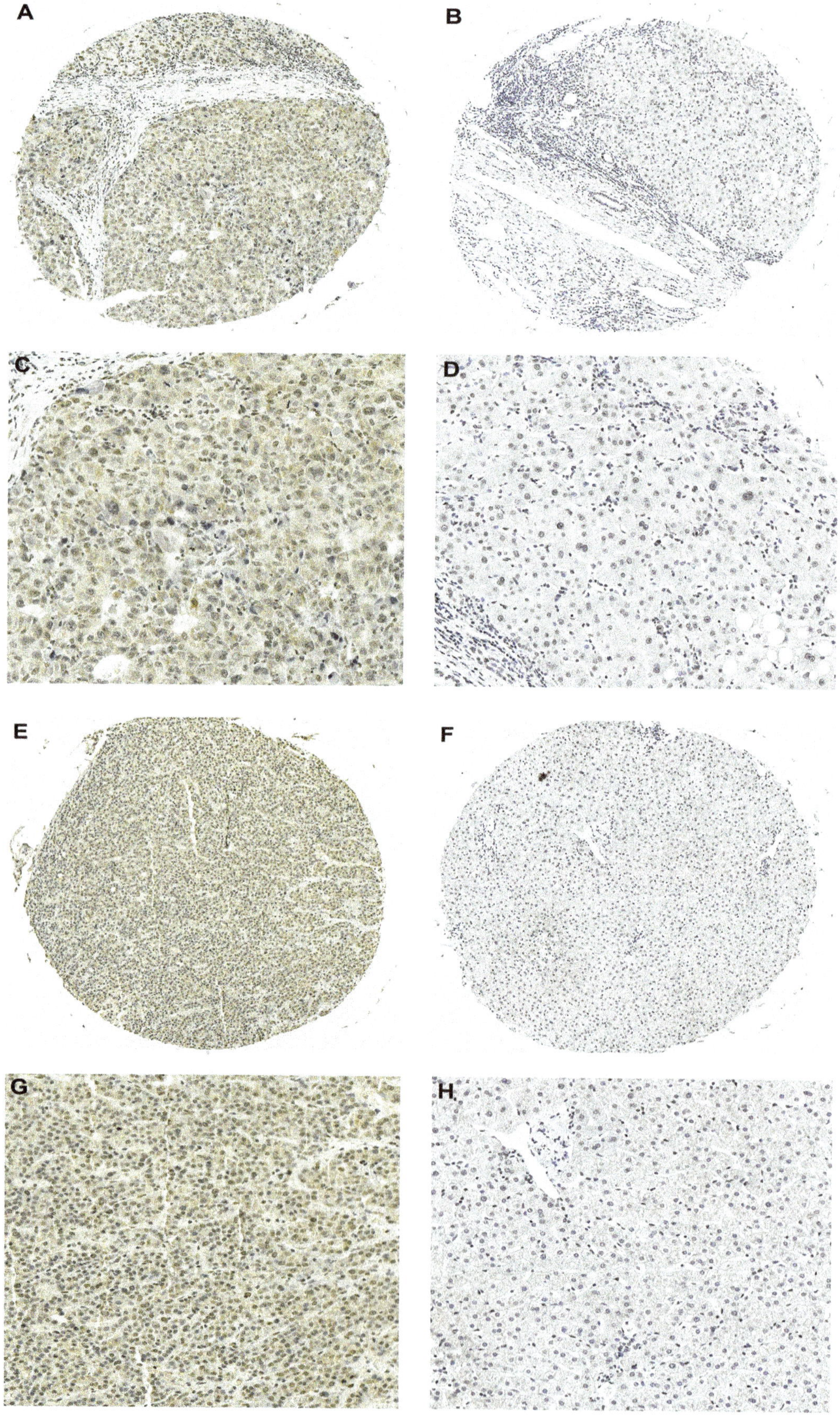
A
B
C
D
E
F
G
H

Figure 2. Immunohistochemical analysis of p-Ser9-GSK-3β expressions in HCCs and the adjacent nontumorous liver tissues. (A-D) Immunohistochemical staining of a paired HCC and nontumoral tissue. HCC cells were strongly positive for p-Ser9-GSK-3β expression in the cytoplasm (A,C). Normal hepatocytes in the nontumoral tissue showed no detectable p-Ser9-GSK-3β expression(B,D). (E-H) Immunohistochemical staining of another paired HCC and nontumoral tissue. HCC cells were strongly positive for p-Ser9-GSK-3β expression in the cytoplasm(E,G). Normal hepatocytes in the nontumoral tissue showed no detectable p-Ser9-GSK-3β expression(F,H). Original magnifications: magnification*50 (A,B,E,F); magnification*100 (C,D,G,H).

GSK-3β, forward: 5′-AACACCAACAAGGGAGCAAA-3′; reverse: 5′-GAGCGTGAGGAGGGATAAGG-3′, 326bp. β-actin, forward: 5′-ACCATGGATGATGATATCGC-3′ and reverse: 5′-ACATGGCTGGGGTGTTGAAG-3′, 386bp. β-actin served as an endogenous control. The expression of the target messenger RNA(mRNA) was quantified relative to that of the β-actin mRNA. A ratio of relative GSK-3β mRNA levels in tumor samples/nontumorous samples of 0.5-fold was defined as under-expression of the gene, whereas a ratio of 2.0-fold was defined as over-expression.

5. Diagnosis of Type 2 diabetes

Diagnosis of diabetes mellitus was based on the 1999 World Health Organization criteria. Patients who were found to have a fasting blood sugar level between 5.6 and 6.1 mmol/L were defined as having impaired fasting glucose and were referred for confirmation of their diabetes status. Those with a fasting blood sugar level of at least 7.0 mmol/L or those diagnosed with Type 2 diabetes before entering the hospital were defined as having Type 2 diabetes and were referred for further diabetic care. Patients with prior diagnosis of Type 1 diabetes were excluded from the study.

6. Follow-up

The follow-up ended on May 2012 and the median follow-up duration was 48.2 months (3.8–114.5 months). Contrast-enhanced CT scan or MRI of the abdomen was carried out once every 3 months in the first two years after surgery, and then once every 6 months thereafter. The diagnostic criteria for HCC recurrence was the same as used for the initial diagnosis.

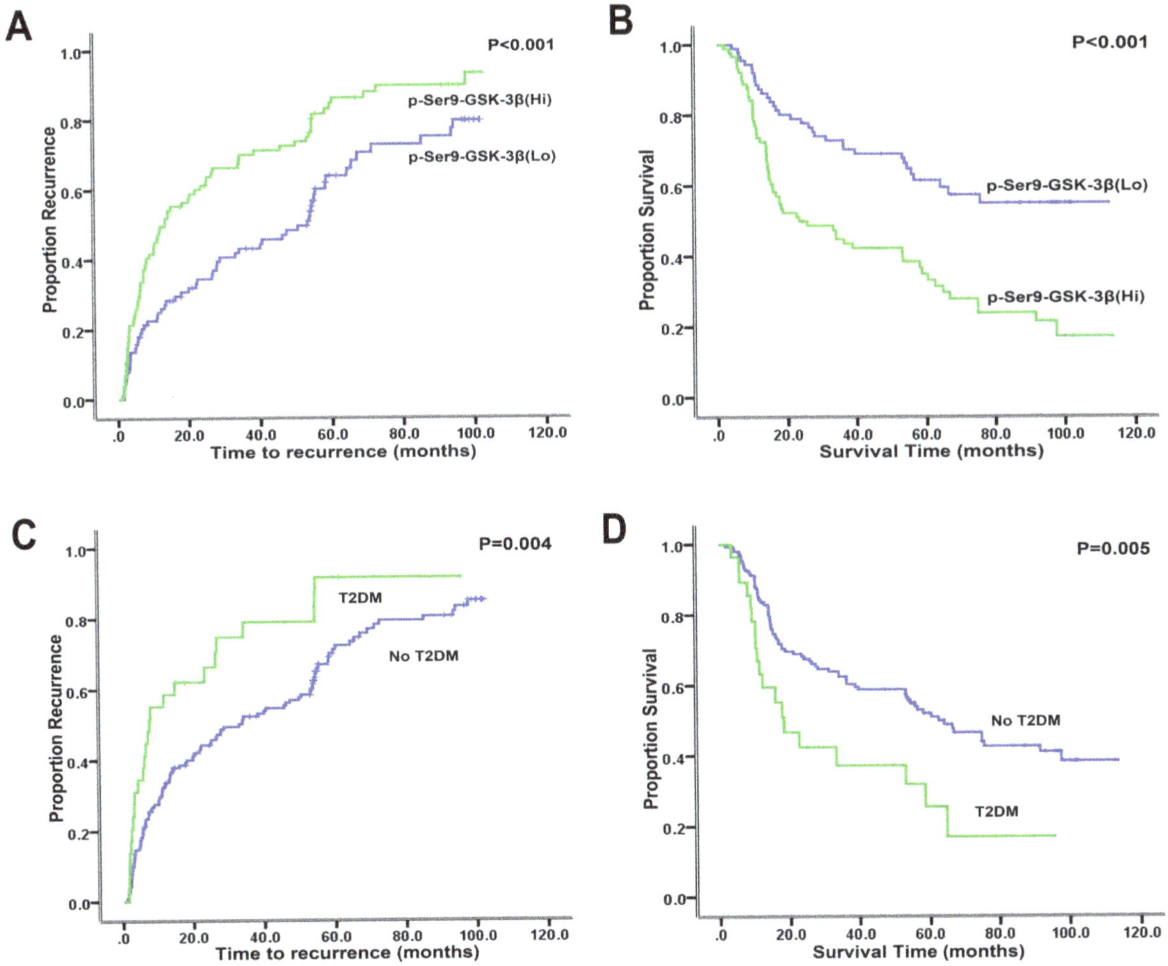

Figure 3. Kaplan-Meier analysis of TTR and OS of patients with HCC. (A,B) Kaplan-Meier curves of the correlation between p-Ser9-GSK-3β expression level and (A) recurrence or (B) overall survival of HCC patients; (C,D) Kaplan-Meier curves of the correlation between T2DM and (A) recurrence or (B) overall survival of HCC patients.

Table 2. Multivariate analysis for overall survival.

Variable	Overall Survival			Overall Survival(exclude T2DM)			Overall Survival(exclude pG)		
	HR	95%CI	P value	HR	95%CI	P value	HR	95%CI	P value
Tumor Size: >5cm/≤5cm	1.742	1.155-2.626	0.008	1.865	1.247-3.032	0.006	1.675	1.192-2.458	0.010
Microvascular Invasion: Yes/No	1.631	1.083-2.457	0.019	1.564	1.102-2.316	0.024	1.725	1.267-2.687	0.013
Tumor Number: Multiple/Solitary	1.823	1.256-3.582	0.017	1.697	1.378-3.214	0.015	1.587	1.145-2.453	0.020
p-Ser9-GSK-3β Expression: High/Low	2.292	1.320-3.978	0.003	2.439	1.577-3.772	0.001	–	–	–
T2DM: Yes/No	1.193	0.708-2.010	0.507	–	–	–	1.815	1.158-3.224	0.008

Abbreviations: pG, p-Ser9-GSK-3β; T2DM, type 2 diabetes mellitus.

7. Statistical analysis

Overall Survival (OS) and Time To Recurrence (TTR) were used as primary endpoints. OS was defined as the interval between hepatectomy and death or the date of last follow-up. TTR was calculated from surgery to the date when recurrence was diagnosed. All statistical calculations were carried out using the SPSS.16.0 software. The $\chi 2$ test or Fisher's exact test were used to compare qualitative variables, while continuous variables were compared using Student's t-test or Mann-Whitney test for variables with an abnormal distribution. Receiver operating characteristic curve analysis was used to determine the optimal cut-offs of continuous variables. Survival curves were calculated by the Kaplan-Meier method and compared using the log-rank test. The Cox proportional hazards model was used to determine the independent factors for tumor recurrence and patient's survival based on the variables selected by univariate analysis. Differences were considered statically significant at $p< 0.05$.

Results

1. Over-expression of GSK-3β and p-Ser9-GSK-3β in HCC samples

We firstly assayed and compared GSK-3β mRNA levels in 60 TTs(tumor tissues) and their matched NTTs(nontumorous tissues) by the way of RT-PCR assay (Fig. 1A, B), in which 50 of 60 (83.3%)specimens showed GSK-3β mRNA over-expression in HCC(tumor/nontumorous ratio>2.0). . We found increased protein expression level of total GSK-3β and p-Ser9-GSK-3β in 46 of 60(76.7%)tumor tissues compared with their normal counterparts by western blotting (Fig. 1C). We then performed immunostaining in the 178 paired HCC samples and found that 89(50.0%)patients were identified as p-Ser9-GSK-3β over-expression (Fig. 2A-H)

2. Association of p-Ser9-GSK-3β expression with T2DM

We examined the association between the expression level of p-Ser9-GSK-3β in the tumor tissues with T2DM and other clinic-pathological characteristics of patients (Table 1). Correlation and regression analysis indicated that the over-expression of p-Ser9-GSK-3β was significantly associated with T2DM, and the correlation coefficient was 0.259 ($P=0.001$).

3. Association of p-Ser9-GSK-3β expression and T2DM with prognosis of HCC patients

Patients with over-expression of p-Ser9-GSK-3β had higher recurrence rates (1-,3-,and 5-year recurrence rates: 49.4%, 70.0% and 84.7% vs. 24.9%, 43.1%, and 63.9%, $P<0.001$), and lower overall survival rates (1-,3-,and 5-year survival rates: 73.6%, 44.8% and 34.9% vs. 88.5%, 72.8% and 61.5%, $P<0.001$) than those with low expression.

T2DM was negatively correlated with 1-,3-, and 5-year survival rates (64.6%, 39.7% and 29% for T2DM vs 84.2%, 62.2% and 51.7% for No T2DM; $P < 0.001$). The 1-,3-, and 5-year cumulative recurrence rates in patients with T2DM were significantly higher than those in patients with No T2DM(58.6%, 78.9% and 91.6% vs 33.1%, 52.4% and 71.2%; $P<0.001$).

Based on Kaplan-Meier survival analysis, the comparisons of p-Ser9-GSK-3β expression levels(high or low) in the 178 patients with HCC were shown in the Fig 3A, B. The comparisons of patients with no T2DM versus T2DM were shown in the Fig 3C, D.

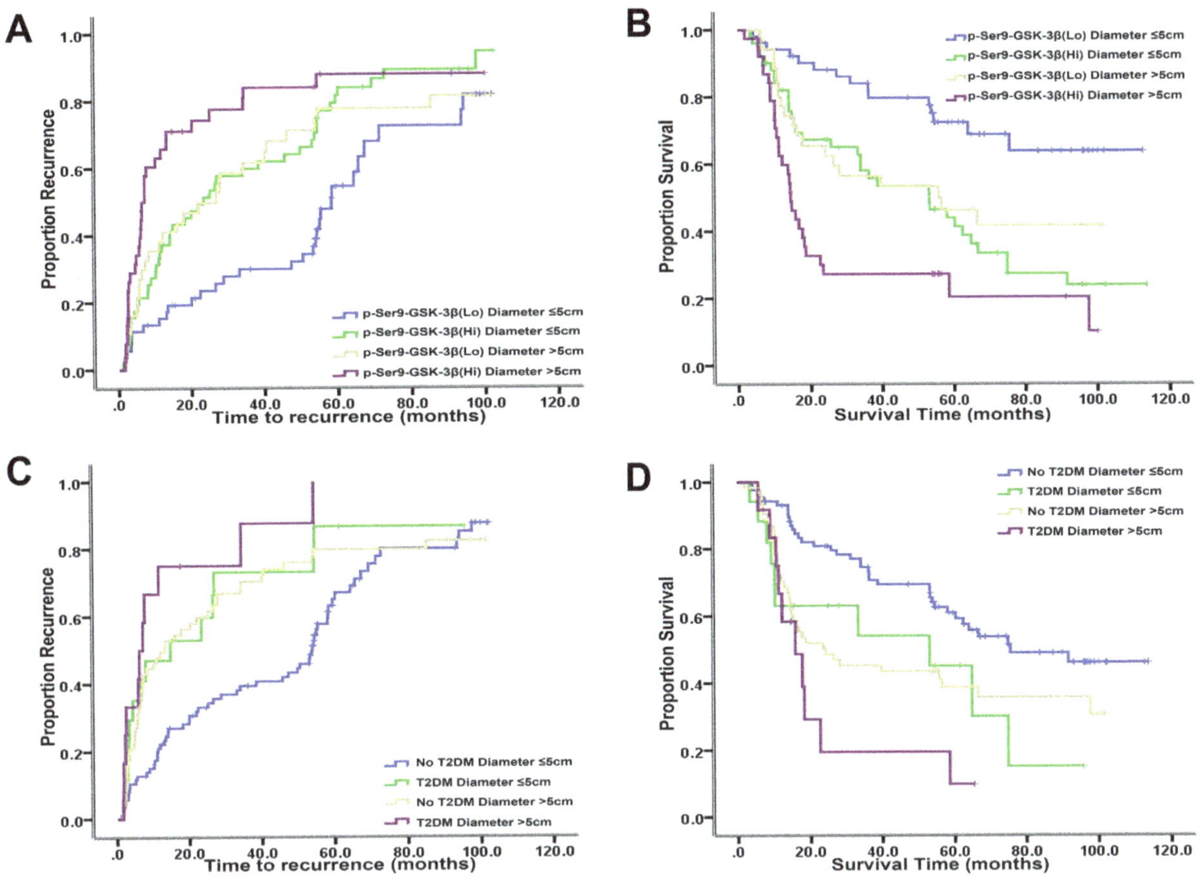

Groups	Survival Comparison (P value)	Recurrent Comparison (P value)	Groups	Survival Comparison (P value)	Recurrent Comparison (P value)
p-Ser9-GSK-3β(Lo) Diameter ≤5cm vs.p-Ser9-GSK-3β(Hi) Diameter ≤5cm	<0.001	0.002	No T2DM Diameter ≤5cm vs.T2DM Diameter ≤5cm	0.028	0.026
p-Ser9-GSK-3β(Lo) Diameter ≤5cm vs.p-Ser9-GSK-3β(Lo) Diameter >5cm	0.017	0.025	No T2DM Diameter ≤5cm vs.No T2DM Diameter >5cm	0.006	0.01
p-Ser9-GSK-3β(Lo) Diameter ≤5cm vs.p-Ser9-GSK-3β(Hi) Diameter >5cm	<0.001	<0.001	No T2DM Diameter ≤5cm vs.T2DM Diameter >5cm	<0.001	<0.001
p-Ser9-GSK-3β(Hi) Diameter ≤5cm vs.p-Ser9-GSK-3β(Lo) Diameter >5cm	0.397	0.699	T2DM Diameter ≤5cm vs.No T2DM Diameter >5cm	0.781	0.77
p-Ser9-GSK-3β(Hi) Diameter ≤5cm vs.p-Ser9-GSK-3β(Hi) Diameter >5cm	0.022	0.037	T2DM Diameter ≤5cm vs.T2DM Diameter >5cm	0.202	0.171
p-Ser9-GSK-3β(Lo) Diameter >5cm vs.p-Ser9-GSK-3β(Hi) Diameter >5cm	0.009	0.056	No T2DM Diameter >5cm vs.T2DM Diameter >5cm	0.125	0.094

Figure 4. Kaplan-Meier analysis of TTR and OS stratified by tumor diameter of HCC patients. (A,B) Kaplan-Meier curves of the correlation between p-Ser9-GSK-3β expression level, tumor diameter divided by 5cm and (A) recurrence or (B) overall survival of HCC patients; (C,D) Kaplan-Meier curves of the correlation between T2DM, tumor diameter divided by 5cm and (C) recurrence or (D) overall survival of HCC patients.

Univariate analysis of 23 survival-related clinic-pathological variables revealed that serum AFP level(P = 0.024), tumor size(P = 0.003), tumor number(P = 0.022), liver cirrhosis(P = 0.038), microvascular invasion(P = 0.011), p-Ser9-GSK-3β expression level(P<0.001), and T2DM(P = 0.006) were statistically correlated with OS of patients with HCC (Table S1).

These significant variables were further subjected to multivariate Cox proportional hazards model, which shown that tumor size(P = 0.008), tumor number(P = 0.032), microvascular invasion(P = 0.019), p-Ser9-GSK-3β expression level(P<0.001) were independent risk factors that could affect the survival of patients with HCC(table 2). We speculated that some interaction or colinearity existed between the variables of p-Ser9-GSK-3β and T2DM. Thus, we further conducted multivariate Cox proportional hazards analysis excluding the variables of p-Ser9-GSK-3β or T2DM respectively (table 2). The results also demonstrated that these two variables were closely related with each other.

4. Stratified analysis of the impact of p-Ser9-GSK-3β expression and T2DM on the prognosis of HCC patients

In the subgroup of tumor size≤5cm, p-Ser9-GSK-3β overexpressing patients had higher recurrence rates(1-,3-,and 5-year recurrence rates: 37.3%, 59.9% and 81.6% vs. 15.4%, 29.9%, and 54.6%, P = 0.002), and lower survival rates(1-,3-,and 5-year survival rates: 82%, 58.1% and 43.9% vs. 94.2%, 83.9% and 72.4%, P<0.001) than those of under-expressing patients.

Similar results were obtained in the tumor size>5 cm subgroup: the 1-,3-,and 5-year recurrence rates were 65.8%, 83.9% and 87.9% vs. 38.3%, 61.6%, and 77.6% in over-expressing and under-expressing patients, respectively, and the 1-,3-,and 5-year survival rates: 62.5%, 27.2% and 20.4% vs. 80%, 56.5% and 46.2%, respectively (P = 0.056, P = 0.009). (Fig 4A,B).

In the subgroup of tumor size≤5cm, patients with T2DM had higher recurrence rates (1-,3-,and 5-year recurrence rates: 47.1%, 73.1% and 86.6% vs. 22.2%, 39.4%, and 65%, P = 0.026), and lower survival rates(1-,3-,and 5-year survival rates: 63%, 54% and 45% vs. 93%, 74.5% and 60.9%, P = 0.028) than those of patients without T2DM.

In the tumor size>5 cm subgroup: the 1-,3-,and 5-year recurrence rates were 75%, 87.5% and 91.7% vs. 48%, 70.3%, and 79.7% in patients with and without T2DM, respectively, and 1-,3-,and 5-year survival rates: 66.7%, 19.4% and 9.7% vs. 71.9%, 45.1% and 38.7%, respectively (P = 0.094, P = 0.125) (Fig 4C,D). There were no significant differences in TTR and OS in the subgroup of tumor size>5cm, due to the limitation of the amount of patients with T2DM.

We then subdivided HCC patients with T2DM, we found that In the subgroup of without T2DM, p-Ser9-GSK-3β over-expressing patients had higher recurrence rates(1-,3-,and 5-year recurrence rates: 45.5%, 64.8% and 83.3% vs. 23.0%, 42.4%, and 57.1%, P = 0.004), and lower survival rates(1-,3-,and 5-year survival rates: 78.4%, 49.3% and 24.4% vs. 87.6%, 72.4% and 60.7%, P<0.001) than those of under-expressing patients. There were no significant differences in TTR(p = 0.308) and OS(p = 0.057) in the subgroup of with T2DM (Figure S1).

Discussion

In the present study, we showed that the total GSK-3β and the p-Ser9-GSK-3β were increased at both mRNA and protein levels in HCC specimens. The over-expression of p-Ser9-GSK-3β was associated with the poor prognosis of patients with HCC after curative resection. We also found that T2DM was related with the poor prognosis of patients with HCC, and the expression level of p-Ser9-GSK-3β was significantly related with T2DM. We speculated that the regulation of GSK-3β might play a significant role in mediating the impact of T2DM on HCC prognosis. To the best of our knowledge, no previous study reported the impact of p-Ser9-GSK-3β expression on the prognosis of HCC and the relationship between the expression of p-Ser9-GSK-3β and T2DM.

GSK-3β was a crucial signaling molecule involved in glycogen synthesis, gene expression, cell migration, cell cycle, cellular architectural pathways and oncogenesis [20,21]. It was a downstream target of insulin and insulin-like growth factor(IGF) receptor-dependent pathways which could result in GSK-3β phosphorylation on the serine 9 residue(p-Ser9-GSK-3β), and subsequent phosphorylation of insulin receptor substrate-1(IRS1) [22,23]. Insulin receptor substrate (IRS) proteins were major docking proteins that mediated insulin/insulin-like growth factor 1 (IGF1) signaling in various insulin-sensitive tissues [24]. Therefore, dysregulation of GSK-3β could result in attenuating insulin signaling, which was thought to induce insulin resistance. Insulin resistance was a major pathophysiological problem underlying the initiation and progression of type II diabetes mellitus (T2DM) [25]. Moreover, Activation of Wnt signaling could lead to GSK-3β inactivation and prevented phosphorylation of β-catenin protein in the cytosol. The increased levels of β-catenin transported to the nuclear, and interacted with transcription factors LEF/TCF (lymphoid enhancer factor/T cell factor) to activate the expression of target genes like c-myc and cyclin D1, and lead to cell proliferation [21,26]. This process was implicated with a wide range of cancers. With respect to HCC, apart from the Wnt-β-catenin pathway, insulin and insulin-like growth factor(IGF) pathways were also implicated with the development and/or progression of HCC [27-29]. GSK-3β was involved in these pathways and recent findings indicated that hyperphosphorylation of Ser9-GSK-3β was a hallmark of hepatocarcinogenesis. And also, GSK-3β was showed as a potential therapeutic target in various cancer involved in pancreatic, colon, renal, prostate, thyroid, ovarian cancer and leukemia [30-37].

Increasing evidence showed that DM was an independent risk factor for the prognosis of patients with HCC [15,38]. We focused on T2DM because type 1 and type 2 DM might have different impacts on HCC prognosis and their pathophysiology mechanisms were different. In this study, our findings showed that T2DM was associated with poor survival of patients with HCC. In the subgroup analysis, T2DM was a significant independent risk factor in early HCC (tumor size< or = 5cm, P = 0.026 for recurrence, P = 0.028 for survival). While in the group of HCC with tumor size>5cm, T2DM showed no significant difference (P = 0.094 for recurrence, P = 0.125 for survival). The mechanism underlying the impact of DM on HCC prognosis was still unclear. Insulin resistance and hyperinsulinemia could result in increasing of IGF-1. Both insulin and IGF-1 promoted proliferation and inhibited apoptosis by receptor-mediated pathways, which may lead to carcinogenesis [39].

This study focused on the impact of p-Ser9-GSK-3β on the prognosis of patients with HCC and the interaction among the expression level of p-Ser9-GSK-3β, T2DM and the prognosis of HCC. Further studies are needed to confirm the interconnection or explain the complex mechanisms among them. We have began a new study aimed at finding this potential mechanism by detecting the expression levels of other related molecules in multiple pathways involved in IGF, NF-kB, PI 3-kinase/Akt and Wnt/β-catenin pathways [40,41].

In conclusion, we firstly reported p-Ser9-GSK-3β was an independent prognostic factor of patients with HCC and it might mediate the influence of type 2 diabetes mellitus on the prognosis of patients with HCC.

Supporting Information

Figure S1 Kaplan-Meier analysis of TTR and OS stratified by T2DM. (A,C) Kaplan-Meier curves of p-Ser9-GSK-3β expression level in the subgroup of without T2DM, (A) overall survival or (C) recurrence of HCC patients; (B,D) Kaplan-Meier curves of p-Ser9-GSK-3β expression level in the subgroup of with T2DM, (B) overall survival or (D) recurrence of HCC patients.

Table S1 Univariate analysis for overall survival.

Author Contributions

Conceived and designed the experiments: GQ FS. Performed the experiments: YL JL LW. Contributed reagents/materials/analysis tools: LW. Contributed to the writing of the manuscript: GQ FS. Performed the statistical analysis: GQ YL.

References

1. Jemal A, Bray F, Center MM, Ferlay J, Ward E, et al. (2011) Global cancer statistics. CA Cancer J Clin 61: 69–90.
2. Duffy JP, Hiatt JR, Busuttil RW (2008) Surgical resection of hepatocellular carcinoma. Cancer J 14: 100–110.
3. Zhang BH, Yang BH, Tang ZY (2004) Randomized controlled trial of screening for hepatocellular carcinoma. J Cancer Res Clin Oncol 130: 417–422.
4. Cadigan KM, Liu YI (2006) Wnt signaling: complexity at the surface. J Cell Sci 119: 395–402.
5. Henriksen EJ, Dokken BB (2006) Role of glycogen synthase kinase-3 in insulin resistance and type 2 diabetes. Curr Drug Targets 7: 1435–1441.
6. Lee J, Kim MS (2007) The role of GSK3 in glucose homeostasis and the development of insulin resistance. Diabetes Res Clin Pract 77 Suppl 1: S49–57.
7. Zeng X, Huang H, Tamai K, Zhang X, Harada Y, et al. (2008) Initiation of Wnt signaling: control of Wnt coreceptor Lrp6 phosphorylation/activation via frizzled, dishevelled and axin functions. Development 135: 367–375.
8. Sutherland C, Leighton IA, Cohen P (1993) Inactivation of glycogen synthase kinase-3 beta by phosphorylation: new kinase connections in insulin and growth-factor signalling. Biochem J 296 (Pt 1): 15–19.
9. Luo J, Chen J, Deng ZL, Luo X, Song WX, et al. (2007) Wnt signaling and human diseases: what are the therapeutic implications? Lab Invest 87: 97–103.
10. Desbois-Mouthon C, Blivet-Van Eggelpoel MJ, Beurel E, Boissan M, Delelo R, et al. (2002) Dysregulation of glycogen synthase kinase-3beta signaling in hepatocellular carcinoma cells. Hepatology 36: 1528–1536.
11. Boissan M, Beurel E, Wendum D, Rey C, Lecluse Y, et al. (2005) Overexpression of insulin receptor substrate-2 in human and murine hepatocellular carcinoma. Am J Pathol 167: 869–877.
12. Hassan MM, Curley SA, Li D, Kaseb A, Davila M, et al. (2010) Association of diabetes duration and diabetes treatment with the risk of hepatocellular carcinoma. Cancer 116: 1938–1946.
13. Poon RT, Fan ST, Wong J (2002) Does diabetes mellitus influence the perioperative outcome or long term prognosis after resection of hepatocellular carcinoma? Am J Gastroenterol 97: 1480–1488.
14. Huo TI, Hsu CY, Huang YH, Hsia CY, Lin HC, et al. (2010) Diabetes mellitus as an independent prognostic predictor and its association with renal dysfunction in patients with hepatocellular carcinoma. Liver Int 30: 198–207.
15. Shau WY, Shao YY, Yeh YC, Lin ZZ, Kuo R, et al. (2012) Diabetes mellitus is associated with increased mortality in patients receiving curative therapy for hepatocellular carcinoma. Oncologist 17: 856–862.
16. Wang P, Kang D, Cao W, Wang Y, Liu Z (2012) Diabetes mellitus and risk of hepatocellular carcinoma: a systematic review and meta-analysis. Diabetes Metab Res Rev 28: 109–122.
17. Bruix J, Sherman M (2005) Management of hepatocellular carcinoma. Hepatology 42: 1208–1236.
18. Wang K, Liu J, Yan ZL, Li J, Shi LH, et al. (2010) Overexpression of aspartyl-(asparaginyl)-beta-hydroxylase in hepatocellular carcinoma is associated with worse surgical outcome. Hepatology 52: 164–173.
19. Edmondson HA, Steiner PE (1954) Primary carcinoma of the liver: a study of 100 cases among 48,900 necropsies. Cancer 7: 462–503.
20. Ali A, Hoeflich KP, Woodgett JR (2001) Glycogen synthase kinase-3: properties, functions, and regulation. Chem Rev 101: 2527–2540.
21. Jope RS, Johnson GV (2004) The glamour and gloom of glycogen synthase kinase-3. Trends Biochem Sci 29: 95–102.
22. Schuppin GT, Pons S, Hugl S, Aiello LP, King GL, et al. (1998) A specific increased expression of insulin receptor substrate 2 in pancreatic beta-cell lines is involved in mediating serum-stimulated beta-cell growth. Diabetes 47: 1074–1085.
23. Sun XJ, Liu F (2009) Phosphorylation of IRS proteins Yin-Yang regulation of insulin signaling. Vitam Horm 80: 351–387.
24. White MF (2006) Regulating insulin signaling and beta-cell function through IRS proteins. Can J Physiol Pharmacol 84: 725–737.
25. Bouche C, Serdy S, Kahn CR, Goldfine AB (2004) The cellular fate of glucose and its relevance in type 2 diabetes. Endocr Rev 25: 807–830.
26. Patel S, Doble B, Woodgett JR (2004) Glycogen synthase kinase-3 in insulin and Wnt signalling: a double-edged sword? Biochem Soc Trans 32: 803–808.
27. Bannasch P, Klimek F, Mayer D (1997) Early bioenergetic changes in hepatocarcinogenesis: preneoplastic phenotypes mimic responses to insulin and thyroid hormone. J Bioenerg Biomembr 29: 303–313.
28. Tanaka S, Sugimachi K, Maehara S, Harimoto N, Shirabe K, et al. (2002) Oncogenic signal transduction and therapeutic strategy for hepatocellular carcinoma. Surgery 131: S142–147.
29. Scharf JG, Braulke T (2003) The role of the IGF axis in hepatocarcinogenesis. Horm Metab Res 35: 685–693.
30. Liao X, Zhang L, Thrasher JB, Du J, Li B (2003) Glycogen synthase kinase-3beta suppression eliminates tumor necrosis factor-related apoptosis-inducing ligand resistance in prostate cancer. Mol Cancer Ther 2: 1215–1222.
31. Shakoori A, Ougolkov A, Yu ZW, Zhang B, Modarressi MH, et al. (2005) Deregulated GSK3beta activity in colorectal cancer: its association with tumor cell survival and proliferation. Biochem Biophys Res Commun 334: 1365–1373.
32. Cao Q, Lu X, Feng YJ (2006) Glycogen synthase kinase-3beta positively regulates the proliferation of human ovarian cancer cells. Cell Res 16: 671–677.
33. Ougolkov AV, Fernandez-Zapico ME, Bilim VN, Smyrk TC, Chari ST, et al. (2006) Aberrant nuclear accumulation of glycogen synthase kinase-3beta in human pancreatic cancer: association with kinase activity and tumor dedifferentiation. Clin Cancer Res 12: 5074–5081.
34. Kunnimalaiyaan M, Vaccaro AM, Ndiaye MA, Chen H (2007) Inactivation of glycogen synthase kinase-3beta, a downstream target of the raf-1 pathway, is associated with growth suppression in medullary thyroid cancer cells. Mol Cancer Ther 6: 1151–1158.
35. Shakoori A, Mai W, Miyashita K, Yasumoto K, Takahashi Y, et al. (2007) Inhibition of GSK-3 beta activity attenuates proliferation of human colon cancer cells in rodents. Cancer Sci 98: 1388–1393.
36. Bilim V, Ougolkov A, Yuuki K, Naito S, Kawazoe H, et al. (2009) Glycogen synthase kinase-3: a new therapeutic target in renal cell carcinoma. Br J Cancer 101: 2005–2014.
37. Miyashita K, Kawakami K, Nakada M, Mai W, Shakoori A, et al. (2009) Potential therapeutic effect of glycogen synthase kinase 3beta inhibition against human glioblastoma. Clin Cancer Res 15: 887–897.
38. Davila JA, Morgan RO, Shaib Y, McGlynn KA, El-Serag HB (2005) Diabetes increases the risk of hepatocellular carcinoma in the United States: a population based case control study. Gut 54: 533–539.
39. Macaulay VM (1992) Insulin-like growth factors and cancer. Br J Cancer 65: 311–320.
40. Hoeflich KP, Luo J, Rubie EA, Tsao MS, Jin O, et al. (2000) Requirement for glycogen synthase kinase-3beta in cell survival and NF-kappaB activation. Nature 406: 86–90.
41. Ban KC, Singh H, Krishnan R, Seow HF (2003) GSK-3beta phosphorylation and alteration of beta-catenin in hepatocellular carcinoma. Cancer Lett 199: 201–208.

2

The miR-545/374a Cluster Encoded in the *Ftx* lncRNA is Overexpressed in HBV-Related Hepatocellular Carcinoma and Promotes Tumorigenesis and Tumor Progression

Qi Zhao[1], Tao Li[2], Jianni Qi[3], Juan Liu[1], Chengyong Qin[1]*

1 Department of Gastroenterology, Provincial Hospital Affiliated to Shandong University, Jinan, China, **2** Department of Infectious Diseases, Provincial Hospital Affiliated to Shandong University, Jinan, China, **3** Central Laboratory, Shandong Provincial Hospital affiliated to Shandong University, Jinan, China

Abstract

Hepatitis B virus (HBV) infection is a major risk factor for hepatocellular carcinoma (HCC). Previous studies have shown several long noncoding RNAs (lncRNAs) play various roles in HCC progression, but no research has focused on the expression pattern of microRNA clusters encoded in lncRNAs. The Ftx gene encodes a lncRNA which harbors 2 clusters of microRNAs in its introns, the miR-374b/421 cluster and the miR-545/374a cluster. To date, no research has focused on the role of the miR-545/374a and miR-374b/421 clusters in HBV-related HCC. In this study, 66 pairs of HBV-related HCC tissue and matched non-cancerous liver tissue specimens were analyzed for the expression of the Ftx microRNA clusters. Our results showed that the miR-545/374a cluster was upregulated in HBV-HCC tissue and significantly correlated with prognosis-related clinical features, including histological grade, metastasis and tumor capsule. Transfection studies with microRNA mimics and inhibitors revealed that miR-545/374a expression promoted in vitro cell proliferation, cell migration and invasion. The wild-type HBV-genome-containing plasmid or full-length HBx protein encoding plasmid was transfected into the Bel-7402 cell line and observed for their influence on miR-545/374a expression. We found that transfection of the HBV genome or HBx alone resulted in an increase in miR-545/374a expression. Next, by monitoring the expression of sera miR-545/374a before and after surgical tumor excision, we found serum miR-545/374a was tumor-derived and exhibited a sharp decrease 25 days after tumor excision. We also examined the gender-based difference in miR-545/374a expression among HCC patients and utilized microRNA target prediction software to find the targets of miR-545/374a. One of these targets, namely estrogen-related receptor gamma (ESRRG) was inversely correlated with miR-545 expression. In conclusion, the overexpression of miR-545/374a cluster located in the Ftx lncRNA is partially responsible for a poor prognosis, and monitoring sera levels of miR-545/374a may be a useful diagnostic marker for HCC.

Editor: Dong-Yan Jin, University of Hong Kong, Hong Kong

Funding: This work was supported by grants from the Shandong Science and Technology Committee of China (2013GG3202192), the Postdoctoral Science Foundation of China (2013M541926), and the Postdoctoral Innovation Project Special Foundation of Shandong Province (201302031). The funders had no role in study design, data collection and analysis, decision to publish, or preparation of the manuscript.

Competing Interests: The authors have declared that no competing interests exist.

* Email: chengyongqin016@gmail.com

Introduction

Hepatocellular carcinoma (HCC) is one of the most frequently occurring cancers worldwide. A variety of risk factors are associated with HCC development, including the following most common risk factors: hepatitis B virus (HBV) infection, hepatitis C virus (HCV) infection, consumption of food contaminated with aflatoxin B1, heavy alcohol intake, and nonalcoholic fatty liver disease [1]. Due to the growing incidence of HCC, intense research efforts are currently being undertaken to understand the cellular and molecular mechanisms of the disease so that novel diagnostic markers and therapeutic strategies can be developed.

The mechanism of HBV induced oncogenesis may involve integration of viral genomic fragments into the human genome. An alternative hypothesis is that HBV produces regulators which participate in cellular pathways that lead to carcinogenesis. However, the exact mechanism by which HBV infection leads to HCC still remains obscure [1]. In this study, we provide evidence that overexpression of a microRNA cluster promotes tumorigenesis and tumor progression in HBV-related HCC.

RNA has become widely suspected as the culprit behind almost every case of epigenetic regulation in a variety of diseases. Only 1% of the mammalian genome carries protein-coding potential, yet 70 to 90% is transcribed to produce a large transcriptome of long noncoding RNA (lncRNA, defined as RNA>100 nucleotides in length) [2]. Clear roles have emerged for several lncRNAs which participate in HCC disease progression [3,4]. Mechanistically, lncRNAs target a site-specific pathway, and may directly interact with chromatin/mRNAs and recruit histone-modifying enzymes to induce epigenetic silencing of target genes [3,5,6]. Interestingly, few studies have reported that some of these self-functional lncRNAs are also acting as microRNA (miRNA) precursors. The lack of experimental data on these miRNAs leaves open questions about their possible relation to malignant tumors.

The *Ftx* transcript is a conserved functional lncRNA encoded within the X-inactivation center (*Xic*). *Ftx* encodes 4 microRNAs in its introns [7]. Intron 12 encodes 1 cluster of 2 microRNAs (miR-374b and miR-421), which is well conserved in different mammalian species. Intron b encodes 1 related cluster of 2 microRNAs (miR-374a and miR-545), which is absent in mouse and rat due to mutational changes (figure 1A). A recent study showed that miR-374a is upregulated in breast cancer tumors and promotes breast cancer metastasis by activating the Wnt/β-catenin signaling pathway [8]. It remains unknown whether the altered expression of miR-374a occurs independently from the other 3 microRNAs or whether the *Ftx* microRNA clusters are regulated as a group. No studies have explored the expression of the other 3 microRNAs and their potential relationship with malignant tumors. This raises a critical question that our research addresses: does *Ftx* microRNA clusters play a role in cancer progression?

Another example of altered microRNA expression occurs in hand-foot-and-mouth disease (HFMD) [9]. In this case miR-545 expression is upregulated, upon enterovirus 71 (EV71) or coxsackievirus 16 (CAV16) infection. Since viral infections can alter miR-545 expression, we explored the possible relationship between *Ftx* microRNA cluster expression and HBV infection.

In this study, the expression profiles of the miR-545/374a cluster and the miR-421/374b cluster derived from the *Ftx* transcript were examined in HBV-related HCC. Based upon correlation analysis with clinical features, the microRNAs were assayed for their ability to regulate tumor progression. *In vitro* cell culture assays were established to confirm the biological function of the microRNAs and potential regulating mechanism(s). Next, we followed a "tissue to serum, preoperative to postoperative" pattern to investigate the diagnostic value of corresponding serum microRNAs. Since *Ftx* plays a major role in mediating X chromosome inactivation, the influence of sex and the expression of sex related target genes were examined.

Methods

1. Specimens

Sixty-six HBV-related HCC patients and 11 hepatic hemangioma patients (negative control) were recruited from February 2012 to January 2013 at the Provincial Hospital Affiliated to Shandong University. For each HBV-related HCC subject, 4 specimens were collected: (1) HCC tissue, (2) matched distal non-cancerous liver tissue, (3) 5 ml venous peripheral blood before surgery, and (4) 5 ml venous peripheral blood 20 days after surgery. Liver tissue and 5 ml venous peripheral blood were also collected from each negative control subject. For the use of materials for research purposes, written informed consent was obtained from each patient. The consent procedure and study protocol were approved by the Medical Institutional Ethical Committee of the Provincial Hospital Affiliated to Shandong University.

2. Clinical features

The samples obtained from HBV-related HCC subjects after surgery were analyzed by pathologists and features including histological grade, metastasis, tumor capsule and cirrhosis were reported. The levels of serum HBsAg and HBeAg were determined quantitatively by an electro-chemiluminescence immunoassay (ECLIA) on the Roche Elecsys 2010 immunoassay analyzer (Roche, Switzerland). The level of serum HBV-DNA was measured using the high-sensitivity fluorescent quantitative PCR Kit (DaAn Gene Co., China) and amplified in a PE 5700 fluorescence PCR apparatus (Perkin-Elmer, Norwalk, USA). α-fetoprotein (AFP), carcino-embryonic (CEA) and γ-glutamyltransferase γ(-GT) were measured by routine laboratory methods. Concrete information is shown in Table 1. No significant differences between the HBV-related HCC group and the negative control group with respect to age were found. However, there were significant differences concerning the gender of the patient and the levels of HBV-DNA, AFP, CEA and γ-GT (data not shown).

3. Cell culture

Human hepatocellular carcinoma cell lines Bel-7402, HepG2 (Keygen Biotech, Nanjing, China), and previously constructed stable HBV positive HepG2.2.15 cells were maintained in HyClone's media containing 10% fetal calf serum, 100 U/ml penicillin, and 100 mg/ml streptomycin at 37°C in a humidified atmosphere containing 5% CO_2. Bel-7402 cells were seeded at a density of 2.0×10^5 cells/mL and starved for 24 hours before transfection.

4. Plasmid transfection

The wild-type HBV genome-containing plasmid (pCDNA3.1-HBV), and the plasmid encoding full-length HBx protein (pIRSE-HBx) were transfected using Lipofectamine 2000 (Invitrogen, CA, USA) according to the manufacturer's protocol. Empty expression vectors were transfected as a negative control. Expression of plasmids in Bel-7402 cell lines was confirmed by high-sensitivity fluorescent quantitative PCR and western blotting.

5. Oligonucleotide transfection

MicroRNA 545 mimics, miR-545 inhibitor, miR-374a mimics, miR-374a inhibitor, and negative control duplex (designated as NC), were all synthesized by GenePharma (Shanghai, China). The sequences are listed in the **Table S1**. Oligonucleotide transfection was performed using Lipofectamine 2000 according to the manufacturer's protocol.

6. MicroRNA/mRNA extraction, reverse transcription, and real-time PCR analysis

The manufacturer's instructions were followed for each kit utilized. The mRNAiso Plus and microRNAiso Plus kits (Takara Bio, China) were separately used for mRNA and miRNA extraction from liver tissue. The MiRCURY RNA Kit (Exiqon, Denmark) was used for microRNA extraction from serum specimens. The PrimeScript RT Reagent Kit and the SYBR Premix Ex Taq (Takara Bio, China) were used separately for first strand cDNA synthesis and mRNA real time PCR [10]. The SYBR II PrimeScript miRNA RT-PCR Kit (Takara Bio, China) was used for microRNA reverse transcription and real time PCR. Beta-actin was used for normalization of mRNA, and U6 was utilized for normalization of microRNA. Specific and universal primers (Takara Bio, China) were used in pairs when amplifying microRNA. The primers are listed in the **Table S1**.

7. Western blotting

Bel-7402 cells were harvested after transfection with pCDNA3.1-HBx for 48 hours. Whole-cell extracts were prepared in lysis buffer as described previously [11]. Equal amounts of protein were subjected to electrophoresis on 10% SDS-polyacrylamide gels and transferred onto nitrocellulose membranes (Schleicher & Schuell BioScience GmbH, Dassel, Germany) by electroblotting. The membranes were incubated with rabbit anti-human

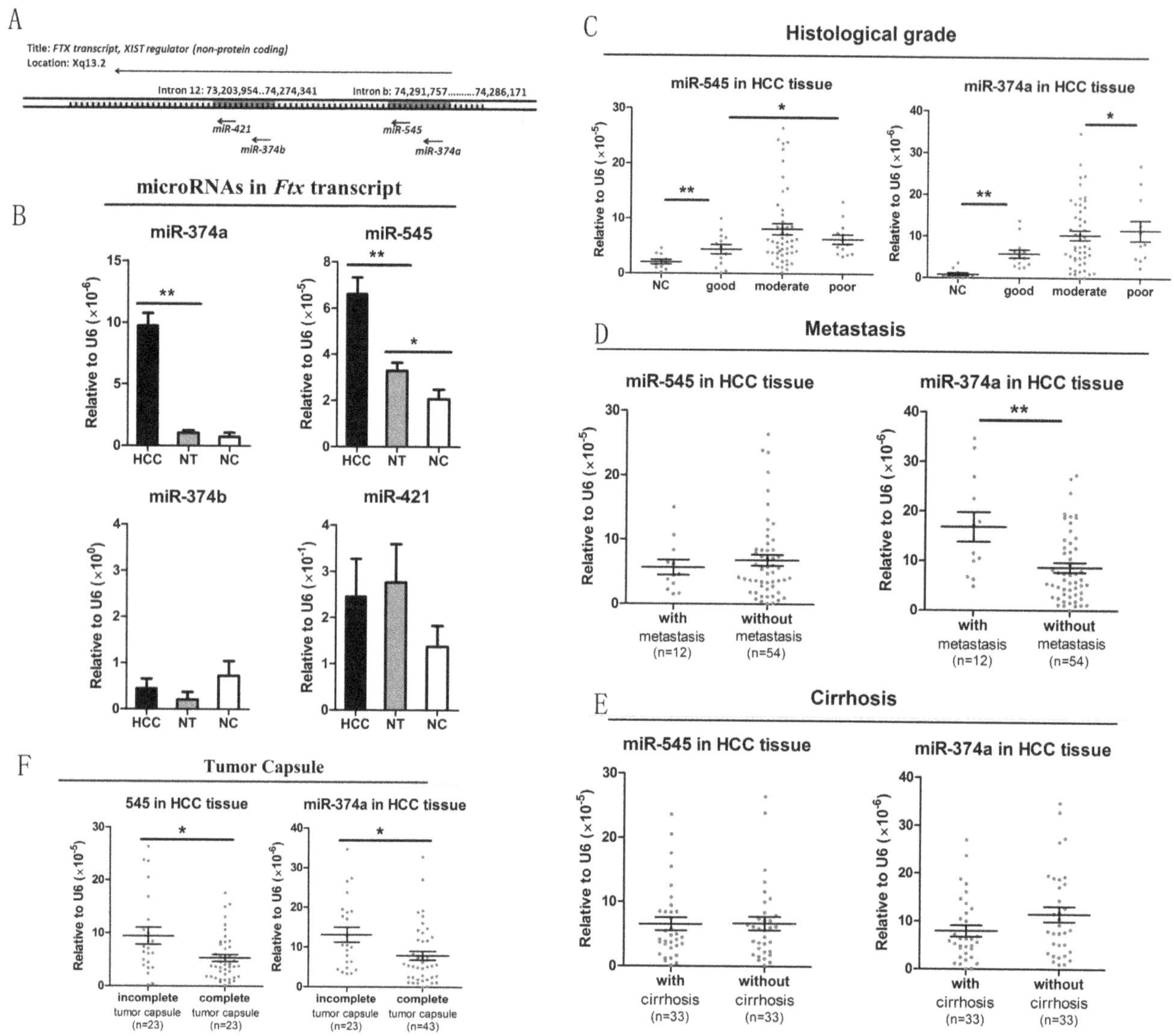

Figure 1. Expression pattern of microRNA clusters within the *Ftx* transcript and their correlation with key clinical features. (A) Genomic location of the Ftx microRNA clusters. Ftx contains a cluster of two microRNAs (miR-374b and miR-421) within intron 12 and a related cluster of two microRNAs (miR-374a and miR-545) within intron b. (B) Expression status of Ftx microRNA clusters (miR-374a, -545, -374b, -421) in human HBV-related hepatocellular carcinoma tissue (HCC; n = 66), matched distal non cancerous liver tissue (NT; n = 66) and negative control (NC; n = 11). The levels of each microRNA were determined by qRT PCR of tissue specimens. The error bars in B represent mean±Std. error. *P<0.05, **P<0.01, t test. (C-F) Analysis of individual microRNA expression patterns with well established prognosis-related clinical features. The levels of each microRNA was determined by qRT PCR of tissue specimens. Pathological examination included histological grade, metastasis, cirrhosis, and tumor capsule as described in the methods. The error bars in C-E represent mean ± Std. deviation. *P<0.05, **P<0.01, t test.

HBx antibody (1:1000 dilution; Abcam, Cambridge, Massachusetts, USA), followed by incubation with mouse anti-rabbit secondary antibodies (1:5000 dilution, Abcam). Protein bands were detected using an enhanced chemiluminescence reagent (Sigma, USA).

8. MTT assay

Approximately 3×10^3 Bel-7402 cells were plated in each well of a 96-well plate. After an overnight incubation, the cells were transfected separately with the NC, miR-545/374a mimics or inhibitor for 6 hours. Twelve hours after the medium was removed, colorimetric 3-(4,5-dimethylthiazol-2-yl)-2,5-diphenyltetrazolium (MTT; Sigma-Aldrich) was added to each well at various times following treatment. The 96-well plates were incubated at 37°C for 3 h. The plates were then centrifuged, and the formazan precipitates were dissolved in 100 ul of dimethyl sulfoxide [12]. The absorbance was measured at 490 nm using a Spectra Max M_2 spectrophotometer (Molecular Devices, Sunnyvale, California, USA).

9. Cell invasion and migration assays

Cell migration and invasion were assayed using a transwell chamber (Millipore, USA) with and without Matrigel (BD, Franklin Lakes, USA), respectively. For the invasion assay, a transwell chamber was placed into a 24-well plate and was coated with 30 ul of Matrigel. In both transwell assays, Bel-7402 cells, 48 hours after transfection, were trypsinized and seeded in chambers at a density of 8×10^4 cells per well. The cells were cultured in 200 ul of RPMI 1640 medium without serum, and 600 μl of RPMI 1640 medium with 10% FBS was added to the

Table 1. Clinicopathological characteristics of patients with HBV-related hepatocellular carcinoma.

Characteristic	No. of patients (N=66)
Age	
<50	25
≥50	41
Sex	
Male	45
Female	21
HBsAg	
Positive	55
Negative	11
HBeAg	
Positive	11
Negative	55
HBV-DNA	
≤1000	17
>1000	49
Cirrhosis	
Positive	33
Negative	33
Histological grade	
Good	13
Moderate	42
Poor	11
Metastasis	
with	12
without	54
Tumor capsule	
Complete	43
Incomplete	23
AFP(ng/ml)	
≤20	36
>20	30
CEA(ng/ml)	
≤10	53
>10	13
γ-GT(U/L)	
≤40	16
>40	50

HBsAg, hepatitis B surface antigen, HBeAg, hepatitis B e antigen, AFP, α-fetoprotein; CEA, carcino-embryonic antigen; γ-GT, γ-glutamyl transpeptidase, NA.

lower chamber. Sixty hours later, migrated cells were fixed with 100% methanol for 30 min. Non-migrated cells were removed by cotton swabs. Next, the cells on the bottom surface of the membrane were stained with crystal violet for 20 min. Cell images were obtained utilizing a phase-contrast microscope (Leica DM4000 B, Germany) [12].

10. Statistics

Data were analyzed with SPSS 16.0 statistical software (SPSS Inc., Chicago, Illinois, USA). The one-Sample Kolmogorov-Smirnov Test was used to confirm the normal distribution of experimental data. To evaluate significant differences between matched HBV-HCC tissue and nontumor tissue, matched serum specimens before and after surgery, paired t tests were performed. Unmatched continuous data were compared using an independent 2-tailed t test. Pearson's correlation (r) was used to measure correlation and logarithmic regression was utilized to derive the equation of the slope. In all cases, $P<0.05$ was considered statistically significant.

Results

The miR-545/374a cluster in the *Ftx* transcript is upregulated in HCC tissue and is significantly correlated with prognosis-related clinical features

To determine the status of the *Ftx* microRNA clusters, we measured the expression of individual microRNAs by quantitative RT-PCR in tissue specimens. As shown in figure 1B, the expression of the miR-545/374a cluster was lower than the miR-421/374b cluster, but showed clear variation in different groups. MicroRNA 545 was significantly upregulated in HCC tissue compared with non cancerous liver tissue (NT) ($HCC=6.60\times10^{-5}$ vs. $NT=3.27\times10^{-5}$; $p=0.003$, paired t test), as well as in NT compared with negative control (NC) ($NC=2.06\times10^{-5}$; $p=0.034$, independent t test). Likewise, miR-374a expression was significantly higher in HCC tissue compared with NT ($HCC=9.73\times10^{-6}$ vs. $NT=1.05\times10^{-6}$; $p=0.000$, paired t test), while no significant difference was found between NT and NC regarding miR-374a expression ($NC=0.73\times10^{-6}$; $p=0.584$, independent t test). On the other hand, the comparatively conserved cluster of miR-374b and miR-421 were highly expressed with large individual difference, but surprisingly showed no significant difference between 66 pairs of matched HCC tissue and corresponding NT. Furthermore, the expression levels of miR-374b and miR-421 did not show any differences between 66 HCC tissues and 11 NC. The result suggests that increased miR-545/374a cluster expression in the *Ftx* transcript may be an estimable event in human HBV-related HCC tumorigenesis.

To investigate the potential role of miR-545/374a in HBV-related HCC, the expression levels of these microRNAs were analyzed with key clinical features associated with tumor progression and disease prognosis. The histological differentiation analysis showed no restrict grade-by-grade variation. However, figure 1C shows that the expression of miR-545 is significantly higher in the poor differentiated group compared to the good differentiated group ($p=0.019$), while the expression of miR-374a is significantly higher in the moderate differentiated group compared to the good differentiated group ($p=0.005$). In addition figure 1F shows that, patients with an incomplete tumor capsule had higher levels of both miR-545 and miR-374a than patients with a complete tumor capsule ($p=0.04$, $p=0.013$). Furthermore, figure 1D shows that patients with distal metastasis had significantly higher miR-374a expression than patients without distal metastasis ($p=0.002$). No significant differences were observed in the miR-545 and miR-374a expression levels with respect to cirrhosis (figure 1E). Likewise, no significant differences were observed for the levels of miR-545 and miR-374a with respect to age (figure S1A). The overall results indicate that high miR-545/374a expression may facilitate tumor invasion and distal metastasis, which may be responsible for a bad prognosis of HBV-HCC patients.

The miR-545/374a cluster promotes HCC cell proliferation, cell migration and invasion

To gain a mechanistic understanding of the biological significance of the upregulated miR-545/374a cluster, the Bel-7402 cell line was transfected with individual microRNA mimics and inhibitors. Nonsense oligonucleotide was transfected as a negative control. The microRNA expression status at 72 h after transfection was monitored by quantitative RT-PCR (Figure 2A). The inhibition rates for miR-545 and miR-374a were 58.6% and 31.3%, respectively.

To determine whether miR-545 and miR-374a have an impact on tumor cell proliferation, we transfected cells with various microRNA mimics and inhibitors (see above) and performed a MTT assay to monitor cell viability. As shown in figure 2B, the proliferation of HCC cells was significantly decreased after transfection with miR-545/374a inhibitors compared to negative control. Overexpression of miR-545/374a (via transfection of the mimics) in the HCC cell line promoted cell proliferation to a small degree. Next, transwell assays were performed using transfected cells (see above) to investigate the effect of miR-545/374a expression on cell migration (figure 2C) and invasion (figure 2D). Both microRNAs enhanced the migration and invasion ability of HCC cell lines, except that inhibition of miR-374a had no statistically significant influence in cell migration assays ($P = 0.102$). We also used wound healing assay to confirm the influence of miR-374a/545 expression on cell migration (Figure S2). Taken together, these results demonstrated that overexpression of the miR-545/374a cluster permits cell proliferation in the HCC cell line, and may exert a promoting effect on cell migration and invasion.

Expression of miR-545/374a is positively regulated by HBV infection and may be induced by HBx expression

In light of previous evidence that the miR-545 expression profile can be altered by viral infection [9], we explored the possibility that overexpression of miR-545/374a might be related to HBV infection. Figure 3A shows that HBeAg positive patients showed a significantly higher level of miR-374a than HbeAg negative patients, and patients with a positive HBV-DNA level had higher expression of both miR-545 and miR-374a compared to patients with a negative HBV-DNA level.

To confirm our hypothesis that miR-545/374a expression might be related to HBV infection, we monitored the expression of miR-545/374a in HBV positive and negative cell lines. Quantitative RT-PCR was used to measure the miR-545/374a expression in the stable HBV positive cell line HepG2.2.15 and its parental HCC cell line HepG2 (figure 3B). A statistically significant increase in miR-545 expression was observed in the HepG2.2.15 cell line compared to the HepG2 cell line ($p = 0.003$), but the data obtained for miR-374a was not statistically significant ($p = 0.057$). Next, the HCC cell line Bel-7402 was transfected with the HBV-genome-containing plasmid (pIRSE-HBV) and empty pIRSE plasmid was utilized as a negative control. The levels of miR-545/374a were then monitored by quantitative RT-PCR. As hypothesized, figure 3C shows that both miR-545 and miR-374a were significantly increased after transfection of the HBV genome encoding plasmid ($p = 0.001$, $p = 0.032$ respectively).

HBx protein is a key regulator of HBV infection. Therefore, we monitored the expression of this protein in 66 HBV-HCC subjects and compared it to the levels of miR-545/374a. The levels of miR-545/374a and HBx mRNA were measured by quantitative RT-PCR. As shown in figure 3D, HBx expression is significantly correlated with miR-545 expression ($r = 0.312$, $p = 0.011$, Pearson's correlation). To investigate whether HBx acts as a potential regulator of the *Ftx* miR-545/374a cluster, an overexpression strategy was conducted via transfection of a HBx expressing plasmid (pCDNA3.1-HBx) into Bel-7402 cells. Figure 3E shows that the HBx protein was overexpressed in pCDNA3.1-HBx transfected cells. Furthermore, the expression level of miR-545/374a was increased in HBx expressing cells compared to negative control cells transfected with empty plasmid ($p = 0.046$, $p = 0.008$). Taken together, these data indicate that the expression of the *Ftx* miR-545/374a cluster is positively regulated by HBV infection, and HBx may be a key regulator in this process.

Serum miR-545/374a are tumor-derived, and their expression are significantly decreased after surgical excision of tumor tissue

Tissue to serum analysis represents the process from mechanism to application. As a first step, the changing tendency of serum microRNAs should be tested to determine if their presence is consistent with their presence in tissue. Figure 4A shows the tissue to serum analysis of miR-545/374a in HBV-HCC subjects. Our study showed that, in 66 HBV-HCC subjects, the expression of miR-545/374a in preoperative period serum is significantly correlated with miR-545/374a expression in HCC tissue ($r = 0.294$, $p = 0.017$; $r = 0.365$, $p = 0.002$; Pearson's correlation). In addition, the expression of miR-545 and miR-374a both showed a statistically significant distinction between sera of HCC patients and sera of negative control patients ($p = 0.030$, $p = 0.000$, independent t test) (figure 4C). These data demonstrated that detection of miR-545/374a in serum may indicate HBV-related HCC occurrence.

To determine the levels of miR-545/374a in sera following surgical excision of tumor tissue, we collected 4 patients' sera repeatedly at different time points after surgery. The miR-545/374a levels were determined by quantitative RT-PCR. The dynamic tendency of individual microRNA levels in the sera samples were recorded as line charts (figure 4B). As the charts show, the sera miR-545 levels show a significant decrease at about 25 days after surgery, while the sera miR-374a levels decrease at approximately 15 days after surgery. Based on these data, we collected the postoperative sera more than 25 days after surgery. The miR-545/374a levels in the sera samples were determined by quantitative RT-PCR. Next, a paired t test was used to compare the microRNA levels between preoperative sera and postoperative sera (figure 4C). The results showed that the miR-545 concentration decreased by 47.3% ($p = 0.001$), while miR-374a similarly decreased by 45.8% ($p = 0.042$), which further confirmed that serum miR-545/374a is tumor-derived. Figure 4D shows the levels of miR-545/374a from the preoperative period to the postoperative period for each patient. As expected, nearly all patients show a reduction in miR-545/374a expression following surgery.

Correlation analysis of preoperative serum miR-545 and miR-374a expression with prognosis/diagnosis related clinical features

The serum levels of miR-545 and miR-374a were examined by quantitative RT-PCR of samples obtained from 66 HBV-HCC subjects and were correlated with prognosis/diagnosis related clinical features. Figure 5A shows that even though miR-545 and miR-374a in each histological grade show significant differences compared to the negative control, there were no statistically significant differences between any two histological grades. Figure 5A also shows that miR-545 and miR-374a showed no

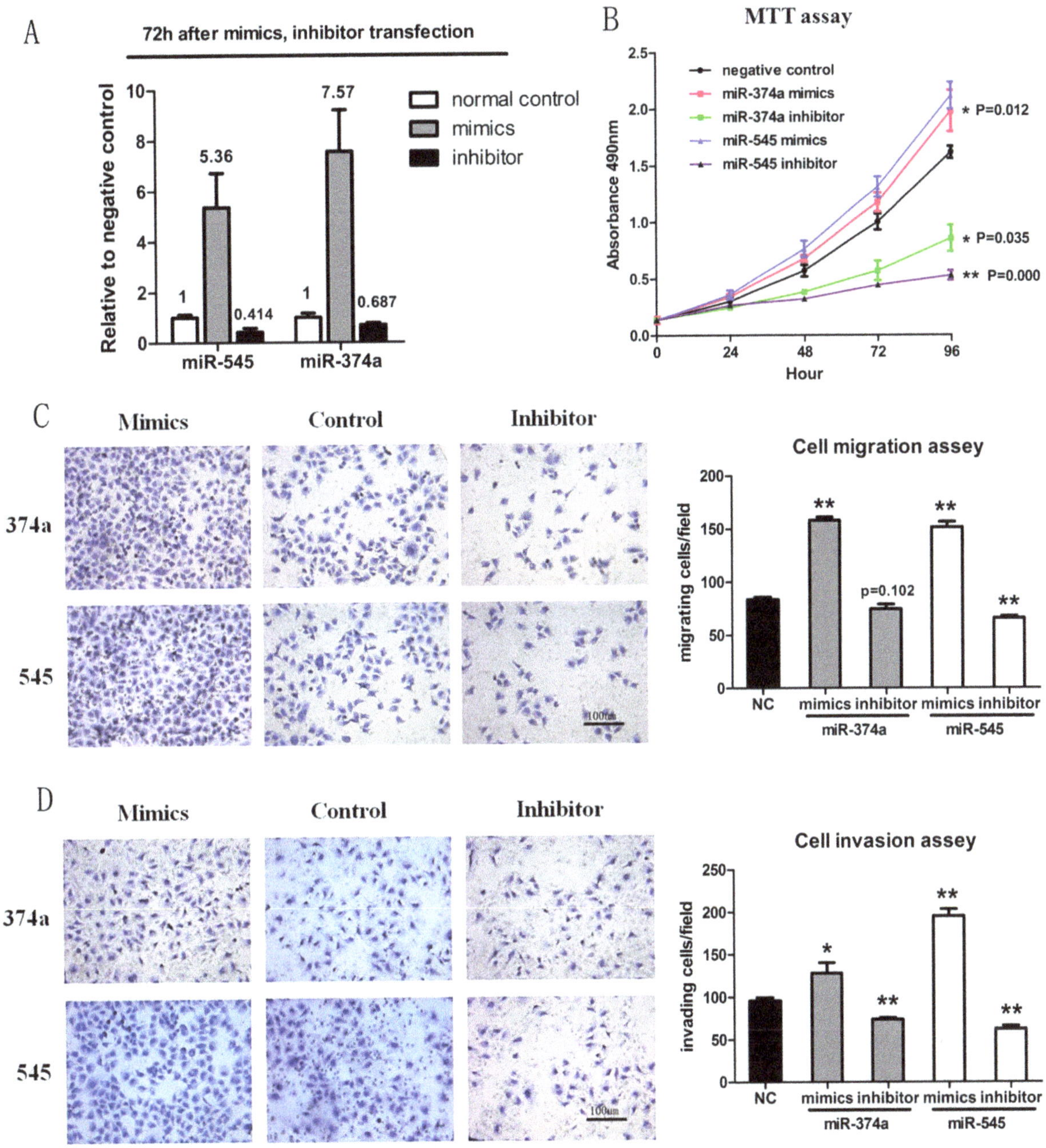

Figure 2. Functional analysis of miR-545 and miR-374a. (A) Expression status of miR-545 and miR-374a following transfection with microRNA mimics and inhibitors. The Bel-7402 cell line was transfected with individual microRNA mimics and inhibitors. Nonsense oligonucleotide was transfected as a negative control. The microRNA expression status at 72 h after transfection was monitored by quantitative RT-PCR. Experiments in A were repeated at least 3 times with similar results, and error bars represent mean ± Std. deviation. (B) Bel-7402 cells were transfected as described in figure 2A and a MTT cell proliferation assay was performed. Experiments in B were repeated at least 3 times with similar results, and error bars represent mean ± Std. deviation. (C) Bel-7402 cells were transfected as described in figure 2A and cell migration assays using transwell membranes were performed. Representative pictures of migration chambers, and average counts from five random microscopic fields are shown. Experiments in C were repeated at least 3 times with similar results, and error bars represent mean ± Std. deviation. (D) Bel-7402 cells were transfected as described in figure 2A and cell invasion assays using Matrigel-coated transwell membranes are shown. Representative pictures of invasion chambers, and average counts from five random microscopic fields are shown. Experiments in D were repeated at least 3 times with similar results, and error bars represent mean ± Std. deviation. *$P<0.05$, **$P<0.01$, t test.

significant differences between patients with or without distal metastasis. Next, 3 previously established clinical features forecasting HCC recurrence (AFP, CEA, and γ-GT) were analyzed along with serum miR-545/374a expression (figure 5B, figure S1B). AFP positive patients (≥20 ng/ml) had a significantly higher miR-545/374a level than AFP negative patients ($p = 0.012$, $p = 0.009$, independent t test) (figure 5B). However, no significant differences in the levels of miR-545/374a were observed for patients expressing CEA or γ-GT (figure S1B).

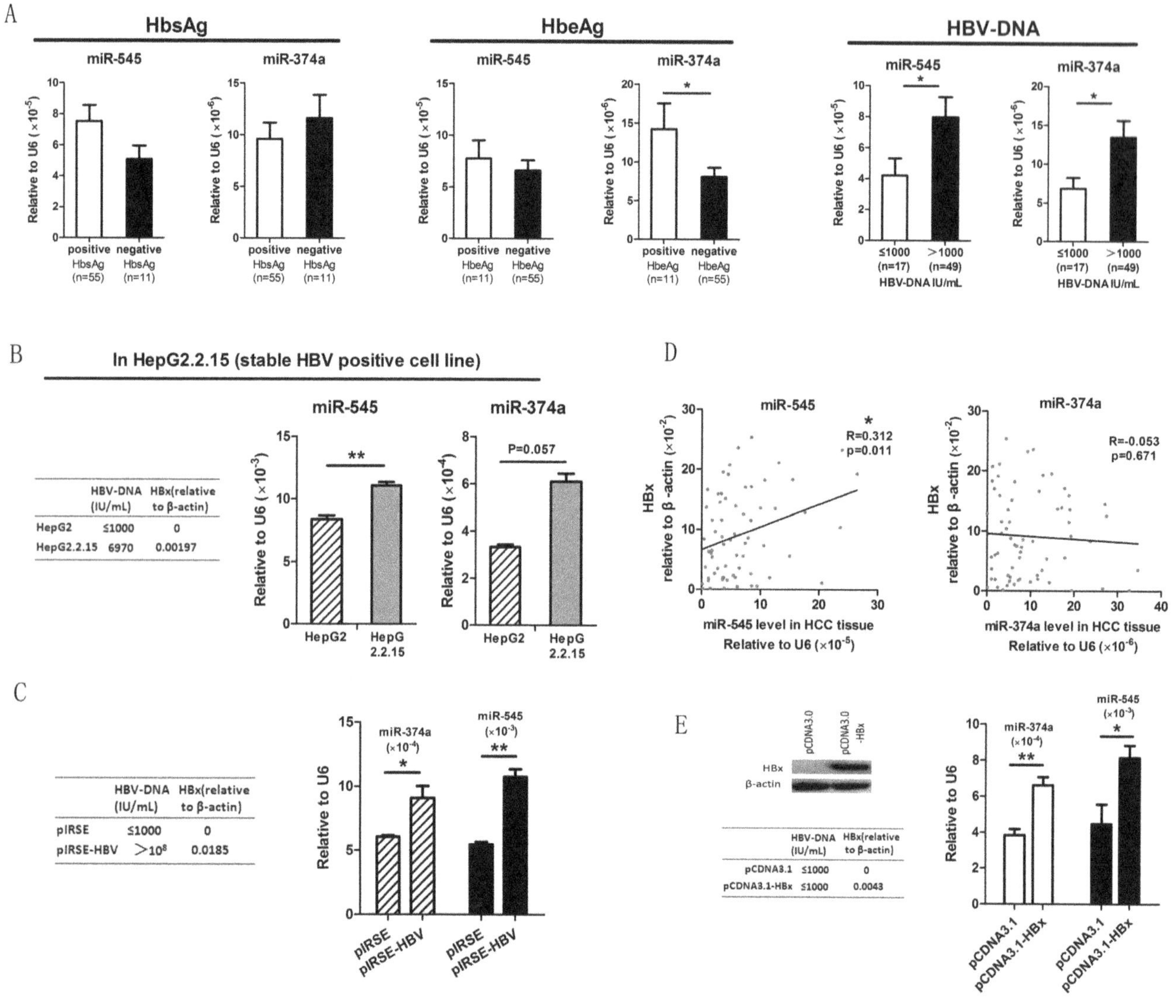

Figure 3. The influence of HBV infection on miR-545/374a cluster expression. (A) HCC subjects were grouped based on clinical HBV indices including HbsAg, HbeAg and HBV-DNA (Mean±Std.deviation, 10.64±9.158; Median, 7.035). The levels of miR-545 and miR-374a were determined by quantitative RT-PCR. Individual microRNA differences were measured by a student-t test between positive and negative groups. The error bars in A represent mean ± Std. deviation. (B) Comparison of microRNA expression levels between the stable HBV positive cell line HepG2.2.15 and its parental HCC cell line HepG2. The levels of miR-545/374a were monitored by quantitative RT-PCR in both cell lines. The error bars in B represent mean ± Std. deviation. (C) Analysis of microRNA expression levels in cells transfected with a HBV encoding plasmid. Cells were transfected with the HBV genome encoding plasmid (pIRSE-HBV) or the empty plasmid (pIRSE). To confirm the effective transfection of the HBV-genome containing plasmid we performed high-sensitive fluorescent quantitative PCR to detect HBV-DNA and quantitative real time PCR to detect HBx protein expression. The expression of miR-374a and miR-545 was measured by quantitative RT-PCR. *$P<0.05$, **$P<0.01$, independent t test. The error bars in C represent mean ± Std. deviation. (D) Analysis of miR-545/374a and HBx expression levels in HBV HCC subjects. The levels of miR-545/374a and HBx mRNA were assayed by quantitative RT-PCR. *$P<0.05$, Pearson's correlation. (E) Analysis of miR-545/374a expression in HBx overexpressing cells. Bel-7402 cells were transfected with a plasmid expressing HBx (pCDNA3.1HBx) or with an empty plasmid (pCDNA3.1). Western blotting and quantitative RT-PCR were used to confirm HBx protein expression after transfection. The levels of miR-545/374a were assayed by quantitative RT-PCR. The error bars in E represent mean ± Std. deviation. *$P<0.05$, **$P<0.01$, independent t test.

MicroRNA 545 and miR-374a are both higher in male HCC patients compared to female HCC patients, and ESRRG may be a target gene of miR-545

To investigate the potential role of miR-545/374a in HBV-HCC, the influence of gender was also evaluated (figure 5C). HCC subjects and negative control subjects were grouped according to gender. The levels of miR-545/374a were then monitored by quantitative RT-PCR of HCC tissue. The expression of both miR-545 and miR-374a were significantly higher in male vs. female HCC subjects (miR-545: male = 6.70, female = 4.34, p = 0.04; miR-374a: male = 9.68, female = 5.26, p = 0.008, independent t test). However, the distinction between male and female is not statistically significant in the negative control group (miR-545: male = 1.91, female = 2.19, p = 0.754; miR-374a: male = 0.37, female = 1.08, p = 0.273, independent t test).

The result is not surprising since the *Ftx* transcript is a positive regulator of *Xist*, the master regulator of the random X chromosome inactivation process [7]. Therefore the *Ftx* transcript

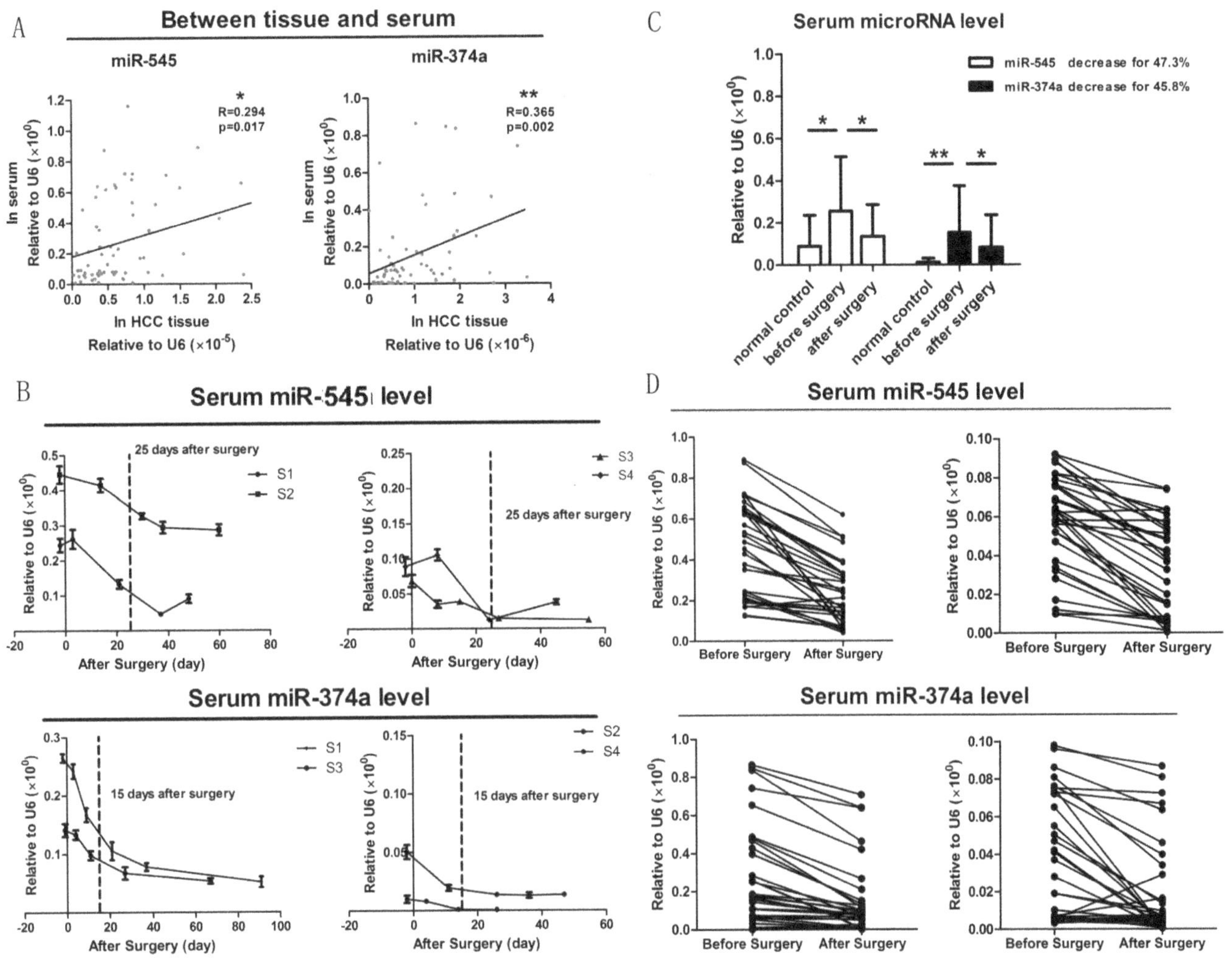

Figure 4. Tissue to serum analysis of miR-545/374a from the preoperative period to the postoperative period. (A) Tissue to serum analysis of miR-545/374a in HBV-HCC subjects. The levels of miR-545/374a in sera and tissue were assayed via quantitative RT-PCR. Pearson's correlations were calculated to measure microRNA expression between HCC tissue and serum. $^*P<0.05$, $^{**}P<0.01$. (B) Sera levels of miR-545/374a after surgical excision of tumor tissue. The sera from 4 representative HBV-related HCC subjects (S1, S2, S3 and S4) were collected at different time points after surgery. Quantitative RT-PCR was utilized to determine the levels of miR-545/374a in the sera samples. The dynamic levels of individual microRNAs in the sera were recorded as line charts. The error bars in B represent mean ± Std. deviation. (C) Pairwise comparison of microRNA levels between 66 pairs of preoperative sera and postoperative sera, and 23 negative control. The levels of miR-545/374a were measured by quantitative RT-PCR. The error bars in C represent Std. error. $^*P<0.05$, $^{**}P<0.01$, t test. (D) The microRNA expression variation from the preoperative period to the postoperative period is shown for each patient.

may be responsible for a gender-based biological phenomenon. To explain the distinct expression between male and female HCC patients, we utilized in silico miRNA target prediction programs (TargetScan and miRanda) to analyze the potential target genes of miR-545 and miR-374a. The following 3 estrogen-related genes were found by this analysis: ESRRA, ESRRG and ARGLU-1. The sequence comprising the miRNA target sites for the 3 genes are shown in figure 5D. The levels of each gene were quantified in 66 HBV-HCC patients. Figure 5E shows the results obtained for ESRRG. Pearson's correlation showed that the ESRRG gene had a reverse correlation with the expression of miR-545 ($r = -0.025$, $p = 0.043$). No statistically significant correlations were observed between miR-545/374a and ESRRA or ARGLU-1 (figure S1C).

Discussion

The *Ftx* gene gives rise to several RNA isoforms through a combination of alternative promoter usage, splicing and termination [7]. The miR-421/374b cluster and the miR-545/374a cluster are located in different introns and are controlled by distinct promoters. Since each microRNA cluster has distinct regulatory elements, it is possible that each cluster is differentially regulated during tumorigenesis. We found this to be the case in HBV-related HCC. Our findings indicated that the miR-545/374a cluster was significantly upregulated in HCC tissue, whereas the miR-421/374b cluster was not differentially regulated in HCC tissue. We then went on to further characterize the expression of the miR-545/374a cluster in HBV-related HCC.

We developed a model to describe the roles of the *Ftx* microRNA cluster in HBV-related HCC (figure 6) [13]. As the model shows, the expression of the miR-545/374a cluster is significantly upregulated in HCC tissue, and correlated with histological differentiation, incomplete tumor capsule formation and distal metastasis. *In vitro* cell transfection assays demonstrated that miR-545/374a may promote HCC cell proliferation, cell

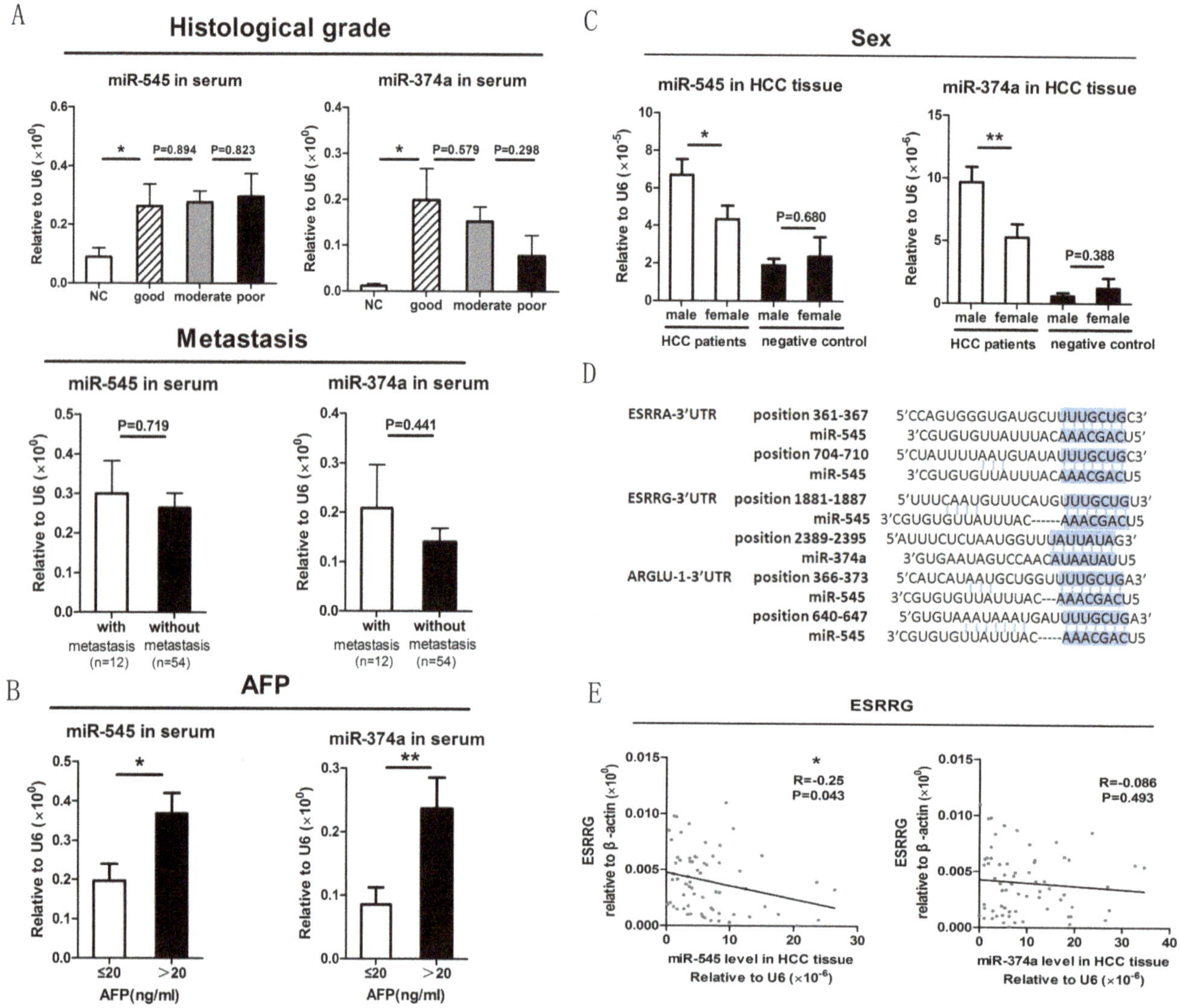

Figure 5. Correlation analysis of preoperative miR-545/374a serum expression with prognosis/diagnosis-related clinical features. (A) Correlation analysis of preoperative miR-545/374a serum levels with the prognosis-related clinical features of histological grade and metastasis. The histological grade was classified by pathological analysis as good, moderate or poor. Sera levels of miR-545/374a were analyzed by quantitative RT-PCR. The error bars in A represent mean ± Std. deviation. (B) Correlation analysis of preoperative miR-545/374a serum levels with the diagnosis-related clinical feature of AFP. The correlation analysis of CEA and γ-GT with the levels of miR-545/374a are shown in figure S1B. The error bars in B represent mean ± Std. deviation. (C) Gender-based investigation of Ftx microRNA cluster expression. HCC subjects and negative control subjects were grouped according to gender. MicroRNA 545 and miR-374a expression in HCC tissue was assayed by quantitative RT-PCR and compared between these groups. The error bars in C represent mean ± Std. deviation.*$P<0.05$, **$P<0.01$, t test. (D) Putative sex-related miR-545 and miR-374a target genes. The sequences comprising the miR-545 and miR-374a target sites are shown. (E) Correlation between HCC tissue miR-545/374a expression and ESRRG gene expression. The levels of miR-545/374a and ESRRG were monitored in 66 HCC tissue samples by quantitative RT-PCR. The correlation analysis of ESRRA and ARGLU-1 with miR-545/374a are shown in figure S1C. *$P<0.05$, Pearson's correlation test.

migration and invasion, thus implicating that overexpression of the miR-545/374a cluster may be responsible for tumor progression and poor prognosis of HCC patients. The correlation of miR-545/374a cluster expression with clinical HBV-related indices including HbeAg and HBV-DNA suggested that the miR-545/374a cluster is positively regulated by HBV infection. *In vitro* cell transfection studies confirmed these findings and showed that miR-545/374a expression may be induced by HBx expression. We also demonstrated that the levels of serum miR-545/374a are higher in HCC subjects compared to negative control patients. Furthermore, we found that serum miR-374a and miR-545 are tumor-derived, and showed a sharp drop in expression within 15 and 25 days after surgical tumor excision, respectively. We also determined that the expression of miR-545/374a correlated with AFP, a previously established clinical feature predicting HCC recurrence.

According to our studies, miR-545 and miR-374a have similar expression patterns and similar biological effects in HBV-related HCC. However, based on their sequence differences, the predicted target genes for each microRNA are different. A study in 2013 demonstrated that miR-374a regulates several target genes mediating the Wnt/β-catenin signaling pathway [8]. Our preliminary biological informative analysis showed that these genes may not be the most probable target genes of miR-545 (data not shown), further indicating that the target genes of miR-545 vs. miR-374a are different. Considering the possibility that miR-545

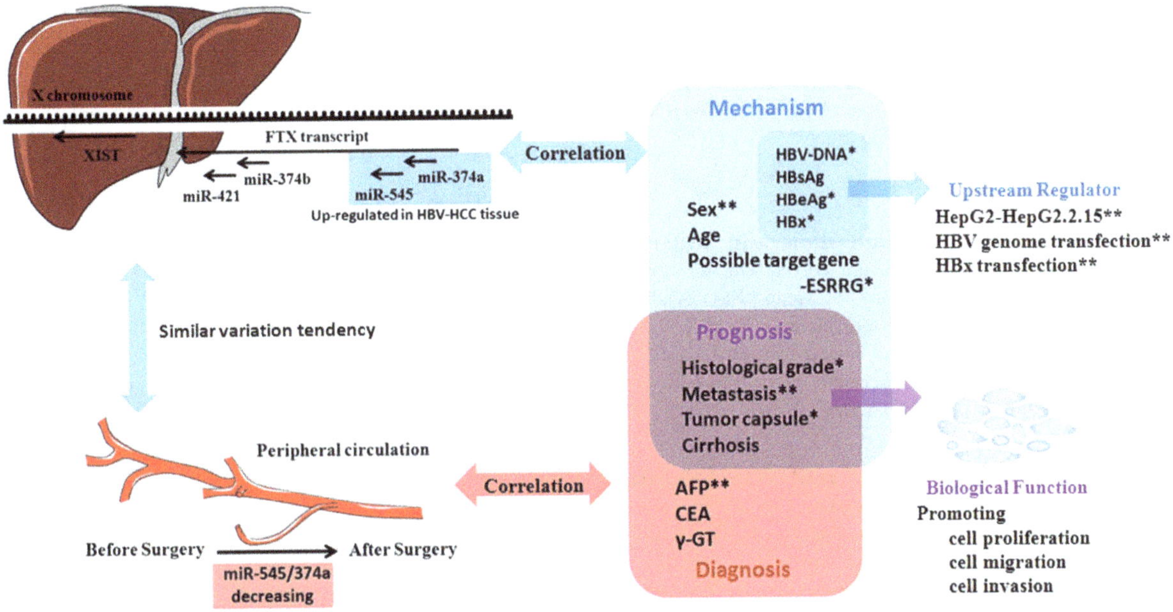

Figure 6. A consolidated model for the role of the miR-545/374a cluster in human HBV related hepatocellular carcinoma. Ftx gene encodes a lncRNA which harbors 2 cluster of microRNAs in its introns, the miR-374a/545 cluster and the miR-374b/421 cluster. In clinical specimens, the miR-545/374a cluster is upregulated in HCC tissue and is significantly correlated with prognosis-related clinical features. Serum miR-545/374a are tumor-derived, and their expression are significantly decreased after surgical excision of tumor tissue. MicroRNA 545 and miR-374a are both higher in male HCC patients compared to female HCC patients, and ESRRG may be a target gene of miR-545. In vitro studies, the miR-545/374a cluster promotes HCC cell proliferation, cell migration and invasion. Expression of miR-545/374a is positively regulated by HBV infection and may be induced by HBx expression.

and miR-374a may have distinct mechanisms which promote tumor progression, we prefer to study them individually rather than studying the cluster as a whole.

From another perspective, now that miR-374a and miR-545 are transcribed off the same promoter, why their abundances are not always correlated (Figure 1C-F, Figure 5A)? It has been suggested that the expression of the intronic miRNAs may be coupled with that of the host mRNA, but differ from each other, especially in the pathological states. These observations point to diverse mechanisms and the existence of additional steps in the posttranscriptional processing of miRNA. Many of the RNA-binding proteins can bind to conserved loop sequences in the miRNA, and therefore, may form part of the gene regulatory network that influence the excision of miRNA in response to intra- or extra-cellular stimuli [14].

We first chose HCC tissue specimens to study the expression of miR-545/374a, and then developed a "from tissue to serum, from preoperative to postoperative" line of study to test the potential prognostic value of miR-545/374a using serum specimens. HCC is a serious condition associated with a high morbidity and mortality, and early detection is the key to effective surgical excision. Since the current biomarkers for HCC, including AFP, CEA and γ-GT, have limited sensitivity and specificity, new biomarkers are needed to improve the diagnosis and management of patients with liver pathologies. It is commonly believed that tumor-derived microRNAs can be released into the peripheral circulation and remain stable under harsh conditions due to protection from RNases [15]. Our results partially support that hypothesis. We found that serum miR-545/374a originated from tumor tissue, and the expression levels of miR-545/374a in HCC patients was higher than in negative control patients. Taken together these data support the hypothesis that serum miR-545/374a may be a potential diagnostic marker for HBV-related HCC. However, serum miR-545/374a may not be useful to predict the prognosis of HCC patients, because there was no significant correlation between serum miR-545/374a expression and a poor prognosis. In contrast, tissue miR-545/374a expression strongly correlated with a poor prognosis of HBV-related HCC patients. Therefore, miR-545/374a based prognosis-predicting may only be useful if tumor tissue is assayed.

We observed a gender-based difference in miR-545/374a expression. Specifically, male HCC patients had a significantly higher expression level of both microRNAs compared to female HCC patients. The distinction was not observed between normal male and female subjects. Based on these findings, we hypothesize that the comparatively small change in miR-545/374a expression in female HCC patients may serve as a protecting mechanism. Through biological analysis and correlation analysis, ESRRG was identified as a potential target gene of miR-545. The estrogen receptor-related receptor (ESRR) family are orphan nuclear receptors, which is closely related to the estrogen receptor family. They can bind to the estrogen response element. Previous researches have found ESRRA, a member of ESRR, can promote p53 gene expression and induce HCC progression in female patients [16], while whether ESRRG have a role in HCC is still unknown. Presently we are amplifying the sample size, especially the female HCC patients. Respective study in female and male patient may better indicate the potential role of ESRRG. Elucidation of the mechanism of miR-545 mediated regulation of ESRRG expression requires further investigation.

Conclusions

In summary, the expression of the miR-545/374a cluster located in the lncRNA *Ftx* is significantly upregulated in HBV-related HCC tissue, and correlated with a poor prognosis of HCC patients. Serum miR-545/374a originated from tumor tissue, and potentially may be utilized as a novel screening and diagnostic marker for HCC occurrence in routine clinical practice. ESRRG is a potential target gene of miR-545 and we hypothesize that this mechanism may be related to the low incidence of HBV-HCC in females, which requires further investigation.

Supporting Information

Figure S1 MicroRNA expression data and different clinical features. (A) No significant correlation is showed concerning patients' age (years, Mean±Std.deviation, 52.73±9.712; Median, 53). Pearson's correlation. (B) HBV-HCC patients are divided into positive and negative groups based on their serum CEA and γ-GT level, however no statistical significance is showed. Independent t test.

Figure S2 Wound healing assay: miR-374a/545 may increase the migration of HCC in vitro. The cells in six-well plate were scratched with pipette tip, incubated at 37°C, 5% CO_2 for 24 hours after being transfected by miroRNA mimics or inhibitor, then monitored by photographing for wounding. Result showed that, cell transfected with miR-374a or 545 mimics exhibit higher migration ability, while inhibition of miR-374a or miR-545 notably delayed healing of wound and inhibited cell migration on the surface of the tissue culture plate.

Table S1 List of the oligonucleotides used in this study.

Table S2 A. The expression of microRNAs in *Ftx* transcript in human tissues. B. The expression of miR-374a/545 in human serum.

Acknowledgments

This work was supported by grants from the Shandong Science and Technology Committee of China (2013GG3202192), the Postdoctoral Science Foundation of China (2013M541926), and the Postdoctoral Innovation Project Special Foundation of Shandong Province (201302031).

Author Contributions

Conceived and designed the experiments: CQ QZ. Performed the experiments: QZ TL JQ. Analyzed the data: QZ JL JQ. Contributed reagents/materials/analysis tools: CQ QZ TL. Wrote the paper: QZ JL.

References

1. Brechot C, Gozuacik D, Murakami Y, Paterlini-Brechot P (2000) Molecular bases for the development of hepatitis B virus (HBV)-related hepatocellular carcinoma (HCC). Semin Cancer Biol 10: 211–231.
2. Lee JT (2012) Epigenetic regulation by long noncoding RNAs. Science 338: 1435–1439.
3. Huang JL, Zheng L, Hu YW, Wang Q (2013) Characteristics of Long Noncoding RNA and Its Relation to Hepatocellular Carcinoma. Carcinogenesis.
4. Xu D, Yang F, Yuan JH, Zhang L, Bi HS, et al. (2013) Long noncoding RNAs associated with liver regeneration 1 accelerates hepatocyte proliferation during liver regeneration by activating Wnt/beta-catenin signaling. Hepatology 58: 739–751.
5. Tsai MC, Manor O, Wan Y, Mosammaparast N, Wang JK, et al. (2010) Long noncoding RNA as modular scaffold of histone modification complexes. Science 329: 689–693.
6. Yang F, Zhang L, Huo XS, Yuan JH, Xu D, et al. (2011) Long noncoding RNA high expression in hepatocellular carcinoma facilitates tumor growth through enhancer of zeste homolog 2 in humans. Hepatology 54: 1679–1689.
7. Romito A, Rougeulle C (2011) Origin and evolution of the long non-coding genes in the X-inactivation center. Biochimie 93: 1935–1942.
8. Cai J, Guan H, Fang L, Yang Y, Zhu X, et al. (2013) MicroRNA-374a activates Wnt/beta-catenin signaling to promote breast cancer metastasis. J Clin Invest 123: 566–579.
9. Cui L, Qi Y, Li H, Ge Y, Zhao K, et al. (2011) Serum microRNA expression profile distinguishes enterovirus 71 and coxsackievirus 16 infections in patients with hand-foot-and-mouth disease. PLoS One 6: e27071.
10. Zhao Q, Fan YC, Zhao J, Gao S, Zhao ZH, et al. (2013) DNA methylation patterns of peroxisome proliferator-activated receptor gamma gene associated with liver fibrosis and inflammation in chronic hepatitis B. J Viral Hepat 20: 430–437.
11. Liu J, Han G, Liu H, Qin C (2013) Suppression of cholangiocarcinoma cell growth by human umbilical cord mesenchymal stem cells: a possible role of Wnt and Akt signaling. PLoS One 8: e62844.
12. Xu X, Li S, Lin Y, Chen H, Hu Z, et al. (2013) MicroRNA-124-3p inhibits cell migration and invasion in bladder cancer cells by targeting ROCK1. J Transl Med 11: 276.
13. Hur K, Toiyama Y, Takahashi M, Balaguer F, Nagasaka T, et al. (2013) MicroRNA-200c modulates epithelial-to-mesenchymal transition (EMT) in human colorectal cancer metastasis. Gut 62: 1315–1326.
14. Shukla GC, Singh J, Barik S (2011) MicroRNAs: Processing, Maturation, Target Recognition and Regulatory Functions. Mol Cell Pharmacol 3: 83–92.
15. Schetter AJ, Leung SY, Sohn JJ, Zanetti KA, Bowman ED, et al. (2008) MicroRNA expression profiles associated with prognosis and therapeutic outcome in colon adenocarcinoma. JAMA 299: 425–436.
16. Li CL, Yeh KH, Liu WH, Chen CL, Chen DS, et al. (2014) Elevated p53 promotes the processing of miR-18a to decrease estrogen receptor-alpha in female hepatocellular carcinoma. Int J Cancer.

Fatty Acid Esters of Phloridzin Induce Apoptosis of Human Liver Cancer Cells through Altered Gene Expression

Sandhya V. G. Nair, Ziaullah, H. P. Vasantha Rupasinghe*

Department of Environmental Sciences, Faculty of Agriculture, Dalhousie University, Truro, Nova Scotia, Canada

Abstract

Phloridzin (phlorizin or phloretin 2′-*O*-glucoside) is known for blocking intestinal glucose absorption. We have investigated the anticarcinogenic effect of phloridzin and its novel derivatives using human cancer cell lines. We have synthesised novel acylated derivatives of phloridzin with six different long chain fatty acids by regioselective enzymatic acylation using *Candida Antarctica* lipase B. The antiproliferative effects of the new compounds were investigated in comparison with the parent compounds, phloridzin, aglycone phloretin, the six free fatty acids and chemotherapeutic drugs (sorafenib, doxorubicin and daunorubicin) using human hepatocellular carcinoma HepG2 cells, human breast adenocarcinoma MDA-MB-231 cells and acute monocytic leukemia THP-1 cells along with normal human and rat hepatocytes. The fatty acid esters of phloridzin inhibited significantly the growth of the two carcinoma and leukemia cells while similar treatment doses were not toxic to normal human or rat hepatocytes. The antiproliferative potency of fatty esters of phloridzin was comparable to the potency of the chemotherapeutic drugs. The fatty acid esters of phloridzin inhibited DNA topoisomerases IIα activity that might induce G_0/G_1 phase arrest, induced apoptosis via activation of caspase-3, and decreased ATP level and mitochondrial membrane potential in HepG2 cells. Based on the high selectivity on cancer cells, decosahexaenoic acid (DHA) ester of phloridzin was selected for gene expression analysis using RT^2PCR human cancer drug target array. Antiproliferative effect of DHA ester of phloridzin could be related to the down regulation of anti-apoptotic gene (BCL2), growth factor receptors (EBFR family, IGF1R/IGF2, PDGFR) and its downstream signalling partners (PI3k/AKT/mTOR, Ras/Raf/MAPK), cell cycle machinery (CDKs, TERT, TOP2A, TOP2B) as well as epigenetics regulators (HDACs). These results suggest that fatty esters of phloridzin have potential chemotherapeutic effects mediated through the attenuated expression of several key proteins involved in cell cycle regulation, DNA topoisomerases IIα activity and epigenetic mechanisms followed by cell cycle arrest and apoptosis.

Editor: Gnanasekar Munirathinam, University of Illinois, United States of America

Funding: HPVR: Discovery Grant program of the Natural Sciences and Engineering Council (NSERC; Grant Number 327056; http://www.nserc-crsng.gc.ca) of Canada and the Atlantic Innovation Funds (AIF) program of the Atlantic Canada Opportunities Agency (ACOA; Grant Number 192020; http://www.acoa-apeca.gc.ca). The funders had no role in study design, data collection and analysis, decision to publish, or preparation of the manuscript.

Competing Interests: The authors have declared that no competing interests exist.

* Email: vrupasinghe@dal.ca

Introduction

Hepatocellular carcinoma (HCC), the most common form of liver cancer, represent the fifth worldwide malignancy and third cause of mortality among cancer related death [1]. In Canada, the incidence of HCC has been increasing over the past several decades [2]. HCC accounts for 71.9% of liver cancers in males and females in Canada. According to Canadian Cancer Statistics in 2013, the incidence rate of liver cancer in Canada has increased by 3.6% per year, and the mortality rate increased by 2.2% per year. The contributing factors of HCC include contact with hepatocarcinogens especially aflatoxin [3], hepatic viral infection and liver cirrhosis [4]. The potential curative treatment options are surgical resection, liver transplantation, and ablation or transarterial embolization [1]. The chemotherapy, oral multi-kinase inhibitor sorafenib (Nexavar) is the most commonly used drug for HCC treatment but the gain in survival is modest [5]. Unavailability of effective treatments and high prevalence rate has led to the search of novel approaches suitable for prevention and treatment of liver cancer. As a result, many phytochemicals have been explored as potential chemopreventive agents that can reverse or suppress hepatocarcinogenic progression.

Flavonoids, one of the major classes of polyphenols, have shown some chemopreventive properties against HCC in a vast number of in vitro [6,7] and in vivo studies [1,8]. Phloridzin (phlorizin or phloretin 2′-*O*-glucoside), a dihydrochalcone, is one of the major phenolic flavonoid glucosides found in apple [9]. The major pharmacological action of phloridzin is inhibition of sodium-dependent glucose linked transporters (SGLT1 and SGLT2) that blocks intestinal glucose absorption and produce renal glycosuria [9]. In addition to their antidiabetic property, phloridzin has other biological activities such as inhibition of lipid peroxidation [10], prevention of bone loss in rats [11] and enhancement of memory in mice [12]. Phloridzin stimulate melanogenesis by increasing tyrosinase gene expression through the cAMP signaling pathway [13]. Phloretin, the aglycone of phloridzin, has been reported to have potent antioxidant activity in peroxynitrite scavenging and the inhibition of lipid peroxidation [14]. Glycosylation at 2-OH decreased the antioxidant activities of phloridzin by 18 times in comparison to phloretin [14]. Phloretin at the concentrations of 100 μM augmented TNFα-related apoptosis-inducing ligand (TRAIL)-induced apoptosis and cytotoxicity in LNCaP prostate cancer cells [15]. However, there is no report on the cancer chemopreventive effects of phloridzin. In an antitumor activity study of apple polyphenols, phloridzin did not affect the proliferation of either transplanted B16 mouse melanoma cells or BALB-MC.E12 mouse mammary tumor cells [16].

In our laboratory, phloridzin was regioselectively acylated with a series of long chain, saturated, mono- and poly-unsaturated, fatty acids by using immobilized lipase B, from *Candida antarctica* (Novozyme 435) [17]. Lipase catalyzed esterification and transesterification of flavonoid glycosides have been reported to increase lipophilicity and improved anticancer effect of the parent compound [18]. Therefore, in this study, we investigated the cytotoxic potential of fatty acid esters of phloridzin on cell proliferation of solid tumours such as hepatocellular carcinoma HepG2 cells and breast adenocarcinoma MDA-MB-231 cells as well as acute monocytes leukemia THP-1 cells. Normal human hepatocytes HP-F and rat hepatocytes RTCP10 were also used to determine the specificity of the esters on cancerous cells. This is the first time these novel fatty acid esters of phloridzin have been tested for antiproliferative effect of cancer cells. In addition to elucidate the cellular and molecular mechanisms of fatty acid esters of phloridzin on HepG2 cells, DNA topoisomerases IIα activity, cell cycle arrest, mitochondrial membrane permeability, caspase 3 activity and associated apoptotic processes were also investigated. Furthermore, we analyzed the effect of decosahexaenoic acid (DHA) ester of phloridzin on expression of 84 genes that targets for anticancer therapeutics and drug development. Our results provided experimental evidence to support further investigation of fatty acid esters of phloridzin especially DHA ester of phloridzin as an effective and safe chemotherapeutic candidate.

Materials and Methods

Test compounds and chemicals

Fatty acid esters of phloridzin (Pz) viz. stearic acid ester of Pz (Pz-stearic acid), oleic acid ester of Pz (Pz-oleic acid), linoleic acid ester of Pz (Pz-linoleic acid), α-linolenic acid ester of Pz (Pz-α-linolenic acid), DHA ester of Pz (Pz-DHA) and eicosapentaenoic acid ester (EPA) of Pz (Pz-EPA) were synthesised in our laboratory as previously reported [17].

Phloridzin, phloretin, caspase 3 colorimetric assay kit, propidium iodide, fatty acids namely oleic acid, stearic acid, linoleic acid, α-linolenic acid, EPA and DHA were purchased from Sigma-Aldrich Canada. Cell Titer 96 Aqueous One solution cell proliferation (MTS) assay, CytoTox 96 non-radioactive cytotoxicity (LDH) assay and CellTiter-Glo luminescent assay kits were purchased from Promega, Madison, WI, USA. Sterile dimethyl sulfoxide (DMSO) (ATCC), GFP-certified apoptosis/necrosis detection kit for microscopy from Enzo Life Sciences, Brockville, ON, Canada; ApoTarget Quick Apoptotic DNA Ladder Detection kit from Invitrogen, Burlington, ON, Canada; DCFDA-Cellular Reactive Oxygen Species detection assay kit form Abcam, Toronto, ON, Canada; and 5′,6,6′-tetrachloro-1,1′,3,3′-tetraethylbenzimidazolylcarbocyanine iodide (JC-1) from Cayman Chemicals, Burlington, ON, Canada were also used for the study.

Cell lines and culture conditions

Human hepatocellular carcinoma cells (HepG2) and THP-1 acute monocytic leukemia cells were purchased from the American Type Culture Collection (ATCC), Manassas, VA, USA (Dalhousie University Biosafety certificate number for use of cell lines is of 2013-10). HepG2 cells were grown in Eagle's modified minimum essential media (EMEM) supplemented with 10% FBS (ATCC) and 1% penicillin-streptomycin (ATCC). THP-1 cells were cultured in RPMI-1640 media supplemented 0.05 mM 2-mercaptoethanol and 10% fetal bovine serum to a final concentration of 10%. MDA-MB-231 breast cancer cells (ATCC HTB-26) were obtained from Cedarlane, Berlington, ON, Canada) and were maintained in DMEM medium (Sigma-Aldrich Canada) supplemented with 100 u/mL penicillin, 100 μg/mL streptomycin, 2 mM L-glutamine, 5 mM HEPES (pH 7.4) and 10% heat-inactivated fetal bovine serum (Invitrogen, Burlington, ON, Canada). Cryopreserved normal human hepatocytes (HP-F), hepatocyte plating medium and hepatocyte maintenance medium were purchased from Zen-Bio, Research Tiangle Park, NC, USA. Normal human hepatocytes plated on 96 well collagen 1 coated cell culture plates (Life Technologies) and maintained in hepatocyte maintenance medium for 24 h to allow for cell recovery and attachment. Rat hepatocytes (RTCP10), thawing media and incubation media were purchased from Life Technologies. Rat hepatocytes were plated in collagen 1 coated 96 well plates (Life Technologies, Burlington, ON, Canada) using thawing media and maintained in incubation medium. All cell types were maintained at 37°C in an incubator under 5% CO_2/95% air atmosphere at constant humidity.

Cells were counted using a hemocytometer (Bright-Line Hemocytometer, Sigma-Aldrich Canada) and were plated according to the number of cells for each experiment in 6, 24 or 96 well format for 24 h prior to addition of test samples. All the test samples were solubilised in sterile filtered DMSO (<0.5% in the culture medium) prior to addition to the culture media. Control cells were also run in parallel and subjected to the same changes in media with <0.5% DMSO.

Cell Proliferation assay

Cell viability was determined by using the MTS assay. In brief, HepG2 cells (5×10^3 cells/100 μL/well), MDA-MB-231 (5×10^3 cells/100 μL/well), THP-1 (25×10^3/100 μL/well), normal human and rat hepatocytes (1×10^4 cells/100 μL/well) were plated in triplicate, in a 96 well sterile flat bottom tissue culture plates. After 24 h incubation, phloridzin fatty esters, phloridzin, phloretin, free fatty acids of respective esters or sorafenib were prepared in media and 100 μL of each treatment was added to each well, each treatment in three replications. Thereby, cells were exposed to various concentrations (0.1, 1, 10, 25, 50, 75, 100 μM) of each treatment. Controls consist of cells with media containing DMSO (<0.5%), test blank wells contained the test compound in media with no cells and blank wells contained media with no cells. After additional 3, 6, 12, 18 or 24 h, 20 μL of the MTS reagent in combination with the electron coupling agent, phenazine methosulfate were added to the wells and cells were incubated in a humidified incubator for 3 h. Absorbance at 490 nm (OD490) was measured by using a Flurostar Optima microplate reader (BMG Labtech, Cary, NC, USA) to obtain the number of viable cells relative to the control population. Percentage of viability of the test compound treated cells are expressed as percentage compared to control (<0.5% DMSO). EC_{50} values (concentration required to reduce cells viability by 50% as compared to control cells) for each test compound was analysed using Graphpad Prism software, La Jolla, CA, USA. The selective index (SI) of the fatty acid esters of phloridzin is defined as the ratio of cytotoxicity (EC_{50} values) on normal HP-F cells to solid cancer HepG2, MDA-MB-231 cells (SI = EC_{50} on HP-F cells/EC_{50} on solid cancer cells). Samples with SI values greater than three were considered to have high selectivity towards cancer cells.

Cytotoxicity assay

Lactate dehydrogenase (LDH) is a stable cytosolic enzyme that is released upon membrane damage in apoptotic/necrotic cells. LDH activity was measured using CytoTox 96 Non-Radioactive Cytotoxicity Assay (Promega, Madison, WI, USA), in which LDH released in culture supernatants is measured with a coupled enzymatic assay, resulting in conversion of a tetrazolium salt into a red formazan product. HepG2 cells (5000/100 μL/well) were seeded and treated with 100 μM of phloridzin fatty acid esters, phloridzin, phloretin, free fatty acids of respective esters or sorafenib prepared in serum free media and incubated (37°C, 5% CO_2) for 6 h. After centrifugation, the supernatant was removed to an assay plate, and the LDH released from the cells into culture medium was measured. The maximal release was obtained after treating control cells with 1% Triton X-100 for 30 min at room temperature. The apoptotic/necrotic percentage was expressed using the formula: (sample value/maximal release) × 100%. Previous studies by the supplier had clearly stated that in HepG2 cells, LDH activity maximum concentration is at 1 to 6 h incubations because LDH activity released from cells has a half-life of approximately 9 h [19]. MTS assay results showed that all the fatty acid esters of phloridzin inhibited 70–80% cell proliferation in 6 h, therefore, we analysed LDH activity after 6 h incubation.

Morphological observation of apoptosis in HepG2 cells

2.5.1. Morphologic observation under inverted phase contrast microscope. HepG2 cells were equally seeded in 24-well flat bottom tissue culture treated plates (BD Biosciences), and then treated with 100 μM of fatty acid esters of phloridzin, phloridzin, phloretin, sorafenib and DMSO (<0.5%) control. After 24 h of treatment, the morphology of HepG2 cells was observed under an inverted phase contrast microscope (Nikon Eclipse E 100, Nikon, Mississauga, ON, Canada) and were captured at 400X magnification using Infinity digital microscopy camera (Lumenera corporation, Ottawa, ON, Canada).

2.5.2. Determination of Apoptosis/Necrosis by Fluorescence Microscopy. HepG2 cells were seeded into Nunc Lab-Tek two chamber slide (Sigma-Aldrich Canada) at a density of 1×10^6 cells/chamber. The attached cells were then treated either with 100 μM fatty acid esters of phloridzin, phloridzin, phloretin, sorafenib or DMSO vehicle (as control) for 24 h. The slides were washed with diluted phosphate buffered saline. After removing the chamber, each slide was added with 50 μL of Dual Detection Reagent containing apoptosis detection reagent (Annexin V-EnzoGold) and necrosis detection reagent (7-AAD) in 1X binding buffer. The samples were incubated at room temperature for 15 min in the dark. After staining, the cells were washed with binding buffer and covered with a glass coverslip. The stained cells were observed under a fluorescence Zeiss Axiovert 200 m inverted microscope (Carl Zeiss, Toronto, ON, Canada) at magnification of ×40 with a filter set for Annexin V-EnzoGold (Ex/Em: 550/570 nm) and 7-AAD (Ex/Em: 546/647 nm).

Analysis of apoptosis by DNA Fragmentation

HepG2 (1×10^5) cells were seeded in 24-well culture plates and were allowed to adhere overnight. Following this, cells were treated either with 100 μM fatty acid esters of phloridzin, phloridzin, phloretin, sorafenib or DMSO vehicle (as control). The plates were re-incubated for another 24 h. DNA fragmentation was detected using ApoTarget Quick Apoptotic DNA Ladder Detection Kit (Invitrogen, Burlington, ON, Canada) according to the manufacturer's protocol. The principle involves detecting the internucleosomal DNA fragments formed during apoptosis. Briefly, floating dead cells and trypsinized adherent cells were collected and centrifuged at 1,000 rpm for 10 min. After washing with diluted phosphate buffered saline, the cells were lysed with 35 μL TE lysis buffer (a kit component). To the lysate, 5 μL of Enzyme A (a kit component) was added and incubated at 37°C for 10 min. Afterwards, 5 μL of Enzyme B (a kit component) was added, gently mixed and incubated at 50°C for 30 min. The DNA was precipitated with the ammonium acetate and absolute ethanol at −20°C. After centrifugation (10 min at 12,000 rpm) and air drying, the DNA pellet was dissolved in 30 μL of DNA suspension buffer. For detecting the DNA ladder, the extracted DNA samples were run on a 1.2% agarose gel containing 0.5 μg/mL gel red in Tris-Borate-EDTA (TBE) buffer. After electrophoresis, the gel image was captured using Gel Doc 100 system (Bio-Rad, Mississauga, ON, Canada).

Assay of Caspase-3 Activity

The activity of caspase 3 enzyme was measured using caspase 3 colorimetric assay kit purchased from Sigma-Aldrich. HepG2 cells (2×10^6 cells/well), grown in 6-well plates, were treated either with 100 μM fatty acid esters of phloridzin, phloridzin, phloretin, sorafenib or DMSO vehicle (as control). Cells were lysed and the protein content of cell lysate was quantified by the BCA protein assay (Thermo Fisher Scientific Inc., Ottawa, ON, Canada). Caspase-3 activity was measured in the 200 μg of cell lysate using the caspase-specific peptide substrate, DEVD (Asp-Glu-Val-Asp), conjugated to reporter p-nitroanaline (ρ-NA) molecules. Cleavage of this peptide by caspase releases the chromophore which is measured colorimetrically at a wavelength of 405 nm as described in the supplier's protocol.

Cell Cycle Analysis

HepG2 cells were plated at 5×10^5 cells per ml in a six-well plate. After 24 h incubation (37°C, 5% CO_2), the cells were treated with 100 μM fatty acid esters of phloridzin, phloridzin, phloretin, sorafenib or DMSO (<0.5%) control prepared in media and incubated for additional 24 h. Following trypsinization, cells were washed and centrifuged at 2000 ×g for 10 min and the pellet re-suspended in 0.5 mL PBS. Fixation was completed by adding 1.2 mL of 70% cold ethanol for 2 h. The fixed cells were washed with PBS and centrifuged at 2000 ×g for 10 min. After suspending cells in 0.3 mL PBS, 8 μL of DNAase free RNAse (10 mg/mL) was added and incubated for 1 h. After adding, 15 μL of propidium iodide (0.5 mg/mL), cells were incubated in 4°C for 30 min. The cells were analyzed for cell cycle using flow cytometer FACS calibur (Beckman Coulter, Fullerton, CA, USA) with an excitation wavelength of 488 nm and emission at 670 nm. DNA content was determined by ModFit software (Verity Software House, Topsham, ME, USA), which provided histograms to evaluate cell cycle distribution.

Mitochondrial Energy Metabolism Assays

ATP level assay. Cellular ATP levels were measured with CellTiter-Glo luminescent assay kit obtained from Promega according to the manufacturer's instructions. HepG2 cells plated on a black walled clear bottom 96-well plate were incubated with 100 μM fatty acid esters of phloridzin, phloridzin, phloretin, sorafenib, free fatty acids or DMSO (<0.5%) control in media. After 24 h, CellTiter-Glo Reagent equal to the volume of cell culture medium present in each well and mixed contents for 2 min on an orbital shaker to induce cell lysis. Luminescence was recorded on Flurostar Optima microplate reader (BMG Labtech) after incubation at room temperature for 10 min to stabilize luminescent signal. The level of ATP in a sample was presented as percentage compared to untreated control.

Mitochondrial membrane potential (MMP). HepG2 cells were seeded in a black walled clear bottom 96-well sterile flat bottom tissue culture plates (BD Biosciences, USA) at a density of 5×10^4 cells/well (100 μL) and incubated in a CO_2 incubator for 24 h at 37°C. Cells were treated with 100 μM fatty acid esters of phloridzin, phloridzin, phloretin, sorafenib, free fatty acids or DMSO (<0.5%) control prepared in media and incubated for 24 h. The staining solution JC-1 was prepared with PBS and 5 μM was added to each well. The cells were further incubated in a CO_2 incubator at 37°C for 1 h. After washing the plate with PBS twice, the fluorescence was measured using a Fluostar Optima microplate reader (BMG Labtech) at 535 nm for JC-1 monomers and at 590 nm for JC-1 aggregates.

Human Topoisomerase IIα (topo IIα) Catalytic Activity

The topo IIα catalytic activity was monitored via electrophoresis using topoisomerase II drug screening kit (TopoGEN, Inc., Columbus, OH, USA). Briefly, 20 μL of reaction mixtures contained 0.5 M Tris-HCl, pH 8.0, 1.5 M NaCl, 100 mM $MgCl_2$, 20 mM ATP, 300 μg BSA/mL and 5 mM dithiothreitol. Supercoiled DNA (pHOT1 DNA), supercoiled provided in the kit was determined to be ideal for this assay because it is small and easy to handle and has a large number of topo IIα recognition elements. After 2 μL (0.25 μg) of pHOT1 DNA was added, followed by the addition of 100 μM fatty acid esters of phloridzin, phloridzin, phloretin, sorafenib or DMSO (<0.5%) control in solvent, the reaction was initiated by adding 4 units (2 μL) of human DNA topo IIα and carried out at 37°C for 30 min. The reaction was terminated by adding 2 μL of 10% sodium dodecyl sulfate (SDS) followed by digestion with 2 μL of proteinase K (50 μg/mL) at 37°C for 15 min to degrade enzyme. After adding 2 μL of loading buffer (0.25% bromophenol blue and 50% glycerol) was added to the mixture, samples were loaded onto 1% agarose gel. Electrophoresis was conducted at 66 V (2 V/cm) for 5 h in TBE buffer using Biorad Electrophoretic Gel System (Bio-Rad, Hercules, CA, USA). Supercoiled DNA (pHOT1 DNA) and relaxed DNA were included in the electrophoresis run as markers for DNA topology. Gels were then stained in 0.5 μg/mL gel red in TBE for 30 min and destained for 15 min in distilled water prior to digital image acquisition using Gel Doc 100 system (Bio-Rad, Hercules, CA, USA).

One unit of topoisomerase II activity was defined as the minimum amount of enzyme required to achieve complete relaxation of 0.5 mg superhelical pHOT1 DNA in 30 min at 37°C. Inhibition of topoisomerase II relaxation activity was investigated by the same procedure using four units of enzyme and 100 μM test compounds. The percent of inhibition was calculated by the following formula:

$$\% \, Inhibition = \frac{(S - S_0)}{(S_{control} - S_0)} \times 100$$

Where $S_{control}$ is the percent of supercoiled DNA in the control lane (without enzyme and test compounds), S_0 is the percent of supercoiled DNA in the lane without test compounds and S is the percent of supercoiled DNA in the lane with test compounds and enzyme.

Real Time RT-PCR analysis

Gene expression profiles were obtained from HepG2 cells treated with DHA esters of phloridzin or sorafenib or DMSO treated control cells. Total RNA extraction was performed using Arum Total RNA minikit (Bio-Rad, Hercules, CA, USA). RNA concentration and purity was determined by measuring the absorbance using a NanoDrop (NanoDrop Technologies, Wilmington, DE, USA). RNA integrity was assessed by formaldehyde agarose gel electrophoresis. RNA (400 ng) was used to synthesize cDNA using RT^2 First Strand kit (SABiosciences, Frederick, MD, USA). RT^2 RNA QC PCR arrays (SABiosciences, Frederick, MD, USA) was used to assess the quality of cDNA samples before characterization with the human cancer drug targets RT^2 profiler PCR array (SABiosciences, Frederick, MD, USA). Gene expression profiles of 84 genes were investigated using the human cancer drug targets RT^2 profiler PCR array (PAHS-507ZD) on a Bio-Rad CFX Connect (Bio-Rad, Hercules, CA, USA) using RT^2 real-time SYBR green PCR master mix (SABiosciences, Frederick, MD, USA). The array also has five reference genes (beta-2-microglobulin (B2M), hypoxanthine phosphoribosyltransferase 1 (HPRT1), ribosomal protein L13a (RPL13A), glyceraldehyde-3-phosphate dehydrogenase (GAPDH), and actin beta (ACTB), three reverse transcription controls (RTCs), three positive PCR controls (PPCs), and one genomic DNA control (GDC), making up to 96 assays. After normalization with RPL13A reference gene, gene expression levels were individually assessed by using the threshold cycle (Ct) values using RT^2 profiler PCR array data analysis software (Microsoft Excel-based program of SABiosciences, Mississauga, ON, Canada). It calculates: 1) ΔCt of each gene = Ct of gene of interest - average Ct of chosen reference genes 2) ΔΔCt for each gene across two groups; ΔΔCt = ΔCt (Pz-DHA ester or sorafenib) - ΔCt (control) & 3) fold-change for each gene from control group to Pz-DHA ester treated group as $2^{(-\Delta\Delta Ct)}$. RT^2 RNA QC PCR data showed no genomic DNA contamination (Ct <35 will indicate least GDC) or presence of impurities in RNA samples based on the Ct value of PPC (Ct should be 20±2 on each array) and showed no inhibition of reverse transcription based on the Ct values of RTC and PPC. Reproducibility was maintained by using three biological replicates from three individual experiments.

Statistical analyses

EC_{50} values were calculated using Graphpad Prism 6 software (GraphPad Software Inc., San Diego CA, USA). Statistical analysis was performed using Statistical Analysis System (SAS, Version 9.2). One-way ANOVA with Tukey's post hoc comparisons at P<0.001 was used for statistical comparisons. All data are presented as a mean value with its standard deviation indicated (Mean ± SD).

Results

Antiproliferative effect of fatty acid esters of phloridzin in various cancer and normal cells

In the present study, the potential cytotoxic effects of fatty acid esters of phloridzin, phloridzin, free fatty acids and phloretin as well as standard commercial cancer drugs were investigated on human hepatocarcinoma (HepG2), breast adenocarcinoma (MDA-MB-231) and acute monocytic leukemia (THP-1) cell lines, primary normal human hepatocytes and rat hepatocytes by using MTS assay. The assay showed that fatty acid esters of phloridzin kills HepG2, MDA-MB-231 and THP-1 cells to a similar extent and in a dose- (Figure 1) and time-dependent manner (Table 1). After 24 h incubation, in HepG2 cells, antiproliferation EC_{50} for stearic acid, oleic acid, linoleic acid, α-linolenic acid, DHA and EPA esters of phloridzin were 37.8, 31.5, 29.2, 53.1, 51.9 and 26.8 μM respectively. EC_{50} were 35.2, 37.9, 32.3, 63.8, 55.5, and 26.5 μM in MDA-MB-231 cells. EC_{50} values of these esters on THP-1 cells were 40.7, 2.1, 6.2, 35.7, 27.3, and 14.8 μM. Although fatty acid esters of phloridzin showed high potency as antiproliferative agent, none of the parent molecule, phloridzin and individual fatty acids showed any effect on cell viability (EC_{50}>100 μM) of HepG2, MDA-MB-231 or THP-1 cells. Interestingly, aglycone phloretin showed a significant antiproliferative effect (EC_{50} 39.6 μM) in THP-1 cells (Table 1).

To evaluate the specificity of fatty acid esters of phloridzin to cancer cells, drug effect on cell viability in normal hepatocytes was quantified by cytotoxicity assay in both normal human (HP-F) and rat (RTCP10) hepatocytes. HP-F cells were treated with 100 μM and lower concentrations of all fatty acid esters of phloridzin, phloridzin, fatty acid, sorafenib and phloretin for 24 h (Table 1). Fatty acid esters of phloridzin did not affect the viability of normal human hepatocytes with EC_{50}>100 μM and are more specific to cancer cell lines (Table 1, Figure 1). In the 100 μM treatment of fatty acid esters of phloridzin for 24 h, fatty acid esters of phloridzin showed least toxicity (>90% viability) in rat hepatocytes also (Figure 1). The most promising and most selective cytotoxic activities were detected in Pz-DHA and Pz-EPA esters. Fatty acid esters of phloridzin except Pz-stearic acid (about 50% viability) also showed much less activity in inhibiting cell viability (>80% viability) of rat hepatocytes than that of cancer cell lines. These results suggest that fatty acid esters of phloridzin may have moderate to minimal side effects. The most promising and most selective cytotoxic activities were detected with Pz-DHA ester. The EC_{50} (μM) and SI values of Pz-DHA in HepG2, MDA-MB-231, THP-1 were 51.9 (SI = 11.2), 55.5 (SI = 10.5), and 27.3 (SI = 21.38), respectively

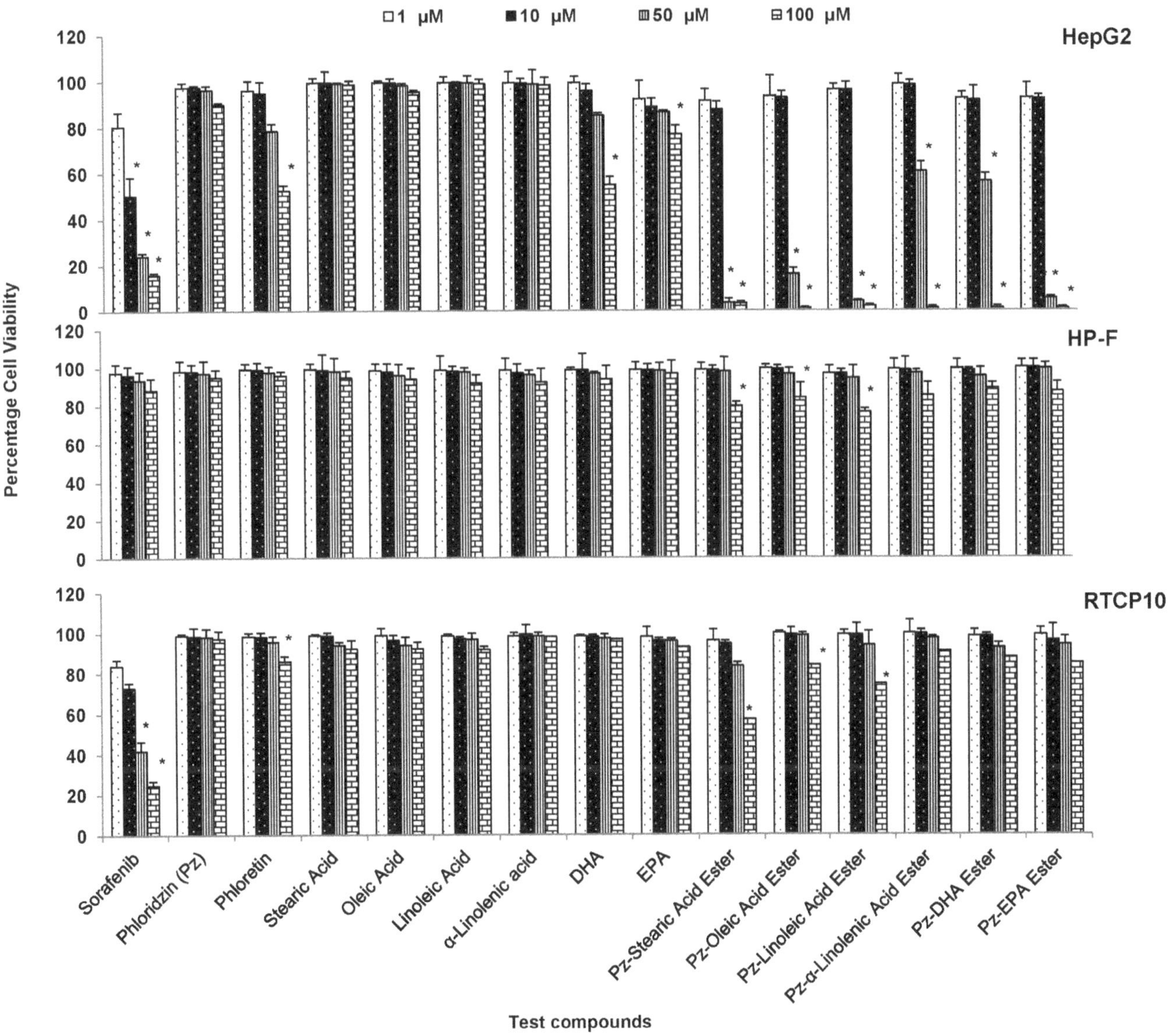

Figure 1. Antiproliferative effect of fatty acid esters of phloridzin on HepG2 and normal cells. Hepatic carcinoma (HepG2) cells and normal human hepatocytes (HP-F) and rat hepatocytes (RTCP10) cells were exposed to test compounds at 1, 10, 50, 100 μM for 24 h. The cell viability was determined using MTS assay. The data presented as the percentage viability relative to vehicle only treated control group. Data are presented as the mean ± SD (n = 3) are representative of at least three separate independent experiments. *P<0.05 significantly different from the vehicle only control group (Tukey HSD, P<0.01).

Table 1. $EC_{50} \pm$ SD values of tested compounds in three human cancer cell lines and a normal cells (HP-F).

		EC_{50} (μM)															
		HepG2					MDA-MB-231					THP-1					HP-F
		3 h	6 h	12 h	18 h	24 h	3 h	6 h	12 h	18 h	24 h	3 h	6 h	12 h	18 h	24 h	24 h
Phloridzin (Pz) Esters	**Pz-Oleic acid ester**	64.6±5.1	60.9±4.9	54.2±4.8	48.5±4.0	37.8±3.1 (4.7)[z]	63.4±5.8	57.4±3.9	50.5±4.1	37.4±2.9	35.2±2.3 (5.1)	95.8±8.1	61.8±5.1	53.8±4.9	41.7±3.8	40.7±2.9 (4.4)	>100
	Pz-Stearic acid ester	53.3±4.5	48.2±3.9	37.6±1.8	34.8±2.0	31.5±2.1 (4.2)	64.8±5.4	61.1±5.5	57.4±4.6	55.7±4.8	37.9±2.1 (3.5)	39.2±3.4	32.3±1.8	23.9±1.7	22.9±1.8	2.1±0.5 (64)	>100
	Pz-Linoleic acid ester	43.3±2.9	40.5±3.1	35.4±2.2	30.8±2.7	29.2±1.9 (4.5)	41.6±2.9	38.8±2.0	38.1±2.5	36.1±2.6	32.3±1.9 (4.1)	36.6±2.1	18.7±1.1	14.7±0.9	13.1±0.9	6.2±0.4 (21.2)	>100
	Pz-α-Linolenic acid ester	76.5±6.0	66.3±5.2	60.5±4.8	55.7±4.1	53.1±3.9 (3.14)	89.9±6.8	83.8±6.7	80.5±7.1	66.1±5.4	63.8±5.1 (3.1)	88.7±6.7	72.4±6.0	41.3±2.8	37.9±2.1	35.7±1.7 (4.67)	>100
	Pz-DHA ester	76.9±5.8	64.4±5.9	56.2±4.9	54.2±3.9	51.9±3.8 (11.2)	131.5±9.9	83.7±7.5	70.2±6.1	62.6±5.1	55.5±4.5 (10.5)	65.8±5.2	49.5±3.8	42.7±3.0	35.8±2.8	27.3±1.2 (21.3)	>100
	Pz-EPA ester	39.4±2.8	37.8±1.9	36.0±2.1	33.1±2.4	26.8±1.8 (7.4)	37.9±2.2	33.6±1.8	32.6±1.8	31.5±2.3	26.5±1.1 (7.5)	27.9±1.5	19.9±1.1	17.0±0.6	15.8±0.8	14.8±0.6 (21.38)	>100
Parent Compounds	**Phloridzin**	>100	>100	>100	>100	>100	>100	>100	>100	>100	>100	>100	>100	>100	>100	>100	>100
	Oleic acid	>100	>100	>100	>100	>100	>100	>100	>100	>100	>100	>100	>100	>100	>100	>100	>100
	Stearic acid	>100	>100	>100	>100	>100	>100	>100	>100	>100	>100	>100	>100	>100	>100	>100	>100
	Linoleic acid	>100	>100	>100	>100	>100	>100	>100	>100	>100	>100	>100	>100	>100	>100	>100	>100
	α-Linolenic acid	>100	>100	>100	>100	>100	>100	>100	>100	>100	>100	>100	>100	>100	>100	>100	>100
	DHA	>100	>100	>100	>100	>100	>100	>100	>100	>100	>100	>100	>100	>100	>100	>100	>100
	EPA	>100	>100	>100	>100	>100	>100	>100	>100	>100	>100	>100	>100	>100	>100	>100	>100
Drugs	**Sorafenib**	67.5±5.2	46.7±3.5	17.3±0.8	13.4±0.9	10.7±0.5											>100
	Doxorubicin						>100	>100	9.6±0.2	5.9±0.3	4.1±0.1						
	Daunorubicin											48.1±2.8	35.2±2.9	12.6±0.8	1.4±0.2	0.02±0.01	
Aglycone of Phloridzin	**Phloretin**	>100	>100	>100	>100	97.20	>100	>100	>100	>100	>100	73.5±5.2	64.1±5.4	60.1±4.2	56.9±3.0	39.6±1.7	

[z] Numbers in the parenthesis are SI values, whereas SI = EC_{50} of HP-F cells/EC_{50} on solid cancer cells.

(Table 1). DHA is a common dietary omega-3 fatty acid and it also possesses antiproliferative properties [20]. Therefore, Pz-DHA ester was selected for gene expression study using human drug target RT^2-PCR array as it showed the strongest cytotoxic effect on cancer cells and was the least toxic on normal cells compared to other fatty acid esters of phloridzin.

HepG2 cells were chosen as the representative cell line for the remainder of this investigation because these liver cancer cells were susceptible to killing by fatty acid esters of phloridzin and it has functionally active p53 protein, competent DNA-repair system, active enzymes for phase-I and -II metabolism which may give a high predictivity for in vivo genotoxicity.

Increase of LDH Leakage by fatty acid esters of phloridzin

Fatty acid esters of phloridzin were evaluated for cytotoxic effects in HepG2 cells (100 μM) using LDH release assay. Incubating the cells with 100 μM of all six fatty esters of phloridzin resulted in significant increase in LDH activity ($P < 0.001$) at 6 h compared to sorafenib, phloridzin and phloretin. Maximum LDH release was showed by pz-EPA ester (82.7±1.5%) and least by phloretin (7.9±0.5%) compared to the positive control (maximum release by 1% Triton-10X treated cells and incubated for 30 min). These results are agreeable with the previous results of MTS cell viability assay (Figure 2).

Morphological evaluation of apoptosis

Apoptotic morphological changes of cells observed under inverted phase contrast microscope. Treatments with fatty acid esters of phloridzin and sorafenib (100 μM for 24 h) showed the distorted membrane structure, shrinkage of the cells and the nucleus as well as condensation of nuclear chromatin into sharply delineated masses. The cell detaches from the plate and its outlines become convoluted and form extensions. These cells showed morphological changes which are characteristic to apoptosis. Phloridzin treated cells have shown no effect and morphology was similar to the control cells (Figure 3).

Apoptosis assessment using Annexin V/7-AAD staining assay

Fluorescence imaging was conducted to visually differentiate between apoptosis induced and necrotic cell death. After incubation of HepG2 cells with 100 μM of fatty acid esters of phloridzin for 24 h, the number of cells remaining as an adherent monolayer was greatly decreased compared to the control cells. In addition, floating cells showed morphological changes, with characteristics similar to apoptosis or necrosis. We co-incubated cells with Annexin V Enzogold (enhanced cyanine), an early marker of phosphatidylserine externalization at the cell membrane and red emitting dye 7-AAD, marker of late apoptosis or necrosis. Upon exposure to fatty acid esters of phloridzin most of the HepG2 cells treated with fluorescent dyes stained green for Annexin V denoting apoptosis and less number of cells stained red for 7-AAD indicating late apoptosis or necrosis. DMSO (<0.5%) control, phloridzin and phloretin treated cells showed less colour indicate less apoptotic death of cells. The results suggested that fatty acid esters of phloridzin induced marked apoptotic and less necrotic morphology in HepG2 cells (Figure 4).

Induction of internucleosomal DNA fragmentation

Internucleosomal DNA fragmentation is a biochemical hallmark of apoptotic cell death. From the agarose gel, DNA samples

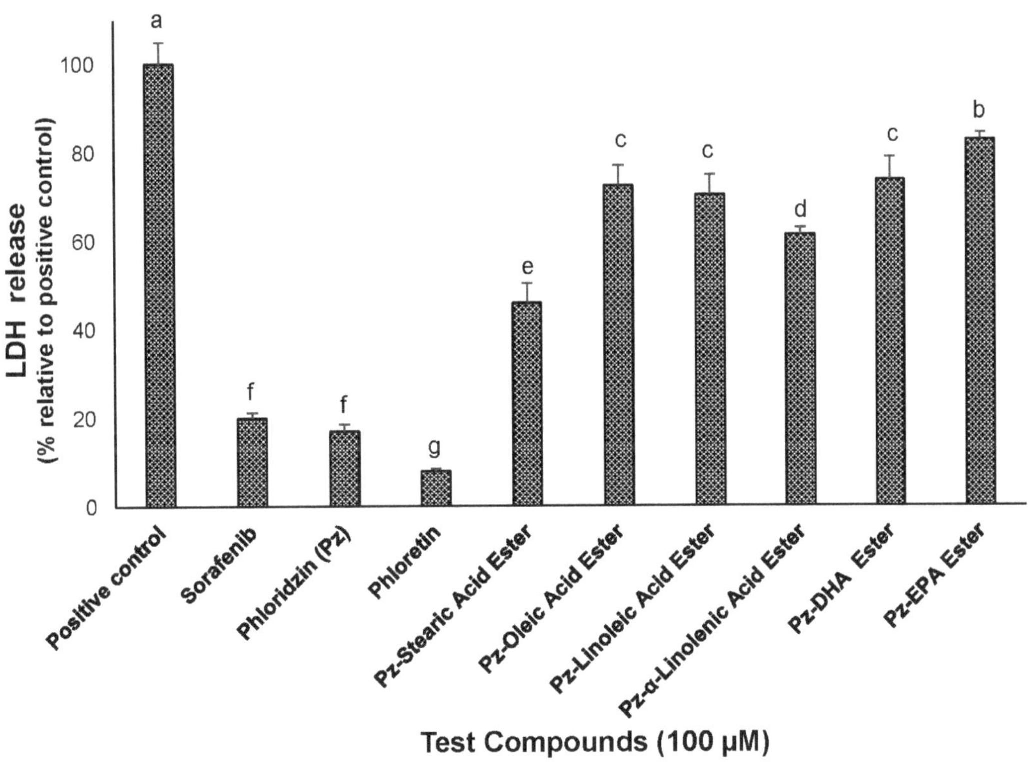

Figure 2. Percentage LDH release relative to control in HepG2 cells. The cells were incubated with 100 μM of fatty acid esters of phloridzin (Pz) in comparison with parent compounds phloridzin, phloretin (aglycone), or liver cancer drug sorafenib for 24 h. Data are presented as the mean ± SD (n = 3) are representative of at least three separate independent experiments. Different letters represent significantly different mean values from other treatments (Tukey HSD, $P < 0.01$).

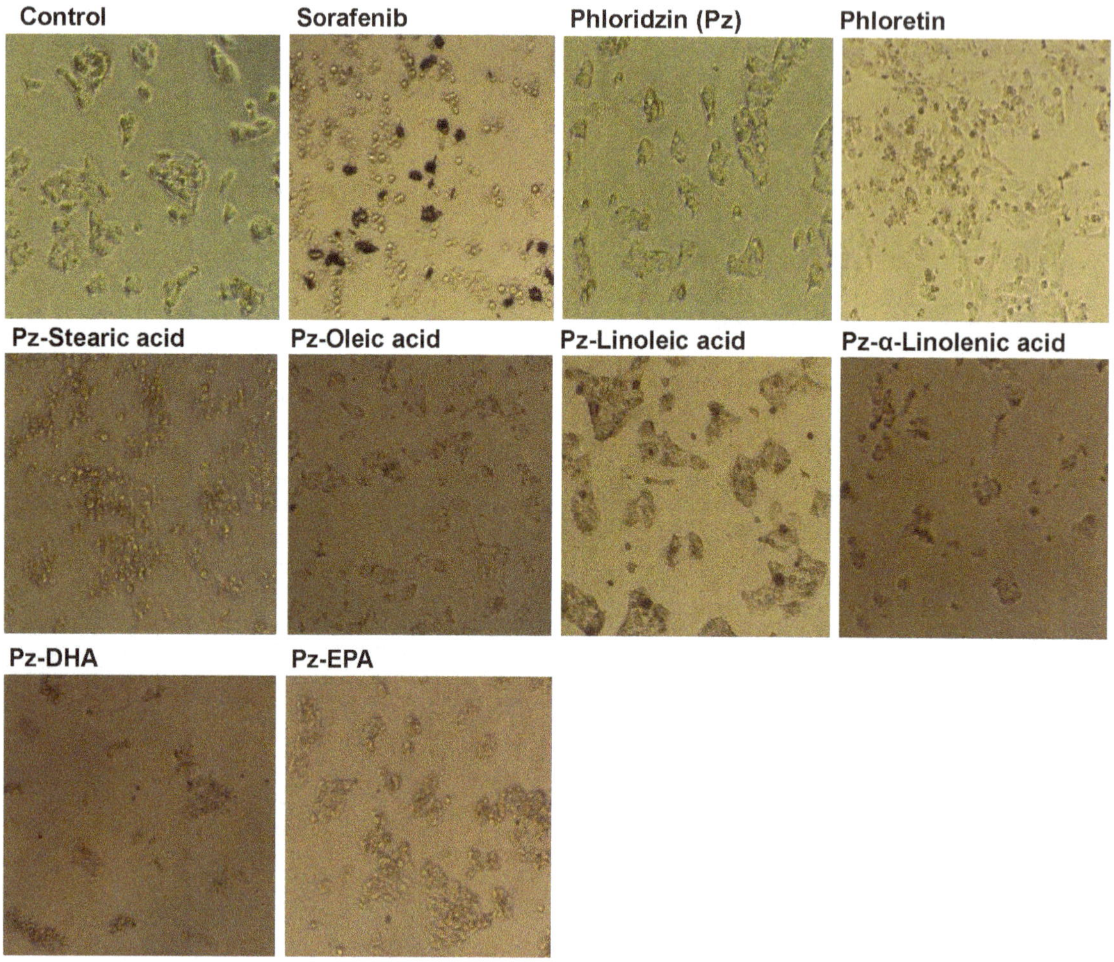

Figure 3. Inverted phase contrast microscopy images of HepG2 cells. The cells were cultured (2×10^4 cells/100 μL) in 96 well plate after incubation with 100 μM of fatty acid esters of phloridzin (Pz) in comparison with parent compounds phloridzin, phloretin (aglycone) or liver cancer drug sorafenib for 24 h. Shown are representative images of three independent experiments.

from the fatty acid esters of phloridzin or sorafenib (100 μM) treated HepG2 cells exhibited intact genomic DNA and clear DNA ladders (Figure 5: Lane 1–7). Treatments with DMSO (< 0.5%) control (C) or free fatty acids of respective esters (Lane 8 to 13) phloridzin (Lane 14) or phloretin (Lane 15) showed only intact genomic DNA and do not marked any DNA laddering or even smearing effect. The pattern of laddering of DNA from fatty acid esters of phloridzin or sorafenib treated cells are characteristic that commonly associated with apoptotic process, in which the DNA is cleaved into fragments of 180–200 base pairs (bp) by the endogenous endonucleases [21] (Figure 5).

Caspases 3 activation

Programmed cell death is associated with induction of caspases which finally lead to the disruption of cellular structures. Incubation of HepG2 cells with fatty esters of phloridzin or sorafenib for 24 h induced a significant ($P<0.001$) increase in caspase 3 activity compared to DMSO treated control at 24 h. These findings emonstrated that the esters induces caspase 3 activation that is required for execution of apoptotic cell death. Phloridzin and phloretin showed enhanced caspase 3 activity but significantly ($P<0.001$) lower than fatty acid esters of phloridzin or the drug (Figure 6).

Fatty acid esters of phloridzin decrease mitochondrial membrane potential and ATP level

We examined whether mitochondrial events were associated with apoptosis induction by fatty acid esters of phloridzin treated cancer cells. Mitochondrial membrane potential, a reliable indicator of mitochondrial dependent apoptosis, is quantified by applying the fluorescent dye JC-1. In the presence of low mitochondrial membrane potential, the dye forms JC-1 monomers. We observed significant ($P<0.05$) reduction in mitochondrial membrane potential in HepG2 cells treated with fatty acid esters of phloridzin, sorafenib and phloretin compared to control and parent compounds (Figure 7). Treatment of HepG2 cells for 24 h with 100 μM fatty acid esters of phloridzin was associated with an >95% decrease in ATP levels (Figure 8). Therefore, we speculate that cellular apoptosis induced by fatty acid esters of phloridzin is a mitochondrial dependent mechanism.

Altered cell cycle phase distributions

As summarized in Figure 9, treatment of HepG2 cells with 100 μM of fatty acid esters of phloridzin resulted in a significantly higher number of cells in the G_0/G_1 phase (52% to 60%) compared with control (48%). Potency of Pz-oleic acid, Pz-α-linolenic acid, Pz-DHA and Pz-EPA esters to induce G_0/G_1 phase

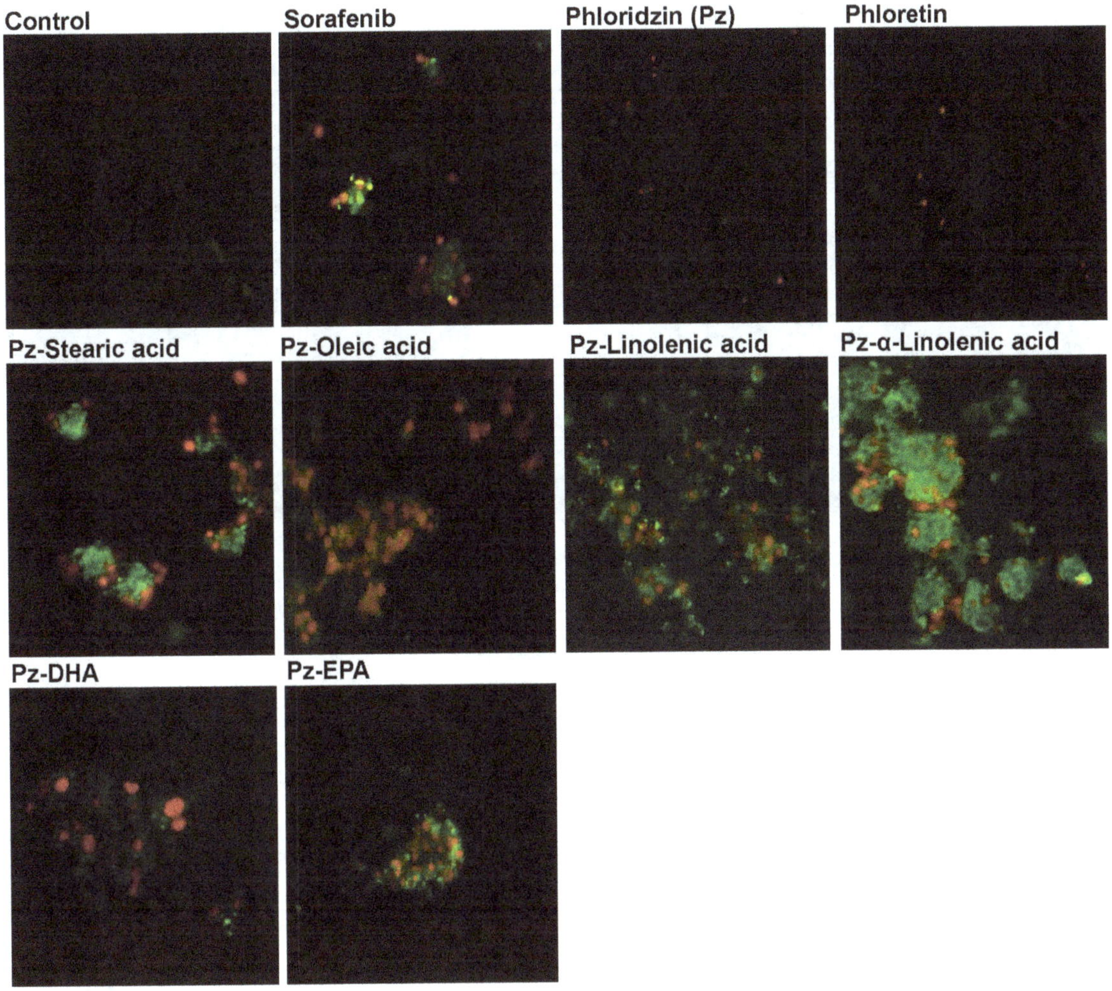

Figure 4. Fluorescent microscopic analysis of apoptotic HepG-2 cells stained with Annexin V-FITC and 7-AAD. The cells were cultures (1×10^5 cells) in chambered slides and incubated with 100 μM of fatty acid esters of phloridzin (Pz) in comparison with parent compounds phloridzin or phloretin (aglycone) or liver cancer drug sorafenib. Green and red color indicates early and late apoptotic cells, respectively. Shown are representative images of three independent experiments.

arrest was similar to prescribed commercial drug sorafenib. As, in each case, there was a concomitant reduction in the number of cells in the S and G_2/M phases. This experiment suggests that fatty acid esters of phloridzin induce G_0/G_1 phase cell cycle arrest in HepG2 cells (Figure 9).

Catalytic inhibition of human DNA Topoisomerase II α

Fatty acid esters of phloridzin, phloridzin, sorafenib as well as phloretin inhibited catalytic activity of human DNA topo IIα. Effect of new compounds on the catalytic activity of DNA topo IIα was evaluated by supercoiled pHOT DNA. As seen in Figure 10, all the test compounds at 100 μM inhibited pHOT DNA relaxation and most of the pHOT DNA remained in supercoiled state. VP-16, an interfacial poison showed linear band and less potent than catalytic inhibition induced by phloridzin fatty acid esters. Inhibition of topo IIα is a good target for anticancer drugs (Figure 10).

Molecular mechanisms of antiproliferative effect of Pz-DHA ester

Molecular pathogenesis of HCC is complex that involves genetic and epigenetic alterations and altered molecular pathways. Based on the least toxicity on normal hepatocytes and high selectivity on cancerous cells, Pz-DHA ester was used for further investigation involving gene expression related to cell growth. According to gene expression studies in HCC, genes responsible for cell proliferation and survival are activation of EGFR signalling, IGF signalling, Ras/MAPK signalling or AKT/mTOR signalling [22]. Evasion of apoptosis due to deregulation of intrinsic or extrinsic pathway is one of the hallmark of liver cancer [22]. To reveal possible molecular mechanisms of the antiproliferative effect of Pz-DHA ester to HepG2 cells, human cancer drug targets RT^2 profiler PCR array was used. This system profiles the expression of 84 actively sought targets for anticancer therapeutics and drug development (http://www.sabiosciences.com/rt_pcr_product/HTML/PAHS-507Z.html). The relative expression of each gene in any two samples (experimental and control) are summarized in the Table 2 revealing genes up- and down-regulated in the experimental sample. In this study, comparing the genes with more than two-fold expression change between Pz-DHA ester treated HepG2 cells with the vehicle treated control, it has shown that the expression of 41 genes was down-regulated and 8 genes up-regulated while the expression of 35 genes were unaffected. Pz-DHA ester treatment down-regulated the expression of some cancer related genes which are

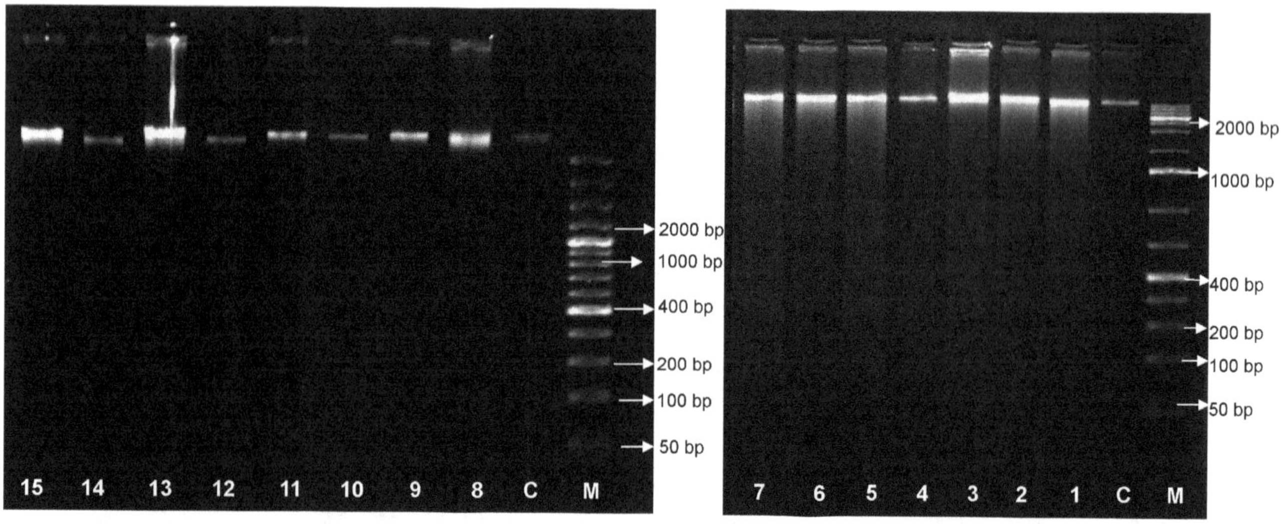

Figure 5. DNA fragmentation of HepG2 cells. DNA were isolated after incubation of HepG2 cells with 100 μM of fatty acid esters of phloridzin (Pz) in comparison with parent compounds phloridzin, free fatty acids, phloretin (aglycone) or liver cancer drug sorafenib for 24 h. Lane M: molecular-weight marker, lane C: control, lane 1–6: stearic acid ester of Pz, oleic acid ester of Pz, linoleic acid ester of Pz, α-linolenic acid ester of Pz, DHA ester of Pz and EPA ester of Pz, lane 7: sorafenib, lane 8–13: stearic acid, oleic acid, linoleic acid, α-linolenic acid, DHA and EPA, lane 14: phloridzin, and lane 15: phloretin. Shown are representative gel images of three independent experiments.

represented as folds in brackets: As shown in Table 2, Pz-DHA ester treatment significantly down regulated ($P<0.05$) the expression of most of cancer promoting genes which are represented as folds in brackets:

1. Apoptosis-related genes: Pz-DHA ester reduced the expression of pro-survival gene BCL2 (−2.8) whereas no significant change was shown on sorafenib treatment. Transcriptional

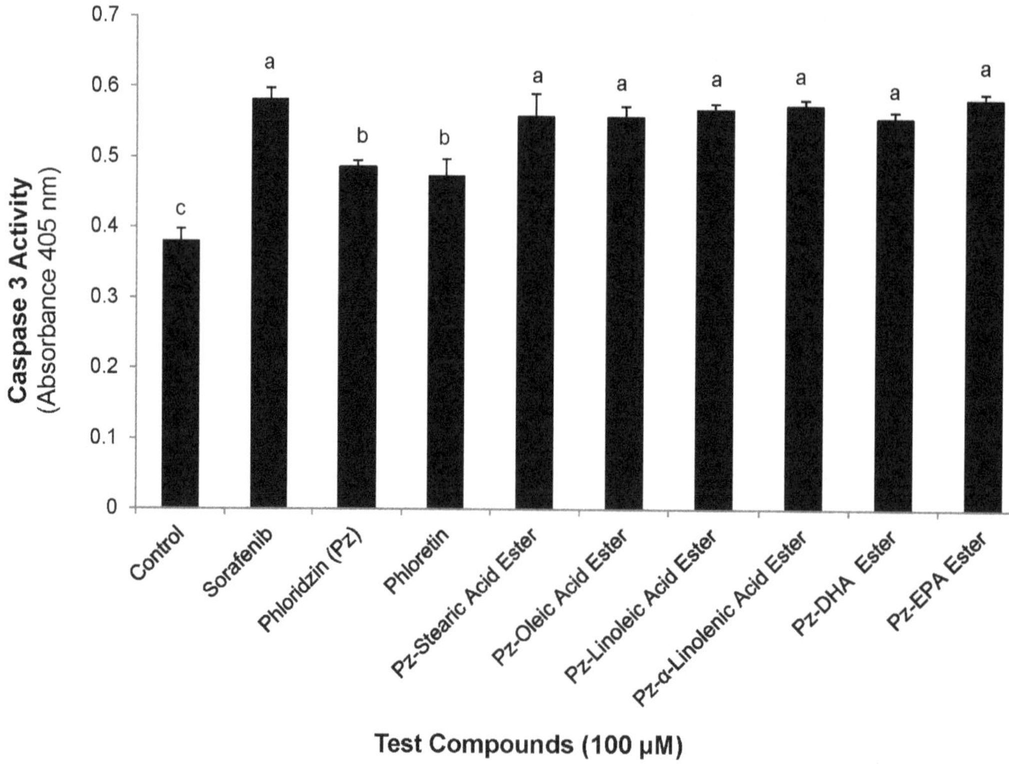

Figure 6. Caspase 3 activity of HepG2 cells. The cells were incubated with 100 μM of fatty acid esters of phloridzin (Pz) in comparison with parent compounds phloridzin, phloretin (aglycone) or standard drug sorafenib for 24 h. Data are presented as the mean ± SD (n = 3) are representative of at least three separate independent experiments. Different letters represent significantly different mean values from other treatments (Tukey HSD, $P<0.01$).

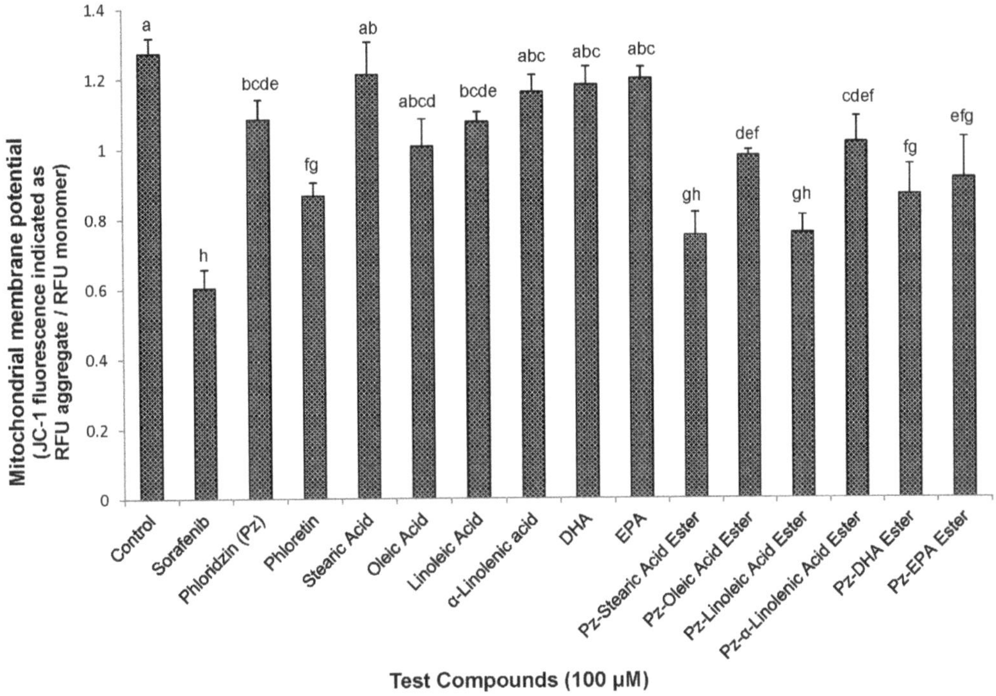

Figure 7. Mitochondrial membrane potential (Δψm) of HepG2 cells measured by JC-1 fluorescence. HepG2 cells were treated with 100 μM of fatty acid esters of phloridzin (Pz) in comparison with parent compounds phloridzin, individual fatty acids, phloretin (aglycone) or liver cancer drug sorafenib for 24 h. The fluorescence of JC-1 monomers was measured at em 535 nm and aggregates at em 590 nm. Data are presented as the mean ± SD (n = 3) are representative of at least three separate independent experiments. Different letters represent significantly different mean values from other treatments (Tukey HSD, P<0.01).

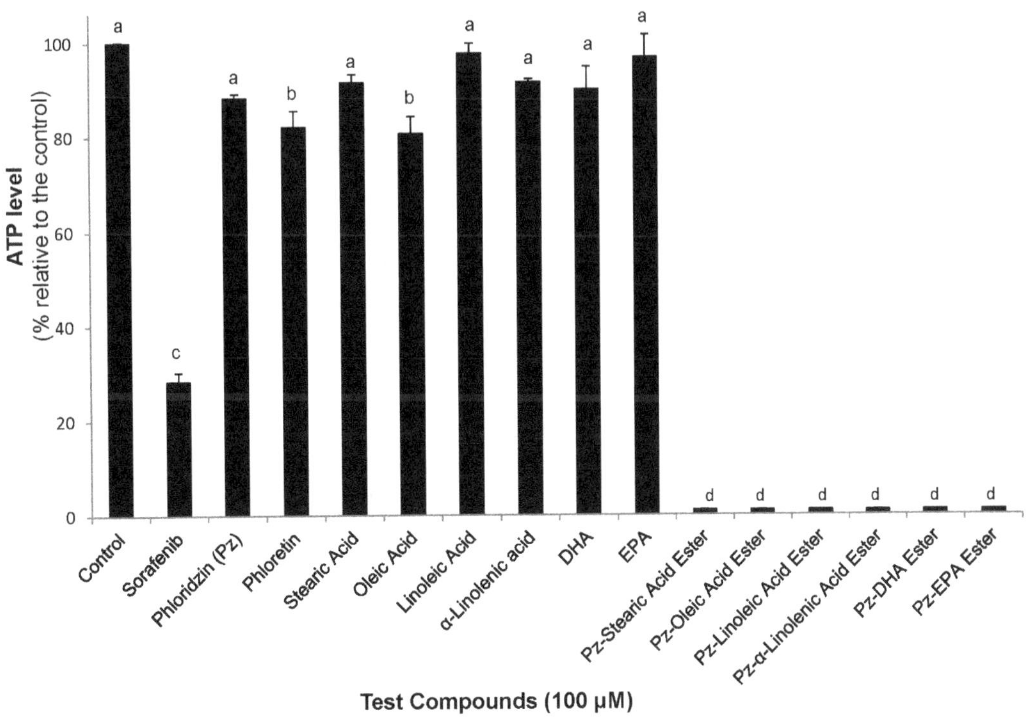

Figure 8. Cellular ATP level in HepG2 cells. The cells were treated with 100 μM of fatty acid esters of phloridzin (Pz) in comparison with parent compounds phloridzin, free fatty acids, phloretin (aglycone) or liver cancer drug sorafenib for 24 h. Cellular ATP content in treated cells is expressed as percentage compared to ATP levels in untreated controls. Data are presented as the mean ± SD (n = 3) are representative of at least three separate independent experiments. Different letters represent significantly different mean values from other treatments (Tukey HSD, P<0.01).

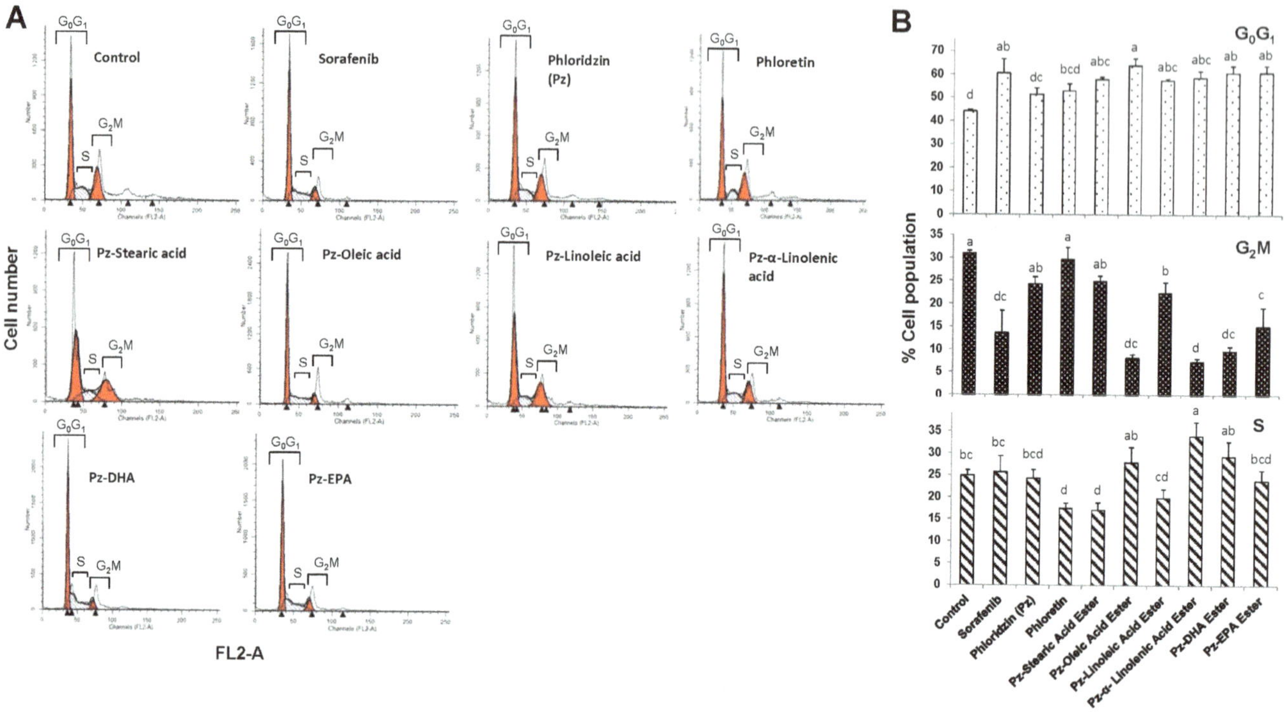

Figure 9. Evaluation of cell cycle in HepG2 cells using the propidium iodide assay. HepG2 cells were treated with 100 μM of fatty acid esters of phloridzin (Pz), pz or phloretin or sorafneib for 24 h, and then cell cycle profile was determined using flow cytometry after staining with PI/ RNase. Representative FACS histograms of nuclear DNA content are shown (A). The DNA content peaks indicating cells in the G_0G_1, S, or G_2/M phase of the cell cycle are marked. The bar chart show the changes in percentages (mean ± SD) of cells in G_0/G_1, S-phase, and G_2/M after treatment (B). Data are presented as the mean ± SD (n = 3) are representative of three separate independent experiments. Different letters represent significantly different mean values from other treatments (Tukey HSD, P<0.01).

activation of NF-κB1 was reduced by Pz-DHA ester (−4.3) or sorafenib (−2.5) treatment.

2. Growth factor receptors and its downstream signalling molecules: Pz-DHA ester reduced the expression of growth factors and receptor genes including IGF1R (−4.2), IGF2 (−2.3), PDGFRB (−16.8), EGFR (−8.9), ERBB2 (−5.7), ERBB3 (−6.1), KDR (−2.8), PDGFRA (−2.8). Pz-DHA esters inhibited PI3K/ AKT/mTOR pathway with reduced expression of AKT1 (−6.1) and AKT2 (−2.8) and its effector GRB2 (−8.6). In parallel, mTOR (−3.6), PIK3C2A (−2.2), IRF5 (−2.3) and TP53 (−7.4) were also down regulated in Pz-DHA treated cells. Inactivation of KRAS (−4.0) on treatment with Pz-DHA ester demonstrated the significant down regulated expression of Ras/MAPK pathway in HepG2 cells. IGFIR (−2.1), IGF2 (−2.8), mTOR (−2.1), PDGFRB (−2.5) and NRAS (−2.4) were down regulated in sorafenib treated HepG2 cells.

3. Cell Cycle: Pz-DHA ester down regulated CDK2 (−2.0) CDK9 (−2.1), telomerase TERT (−5.6), Topoisomerases TOP2A (−2.7) and TOP2B (−2.3) and PARP1 (−5.4). Treatment with sorafenib reduced the expression of MDM4 (−2.3), TOP2B (−2.2) and PARP1 (−3.0) in HepG2 cells.

4. Protein kinases: Overexpression of protein kinases plays a major role in development and progression of HCC. AURKB (−2.0), PLK1 (−2.9), PRKCA (−8.1), PRKCD (−2.1) and PRKCE (−5.6) were down regulated on Pz-DHA ester treatment.

5. Histone deacetylases: HDAC1 (−2.6), HDAC11 (−20.1), HDAC4 (−4.1), HDAC6 (−5.4) and HDAC7 (−6.0) were down regulated by Pz-DHA ester.

The gene significantly up regulated in expression on Pz-DHA ester and sorafenib treatment is FLT1 (16.5).

Discussion

The present work demonstrated the cytotoxicity and selectivity of novel fatty acid esters of phloridzin towards three human cancer cells, hepatocellular carcinoma, breast cancer and acute monocytes leukemia as compared to normal hepatocytes. The cytotoxic effect was drawn on the basis of lower EC_{50} values (<40 μM) and higher SI values (>3) that were obtained for the fatty acid esters of phloridzin. Based on literature to date [16] and present study, phloridzin have no inhibitory effect on cancer cells where as its aglycone, phloretin demonstrated anticancer property. This is agreeable with previous studies that phloretin augmented TRAIL-induced apoptosis and cytotoxicity in prostate cancer cells [15]. To our knowledge, this is the first study that has examined and demonstrated that fatty acid esters of phloridzin induce apoptosis in cancer cells. Fatty acid esters of phloridzin were synthesized in our laboratory by regioselective enzymatic acylation of phloridzin with six different long chain saturated, mono- and poly-unsaturated fatty acids. This study revealed that fatty acid esters of phloridzin were distinctly more potent inhibitors of the growth of solid tumors such as HCC, breast adenocarcinoma, and leukemia than their corresponding parent molecules, phloridzin and the six free fatty acids. Our results are in accordance with previous observations that chemically synthesized polyphenol, acetyl resveratrol analogues can inhibit growth of DU-145 human prostate cancer cells higher than that of resveratrol [23].

The antiproliferative effect suggests that the esterification of 6′-OH of glucose moiety of phloridzin with acyl side chains changed the bioactivity of phloridzin. This conformational change could lead to important modifications in the lipophilicity of the phloridzin molecule that modifies cellular permeability, uptake

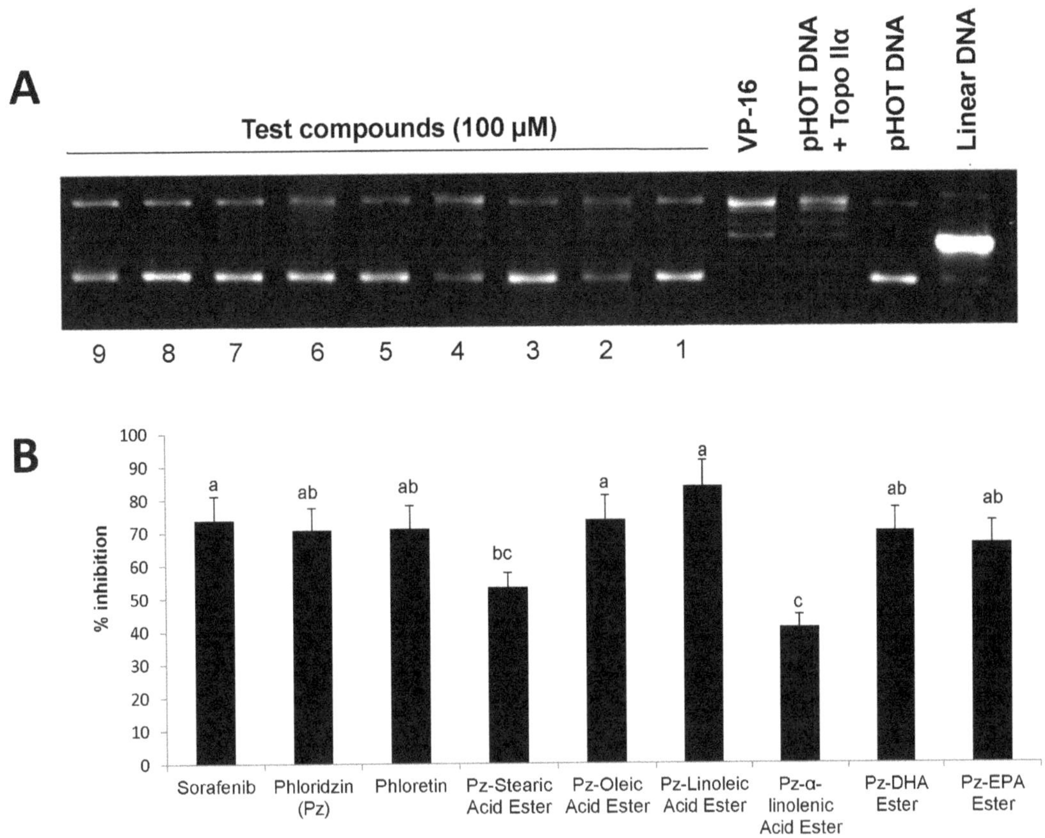

Figure 10. Activity of human topoisomerase II of HepG2 cells. The cells were incubated with 100 μM of fatty acid esters of phloridzin (Pz) in comparison with parent compounds phloridzin, phloretin (aglycone) or sorafenib for 24 h. A. Lanes 1 Pz-oleic acid, lane 2: Pz-stearic acid, lane 3: Pz-linoleic acid, lane 4: Pz-α-linolenic acid, lane 5: Pz-DHA, lane 6: Pz-EPA, lane 7: phloridzin, lane 8: sorafenib, and lane 9: phloretin. The data are representative of three separate, independent experiments. B. Percentage inhibition.

and/or interactions with membrane bound receptors. Synthetic derivatives of phloridzin formed by modification of sugar hydroxyl groups by esterification were shown to increase lipophilicity and antioxidant properties [24]. Furthermore, other studies have showed that the acetylation can enhance biological activities and bioavailability of epigallocatechin-3-gallate [25]. To demonstrate that acylation increases the bioavailability of fatty acid esters of phloridzin, in vivo studies need to be conducted to understand the stability and half-life of the novel esters in the intestine and plasma. Traditionally, medical oncologists have favoured intravenous drug therapy to treat most cancer patients. In an effort to overcome the obstacle of bioavailability, intravenous delivery of fatty acid esters of phloridzin is a major consideration that possibly yields greater bioavailability and therapeutic results than that of oral administration.

Our in vitro results demonstrated that fatty acid esters of phloridzin inhibit the growth of tumorigenic liver cells through the induction of apoptosis which are marked by induction of G_0/G_1 arrest, activation of caspase 3 that resulted in subsequent DNA fragmentation. Fatty acid esters of phloridzin treatment led to a loss of $\Delta\psi m$, suggesting that these compounds induce apoptosis, at least in part, through the mitochondrial pathway. Evidence can be found in literature on proapoptotic properties of synthetic analogues of polyphenols on cancer cells [26]. Chemotherapeutic agents that supress the proliferation of malignant cells by inducing apoptosis postulate a mechanism of their chemopreventive action [27]. Sorafenib has been reported to induce apoptosis and tumour necrosis in HCC [28]. Based upon previous studies, inhibition of topo IIα is a good target for anticancer drug in HCC [29,30]. After topo IIα inhibition, apoptosis is the most efficient death pathway in human tumorigenic cells [31,32]. In a cell-free screening experiment in this study, fatty acid esters of phloridzin, sorafenib, phloretin or phloridzin stopped the formation of cleavage complex and acted as catalytic inhibitor of topo IIα. Moreover, TOP2A transcriptional inhibition on Pz-DHA treatment correlates positively with catalytic inhibition of topo IIα in in vitro study. Phloretin was reported to inhibit DNA topo IIα unknotting activity and act as catalytic inhibitor of topo IIα enzyme [33].

Among the tested six novel esters, Pz-DHA ester had the greatest potential and efficacy as a chemotherapeutic agent. Thus, we have characterized the molecular mechanism and efficacy of Pz-DHA ester as a therapeutic for the treatment of HCC. Targeting with inhibitors directed at receptors and its different downstream signaling pathways is proven to be a more effective approach in anticancer therapy [34]. We found that programmed cell death results in part from the differential regulation of distinct signalling pathways in HepG2 cells evoked by the Pz-DHA ester. It is well known that growth factor receptors particularly epidermal growth factor receptor (EGFR) and insulin-like growth factor/IGF-1 receptor and their downstream signalling pathways activation is a key for diverse cellular processes such as cell proliferation, antiapoptosis and invasive behavior of tumor cells [35]. Activation of EGFR family induces a cascade of downstream signaling through PI3K/AKT/mTOR and mitogen-activated protein kinase (MAPK) resulting in cellular proliferation and

Table 2. Genes with altered expressions in HepG2 cells treated with DHA ester of phloridzin or sorafenib.

Mechanism	Gene	Fold change of gene expression relative to control [z]	
		Phloridzin-DHA	Sorafneib
Apoptosis	BCL2	−2.8	
PI-3 Kinases & Phosphatases	mTOR	−3.6	−2.1
	PIK3C2A	−2.2	
Growth Factors & Receptors	EGFR	−8.9	−2.0
	ERBB2	−5.7	
	ERBB3	−6.1	
	FLT1	+16.5	+5.5
	IGF1R	−4.2	−2.1
	IGF2	−2.3	−2.8
	KDR	−2.8	+2.0
	PDGFRA	−2.8	
	PDGFRB	−16.8	−2.5
Receptor Tyrosine Kinase Signaling	AKT1	−6.1	
	AKT2	−2.8	
	GRB2	−8.6	+2.0
Cell Cycle	CDK2	−2.0	
	CDK9	−2.1	
	MDM4	−2.1	−2.3
	TERT	−5.6	
Topoisomerases, Type II	TOP2A	−2.7	
	TOP2B	−2.3	−2.2
Transcription Factors	IRF5	−2.3	
	NF−κB	−4.3	−2.5
	TP53.	−7.4	
Protein Kinases	AURKB	−2.0	
	PLK1	−2.9	
	PRKCA	−8.1	
	PRKCD	−2.1	
	PRKCE	−5.6	
RAS Signaling	KRAS	−4.0	
	NRAS		−2.4
Histone Deacetylases	HDAC1	−2.6	
	HDAC11	−20.1	
	HDAC4	−4.1	
	HDAC6	−5.4	
	HDAC7	−6.0	
Poly ADP-Ribose Polymerases	PARP1	−5.4	−3.0

[z] Only the fold changes greater (+ or up-regulation) or lower (− or down-regulation) than 2-fold are presented.

differentiation [36]. Indeed, the fact that Pz-DHA ester treatment caused down regulation of the expression levels of EGFR, ERBB2, ERBB3, IGF and IGF-1R and its downstream signalling members PI3KC2A, AKT1, AKT2 and mTOR expression that had attributed to increased apoptotic cell death via caspase 3 signaling [36,37]. Down-regulation of Grb2 adapter and Ras/Raf/MEK/ERK pathway by Pz-DHA ester contribute to the profound effect on proliferative and apoptotic pathways in HepG2 cells [38,39]. In addition, transcription activity of nuclear factor kappa B (NF-κB) is known to be essential in cell proliferation and apoptosis via gene regulation. We found that Pz-DHA ester possessing the ability to suppress the expression of Protein Kinase C that down regulated NF-κB, PI3K/Akt/mTOR as well as MAPK pathway. In addition, our findings indicate that following Pz-DHA ester treatment down regulation of numerous gene expression via, cyclin-dependent kinases (CDK) such as CDK2 and CDK9 that contributes to cell cycle arrest in G_0G_1 phase that block entrance to other phase or mitosis in HepG2 cells [40]. The present study uncovered that Pz-DHA ester is very effective in inhibiting cancer associated enzyme telomerase along with cell cycle machinery.

Studies reported that inhibition of telomerase by polyphenols might provide a plausible explanation for up-regulation of procaspase expressions [41] and the antiproliferative effects of dietary polyphenols [42].

Up-regulation of antiapoptotic proteins is one of the mechanisms employed by cancer cells to evade apoptosis [43]. Targeting the anti-apoptotic Bcl-2 family of proteins can improve apoptosis and thus overcome drug resistance to cancer chemotherapy [44]. In this study, we demonstrated that Bcl-2 down-regulation by Pz-DHA ester mediates mitochondrial membrane damage and apoptosis. It is notable that Bcl-2 protein regulates NF-κB pathway activation that increases the antiapoptotic threshold of cells by suppressing the initiation of caspase-8 activation [45]. Based upon these results, down-regulation of NF-κB and decreased expression of Bcl-2 on Pz-DHA ester treatment induces intrinsic apoptosis and facilitate elimination of transformed cells during hepatocellular carcinogenesis.

Epigenetic deregulations, in particular histone acetylation, play important roles in the pathogenesis and progression of HCC. Pz-DHA ester inhibited the best characterized and probably biologically most relevant histone deacetylases which are commonly dysregulated in cancer [46]. Several polyphenols including EGCG and resveratrol, are known to possess potent HDAC inhibitory activity [47]. HepG2 cells express a wild-type p53 protein [48] and p53 protein over-expression in tumors with wild-type gene has been found in several other studies [48]. It is worthy to note that Pz-DHA ester down-regulated TP53 is unexpected in an antineoplastic treatment. This may be reflective of the complex cellular response to the various signalling pathways by the ester.

In conclusion, this study demonstrated that the chemotherapeutic potential of six saturated, mono- and poly-unsaturated fatty acid esters of phloridzin. In addition to the substantial inhibitory effect against liver cancer cells, Pz-DHA ester had relatively low toxicity towards normal cells. Low toxicity was evident in normal human and rat hepatocytes treated with Pz-DHA ester compared with standard drug sorafenib. Pz-DHA ester also has potential impact on multimolecular targets and pathways that led to apoptosis compared to sorafenib. The HepG2 cell growth inhibition mechanism of these novel compounds is related to inhibition of topo IIα and triggered DNA damage, cell cycle arrest and apoptosis. DHA ester of phloridzin has the greatest potential and efficacy as a chemotherapeutic agent. The anti-proliferative properties of the ester seem to be through a mechanism that down regulate key signalling pathways including PI3K/AKT/mTOR. However, additional studies on Western blot analysis to confirm RT-PCR findings, caspase pathways, expression profiling and in vivo experiments are required to confirm the anti-cancer activity of these novel fatty acid esters of phloridzin.

Acknowledgments

We are grateful to staff of the cellular and molecular digital imaging facility of the Faculty of Medicine, Dalhousie University for facilitating their services. We greatly appreciate critical review of this manuscript by Dr. Robin Robinson, Professor Emeritus of Faculty of Agriculture, Dalhousie University.

Author Contributions

Conceived and designed the experiments: HPVR SVGN. Performed the experiments: SVGN Z. Analyzed the data: SVGN HPVR. Contributed reagents/materials/analysis tools: HPVR. Contributed to the writing of the manuscript: SVGN HPVR Z. Principal investigator and lead scientist: HPVR.

References

1. Stagos D, Amoutzias GD, Matakos A, Spyrou A, Tsatsakis AM, et al. (2012) Chemoprevention of liver cancer by plant polyphenols. Food and Chemical Toxicology 50: 2155–2170.
2. Pocobelli G, Cook LS, Brant R, Lee SS (2008) Hepatocellular carcinoma incidence trends in Canada: analysis by birth cohort and period of diagnosis. Liver Int 28: 1272–1279.
3. Wild CP, Montesano R (2009) A model of interaction: aflatoxins and hepatitis viruses in liver cancer aetiology and prevention. Cancer Lett 286: 22–28.
4. Pang R, Tse E, Poon RT (2006) Molecular pathways in hepatocellular carcinoma. Cancer Lett 240: 157–169.
5. Horgan AM, Dawson LA, Swaminath A, Knox JJ (2012) Sorafenib and radiation therapy for the treatment of advanced hepatocellular carcinoma. J Gastrointest Cancer 43: 344–348.
6. Granado-Serrano AB, Martin MA, Bravo L, Goya L, Ramos S (2012) Quercetin modulates Nrf2 and glutathione-related defenses in HepG2 cells: Involvement of p38. Chem Biol Interact 195: 154–164.
7. Huang SP, Chen JC, Wu CC, Chen CT, Tang NY, et al. (2009) Capsaicin-induced apoptosis in human hepatoma HepG2 cells. Anticancer Res 29: 165–174.
8. Glauert HP, Calfee-Mason K, Stemm DN, Tharappel JC, Spear BT (2010) Dietary antioxidants in the prevention of hepatocarcinogenesis: a review. Mol Nutr Food Res 54: 875–896.
9. Ehrenkranz JR, Lewis NG, Kahn CR, Roth J (2005) Phlorizin: a review. Diabetes Metab Res Rev 21: 31–38.
10. Ridgway T, O'Reilly J, West G, Tucker G, Wiseman H (1997) Antioxidant action of novel derivatives of the apple-derived flavonoid phloridzin compared to oestrogen: relevance to potential cardioprotective action. Biochem Soc Trans 25: 106S.
11. Puel C, Quintin A, Mathey J, Obled C, Davicco MJ, et al. (2005) Prevention of bone loss by phloridzin, an apple polyphenol, in ovariectomized rats under inflammation conditions. Calcif Tissue Int 77: 311–318.
12. Boccia MM, Kopf SR, Baratti CM (1999) Phlorizin, a competitive inhibitor of glucose transport, facilitates memory storage in mice. Neurobiol Learn Mem 71: 104–112.
13. Jung E, Lee J, Huh S, Lee J, Kim YS, et al. (2009) Phloridzin-induced melanogenesis is mediated by the cAMP signaling pathway. Food Chem Toxicol 47: 2436–2440.
14. Rezk BM, Haenen GR, van der Vijgh WJ, Bast A (2002) The antioxidant activity of phloretin: the disclosure of a new antioxidant pharmacophore in flavonoids. Biochem Biophys Res Commun 295: 9–13.
15. Szliszka E, Czuba ZP, Mazur B, Paradysz A, Krol W (2010) Chalcones and dihydrochalcones augment TRAIL-mediated apoptosis in prostate cancer cells. Molecules 15: 5336–5353.
16. Miura T, Chiba M, Kasai K, Nozaka H, Nakamura T, et al. (2008) Apple procyanidins induce tumor cell apoptosis through mitochondrial pathway activation of caspase-3. Carcinogenesis 29: 585–593.
17. Ziaullah, Bhullar KS, Warnakulasuriya SN, Rupasinghe HP (2013) Biocatalytic synthesis, structural elucidation, antioxidant capacity and tyrosinase inhibition activity of long chain fatty acid acylated derivatives of phloridzin and isoquercitrin. Bioorg Med Chem 21: 684–692.
18. Danihelová M, Viskupičová J, Šturdík E (2012) Lipophilization of flavonoids for their food, therapeutic and cosmetic applications. Acta Chimica Slovaca. 59.
19. Riss TL, Moravec RA (2004) Use of multiple assay endpoints to investigate the effects of incubation time, dose of toxin, and plating density in cell-based cytotoxicity assays. Assay Drug Dev Technol 2: 51–62.
20. Schley PD, Jijon HB, Robinson LE, Field CJ (2005) Mechanisms of omega-3 fatty acid-induced growth inhibition in MDA-MB-231 human breast cancer cells. Breast Cancer Res Treat 92: 187–195.
21. Zhivotosky B, Orrenius S (2001) Assessment of apoptosis and necrosis by DNA fragmentation and morphological criteria. Curr Protoc Cell Biol Chapter 18: Unit 18.13.
22. Llovet JM, Bruix J (2008) Molecular targeted therapies in hepatocellular carcinoma. Hepatology 48: 1312–1327.
23. Cardile V, Lombardo L, Spatafora C, Tringali C (2005) Chemo-enzymatic synthesis and cell-growth inhibition activity of resveratrol analogues. Bioorg Chem 33: 22–33.
24. Baldisserotto A, Malisardi G, Scalambra E, Andreotti E, Romagnoli C, et al. (2012) Synthesis, antioxidant and antimicrobial activity of a new phloridzin derivative for dermo-cosmetic applications. Molecules 17: 13275–13289.
25. Lambert JD, Sang S, Hong J, Kwon SJ, Lee MJ, et al. (2006) Peracetylation as a means of enhancing in vitro bioactivity and bioavailability of epigallocatechin-3-gallate. Drug Metab Dispos 34: 2111–2116.
26. Chen D, Wan SB, Yang H, Yuan J, Chan TH, et al. (2011) EGCG, green tea polyphenols and their synthetic analogs and prodrugs for human cancer prevention and treatment. Adv Clin Chem 53: 155–177.

27. Brown EM, Gill CI, McDougall GJ, Stewart D (2012) Mechanisms underlying the anti-proliferative effects of berry components in in vitro models of colon cancer. Curr Pharm Biotechnol 13: 200–209.
28. Gu FM, Li QL, Gao Q, Jiang JH, Huang XY, et al. (2011) Sorafenib inhibits growth and metastasis of hepatocellular carcinoma by blocking STAT3. World J Gastroenterol 17: 3922–3932.
29. Topcu Z (2001) DNA topoisomerases as targets for anticancer drugs. J Clin Pharm Ther 26: 405–416.
30. Larsen AK, Escargueil AE, Skladanowski A (2003) From DNA damage to G2 arrest: the many roles of topoisomerase II. Prog Cell Cycle Res 5: 295–300.
31. Watanuki A, Ohwada S, Fukusato T, Makita F, Yamada T, et al. (2002) Prognostic significance of DNA topoisomerase IIalpha expression in human hepatocellular carcinoma. Anticancer Res 22: 1113–1119.
32. El-Awady RA, Ali MM, Saleh EM, Ghaleb FM (2008) Apoptosis is the most efficient death-pathway in tumor cells after topoisomerase II inhibition. Saudi Med J 29: 558–564.33.
33. Constantinou A, Mehta R, Runyan C, Rao K, Vaughan A, et al. (1995) Flavonoids as DNA topoisomerase antagonists and poisons: structure-activity relationships. J Nat Prod 58: 217–225.
34. Faivre S, Djelloul S, Raymond E (2006) New paradigms in anticancer therapy: targeting multiple signaling pathways with kinase inhibitors. Semin Oncol 33: 407–420.
35. Breuhahn K, Longerich T, Schirmacher P (2006) Dysregulation of growth factor signaling in human hepatocellular carcinoma. Oncogene 25: 3787–3800.
36. Olsen SK, Brown RS, Siegel AB (2010) Hepatocellular carcinoma: review of current treatment with a focus on targeted molecular therapies. Therap Adv Gastroenterol 3: 55–66.
37. Zhou Q, Lui VWY, Yeo W (2011) Targeting the PI3K/Akt/mTOR pathway in hepatocellular carcinoma. Future Oncology 7: 1149–1167.
38. Roberts PJ, Der CJ (2007) Targeting the Raf-MEK-ERK mitogen-activated protein kinase cascade for the treatment of cancer. Oncogene 26: 3291–3310.
39. Chappell WH, Steelman LS, Long JM, Kempf RC, Abrams SL, et al. (2011) Ras/Raf/MEK/ERK and PI3K/PTEN/Akt/mTOR inhibitors: Rationale and importance to inhibiting these pathways in human health. Oncotarget 2: 135–64.
40. Shapiro GI (2006) Cyclin-dependent kinase pathways as targets for cancer treatment. J Clinical Oncology 24: 1770–1783.
41. Zhang RG, Fang DC, Ning XY, Wang GA (2007) [Mechanisms of human telomerase reverse transcriptase RNAi which increases hepatocellular carcinoma cell apoptosis induced by TRAIL]. Zhonghua Gan Zang Bing Za Zhi 15: 32–36.
42. Naasani I, Oh-Hashi F, Oh-Hara T, Feng WY, Johnston J, et al. (2003) Blocking telomerase by dietary polyphenols is a major mechanism for limiting the growth of human cancer cells in vitro and in vivo. Cancer Res 63: 824–830.
43. Fulda S (2010) Evasion of apoptosis as a cellular stress response in cancer. Int J Cell Biol 2010: 370835.
44. Kang NJ, Shin SH, Lee HJ, Lee KW (2011) Polyphenols as small molecular inhibitors of signaling cascades in carcinogenesis. Pharmacology Therapeutics 130: 310–324.
45. Saitou Y, Shiraki K, Yamanaka T, Miyashita K, Inoue T, et al. (2005) Augmentation of tumor necrosis factor family-induced apoptosis by E3330 in human hepatocellular carcinoma cell lines via inhibition of NF kappa B. World J Gastroenterol 11: 6258–6261.
46. Delcuve GP, Khan DH, Davie JR (2012) Roles of histone deacetylases in epigenetic regulation: emerging paradigms from studies with inhibitors. Clin Epigenetics 4: 5.
47. Link A1, Balaguer F, Goel A (2010) Cancer chemoprevention by dietary polyphenols: promising role for epigenetics. Biochemical Pharmacology 80: 1771–92.
48. Hsu IC, Tokiwa T, Bennett W, Metcalf RA, Welsh JA, et al. (1993) p53 gene mutation and integrated hepatitis B viral DNA sequences in human liver cancer cell lines. Carcinogenesis 14: 987–992.

4

Anti-Tumor Effect of a Novel Soluble Recombinant Human Endostatin: Administered as a Single Agent or in Combination with Chemotherapy Agents in Mouse Tumor Models

Zhihua Ren[1,3]⁹, Yanan Wang[2]⁹, Wenhong Jiang[1], Wei Dai[3,4]*, Yongping Jiang[1,3]*

1 Biopharmagen Corp., Suzhou, China, **2** Department of Laboratory Diagnosis, Suzhou Municipal Hospital Affiliated Nanjing Medical University, Suzhou, China, **3** Biopharmaceutical R&D Center, Chinese Academy of Medical Sciences & Peking Union Medical College, Suzhou, China, **4** Department of Environmental Medicine, New York University Langone Medical Center, Tuxedo, New York, United States of America

Abstract

Background: Angiogenesis has become an attractive target in cancer treatment. Endostatin is one of the potent anti-angiogenesis agents. Its recombinant form expressed in the yeast system is currently under clinical trials. Endostatin suppresses tumor formation through the inhibition of blood vessel growth. It is anticipated that combined therapy using endostatin and cytotoxic compounds may exert an additive effect. In the present study, we expressed and purified recombinant human endostatin (rhEndostatin) that contained 3 additional amino acid residues (arginine, glycine, and serine) at the amino-terminus and 6 histidine residues in its carboxyl terminus. The recombinant protein was expressed in *E. Coli* and refolded into a soluble form in a large scale purification process. The protein exhibited a potent anti-tumor activity in bioassays. Furthermore, rhEndostatin showed an additive effect with chemotherapy agents including cyclophosphamide (CTX) and cisplatin (DDP).

Methods: rhEndostatin cDNA was cloned into PQE vector and expressed in *E. Coli*. The protein was refolded through dialysis with an optimized protocol. To establish tumor models, nude mice were subcutaneously injected with human cancer cells (lung carcinoma A549, hepatocellular carcinoma QGY-7703, or breast cancer Bcap37). rhEndostatin and/or DDP was administered peritumorally to evaluate the rate of growth inhibition of A549 tumors. For the tumor metastasis model, mice were injected intravenously with mouse melanoma B16 cells. One day after tumor cell injection, a single dose of rhEndostatin, or in combination with CTX, was administered intravenously or at a site close to the tumor.

Results: rhEndostatin reduced the growth of A549, QGY-7703, and Bcap37 xenograft tumors in a dose dependent manner. When it was administered peritumorally, rhEndostatin exhibited a more potent inhibitory activity. Furthermore, rhEndostatin displayed an additive effect with CTX or DDP on the inhibition of metastasis of B16 tumors or growth of A549 tumors.

Conclusion: Soluble rhEndostatin exhibits a potent anti-tumor activity in mouse xenograft models and it also has an additive effect with CTX and DDP, implying possible applications in clinical settings.

Editor: Irina V. Lebedeva, Columbia University, United States of America

Funding: This study was supported in all by the Key State projects of China (2011ZX09401-027) and (2011ZX09102-010-04). The funders had no role in study design, data collection and analysis, decision to publish, or preparation of the manuscript.

Competing Interests: Zhihua Ren, Wenhong Jiang and Yongping Jiang are employed by Biopharmagen Corp. There are no patents, products in development or marketed products to declare.

* Email: wei.dai@nyumc.org (WD); yjiang@biopharmagen.com (YK)

⁹ These authors contributed equally to this work.

Introduction

Angiogenesis plays a key role in promoting growth, invasion and metastasis of tumors [1,2,3]. It has become an attractive target for tumor therapy. Endostatin, a cleaved product of the carboxyl-terminal domain of collagen XVIII, was originally found in conditioned media from a murine endothelial tumor cell line (hemangio-endothelioma). It was reported that endostatin inhibits endothelial cell proliferation and migration both in vivo and in vitro, thus inhibiting tumor growth [4,5]. Endostatin has been evaluated in clinical trials. In a Phase I clinical study, Endostatin was reported to be safe and well tolerated in advanced cancer patients, demonstrating some antitumor activities [6,7]. Of the 74 patients' cohort, minor responses have been found in 2 patients (40% and 17% reduction in tumor volume for 22 and 11 months, respectively), and mixed responses in 2 patients for 14 or 5 months; In addition, 8 patients were reported to have stable disease for more than 3 months [8]. Furthermore, independent studies have shown that Endostatin decreases blood flow in tumors in a dose-dependent manner as measured by positron emission tomography scan [9,10] and that it induces apoptosis in tumor cells [11,12].

Endostatin that was used in previous clinical studies was expressed in yeast [13,14], which makes the preparation costly and laborious. Endostatin has no direct cytotoxicity against tumor cells. The anti-tumor effect of endostatin stems from its ability to inhibit neo-angiogenesis around tumors, thus preventing tumor growth and progression. while it shows no direct cytotoxicity against tumor cells [15]. It has been reported that endostatin-mediated inhibition of angiogenesis was most effective when it is combined with other therapies, especially chemotherapy [16,17,18].

The conventional chemotherapy agents, such as cyclophosphamide (CTX) and cisplatin (DDP), directly target tumor cells and induce cytotoxicity. However, the efficacy of chemotherapy agents is often compromised due to their adverse side effects such as myelosuppression and development of drug resistance [19,20]. It is believed that a combination of anti-angiogenesis agents and chemotherapy agents will significantly enhance the therapeutic efficacy and reduce side effects [17,21]. In this study, we expressed rhEndostatin with additional arginine, glycine, and serine residues at the N-terminus using the prokaryotic expression system. The added amino acid residues were expected to enhance the binding affinity of target molecule to the cellular receptor [22]. rhEndostatin also contained 6-histidine residues at the caboxyl terminus for affinity purification. We also developed and optimized a protocol for efficient refolding of bioactive rhEndostatin in a large scale. We demonstrated that rhEndostatin exhibited a potent bioactivity and was capable of synergizing with CTX and DDP in suppression of tumor cell growth. Our combined studies strongly suggest that rhEndostatin can be developed as a therapeutical agent for the treatment of various malignancies.

Materials and Methods

Ethics Statement

All research involving animals was conducted according to relevant national and international guidelines. Male BALB/c nude mice, weight 16.0~25.1 g were purchased from SLAC Company (Shanghai, China). The experiment protocols were approved by the Institutional Animal Care and Use Committees of Soochow University (IACUC permit number: SYXK(Su) 2012-0045), and were in accordance with the Guidelines for the Care and Use of Laboratory Animals (National Research Council, People's Republic of China, 2010). We further attest that all efforts were made to ensure minimal suffering.

Cell lines and reagents

Human A549 lung carcinoma cell line [23], human umbilical vein endothelial cells (HUVEC) [4,24], and mouse B16 melanoma cell line [25] were purchased from ATCC (Manassas, VA, USA). Human hepatocellular carcinoma cell line QGY-7703 [26], and human breast cancer cell line Bcap37 [27] were from Shanghai Institute of Cell Biology (Shanghai, China). Restriction enzyme BamHI and HindIII were purchased from New England Biolabs (Ipswich, MA, USA). The PQE60 plasmid, *E.Coli* M15 and Ni-NTA purification kit were obtained from QIAGEN (Valencia, CA, USA). Isopropyl-1-thio-ß- D-galactopyranoside (IPTG) was from Bio-Basic Inc (Amherst, NY, USA) to induce rhEndostatin expression in bacteria. Guanidine Hydrochloride was from Amresco Inc (Solon, OH, USA). Urea was from Shanghai Experimental Reagent Inc (Shanghai, China). M199 medium and RPMI 1640 medium were from Gibco (Grand Island, NY, USA). Fetal bovine serum was from Hyclone (Logan, UT, USA). Basic fibroblast growth factor (bFGF) and vascular endothelial growth factor (VEGF) were from R&D systems (Minneapolis, MN, USA). MTT was from Cell Biolabs (San Diego, CA, USA). DMSO was from Sigma Aldrich (St. Louis, MO, USA). Cisplatin (DDP) was purchased from Shandong Qilu Pharmaceutical Co., Ltd (Shandong, China), and Cyclophosphamide (CTX) was from Shanghai Hualian Pharmaceutical Co, Ltd (Shanghai, China).

Sequence Modified rhEndostatin and Expression of rhEndostatin in *E.Coli*

Human endostatin mRNA was extracted from Chinese embryo hepatocytes and cDNA was obtained by reverse transcription-polymerase chain reaction (RT-PCR). The amplified products were fractionated on agarose gels, and then ligated to plasmid PQE60, after been digested with restriction enzyme BamHI and HindIII. Mutant rhEndostatin was made by adding CGAGGUUCC after the starting codon of AUG, and ligating CACCACCACCACCACCAC before the stop codon. The PQE60 plasmid expressing mutant rhEndostatin was transformed into *E.Coli* M15, in a form as inclusion body.

rhEndostatin purification and refolding in large scale

The inclusion body was collected from IPTG induced bacteria lysate and dissolved with Guanidine Hydrochloride (6 Mol). Ni-NTA Purification System has been employed to purify poly-histidine-containing rhEndostatin as previously described [28]. The purified rhEndostatin protein were then diluted with a phosphate buffer containing 8 Mol of Urea (PH 4.5) to 0.3 mg/ml, and the refolding protein was obtained by a series of dialysis procedure with optimized buffer conditions at 4°C.

rhEndostatin inhibits human umbilical vein endothelial cell proliferation in vitro

Primary human umbilical vein endothelial cells (HUVEC) at 2–5 passages were suspended in M199 basal medium supplemented with 10% heat-inactivated fetal bovine serum, and then plated in 96-well culture plates at 5×10^3 cells per 100 µl/well. Cells were incubated with rhEndostatin at various concentrations (0.1, 0.2, 0.5, 1, 2, 5, 8, 16 µg/ml) in bFGF(5 ng/ml) supplemented M199 medium or basal medium alone at 200 µl volume for 72 hours at 37°C. 20 µl of MTT(5%) was added to each well at 4 hours before the end of treatment, and then aspirated carefully. Cells were further incubated with 100 µl of DMSO for 15 minutes on the shaker, and optical density (OD) value was read at 570 nm wave length with the microplate reader (Bio-Rad, Hercules, CA. USA).

Inhibition of chick embryo chorioallantoic membrane (CAM) angiogenesis by rhEndostatin

Chick embryonic chorioallantoic membrane assay was employed for evaluating the anti-angiogenesis activity of rhEndostatin. All procedures were carried out in a biosafety hood under sterile conditions. Briefly, fertilized eggs were incubated for 7 days at 37°C and 60% humidity. A window was made on the top of each egg after 2 days' incubation. Chick embryonic chorioallantoic membrane was exposed by tearing up the egg membrane with a tip. A filter paper disc of 5 mm diameter containing 20 µl of rhEndostatin (0.3 mg/mL) or saline was gently implanted, and changed every day for 10 days. The membrane was cut around the air sac, which was turned upside down and observed and photographed by a stereomicroscope. The number of blood vessel branch points was counted, and the vessel density was calculated according to the size of area where the blood vessel distributed to evaluate the anti-angiogenesis activity.

In vitro anti-tumor study on rhEndostatin

All tumor cell lines (human A549 lung carcinoma cell line and mouse B16 melanoma cell line, human hepatocellular carcinoma cell line QGY-7703, and human breast cancer cell line Bcap37) were maintained in RPMI 1640 supplemented with 10% FBS. Human umbilical vein endothelial cells were cultured in RPMI 1640 supplemented with 2% FBS and 10 ng/mL each of VEGF and b-FGF. In vitro activity assay on rhEndostatin was performed as O'Reilly MS et al. described [4], with minor modifications.

Animals

Male BALB/c nude mice, at 4–6 weeks of age, with an average weight of 20.5±1.2 g (16.0~25.1 g) were employed in our studies. A total of 50 mice were involved in each of the following anti-tumor studies with single rhED treatment, including hepatocellular carcinoma QGY-7703, A549 lung carcinoma, or Bcap37 breast cancer, which were further divided into 5 groups, randomly. To evaluate the combination effects with CTX or DDP, a total of 160 nude mice (N = 10 in each treatment group) were selected. Another 60 nude mice (N = 10 each) were used to analyze if local rhEndostatin delivery will improve the tumor inhibition rate, in A549 lung carcinoma and Bcap37 breast cancer models. Animals were housed in individual stainless steel cages in a SPF facility in Soochow University, with a regulated temperature of 24±2°C, relative humidity of 50±10%, and a 12-h light cycle. Animals were sacrificed by Carbon dioxide (CO_2) inhalation at 24 hours post the final treatment. Tumor tissues and organs were collected after euthanasia.

Tumor-bearing mouse studies

The inhibition capabilities of rhEndostatin to tumor growth and tumor metastasis were evaluated. The tumor-bearing mouse model was generated by injecting BALB/c strain nude mice subcutaneously with $6\times10^6/100$ µl of each tumor cells, including human A549 lung carcinoma, human hepatocellular carcinoma QGY-7703 and human breast cancer Bcap37 cells. When the tumors volume were about of 170 mm^3, approximately 15 days after implantation, either rhEndostatin alone, or in combination with DDP were delivered to the animal model either intravenously or subcutaniously at the site close to the inoculated tumor, to evaluate the inhibition rate of tumor growth. Whereas rhEndostatin alone or along with CTX was given intraperitoneally to observe the metastatic rate of tumor. The mice from control group were received injections of phosphate-buffered saline (PBS) at the same volume intravenously. The mice were evaluated for tumor growth at every other day. The formula, width^2×length×0.52, was applied to estimate the volume of a spheroid as described [5]. The formula, [(tumor volume of control-tumor volume of treatment)/tumor volume of control]×100%, was used to calculate the inhibition rate of tumor growth [5]. For the estimation of the metastasis inhibition rate, tumor-bearing mice were sacrificed by carbon dioxide asphyxiation, and evaluation was calculated with following formula: [(numbers of tumor colonies in lung of control mice numbers of tumor colonies in lung of treatment mice)/numbers of tumor colonies in lung of control mice]×100%. All procedures involving animals were done in accordance with national and international laws and policies.

Statistical analysis

Comparison of variables was performed using One-Way ANOVA in SPSS program (SPSS). A statistically significant difference was defined as $P<0.05$.

Results

Expression, refolding, and purification of rhEndostatin in *E. coli*

Modified rhEndostatin was expressed in *E. coli* using a pQE vector expression system. Following the addition of IPTG, rhEndostatin was highly induced (Figure 1A). Harvested from 40-L bio-reactor, about 1.5 g/L of rhEndostatin inclusion body was collected. The rhEndostatin was purified by affinity purification with nickel (Ni) resin followed by size-exclusion chromatography, and then the denatured protein underwent an optimized refolding procedure to gain a refolding rate of over 80%. Eventually, about 200 mg/L of purified rhEndostatin with bioactivity was generated. SDS-PAGE analysis revealed that rhEndostatin was purified to homogeneity and remained intact (Figure 1A). Immunoblotting showed that the commercial available rhEndostatin antibody detected IPTG-induced sequence-modified- rhEndostatin in the total bacterial lysates as well as its purified form (Figure 1B), suggesting that the amino acids addition did not significantly change the overall conformation of the protein. Protein sequencing analysis confirmed that the purified protein was the modified form of rhEndostatin with the addition of arginine, glycine, and serine residues at the amino-terminus (data not shown).

Anti-angiogenesis assay on rhEndostatin in vitro and in vivo

To determine whether rhEndostatin could inhibit the growth of endothelial cells in vitro, HUVECs had been treated with rhEndostatin at the dose range from 0.1 to 16 µg/ml. Cell variability has been evaluated by MTT assay. rhEndostatin

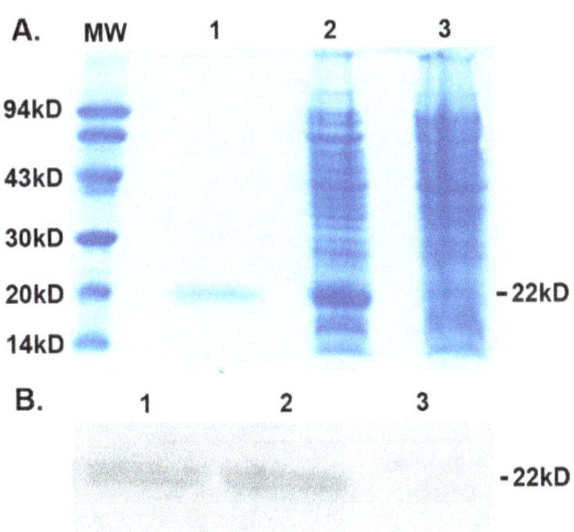

Figure 1. SDS-PAGE and immunoblotting of expression and purified rhEndostatin. A. SDS-PAGE of rhEndostatin. Lane 1: Pre-stained molecular weight markers; Lane 2: Purified rhEndostatin; Lane 3: Induced bacterial lysates; Lane 4: Non-induced bacterial lysates. (B). Immunoblotting of rhEndostatin. Lane 1: Purified rhEndostatin Lane 2: Whole bacterial cell lysates after IPTG induction; Lane 3: Non-induced bacterial lysates.

remarkably inhibited HUVEC proliferation in a dose depended manner (figure 2). rhEndostatin significantly inhibited HUVECs growth at the concentration above 0.2 μg/ml compared with the saline vehicle control. *In vivo* anti-angiogenic effect was investigated on a chicken embryonic chorioallantoic membrane assay (CAMs). CAMs vascularization was inhibited by rhEndostatin at 6 μg/disc for 10 days incubation. Figure 3B showed a normal looking of vascularization of untreated CAMs with primary, secondary and tertiary vessels and dendritic branching. On the contrary, CAMs treated with rhEndostatin demonstrated a distorted vasculature or the absence of blood vessels (Figure 3A).

Antitumor efficacy of rhEndostatin administered as a single agent

We first studied the anti-tumor bioactivity of rhEndostatin both in vitro and in vivo. rhEndostatin had no effect on the growth of any kind of tumor cells in vitro (data not shown). In the *in vivo* study, tumor cells were implanted subcutaneously, and measurable solid tumors were developed approximately 14 days post implantation at the injection site in all mice. Administration of rhEndostatin alone significantly delayed the growth of human A549 lung carcinoma, human hepatocellular carcinoma QGY-7703 and human breast cancer Bcap37 (Figure 4A, B, C), by 45% -35% at a high to medium dosage, compared with PBS vehicle control. Moreover, subcutaneous administration of rhEndostatin peritumorally exhibited a higher inhibition rate on day 30 post treatment than that by intravenous injection (Figure 5). Endostar, a version of commercially available endostatin, also exhibited an inhibitory activity toward A549 xenograft tumors. Although no statistically significant difference was observed between Endostar and rhEndostatin in blocking tumor growth, on day 9 rhEndostatin appeared to be more efficacious in reducing the tumor size (Figure S1).

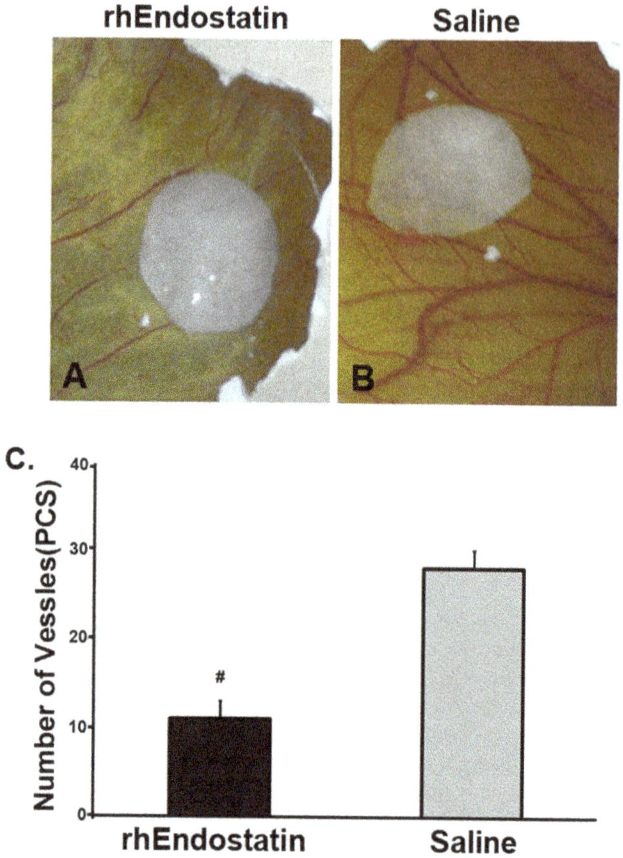

Figure 3. ***In vivo* inhibition of angiogenesis using chicken embryo CAMs.** Treated with rhEndostatin at 6 μg/disc (**A**), or treated with saline vehicle control disc (**B**) the vessels numbers were calculated(n = 8, each) in CAMs assay after 10 days treatment, and data were presented as mean±SD. # indicated $P<0.05$. (**C**).

rhEndostatin administered in combination with CTX

B16 melanoma metastasis model was employed to assay the additive effect of rhEndostatin with CTX. As shown in Figure 6, intravenously administration of three dosages of rhEndostatin (10 mg/kg/day, 5 mg/kg/day, and 2.5 mg/kg/day, respectively) for successive 15 days significantly inhibited the metastasis of B16 melanoma, with the inhibition rate of 34.87%, 29.66% and 29.26%, respectively. Furthermore, rhEndostatin and CTX exhibited an additive effect. CTX (15 mg/kg/day) administered alone in the first 7 days inhibited the metastasis by 59.32%, whereas rhEndostatin, which was intravenously injected at the dosage of 10 mg/kg/day, 5 mg/kg/day, and 2.5 mg/kg/day for successive 15 days, increased the inhibition rate to 77.15%, 70.94%, and 65.93%, respectively.

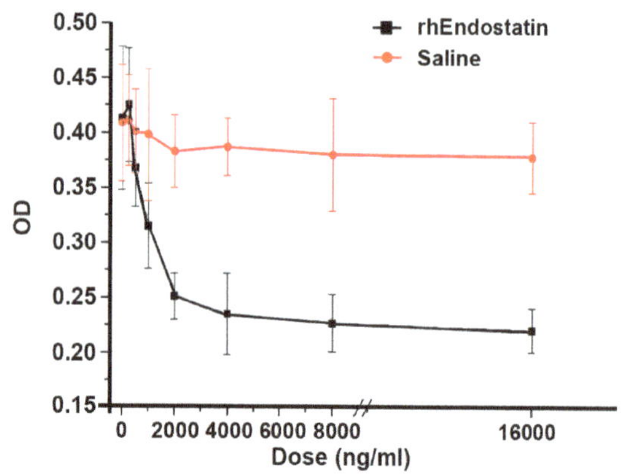

Figure 2. The inhibition effect of rhEndostatin on the growth of HUVEC *in vitro*. HUVECs were planted in fibronectin coated 96-well microtiterplates at 5×10^3cells per well with bFGF supplemented M199 medium. rhEndostatin was applied at the dosage of 0.1, 0.2, 0.5, 1.0, 2.0, 4.0, 8.0, 16 μg/ml, as described before. All the treatments were triplicated. The OD value were shown as mean ± SD. Treatment with 2 μg/mL of rhEndostatin and above significantly inhibited HUVEC proliferation compared to saline vehicle control.

rhEndostatin used in combination with DDP

A nude mouse model with xenograft tumors (A549 cells) was used to evaluate the additive effect of rhEndostatin with DDP. As shown in Figure 7, three dosages of rhEndostatin, 5 mg/kg/day, 10 mg/kg/day, and 15 mg/kg/day, were administered peritumorally, twice a day for successive 15 days. Significant inhibition of tumor growth was observed with the inhibition rate of 28.79%, 28.88% and 32.43% (N = 10, each), respectively. Furthermore, an additive effect was also exhibited when rhEndostatin administered in combined with DDP. DDP (3 mg/kg/day) administered alone by i.p. in the first 7 days suppressed the tumor volume by 45.19%. After the first 7 days treatment, DDP (3 mg/kg/day), was administered in combination with rhEndostatin at the dose of 5 mg/kg/day, 10 mg/kg/day, and 15 mg/kg/day, respectively, for another 15 days successively. The inhibition rate was increased to 54.24%, 47.26%, and 60.66%, respectively.

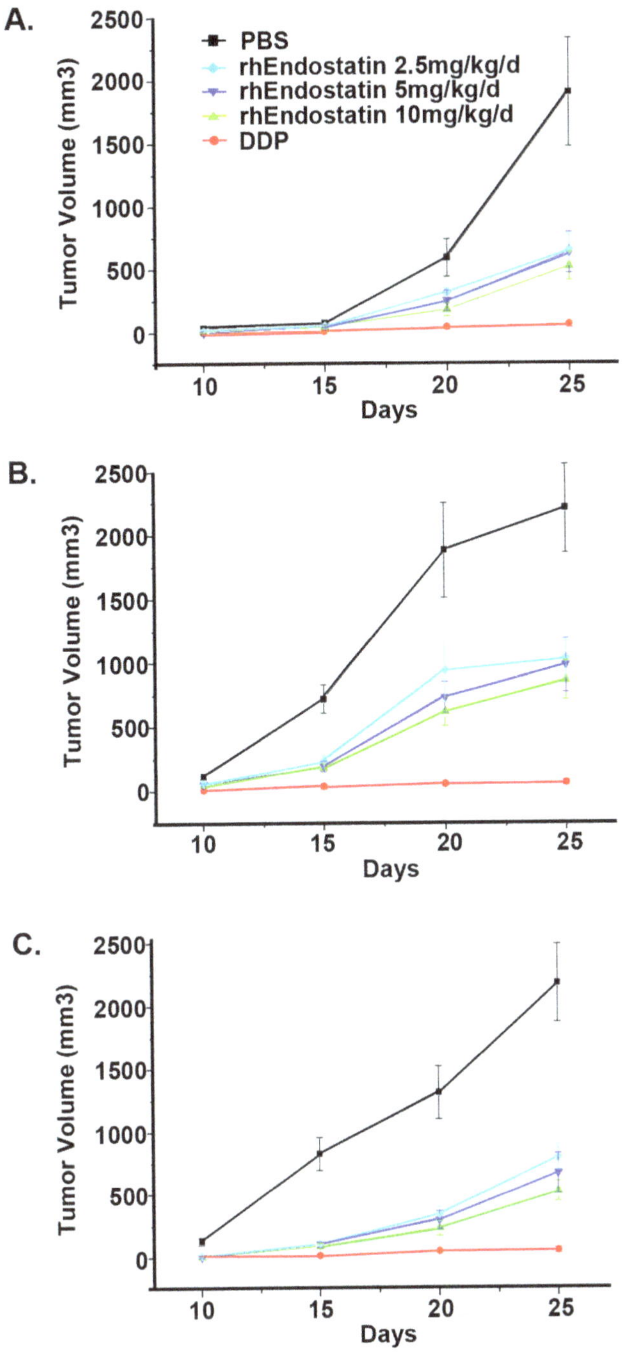

Figure 4. Inhibition of human tumor growth by administrating rhEndostatin intravenously. Hepatocellular carcinoma QGY-7703(A), A549 lung carcinoma(B), or Bcap37 breast cancer cells(C), were implanted to nude mice at the dosage of 6×10^6 cells each, subcutaneously. Tumor-bearing mice were treated with either DDP (2 mg/kg/day) for successively 7 days(●), or rhEndostatin 10 mg/kg/day(▲), rhEndostatin 5 mg/kg/day(▼), and rhEndostatin 2.5 mg/kg/day(□) for successively 15 days. PBS(■) was injected as the vehicle control. Results were presented as mean±SD (n = 10, each). Mice administered with rhEndostatin i.v. exhibited a significant reduction in tumor volume, compared with that in vehicle control group.

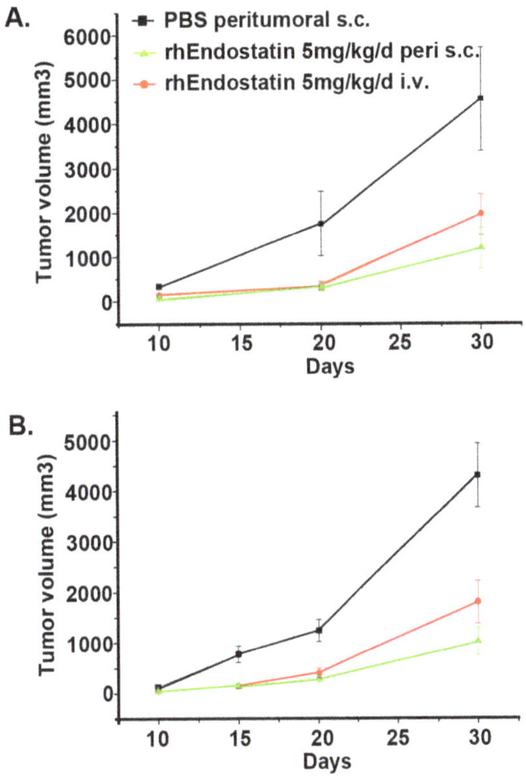

Figure 5. Inhibition of human tumor growth by administrating rhEndostatin s.c. peritumorally. Either A549 lung carcinoma cells (A), or Bcap37 breast cancer cells(B) were implanted to nude mice of 6×10^6 tumor cells each, subcutaneously. Tumor-bearing mice were then treated for successively 15 days with rhEndostatin (5 mg/kg/day) intravenously (●), or at the site close to the tumor (▲). PBS was injected as the vehicle control at the site close to the tumor (■). Results were presented as mean±SD(n = 10). Tumor volume was measured every other day, and the data indicated an enhanced reduction in tumor volume, when administered rhEndostatin s.c. peritumorally.

Discussion

Angiogenesis is critical for growth, invasion and metastasis of solid tumors. Most solid tumors begin as avascularized malignant cells [29,30,31,32]. Without further vascularization, solid tumors cannot grow beyond 1–2 mm^2 [33]. And there is a close correlation between microvessel counts and metastatic cancer. The mean microvessel count within biopsy tissue for the metastatic group is 76.8 vessels per field compared with 39.2 for those without metastasis ($P<0.0001$) [34]. Endostatin is first reported by O'Reilly MS as a potent angiogenesis inhibitor [35]. Several studies subsequently reported the anti-angiogenesis and anti-tumor activity of endostatin [4,5,36,37]. Most of them employed endostatin which expressed in eukaryotic cells, or administered directly in the form of inclusion body, which leads to a limited yield rate as well as a low antitumoral bioactivity. The yeast expression system for the generation of rhEndostatin is characterized as a relative high cost, a low yield (with 10–20 mg/L of soluble protein produced [38]), and an unstable structure with a common feature of 2–4 amino acid residues truncated from the N-terminus of rhEndostatin. These shortcomings have limited the application of rhEndostatin in the clinical practice. The reported *E. Coli* expression system for rhEndostatin, on the other hand, has several salient features including low cost and a high expression rate; however, the refolding efficiency was low (less than 1% [39]).

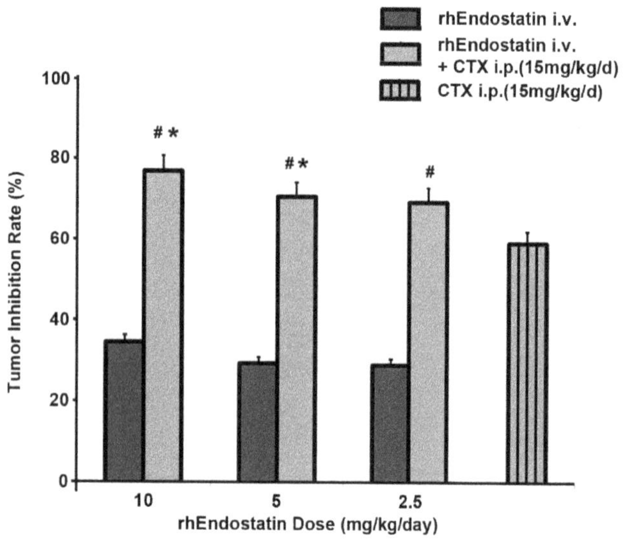

Figure 6. Additive effect of rhEndostatin with CTX on the metastasis of B16 melanoma. Nude mice (n = 10, each) were inoculated with 2.5×10^5 tumor cells intravenously to establish a metastasis model. Mice were either administered i.v. with rhEndostatin alone at 10 mg/kg/day, 5 mg/kg/day, or 2.5 mg/kg/day for 15 days successively, or combined treated with CTX at the dosage of 15 mg/kg/d for successively 7 days, then intravenously administered with rhEndostatin at 10 mg/kg/day, 5 mg/kg/day, or 2.5 mg/kg/day for successively 15 days. The mice were sacrificed to count the metastasis colony in the lung on day 25 post inoculation. The formula, [(mean colony of PBS control- mean colony of treated mice)/mean colony of PBS control]×100, was used to calculate the inhibition rate of metastasis. #: $P<0.05$ vs mice administered with single rhEndostatin treatment at the same dose, respectively; *: $P<0.05$ vs mice treated with CTX alone, at the dosage of 15 mg/kg/day.

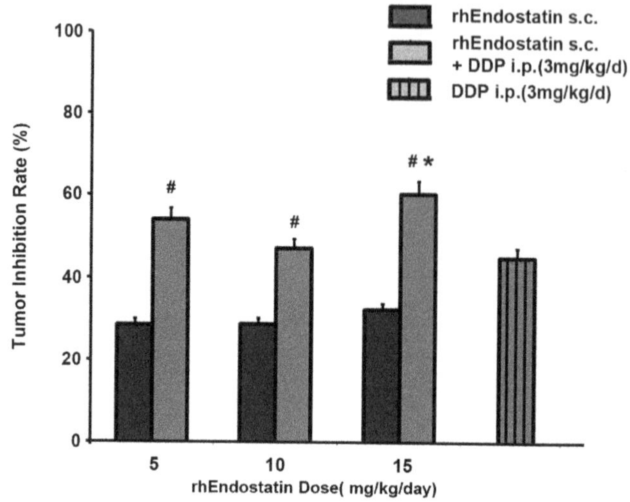

Figure 7. Additive inhibition effect of rhEndostatin with DDP on the growth of A549 lung cancer. Nude mice (n = 10, each) were inoculated with 6×10^6 tumor cells subcutanously to establish the tumor-bearing model. The animals were either administered peritumorally with rhEndostatin alone at 5 mg/kg/day, 10 mg/kg/day, and 15 mg/kg/day for 15 days, successively, or combined with DDP treatment at 3 mg/kg/d every other day for 15 days. The tumor volume was measured every other day, and the formula, [(tumor volume of control-tumor volume of treatment)/tumor volume of control]×100%, was used to calculate the inhibition rate of tumor growth. #: $P<0.05$ vs mice administered with single rhEndostatin treatment at the same dose, respectively; *: $P<0.05$ vs mice treated with DDP alone at 3 mg/kg/day.

Therefore, our strategy focused on the optimization of refolding and purification procedure, in order to provide a sufficient amount of soluble form of rhEndostatin which can be potentially used for clinical trials. Our current study is among the very few that use rhEndostatin expressed in *E. Coli* and refolds into a soluble form with an optimized dialysis procedure (patent pending), which yields about 100 mg/L of soluble protein with a purity of 99%. Structural integrity of rhEndostatin is evaluated by protein sequencing, and anti-angiogenic and antitumor activities are also determined, which yields a comparable result as compared with the commercially available Endostar.

In order to achieve an optimal tumor inhibition and regression, researchers have demonstrated that it is critical to continuously elevate endostatin levels in blood circulation [40,41]. A short half-life of 2 h of endostatin has been reported, which requires a more frequent drug administration in addition to escalating drug doses to achieve the effective plasma concentration. Our modified rhEndostatin contains 3 additional amino acid residues (arginine, glycine, and serine) at the amino-terminus, which appears to increase the overall positive charge of protein, which may in turn enhance its affinity to the cognate receptor molecule, as previously reported [42,43,44]. Thus, it is not surprising that a prolonged half-life and better antitumoral activity were observed. Future studies will be focused on pharmacokinetics on non-human primates. In addition, 6 histidine residues are included in the carboxyl terminus of rhEndostatin, which are used for affinity purification. At present, we are not sure whether the addition of these residues would affect the activity of rhEndostatin.

Previous studies showed that endostatin has an additive effect with chemotherapy agents towards various types of tumors [45,46,47] with little toxicity [5,7,12]. Endostar has been approved for clinical trials in China. Preclinical studies indicated that the combination of Endostar with chemotherapy is more effective to inhibit lung tumor growth and metastases [48,49]. Most recently, clinical data from multiple institutes suggest that the strategy to combine Endostar and chemotherapy agents can dramatically improve outcomes of cancer patients [50,51,52]. Similar results have been observed in our preclinical models that the rhEndostatin exhibits a potent antitumor activity against homogeneic and allogeneic tumors in mice alone or in combination with CTX, as well as DDP. The commercially available Endostar is also included in our study. The tumor inhibition rate by Endostar and rhED are about 22% and 28%, respectively. On the other hand, no significant difference has been found between these two factors. Furthermore, our studies reveal that an enhanced tumor inhibitory activity can be achieved when rhEndostatin is administered peritumorally, implying that the route of drug delivery may affect its bioactivity. It has been shown that endostatin binds to the blood vessels when it is administered systemically, resulting in the decreased angiogenic protein concentration around the tumor microenvironment [53]. Angiogenesis inhibitors are most effective when administered in a way which maintains a stable concentration in the circulation [54]. Local administration of rhEndostatin may help to maintain an effective concentration around tumors.

A combination of endostatin with chemotherapy agents is currently employed to improve the therapeutic efficacy. However, its application is often hampered by either non-overlapping or overlapping toxicities [10,55]. Moreover, due to unstable genome, tumor cells frequently develop multi-drug resistance to various chemotherapies [56]. While Endostatin exerts a cytostatic effect on endothelium, which is less prone to the development of drug resistance [55,57]. In the present study, we have demonstrated that a combination of conventional chemotherapy agent, CTX, with rhEndostatin exhibits an additive effect on the metastasis of B16 melanoma. Our research data also confirm that a combination of cytotoxic antitumor drug, DDP, with rhEndostatin results in an additive effect on growth inhibition of A549 xenograft tumors. This combination strategy aims at multiple targets of tumor development, thus enhancing the therapeutic efficacy and reducing the toxicity of chemotherapy and occurrence of drug resistance.

Our current study demonstrates that prokaryotically expressed, soluble rhEndostatin exhibits a potent anti-tumor effect. rhEndostatin that is administered peritumorally achieved a better anti-tumor activity than that achieved by intravenous injection. Moreover, rhEndostatin displays increased tumor inhibition in A549 tumor cell xenografts in mice when it is combined with DDP. Furthermore, rhEndostatin exhibits an additive effect with CTX on inhibition of metastasis of B16 melanoma. Our preclinical studies strongly suggest that rhEndostatin can be further explored for clinical trials for eventual applications in the clinic.

Supporting Information

Figure S1 Inhibition of human A549 lung carcinoma growth by administrating rhEndostatin or Endostar. A549 lung carcinomas were implanted to nude mice at the dosage of 6×10^6 cells each, subcutaneously. Tumor-bearing mice were treated peritumorally with either Endostar (▲, 5 mg/kg/day) or rhEndostatin (■, 5 mg/kg/day), for successively 15 days. PBS (◆)was injected at the same volume as the vehicle control. The tumor volume was measured on day 0, 3, 6, 9, 12, 15 post injections. Results were presented as mean±SD (n = 10, each).

Checklist S1 ARRIVE Guidelines.

Acknowledgments

We thank co-workers in the laboratory for the valuable discussions and suggestions. The authors read and approved the manuscript.

Author Contributions

Conceived and designed the experiments: YJ ZR WD. Performed the experiments: YW WJ ZR YJ. Analyzed the data: YW ZR YJ WD. Contributed reagents/materials/analysis tools: YW. Contributed to the writing of the manuscript: YJ ZR WD.

References

1. Folkman J (2002) Role of angiogenesis in tumor growth and metastasis. Semin Oncol 29: 15–18.
2. Zetter BR (1998) Angiogenesis and tumor metastasis. Annu Rev Med 49: 407–424.
3. Rao JS, Gondi C, Chetty C, Chittivelu S, Joseph PA, et al. (2005) Inhibition of invasion, angiogenesis, tumor growth, and metastasis by adenovirus-mediated transfer of antisense uPAR and MMP-9 in non-small cell lung cancer cells. Mol Cancer Ther 4: 1399–1408.
4. O'Reilly MS, Boehm T, Shing Y, Fukai N, Vasios G, et al. (1997) Endostatin: an endogenous inhibitor of angiogenesis and tumor growth. Cell 88: 277–285.
5. Boehm T, Folkman J, Browder T, O'Reilly MS (1997) Antiangiogenic therapy of experimental cancer does not induce acquired drug resistance. Nature 390: 404–407.
6. Mundhenke C, Thomas JP, Wilding G, Lee FT, Kelzc F, et al. (2001) Tissue examination to monitor antiangiogenic therapy: a phase I clinical trial with endostatin. Clin Cancer Res 7: 3366–3374.
7. Eder JP, Jr., Supko JG, Clark JW, Puchalski TA, Garcia-Carbonero R, et al. (2002) Phase I clinical trial of recombinant human endostatin administered as a short intravenous infusion repeated daily. J Clin Oncol 20: 3772–3784.
8. Kulke MH, Bergsland EK, Ryan DP, Enzinger PC, Lynch TJ, et al. (2006) Phase II study of recombinant human endostatin in patients with advanced neuroendocrine tumors. J Clin Oncol 24: 3555–3561.
9. Sun L, Ye HY, Zhang YH, Guan YS, Wu H (2007) Epidermal growth factor receptor antibody plus recombinant human endostatin in treatment of hepatic metastases after remnant gastric cancer resection. World J Gastroenterol 13: 6115–6118.
10. Plum SM, Hanson AD, Volker KM, Vu HA, Sim BK, et al. (2003) Synergistic activity of recombinant human endostatin in combination with adriamycin: analysis of in vitro activity on endothelial cells and in vivo tumor progression in an orthotopic murine mammary carcinoma model. Clin Cancer Res 9: 4619–4626.
11. Roy Choudhury S, Karmakar S, Banik NL, Ray SK (2012) Targeting angiogenesis for controlling neuroblastoma. J Oncol: 782020.
12. Herbst RS, Mullani NA, Davis DW, Hess KR, McConkey DJ, et al. (2002) Development of biologic markers of response and assessment of antiangiogenic activity in a clinical trial of human recombinant endostatin. J Clin Oncol 20: 3804–3814.
13. Dhanabal M, Ramchandran R, Volk R, Stillman IE, Lombardo M, et al. (1999) Endostatin: yeast production, mutants, and antitumor effect in renal cell carcinoma. Cancer Res 59: 189–197.
14. Boehm T, Pirie-Shepherd S, Trinh LB, Shiloach J, Folkman J (1999) Disruption of the KEX1 gene in Pichia pastoris allows expression of full-length murine and human endostatin. Yeast 15: 563–572.
15. Dome B, Hendrix MJ, Paku S, Tovari J, Timar J (2007) Alternative vascularization mechanisms in cancer: Pathology and therapeutic implications. Am J Pathol 170: 1–15.
16. Morioka H, Weissbach L, Vogel T, Nielsen GP, Faircloth GT, et al. (2003) Antiangiogenesis treatment combined with chemotherapy produces chondrosarcoma necrosis. Clin Cancer Res 9: 1211–1217.
17. Ma J, Waxman DJ (2008) Combination of antiangiogenesis with chemotherapy for more effective cancer treatment. Mol Cancer Ther 7: 3670–3684.
18. Kaya M, Wada T, Nagoya S, Yamashita T (2007) Prevention of postoperative progression of pulmonary metastases in osteosarcoma by antiangiogenic therapy using endostatin. J Orthop Sci 12: 562–567.
19. Kerbel RS, Viloria-Petit A, Klement G, Rak J (2000) 'Accidental' anti-angiogenic drugs. anti-oncogene directed signal transduction inhibitors and conventional chemotherapeutic agents as examples. Eur J Cancer 36: 1248–1257.
20. Klement G, Baruchel S, Rak J, Man S, Clark K, et al. (2000) Continuous low-dose therapy with vinblastine and VEGF receptor-2 antibody induces sustained tumor regression without overt toxicity. J Clin Invest 105: R15–24.
21. Cabebe E, Wakelee H (2007) Role of anti-angiogenesis agents in treating NSCLC: focus on bevacizumab and VEGFR tyrosine kinase inhibitors. Curr Treat Options Oncol 8: 15–27.
22. Jiang Y, Jiang W, Qiu Y, Dai W Effect of a structurally modified human granulocyte colony stimulating factor, G-CSFa, on leukopenia in mice and monkeys. J Hematol Oncol 4: 28.
23. Giard DJ, Aaronson SA, Todaro GJ, Arnstein P, Kersey JH, et al. (1973) In vitro cultivation of human tumors: establishment of cell lines derived from a series of solid tumors. J Natl Cancer Inst 51: 1417–1423.
24. Hoshi H, McKeehan WL (1984) Brain- and liver cell-derived factors are required for growth of human endothelial cells in serum-free culture. Proc Natl Acad Sci U S A 81: 6413–6417.
25. Briles EB, Kornfeld S (1978) Isolation and metastatic properties of detachment variants of B16 melanoma cells. J Natl Cancer Inst 60: 1217–1222.
26. Luo D, Cheng SC, Xie H, Xie Y (1999) Chemosensitivity of human hepatocellular carcinoma cell line QGY-7703 is related to bcl-2 protein levels. Tumour Biol 20: 331–340.
27. Xiong X, Sui M, Fan W, Kraft AS (2007) Cell cycle dependent antagonistic interactions between paclitaxel and carboplatin in combination therapy. Cancer Biol Ther 6: 1067–1073.
28. Song SJW, Jiang Y (2012) Large-scale production, refolding, and purification of a novel recombinant human granulocyte colony stimulating factor. Chinese Journal of Biomedical Engineering 31: 552–557.
29. Folkman J (1996) New perspectives in clinical oncology from angiogenesis research. Eur J Cancer 32A: 2534–2539.
30. Saphir A (1997) Angiogenesis: the unifying concept in cancer? J Natl Cancer Inst 89: 1658–1659.
31. Hagedorn M, Bikfalvi A (2000) Target molecules for anti-angiogenic therapy: from basic research to clinical trials. Crit Rev Oncol Hematol 34: 89–110.
32. Harris AL (1998) Anti-angiogenesis therapy and strategies for integrating it with adjuvant therapy. Recent Results Cancer Res 152: 341–352.
33. Brem H, Folkman J (1975) Inhibition of tumor angiogenesis mediated by cartilage. J Exp Med 141: 427–439.

34. Weidner N, Carroll PR, Flax J, Blumenfeld W, Folkman J (1993) Tumor angiogenesis correlates with metastasis in invasive prostate carcinoma. Am J Pathol 143: 401–409.
35. O'Reilly MS, Holmgren L, Shing Y, Chen C, Rosenthal RA, et al. (1994) Angiostatin: a circulating endothelial cell inhibitor that suppresses angiogenesis and tumor growth. Cold Spring Harb Symp Quant Biol 59: 471–482.
36. O'Reilly MS, Holmgren L, Chen C, Folkman J (1996) Angiostatin induces and sustains dormancy of human primary tumors in mice. Nat Med 2: 689–692.
37. Boehm T, O'Reilly M S, Keough K, Shiloach J, Shapiro R, et al. (1998) Zinc-binding of endostatin is essential for its antiangiogenic activity. Biochem Biophys Res Commun 252: 190–194.
38. Dhanabal M, Volk R, Ramchandran R, Simons M, Sukhatme VP (1999) Cloning, expression, and in vitro activity of human endostatin. Biochem Biophys Res Commun 258: 345–352.
39. Folkman J (1995) Seminars in Medicine of the Beth Israel Hospital, Boston. Clinical applications of research on angiogenesis. N Engl J Med 333: 1757–1763.
40. Capillo M, Mancuso P, Gobbi A, Monestiroli S, Pruneri G, et al. (2003) Continuous infusion of endostatin inhibits differentiation, mobilization, and clonogenic potential of endothelial cell progenitors. Clin Cancer Res 9: 377–382.
41. Kisker O, Becker CM, Prox D, Fannon M, D'Amato R, et al. (2001) Continuous administration of endostatin by intraperitoneally implanted osmotic pump improves the efficacy and potency of therapy in a mouse xenograft tumor model. Cancer Res 61: 7669–7674.
42. Scheer A, Costa T, Fanelli F, De Benedetti PG, Mhaouty-Kodja S, et al. (2000) Mutational analysis of the highly conserved arginine within the Glu/Asp-Arg-Tyr motif of the alpha(1b)-adrenergic receptor: effects on receptor isomerization and activation. Mol Pharmacol 57: 219–231.
43. Hawtin SR, Simms J, Conner M, Lawson Z, Parslow RA, et al. (2006) Charged extracellular residues, conserved throughout a G-protein-coupled receptor family, are required for ligand binding, receptor activation, and cell-surface expression. J Biol Chem 281: 38478–38488.
44. Joseph MK, Solomon LR, Petros AM, Cai J, Simmer RL, et al. (2004) Divergence of Genbank and human tumor Bcl-2 sequences and implications for binding affinity to key apoptotic proteins. Oncogene 23: 835–838.
45. Wu Y, Yang L, Hu B, Liu JY, Su JM, et al. (2005) Synergistic anti-tumor effect of recombinant human endostatin adenovirus combined with gemcitabine. Anticancer Drugs 16: 551–557.
46. Jia Y, Liu M, Huang W, Wang Z, He Y, et al. Recombinant human endostatin endostar inhibits tumor growth and metastasis in a mouse xenograft model of colon cancer. Pathol Oncol Res 18: 315–323.
47. Huang X, Wong MK, Zhao Q, Zhu Z, Wang KZ, et al. (2001) Soluble recombinant endostatin purified from Escherichia coli: antiangiogenic activity and antitumor effect. Cancer Res 61: 478–481.
48. Dong XP, Xiao TH, Dong H, Jiang N, Zhao XG Endostar combined with cisplatin inhibits tumor growth and lymphatic metastasis of lewis lung carcinoma xenografts in mice. Asian Pac J Cancer Prev 14: 3079–3083.
49. Fu XH, Li J, Zou Y, Hong YR, Fu ZX, et al. Endostar enhances the antineoplastic effects of combretastatin A4 phosphate in an osteosarcoma xenograft. Cancer Lett 312: 109–116.
50. Xu M, Xu CX, Bi WZ, Song ZG, Jia JP, et al. Effects of endostar combined multidrug chemotherapy in osteosarcoma. Bone 57: 111–115.
51. Cui C, Mao L, Chi Z, Si L, Sheng X, et al. A phase II, randomized, double-blind, placebo-controlled multicenter trial of Endostar in patients with metastatic melanoma. Mol Ther 21: 1456–1463.
52. Zhang LP, Liao XY, Xu YM, Yan LJ, Yan GF, et al. Efficacy and safety of endostar(R) combined with chemotherapy in patients with advanced soft tissue sarcomas. Asian Pac J Cancer Prev 14: 4255–4259.
53. Calvo A, Feldman AL, Libutti SK, Green JE (2002) Adenovirus-mediated endostatin delivery results in inhibition of mammary gland tumor growth in C3(1)/SV40 T-antigen transgenic mice. Cancer Res 62: 3934–3938.
54. Kerbel R, Folkman J (2002) Clinical translation of angiogenesis inhibitors. Nat Rev Cancer 2: 727–739.
55. Brandwijk RJ, Dings RP, van der Linden E, Mayo KH, Thijssen VL, et al. (2006) Anti-angiogenesis and anti-tumor activity of recombinant anginex. Biochem Biophys Res Commun 349: 1073–1078.
56. Abdollahi A, Hlatky L, Huber PE (2005) Endostatin: the logic of antiangiogenic therapy. Drug Resist Updat 8: 59–74.
57. Prokopiou EM, Ryder SA, Walsh JJ Tumour vasculature targeting agents in hybrid/conjugate drugs. Angiogenesis 16: 503–524.

5

Hepatic Resection is Safe and Effective for Patients with Hepatocellular Carcinoma and Portal Hypertension

Jian-Hong Zhong[1]☯, Hang Li[2]☯, Nan Xiao[3]☯, Xin-Ping Ye[4], Yang Ke[1], Yan-Yan Wang[1], Liang Ma[1], Jie Chen[1], Xue-Mei You[1], Zhi-Yuan Zhang[1], Shi-Dong Lu[1], Le-Qun Li[1]*

1 Hepatobiliary Surgery Department, Affiliated Tumor Hospital of Guangxi Medical University, Nanning, PR China, **2** Ultrasound Department, Affiliated Tumor Hospital of Guangxi Medical University, Nanning, PR China, **3** Department of General Surgery Education, Guangxi Medical University, Nanning, PR China, **4** Hepatobiliary Surgery Department, the First Affiliated Hospital of Guangxi Medical University, Nanning, PR China

Abstract

Background & Aims: Official guidelines do not recommend hepatic resection (HR) for patients with hepatocellular carcinoma (HCC) and portal hypertension (PHT). This study aims to investigate the safety and efficacy of HR for patients with HCC and PHT.

Methods: Mortality and survival after HR were analyzed retrospectively in a consecutive sample of 1738 HCC patients with PHT (n = 386) or without it (n = 1352). To assess the robustness of findings, we repeated the analysis using propensity score-matched analysis. We also comprehensively searched the PubMed database for studies evaluating the efficacy and safety of HR for patients with HCC and PHT.

Results: The 90-day mortality rate was 6.7% among those with PHT and 2.1% among those without it ($P<.001$). Patients without PHT had a survival benefit over those with PHT at 1, 3, and 5 years (96% vs 90%, 75% vs 67%, 54% vs 45%, respectively; $P=.001$). In contrast, PHT was not associated with worse short- or long-term survival when only propensity score-matched pairs of patients and those with early-stage HCC or those who underwent minor hepatectomy were included in the analysis (all $P>.05$). Moreover, the recurrence rates were similar between the two groups. Consistent with our findings, all 9 studies identified in our literature search reported HR to be safe and effective for patients with HCC and PHT.

Conclusions: HR is safe and effective in HCC patients with PHT and preserved liver function. This is especially true for patients who have early-stage HCC or who undergo minor hepatectomy.

Editor: Devanand Sarkar, Virginia Commonwealth University, United States of America

Funding: This work was supported by the Self-raised Scientific Research Fund of the Ministry of Health of Guangxi Province (no. Z2012345 and Z2014241) and Youth Science Foundation of Guangxi Medical University (no. GXMUYSF201302) to JHZ; and Guangxi Natural Science Foundation (no. 2011GXNSFD018032) and the HCC Bridge Study (no. CA182023) to LQL. The funders had no role in study design, data collection and analysis, decision to publish, or preparation of the manuscript.

Competing Interests: The authors have declared that no competing interests exist.

* Email: zhongjianhong66@163.com

☯ These authors contributed equally to this work.

Background

Hepatocellular carcinoma (HCC) is associated with poor prognosis. Risk factors of HCC include infection with hepatitis B virus (HBV) or hepatitis C virus (HCV) and chronic heavy alcohol consumption, which leads to liver cirrhosis [1]. Thus cirrhosis is common among HCC patients; in China, for example, it occurs in approximately 80% of HCC patients [2,3]. Another common comorbidity of HCC is clinically significant portal hypertension (PHT), which occurs in 25–55% of patients with both HCC and cirrhosis [4–6]. PHT correlates with the severity of cirrhosis, and it can complicate HCC treatment by increasing the risk of perioperative hemorrhage and liver failure.

Hepatic resection (HR) is a widely used radical therapy for HCC. Although HR is often suitable for HCC patients with cirrhosis, it is widely regarded as unsuitable for HCC patients with PHT [7,8] because of the potential for postoperative hepatic decompensation [9]. In fact, the absence of PHT is the best predictor of excellent HR outcomes [7,8]. Guidelines of the American and European Associations for the Study of Liver Disease do not recommend HR as an option for HCC patients with PHT [10,11]. Several studies, however, have reported that HCC patients with and without clinically significant PHT showed similar short- and long-term outcomes after HR [12–14]. This controversy is important to resolve because more than 25% of cirrhotic patients with HCC also present with PHT [4–6].

The present study aimed to address the safety and efficacy of HR for HCC patients with PHT using a population from Guangxi province of China, where the population shows the highest HCC incidence in the world [4]. Subgroup analyses were conducted based on tumor stage and extent of hepatectomy. To complement this clinical study, we searched the PubMed database for studies evaluating the efficacy of HR for HCC patients with PHT. Our goal was to clarify the indications for HR in patients with or without PHT.

Patients and Methods

Ethics statement

This study was approved by the Institutional Review Board of Guangxi Medical University, and it was conducted in accordance with the Declaration of Helsinki and current ethical guidelines. Written consent was given by the patients for their information to be stored in hospital databases and used for research. The hospital records data were de-identified and analyzed anonymously.

Patients

Retrospective analysis was carried out on medical records of patients diagnosed with HCC who had been included in prospective databases at the Tumor Hospital and First Affiliated Hospital of Guangxi Medical University, the two major hospitals in Guangxi province. We planned to investigate the safety and efficacy of HR in patients with HCC and concomitant PHT by comparing survival data for patients with or without PHT. Patients were included in this analysis if they satisfied the inclusion criteria (Table 1). Curative resection was defined as any operation in which all tumors were resected macroscopically. Patients who satisfied the inclusion criteria were divided into two groups based on the presence or absence of PHT.

Definitions

PHT. Since venous pressure is not routinely measured directly in most of the included patients, we defined PTH indirectly as the presence of gastric and/or esophageal varices detectable by endoscopy and/or computed tomography (CT), the presence of splenomegaly (pedicle rib unit >5) with a platelet count of <100,000/mm^3, or the presence of hypertensive gastropathy [15,16]. One of the three criterias exist implys the presence of PHT.

Major and minor hepatectomy. Major hepatectomy was defined as the resection of three or more Couinaud segments; minor hepactectomy, as the resection of fewer than three segments [17]. The decision whether to perform major or minor hepatectomy was based on the location and diameter of HCC and liver function tests.

Mortality and Morbidity. Postoperative mortality was analyzed as death within 30 and 90 days after surgery. Postoperative complications were assessed using the Clavien-Dindo classification [18].

Tumor Stage. Tumor stages were defined as before [4,19].

Diagnosis of HCC

Tumor status was assessed by ultrasonography, CT scanning, magnetic resonance imaging, and/or hepatic angiography. Since our centers did not begin using the indocyanine green test until 2010, data for this test were not used in our analysis. Vascular invasion was defined by the presence of a thrombus adjacent to the tumor in the portal and hepatic veins with vague boundaries confirmed using at least two imaging modalities [20]. In all patients, diagnosis of HCC was confirmed by histopathological examination of surgical samples.

Treatment and follow-up

The indications for HR at our centers have already been published [4,21,22]. In brief, surgery was indicated when ascites and hepatic encephalopathy were absent. HR was not carried out in patients with intermediate or advanced cirrhosis and with Child-Pugh B or C liver function. Adequate remnant liver volume, as determined by volumetric CT, was 30% for HCC patients without cirrhosis, and >50% for HCC patients with chronic hepatitis, cirrhosis, or severe fatty liver. Patients who satisfied the indication for HR were treated by HR unless the patient requested other treatment modality.

Endoscopy was routinely carried out before HR. Intraoperative ultrasound was routinely performed to determine tumor location and assess the vascular anatomy of the liver. To minimize perioperative blood loss, Pringle's maneuver was carried out intermittently, each time for less than 20 minutes, with a clamp-free interval of 5 min. In most cases, the resection margin was more than 1 cm. Adequate drainage was monitored. Splenectomy, splenic embolization, and endoscopic treatments such as variceal band ligation and sclerotherapy were not performed. None of the patients underwent preoperative portal vein embolization or received portosystemic shunts before or during HR. None of the patients in our study was treated as an emergency.

After HR, all patients were periodically examined at follow-up to detect possible recurrence of HCC using liver function tests, measurement of serum alpha-fetoprotein (AFP), abdominal ultrasonography, and chest radiography. These follow-up visits were conducted every 2–3 months during the first postoperative year and every 6 months thereafter. Postoperative enhanced CT was performed every 6 months [21].

Recurrence was diagnosed on the basis of two concurring imaging techniques or the combination of increased AFP and consistent ultrasonography or CT findings, and defined as the appearance of a new lesion with radiologic features characteristic of HCC. In patients who showed recurrence or resectable extrahepatic metastasis after initial treatment, HR was performed if it was judged feasible on the basis of liver function and remnant liver volume, which were evaluated according to the same criteria as those used at the time of initial resection. If HR could not be performed because of poor liver function or other unfavorable

Table 1. Inclusion Criteria for Retrospective Analysis of HR Outcomes in HCC Patients with and without PHT.

	Inclusion criteria
a.	Patients underwent initial hepatic resection at one of our two liver centers
b.	Patients had cirrhosis but with Child-Pugh A liver function and underwent potentially curative hepatic resection, regardless of tumor size, tumor number, macrovascular invasion
c.	Patients showed no evidence of metastasis to the lymph nodes and/or distant metastases on the basis of preoperative imaging results and perioperative findings
d.	Patients suffered no malignancy other than HCC for 5 years prior to the initial HCC treatment

factors, then transarterial chemoembolization, radiofrequency ablation, or sorafenib therapy were applied [4].

Statistical analysis

All demographic and clinicopathological data had been prospectively collected in computer databases prior to this retrospective analysis. Continuous data were expressed as median (range). The statistical significance of differences in continuous data was analyzed using the Mann-Whitney *U* test, and the significance of differences between categorical data was assessed with the chi-squared test. Survival curves were estimated using the Kaplan-Meier method and compared using the log-rank test. Multivariate analysis to identify independent prognostic factors was carried out using the Cox proportional hazards model. For all tests, a two-tailed P value<0.05 was considered statistically significant. All statistical analyses were performed using the SPSS 19.0 statistical package (IBM, USA).

Propensity score analysis

In order to reduce confounding and selection bias, propensity score analysis was conducted using logistic regression to create propensity scores for HCC patients with or without PHT [23]. Clinical variables already proposed as important for HR outcomes [4,21] were assembled into a logistic regression model, which was used to generate propensity scores for each patient along a continuous range from 0 to 1. The one-to-one nearest-neighbor matching method was used to generate pairs of patients in which one had PHT and the other did not [4,21].

Literature review

We comprehensively searched the PubMed database using the following medical subject headings (MeSH): "*hepatocellular carcinoma* or *liver cancer* or *liver carcinoma*" and "*liver resection* or *hepatic resection* or *hepatectomy* or *surgery*" and "*portal hypertension* or *portal venous pressure*". Manual searching of relevant references and review articles was also performed. Studies were included in our review if they (a) evaluated the efficacy of HR for primary HCC patients with PHT and provided survival data, (b) were published in English and (c) were published between January 2000 and February 2014. Studies evaluating HR to treat recurrent HCC were excluded. In the case of multiple studies based on the same population, we selected the study with the largest number of participants.

Results

Characteristics of the study population

Between January 2007 and December 2010, a total of 5257 patients with HCC were prospectively registered in the databases of our centers. Based on the inclusion criteria, 386 HCC patients with PHT and 1352 patients without PHT were included in the present study. Baseline demographic and clinicopathological data for the 1738 patients (Table 2) showed that more than 90% had HBV-related HCC, whereas less than 2.6% of patients were infected with HCV.

Patients with PHT had worse liver function, i.e. lower platelet count and albumin concentration, longer prothrombin time, and higher concentrations of alanine aminotransferase and bilirubin (all P<.05). More patients with PHT underwent minor hepatectomy (P<.001).

Anatomic HR was the preferred surgical procedures. Most patients with multiple tumors underwent two or more concomitant HR. The feasibility of anatomic HR was significantly lower in the PHT group than in the non-PHT group. However, the surgical time and blood loss were similar between the two groups.

Morbidity and mortality in the entire study population

Patients with PHT had a significantly higher morbidity rate (31%) than those without PHT (23%, P = .004). However, most of the complications were grade I or II (Table 3). Patients with or without PHT showed similar 30-day mortality (2.3% vs 1.0%, P = .051), while patients with PHT showed significantly higher 90-day mortality (6.7% vs 2.1%, P<.001).

Among patients who underwent minor hepatectomy, 90-day mortality was similar between those who had PHT (4/147, 2.7%) and those who did not (2/379, 0.5%; P = .07). Among patients who underwent major hepatectomy, 90-day mortality was higher among those with PHT (22/239 or 9.2% vs 26/973 or 2.7%; P<.001).

Survival analysis in the entire study population

During a median follow-up of 39.3 months (range, 1–152.4), 198 patients with PHT (51.3%) died, compared to 549 patients without PHT (40.6%). These included 582 (78%) patients died of HCC recurrence, 38 (5%) died of liver failure without evidence of recurrence, and 127 (17%) died of other diseases. Median survival time was 69.2 months in patients without PHT, compared to 48.1 months in patients with PHT (P<.001). Overall survival (OS) at 1, 3, and 5 years was 90%, 67%, and 45% for patients with PHT, and 96%, 75%, and 54% for patients without (P = .001; Fig. 1A).

However, cumulative recurrence rates were similar between the PHT group and non-PHT group at 1 year (30% vs 28%), 3 years (50% vs 46%), and 5 years (60% vs 55%; P = .11). Moreover, the sizes and number of recurrent tumors, and the proportion of patients with recurrence in whom a second HR was indicated were similar between the two groups (Table 4). OS in each group was better among the patients with recurrence who underwent a second HR as compared with those who did not.

Univariate analysis identified the following prognostic risk factors in the total population: tumor number ≥3, serum AFP ≥400 ng/mL, serum albumin <4 g/dL, serum alanine aminotransferase >80 U/L, serum bilirubin >1.2 mg/dL, macrovascular invasion, major hepatectomy, and PHT. All these factors, except serum albumin, were also identified in multivariate Cox proportional hazard modeling as independent predictors of poor prognosis (Table 5).

Subgroup analysis by Barcelona group tumor stage

We examined whether the efficacy of HR depended on tumor stage. Among the 455 patients with early-stage HCC (26% of the total), patients with and without PHT had similar OS at 1 year (96% vs 99%), 3 years (80% vs 89%), and 5 years (63% vs 75%) (P = .108; Fig. 2A). However, among the 824 patients with intermediate-stage HCC (47%), patients with PHT had significantly worse OS than those without PHT at 1 year (94% vs 97%), 3 years (69% vs 77%), and 5 years (45% vs 56%) (P = .004; Fig. 2B). Similar results were observed among the 459 patients with advanced-stage HCC (27%), which was defined as HCC with macrovascular invasion: patients with PHT had significantly worse OS at 1 year (78% vs 91%), 3 years (43% vs 60%), and 5 years (20% vs 34%) (P = .001; Fig. 2C).

Subgroup analysis by major or minor hepatectomy

Of our 1738 patients, 1212 (70%) underwent major hepatectomy. Their OS was significantly lower if they had PHT: 88% vs 95% (1 year), 59% vs 73% (3 years), and 30% vs 50% (5 years)

Table 2. Preoperative Clinicopathological Data of Patients with HCC and Child-Pugh A Liver Function who Underwent HR.

Variable	Before propensity matching			After propensity matching		
	Without PHT (n = 1352)	With PHT (n = 386)	*P* value	Without PHT (n = 224)	With PHT (n = 224)	*P* value
Median age in yr (range)	53 (19–80)	46 (17–90)	<.001	53 (19–76)	51 (19–82)	.472
Gender, M/F (%)	1221 (90.3)/131 (9.7)	344 (89.1)/42 (10.9)	.529	198 (88.4)/26 (11.6)	201 (89.7)/23 (10.3)	.650
Median tumor size in cm (range)	6.3 (2.0–18.0)	6.0 (1.0–21.0)	.060	6.0 (2.0–28.0)	6.0 (1.0–20.0)	.703
No. (%) of patients with <3/≥3 tumors	1247 (92)/105 (8)	347 (90)/39 (10)	.241	207 (92)/17 (8)	202 (90)/22 (10)	.402
No. (%) of patients +/− for hepatitis B surface antigen	1230 (91)/120 (9)	351 (91)/35 (9)	.735	199 (89)/25 (11)	199 (89)/25 (11)	.000
No. (%) of patients positive for hepatitis C antibody	31 (2.3)	10 (2.6)	.861	7 (3.1)	6 (2.7)	.778
Serum AFP, n (%)						
≥400 ng/mL	610 (45)	174 (45)	.988	101 (45)	103 (46)	.850
<400 ng/mL	742 (55)	212 (55)		123 (55)	121 (54)	
Median platelet count, $\times 10^3$ μ/L (range)	210 (68–528)	158 (46–533)	<.001	173 (48–600)	168 (46–533)	.504
Median prothrombin time, s (range)	12 (2–32)	14 (6–28)	<.001	14 (5–32)	14 (6–24)	.647
Median albumin, g/dL (range)	3.9 (2.3–6.2)	3.8 (2.2–5.0)	<.001	3.8 (2.8–4.9)	3.8 (2.7–5.0)	.370
Median alanine aminotransferase, U/L (range)	48 (12–185)	65 (18–260)	<.001	58 (15–185)	61 (18–220)	.879
Median total bilirubin, mg/dL (range)	0.9 (0.1–4.7)	1.2 (0.3–12.9)	<.001	1.1 (0.2–4.7)	1.1 (0.3–4.1)	.175
BCLC tumor stage, n (%)						
Early	339 (25)	116 (30)	.069	63 (28)	72 (32)	.354
Intermediate	650 (48)	174 (45)	.303	98 (44)	92 (41)	.650
Advanced (macrovascular invasion)	363 (27)	96 (25)	.521	63 (28)	60 (27)	.751
Major hepatectomy, n (%)	973 (72)	239 (62)	<.001	155 (69)	146 (65)	.370
30-day mortality, n (%)	13 (1.0)	9 (2.3)	.051	4 (1.8)	4 (1.8)	.000
90-day mortality, n (%)	28 (2.1)	26 (6.7)	<.001	7 (3.1)	6 (2.1)	.780
Postoperative complications, n (%)	311 (23)	120 (31)	.004	47 (21)	63 (28)	.080
Median survival time in mos. (range)	69 (1–152)	48 (1–132)	<.001	64 (1–129)	47 (1–106)	<.001

AFP, α-fetoprotein; BCLC, Barcelona Clinic Liver Cancer; PHT, portal hypertension.

Table 3. Postoperative Complications in HCC Patients with or without PHT After HR, Assessed Using the Clavien-Dindo Classification Scheme.

Grade	No. (%) of patients		*P* value
	Without PHT (n = 1352)	With PHT (n = 386)	
I	252 (18.6)	104 (26.9)	.007
II	181 (13.4)	67 (17.4)	
III-a	81 (6.0)	30 (7.8)	
III-b	55 (4.1)	21 (5.5)	
IV-a	30 (2.2)	30 (7.8)	
IV-b	51 (3.8)	16 (4.1)	
V	28 (2.1)	26 (6.7)	

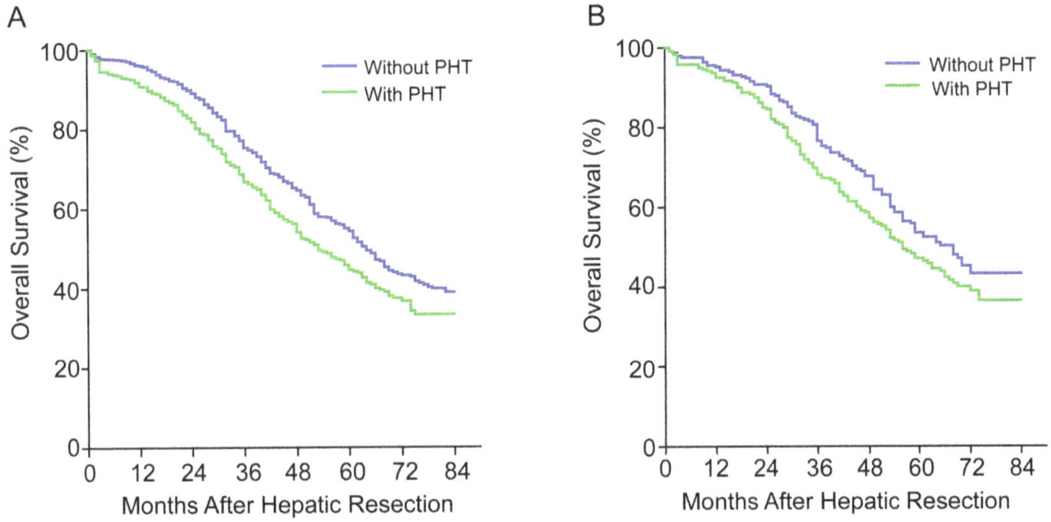

Figure 1. Overall survival curves of the population undergoing HR for HCC with and without PHT. (A) Total population ($P<.001$). (B) Propensity score-matched population ($P=.061$).

($P<.001$; Fig. 2D). However, among the 526 (30%) patients who underwent minor resection, PHT was not associated with worse OS: 1 year, 95% vs 98%; 3 years, 77% vs 87%; and 5 years, 59% vs 71% ($P=.064$; Fig. 2E).

Characteristics and survival analysis of propensity-matched patients

Propensity score analysis based on variables associated with prognosis identified 224 matched pairs of patients. When only these pairs were considered, no significant baseline difference between the two groups was observed (Table 2). Patients selected in the propensity-matching model with PHT did not show significantly worse survival than did those without PHT ($P=.061$; Fig. 1B). The 1, 3, and 5 years OS was 92%, 68%, and 46% for patients with PHT, and 95%, 76%, and 52% for patients without PHT. Cumulative recurrence rates at 1 (26% vs 29%), 3 (45% vs 51%), and 5 years (56% vs 65%) were similar between patients with and without PHT ($P=.21$).

Patients with and without PHT had similar morbidity (28% vs 21%, $P=.08$), 30-day mortality (1.8% vs 1.8%, $P=1.00$), and 90-day mortality (2.1% vs 3.1%, $P=.78$). The multivariate Cox proportional hazards model identified tumor number (≥3), serum AFP (≥400 ng/mL), macrovascular invasion, major hepatectomy, and PHT as mortality risk factors (Table 5).

Literature review

A comprehensive search of the PubMed database identified 9 studies that satisfied the inclusion criteria; they examined HCC patients with and without PHT who were treated by HR in Italy [5,12–14,24], Korea [25], and Japan [26–28] and who had been recruited between 1982 and 2012 (Table 6). Hospital mortality at 3 months was less than 5% for patients without PHT, while it was more than 6% for patients with PHT. Interestingly, the study [28] that recruited patients starting in 1982 reported 1-month mortality as high as 12.9%, while the study [12] that recruited patients starting in 1985 reported 2-month mortality of 11.1%. The downward trend of mortality reflects the improvement of surgical techniques.

The 5-year OS after HR ranged from 29% to 75% for patients with HCC and PHT, and 31% to 79% for patients without PHT (Table 6). In 6 studies, median survival was significantly longer for patients without PHT [5,12,14,24–26], while 3 studies found

Table 4. Characteristics and treatment modalities for recurrence.

Variable		Without PHT (n = 1352)	With PHT (n = 386)	*P* value
Number of recurrence		798 (59%)	248 (64%)	.064
Median tumor size in cm (range)		1.4 (0.7–3.8)	1.3 (0.8–3.6)	.156
Site of recurrence	Extrahepatic	200 (25%)	22 (9%)	<.001
	Intrahepatic	598 (75%)	226 (91%)	
Tumor number of intraheaptic recurrence	Single	310 (41%)	94 (38%)	.396
	Multiple	447 (59%)	154 (62%)	
Treatment for recurrence	Second resection	311 (39%)	87 (35%)	.276
	Transarterial chemoembolization	479 (60%)	156 (63%)	
	Radiofrequency ablation	8 (1%)	5 (2%)	

Table 5. Multivariate Analysis of Clinicopathological Factors Predictive of Poor Overall Survival.

Variable	Before propensity matching			After propensity matching		
	Hazard ratio	95% confidence interval	*P* value	Hazard ratio	95% confidence interval	*P* value
Tumor number≥3	1.543	1.233–1.931	<.001	1.543	1.045–2.277	.029
α-fetoprotein≥400 ng/mL	1.321	1.171–1.491	<.001	1.263	1.015–1.572	.037
Albumin<4 g/dL	0.880	0.776–1.026	.120	0.902	0.715–1.138	.386
Alanine aminotransferase>80 U/L	1.196	1.007–1.421	.041	0.978	0.756–1.265	.866
Bilirubin>1.2 mg/dL	1.161	1.010–1.334	.035	0.950	0.757–1.191	.654
Macrovascular invasion	1.541	1.341–1.769	<.001	1.415	1.100–1.821	.007
Major hepatectomy	1.232	1.142–1.662	.021	1.025	1.080–1.523	.046
Portal hypertension	1.830	1.554–2.154	<.001	1.609	1.285–2.013	<.001

similar median survival between the two patient groups [13,27,28]. All 9 studies identified in our review explicitly concluded that PHT should not be considered an absolute contraindication for HR in cirrhotic patients [5,12–14,24–28].

Discussion

Historically HR has been applied with caution to HCC patients because of concerns about morbidity and mortality; indeed mortality rates with HR used to exceed 10%. However, recent improvements in surgical technique and perioperative care have improved HR outcomes even as the procedure has been extended to more high-risk patients; some major liver centers now report hospital mortality below 5% [29,30]. Nevertheless selecting patients for HR remains important. For example, PHT may increase the risk of perioperative hemorrhage, impair liver regeneration, and increase the risk of liver failure, leading the American and European Associations for the Study of Liver Disease to classify PHT as a contraindication to HR. These guidelines are based on Barcelona group studies of very small sample size [7,8], and they conflict with larger studies showing that HCC patients with and without clinically significant PHT show similar short- and long-term outcomes after HR [12–14]. Given the high frequency of PHT among HCC patients in China [4] and elsewhere [11], it is important to resolve this lack of consensus on whether HR is safe and effective for such patients.

In this clinical study of a large cohort of patients from a region in which more than 77% of HCC is associated with cirrhosis [4], OS for HCC patients with PHT after HR was 67% at 3 years and 45% at 5 years. OS at 1, 3, and 5 years for both the two groups was similar to survival results reported by studies that we identified in a comprehensive review of PubMed. In contrast to our results, some of those previous studies found similarly good OS in patients with and without PHT (Table 6).

Our previous study reported that HR of patients with intermediate- and advanced-stage HCC and PHT gave better survival than transarterial chemoembolization [4], and another study reported that HR was associated with longer survival and time to recurrence than radiofrequency ablation [31]. For Child-Pugh A cirrhotic patients with a single HCC up to 5 cm, HR offers a similar 5-year OS to liver transplantation, even for patients with PHT [32,33]. However, the liver donation is shortage in most countries. In this way, we take a different position from that of the American and European guidelines, recent seminars [11,34,35] and consensus statements of the Asian Pacific Association for the Study of the Liver [36], the Japan Society of Hepatology [37], and the American Hepato-Pancreato-Biliary Association [38].

Though we argue for expanding HR to HCC patients with PHT, we emphasize that patient selection remains critical for success. The two most important selection criteria in our study were preoperative Child-Pugh A liver function and >50% postoperative residual liver volume. Careful application of these rigorous selection criteria may explain why patients with and without PHT showed similar OS after being stratified by Barcelona group tumor stage or extent of hepatectomy. It may also explain why 90-day mortality was similar between patients with and without PHT who underwent minor resection. Our findings suggest that as long as appropriate inclusion criteria are strictly applied, there is no absolute contraindication of HR for treating HCC patients with PHT.

Indeed, we suggest that our strict selection process explains why the mortality of our population of patients with PHT and early-, intermediate- or advanced-stage HCC was 6.7% (26/386), whereas the mortality of an earlier group of patients we studied with PHT and intermediate- or advanced-stage HCC was 10.3% (17/166) [4]. The present cohort was recruited over the period from 2007 to 2010, while the earlier cohort was recruited from 2000 to 2007. This suggests gradual improvement in mortality over time. In fact, some liver centers have reported zero perioperative mortality during HR of HCC patients [30,39]. These findings provide further support for our suggestion that, largely due to improvements in surgical technique and medical care, HR is safe for HCC patients with PHT, especially for those with early-stage HCC and those undergoing minor resection.

Some studies suggest that PHT is an independent risk factor of morbidity and mortality [4,8,40,41]. The main risks of HR in patients with PHT are liver failure, varices rupture, and coagulation disorders caused by thrombocytopenia. Patients with PHT tended to have poorer preoperative liver function than those without PHT (Table 2), even though all our patients had Child-Pugh A liver function. Patients with PHT showed a higher morbidity rate (31%) than those without PHT (23%); nevertheless, most postoperative complications were Clavien-Dindo grade I or II. Of the 26 patients who died within 90 days of HR in the PHT group, 15 underwent major hepatectomy and died from postoperative liver failure, 5 died from varices rupture, and 3 died from thrombocytopenia. The remaining 3 patients had concurrent liver failure and varices rupture. Therefore we recommend selecting patients with PHT carefully for major hepatectomy, especially when preoperative liver function is unsatisfactory, regardless of

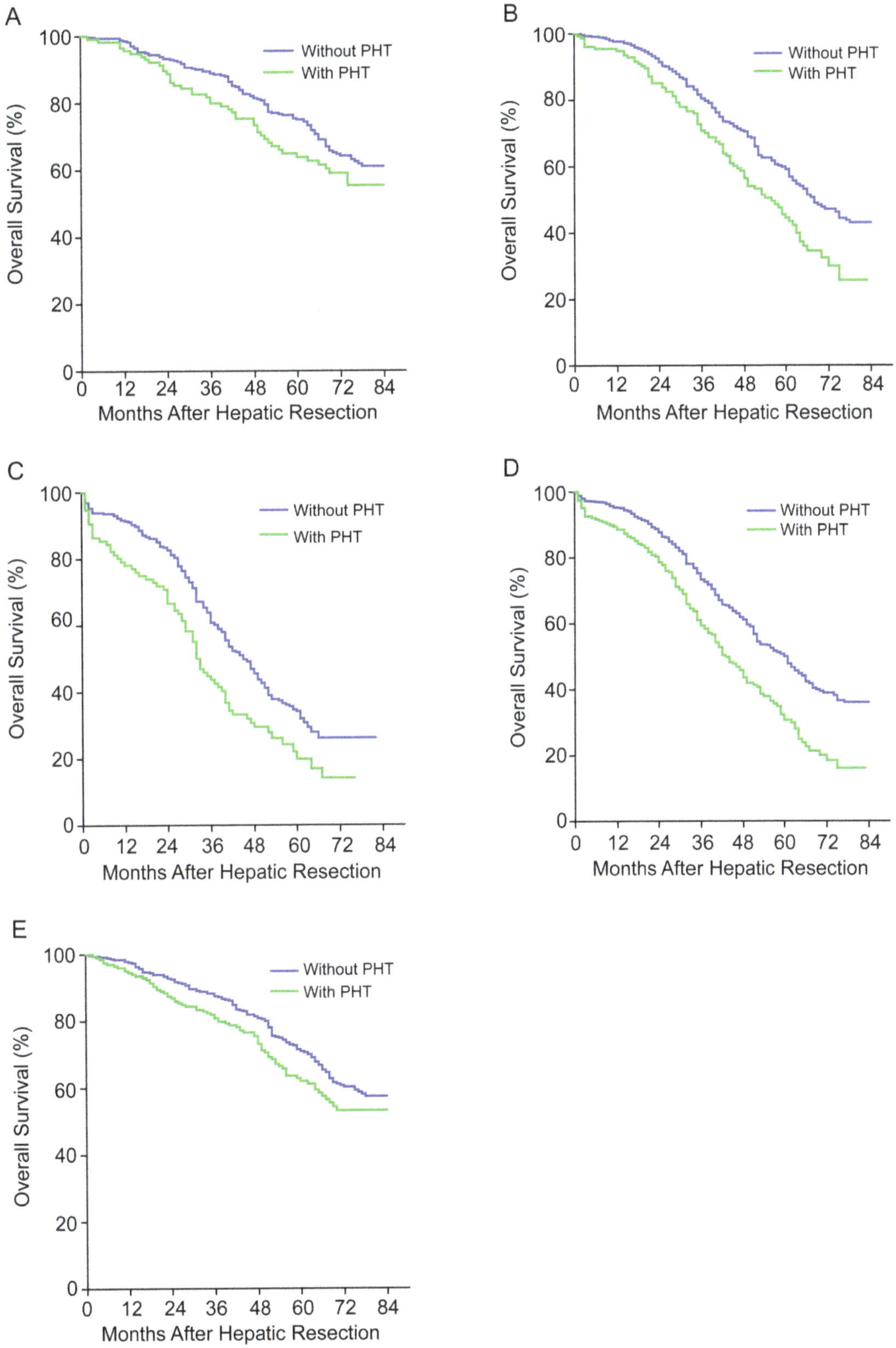

Figure 2. Overall survival curves of subgroup analysis. (A) Early-stage HCC (P = .108). (B) Intermediate-stage HCC (P = .004). (C) Advanced-stage HCC (P = .001). (D) Major hepatectomy (P<.001). (E) Minor hepatectomy (P = .064).

Table 6. Characteristics and Outcomes of Patients with PHT Following Curative Resection of HCC, Based on a Literature Review.

Study	Patient origins	Recruitment period	N (no PHT/PHT)	Without PHT (%)				With PHT (%)			
				Mortality	1 yr OS	3 yr OS	5 yr OS	Mortality	1 yr OS	3 yr OS	5 yr OS
Capussotti et al[12]	Italy	1985–2003	118/99	5.1 (2 m)	76	62	40	11.1 (2 m)	71	45	29
Choi et al[24]	Korea	1996–2006	53/47	1.9 (1 m)	92	79	79	6.4 (1 m)	77	48	38
Cucchetti et al[5]	Italy	1997–2007	152/89	-	-	73	62	-	-	62	52
Giannini et al[13]	Italy	1987–2008	70/42	-	98	82	60	-	100	87	75
Hidaka et al[25]	Japan	1997–2009	129/48*	-	92	78	64	-	73	49	31
Ishizawa et al[26]	Japan	1994–2004	250/136	-	-	81 and 62†	71 and 31†	-	-	71 and 59†	56 and 41†
Kawano et al[27]	Japan	1982–2003	103/31	8.7 (1 m)	-	-	48	12.9 (1 m)	-	-	70
Ruzzenente et al[14]	Italy	1995–2008	91/44	3.3 (3 m)	-	68	61	13.6 (3 m)	-	49	45
Santambrogio et al[23]	Italy and France	1997–2012	160/63	1.9 (3 m)	-	80	65	6.3 (3 m)	-	66	48
This study	China	2007–2010	1352/386	2.1 (3 m)	98	81	60	6.7 (3 m)	91	72	37

* patients were divided into a group with high portal venous pressure ($\geq$20 cmH_2O) and a group with low portal venous pressure (<20 cmH_2O);
† Child-Pugh class A cirrhosis and Child-Pugh class B cirrhosis.

whether the expected remnant liver volume is more than 50%. Major hepatectomy may, in fact, aggravate PHT because it reduces the hepatic parenchymal mass. For HCC patients whose PHT poses a problem for HR, alternative therapies or a reduction in the extent of hepatectomy may be preferable.

In HCC patients with severe gastric and/or esophageal varices, it may be possible to reduce the rate of varices rupture by using preoperative endoscopic treatments and/or splenectomy with or without devascularization of the abdominal esophagus and the upper part of the stomach [27].

Platelet count less than 150,000/mm^3 is independently associated with increased major complications and mortality [15,29]. Preoperative platelet transfusion was performed in the 3 patients who ultimately died from thrombocytopenia; these outcomes may reflect the difficulties of controlling coagulation disorders effectively once the patient has been discharged. In our experience, HR should be selected with caution when preoperative platelet counts are less than 75,000/mm^3.

Preoperative hepatic venous pressure gradient (HVPG) was not routinely assessed in patients with PHT. HVPG correlates with the severity of PHT [42]. Elevated HVPG (median levels of 11–12 mmHg) is associated with postoperative liver dysfunction and mortality after HR in patients with HCC and cirrhosis [38,42,43], independently of esophageal varices, splenomegaly and thrombocytopenia [39]. In one of those studies [40], 26 patients were diagnosed with PHT using indirect methods, but only 18 of these had an HVPG $\geq$10 mmHg, which Barcelona group studies[7,8] have proposed as the cut-off when HPVG becomes an independent risk predictor of liver dysfunction. This suggests that some patients diagnosed with PHT by indirect methods do not fulfill the Barcelona group cut-off, highlighting the need for direct measurement of preoperative HVPG measurement in patients with clinically significant PHT.

Our multivariate Cox modeling to identify prognostic factors in HCC patients with or without PHT led to similar conclusions as previous studies: patients with high preoperative AFP [4], alanine aminotransferase [21] and bilirubin levels [8], multinodularity [44], macrovascular invasion [4], history of major resection [45], and PHT [41] had significantly worse outcomes than did other patients after HR. However, when this analysis was repeated using propensity-matched patient pairs, elevated alanine aminotransferase and bilirubin were not identified as risk factors. Elevated AFP can be a useful prognostic marker in patients with HCC who do not show any well-established risk factors. Multinodularity and macrovascular invasion are risk factors presumably because they have been linked to the emergence of *de novo* tumors and HCC recurrence, respectively [34,46,47]. Our finding of PHT as an independent risk predictor may explain the high 90-day mortality (6.7%) among patients with PHT. When we repeated the multivariate analysis after excluding 73 patients who survived fewer than 20 months after surgery, PHT remained a significant risk factor. PHT may be such a strong risk factor at least in part because it so often co-occurs with severe cirrhosis, which on its own is an independent risk factor for carcinogenesis.

Even though our patients came from the region with the highest incidence of HCC in the world [4], we believe our results are generalizable to other populations because our findings are consistent with an extensive literature review in which we identified studies of patient populations in several other countries.

Conclusions

Our clinical studies at two large liver care centers together with our literature review strongly suggest that HR is safe and effective for HCC patients with PHT and preserved liver function, especially for those with Barcelona group early-stage HCC and those who undergo minor hepatectomy.

Author Contributions

Conceived and designed the experiments: JHZ. Performed the experiments: JHZ LQL YK. Analyzed the data: JHZ LM YK HL YYW JC ZYZ SDL. Contributed reagents/materials/analysis tools: JHZ XMY NX XPY. Wrote the paper: JHZ.

References

1. Zhong JH, Ma L, Wu LC, Zhao W, Yuan WP, et al. (2012) Adoptive immunotherapy for postoperative hepatocellular carcinoma: a systematic review. Int J Clin Pract 66: 21–27.
2. Chen XP, Qiu FZ, Wu ZD, Zhang ZW, Huang ZY, et al. (2006) Long-term outcome of resection of large hepatocellular carcinoma. Br J Surg 93: 600–606.
3. Zhou XD, Tang ZY, Ma ZC, Wu ZQ, Fan J, et al. (2003) Surgery for large primary liver cancer more than 10 cm in diameter. J Cancer Res Clin Oncol 129: 543–548.
4. Zhong JH, Ke Y, Gong WF, Xiang BD, Ma L, et al. (2014) Hepatic Resection Associated With Good Survival for Selected Patients With Intermediate and Advanced-Stage Hepatocellular Carcinoma. Ann Surg. 260: 329–340.
5. Cucchetti A, Ercolani G, Vivarelli M, Cescon M, Ravaioli M, et al. (2009) Is portal hypertension a contraindication to hepatic resection? Ann Surg 250: 922–928.
6. Alswat KA, Sanai FM, Altuwaijri M, Albenmousa A, Almadi M, et al. (2013) Clinical characteristics of patients with hepatocellular carcinoma in a middle eastern population. Hepat Mon 13: e7612.
7. Bruix J, Castells A, Bosch J, Feu F, Fuster J, et al. (1996) Surgical resection of hepatocellular carcinoma in cirrhotic patients: prognostic value of preoperative portal pressure. Gastroenterology 111: 1018–1022.
8. Llovet JM, Fuster J, Bruix J (1999) Intention-to-treat analysis of surgical treatment for early hepatocellular carcinoma: resection versus transplantation. Hepatology 30: 1434–1440.
9. El-Serag HB, Marrero JA, Rudolph L, Reddy KR (2008) Diagnosis and treatment of hepatocellular carcinoma. Gastroenterology 134: 1752–1763.
10. Bruix J, Sherman M (2011) Management of hepatocellular carcinoma: an update. Hepatology 53: 1020–1022.
11. European Association For The Study Of The Liverl; European Organisation For Research And Treatment Of Cancer (2012) EASL-EORTC clinical practice guidelines: management of hepatocellular carcinoma. J Hepatol 56: 908–943.
12. Capussotti L, Ferrero A, Vigano L, Muratore A, Polastri R, et al. (2006) Portal hypertension: contraindication to liver surgery? World J Surg 30: 992–999.
13. Giannini EG, Savarino V, Farinati F, Ciccarese F, Rapaccini G, et al. (2013) Influence of clinically significant portal hypertension on survival after hepatic resection for hepatocellular carcinoma in cirrhotic patients. Liver Int 33: 1594–1600.
14. Ruzzenente A, Valdegamberi A, Campagnaro T, Conci S, Pachera S, et al. (2011) Hepatocellular carcinoma in cirrhotic patients with portal hypertension: is liver resection always contraindicated? World J Gastroenterol 17: 5083–5088.
15. Maithel SK, Kneuertz PJ, Kooby DA, Scoggins CR, Weber SM, et al. (2011) Importance of low preoperative platelet count in selecting patients for resection of hepatocellular carcinoma: a multi-institutional analysis. J Am Coll Surg 212: 638–648.
16. de Franchis R (2005) Evolving consensus in portal hypertension. Report of the Baveno IV consensus workshop on methodology of diagnosis and therapy in portal hypertension. J Hepatol 43: 167–176.
17. Belghiti J, Clavien PA, Gadzijev E, Garden JO, Lau WY, et al. (2000) The Brisbane 2000 terminology of liver anatomy and resections. HPB (Oxford) 2: 333–339.
18. Dindo D, Demartines N, Clavien PA (2004) Classification of surgical complications: a new proposal with evaluation in a cohort of 6336 patients and results of a survey. Ann Surg 240: 205–213.
19. Torzilli G, Belghiti J, Kokudo N, Takayama T, Capussotti L, et al. (2013) A snapshot of the effective indications and results of surgery for hepatocellular carcinoma in tertiary referral centers: is it adherent to the EASL/AASLD recommendations?: an observational study of the HCC East-West study group. Ann Surg 257: 929–37.
20. Kikuchi LO, Paranagua-Vezozzo DC, Chagas AL, Mello ES, Alves VA, et al. (2009) Nodules less than 20 mm and vascular invasion are predictors of survival in small hepatocellular carcinoma. J Clin Gastroenterol 43: 191–195.
21. Zhong JH, Xiang BD, Gong WF, Ke Y, Mo QG, et al. (2013) Comparison of long-term survival of patients with BCLC stage B hepatocellular carcinoma after liver resection or transarterial chemoembolization. PLoS One 8: e68193.
22. Ke Y, Ma L, You XM, Huang SX, Liang YR, et al. (2013) Antiviral therapy for hepatitis B virus-related hepatocellular carcinoma after radical hepatectomy. Cancer Biol Med 10: 158–164.
23. D'Agostino RB Jr (1998) Propensity score methods for bias reduction in the comparison of a treatment to a non-randomized control group. Stat Med 17: 2265–2281.
24. Santambrogio R, Kluger MD, Costa M, Belli A, Barabino M, et al. (2013) Hepatic resection for hepatocellular carcinoma in patients with Child-Pugh's A cirrhosis: is clinical evidence of portal hypertension a contraindication? HPB (Oxford) 15: 78–84.
25. Choi GH, Park JY, Hwang HK, Kim DH, Kang CM, et al. (2011) Predictive factors for long-term survival in patients with clinically significant portal hypertension following resection of hepatocellular carcinoma. Liver Int 31: 485–493.
26. Hidaka M, Takatsuki M, Soyama A, Tanaka T, Muraoka I, et al. (2012) Intraoperative portal venous pressure and long-term outcome after curative resection for hepatocellular carcinoma. Br J Surg 99: 1284–1289.
27. Ishizawa T, Hasegawa K, Aoki T, Takahashi M, Inoue Y, et al. (2008) Neither multiple tumors nor portal hypertension are surgical contraindications for hepatocellular carcinoma. Gastroenterology 134: 1908–1916.
28. Kawano Y, Sasaki A, Kai S, Endo Y, Iwaki K, et al. (2008) Short- and long-term outcomes after hepatic resection for hepatocellular carcinoma with concomitant esophageal varices in patients with cirrhosis. Ann Surg Oncol 15: 1670–1676.
29. Poon RT, Fan ST, Lo CM, Liu CL, Lam CM, et al. (2004) Improving perioperative outcome expands the role of hepatectomy in management of benign and malignant hepatobiliary diseases: analysis of 1222 consecutive patients from a prospective database. Ann Surg 240: 698–708; discussion 708–610.
30. Jarnagin WR, Gonen M, Fong Y, DeMatteo RP, Ben-Porat L, et al. (2002) Improvement in perioperative outcome after hepatic resection: analysis of 1,803 consecutive cases over the past decade. Ann Surg 236: 397–406; discussion 406–397.
31. Hasegawa K, Kokudo N, Makuuchi M, Izumi N, Ichida T, et al. (2013) Comparison of resection and ablation for hepatocellular carcinoma: a cohort study based on a Japanese nationwide survey. J Hepatol 58: 724–729.
32. Margarit C, Escartín A, Castells L, Vargas V, Allende E, et al. (2005) Resection for hepatocellular carcinoma is a good option in Child-Turcotte-Pugh class A patients with cirrhosis who are eligible for liver transplantation. Liver Transpl 11: 1242–1251.
33. Li C, Zhu WJ, Wen TF, Dai Y, Yan LN, et al. (2014) Child-Pugh A Hepatitis B-Related Cirrhotic Patients with a Single Hepatocellular Carcinoma Up to 5 cm: Liver Transplantation vs. Resection. J Gastrointest Surg 18: 1469–1476.
34. Forner A, Llovet JM, Bruix J (2012) Hepatocellular carcinoma. Lancet 379: 1245–1255.
35. de Lope CR, Tremosini S, Forner A, Reig M, Bruix J (2012) Management of HCC. J Hepatol 56 Suppl 1: S75–87.
36. Omata M, Lesmana LA, Tateishi R, Chen PJ, Lin SM, et al. (2010) Asian Pacific Association for the Study of the Liver consensus recommendations on hepatocellular carcinoma. Hepatol Int 4: 439–474.
37. Kudo M, Izumi N, Kokudo N, Matsui O, Sakamoto M, et al. (2011) Management of hepatocellular carcinoma in Japan: Consensus-Based Clinical Practice Guidelines proposed by the Japan Society of Hepatology (JSH) 2010 updated version. Dig Dis 29: 339–364.
38. Jarnagin W, Chapman WC, Curley S, D'Angelica M, Rosen C, et al. (2010) Surgical treatment of hepatocellular carcinoma: expert consensus statement. HPB (Oxford) 12: 302–310.
39. Imamura H, Seyama Y, Kokudo N, Maema A, Sugawara Y, et al. (2003) One thousand fifty-six hepatectomies without mortality in 8 years. Arch Surg 138: 1198–1206; discussion 1206.
40. Boleslawski E, Petrovai G, Truant S, Dharancy S, Duhamel A, et al. (2012) Hepatic venous pressure gradient in the assessment of portal hypertension before liver resection in patients with cirrhosis. Br J Surg 99: 855–863.
41. Figueras J, Llado L, Ruiz D, Ramos E, Busquets J, et al. (2005) Complete versus selective portal triad clamping for minor liver resections: a prospective randomized trial. Ann Surg 241: 582–590.
42. Chen X, Zhai J, Cai X, Zhang Y, Wei L, et al. (2012) Severity of portal hypertension and prediction of postoperative liver failure after liver resection in patients with Child-Pugh grade A cirrhosis. Br J Surg 99: 1701–1710.
43. Stremitzer S, Tamandl D, Kaczirek K, Maresch J, Abbasov B, et al. (2011) Value of hepatic venous pressure gradient measurement before liver resection for hepatocellular carcinoma. Br J Surg 98: 1752–1758.
44. Wu JC, Huang YH, Chau GY, Su CW, Lai CR, et al. (2009) Risk factors for early and late recurrence in hepatitis B-related hepatocellular carcinoma. J Hepatol 51: 890–897.
45. Hsieh CB, Chung KP, Chu CM, Yu JC, Hsieh HF, et al. (2011) Appropriate liver resection type for patients with the American joint committee on cancer classification T1 and T2 hepatocellular carcinoma. Eur J Surg Oncol 37: 497–504.
46. Zhong JH, Li H, Li LQ, You XM, Zhang Y, et al. (2012) Adjuvant therapy options following curative treatment of hepatocellular carcinoma: a systematic review of randomized trials. Eur J Surg Oncol 38: 286–295.
47. Zhong JH, Ma L, Li LQ (2014) Postoperative therapy options for hepatocellular carcinoma. Scand J Gastroenterol 49: 649–661.

6

Comparison of Hepatocellular Carcinoma miRNA Expression Profiling as Evaluated by Next Generation Sequencing and Microarray

Yoshiki Murakami[1]*, Toshihito Tanahashi[2,3], Rina Okada[3], Hidenori Toyoda[4], Takashi Kumada[4], Masaru Enomoto[1], Akihiro Tamori[1], Norifumi Kawada[1], Y-h Taguchi[5], Takeshi Azuma[3]

1 Department of Hepatology, Osaka City University Graduate School of Medicine, Osaka, Japan, **2** Department of Medical Pharmaceutics, Kobe Pharmaceutical University, Kobe, Japan, **3** Division of Gastroenterology, Department of Internal Medicine, Kobe University Graduate School of Medicine, Kobe, Japan, **4** Department of Gastroenterology, Ogaki Municipal Hospital, Ogaki, Japan, **5** Department of Physics, Chuo University, Tokyo, Japan

Abstract

MicroRNA (miRNA) expression profiling has proven useful in diagnosing and understanding the development and progression of several diseases. Microarray is the standard method for analyzing miRNA expression profiles; however, it has several disadvantages, including its limited detection of miRNAs. In recent years, advances in genome sequencing have led to the development of next-generation sequencing (NGS) technologies, which significantly advance genome sequencing speed and discovery. In this study, we compared the expression profiles obtained by next generation sequencing (NGS) with the profiles created using microarray to assess if NGS could produce a more accurate and complete miRNA profile. Total RNA from 14 hepatocellular carcinoma tumors (HCC) and 6 matched non-tumor control tissues were sequenced with Illumina MiSeq 50-bp single-end reads. Micro RNA expression profiles were estimated using miRDeep2 software. As a comparison, miRNA expression profiles for 11 out of 14 HCCs were also established by microarray (Agilent human microRNA microarray). The average total sequencing exceeded 2.2 million reads per sample and of those reads, approximately 57% mapped to the human genome. The average correlation for miRNA expression between microarray and NGS and subtraction were 0.613 and 0.587, respectively, while miRNA expression between technical replicates was 0.976. The diagnostic accuracy of HCC, p-value, and AUC were 90.0%, 7.22×10^{-4}, and 0.92, respectively. In summary, NGS created an miRNA expression profile that was reproducible and comparable to that produced by microarray. Moreover, NGS discovered novel miRNAs that were otherwise undetectable by microarray. We believe that miRNA expression profiling by NGS can be a useful diagnostic tool applicable to multiple fields of medicine.

Editor: Max Costa, New York University School of Medicine, United States of America

Funding: The authors have no support or funding to report.

Competing Interests: The authors declare that they have no competing interests.

* Email: m2079633@med.osaka-cu.ac.jp

Introduction

MicroRNAs (miRNAs) are an abundant class of small (19–24 nt) and highly conserved, non-coding RNA. They act as post-transcriptional regulators of gene expression, altering mRNA transcription and translation by hybridizing to the untranslated regions (UTRs) of certain subsets of mRNAs [1] [2]. Since their initial discovery in *Caenorhabditis elegans* in 1993 [3], researchers have gained much insight into the prevalence of miRNAs in other species. The latest miRBase database (release 20) contains 1827 precursor miRNAs and 2578 mature miRNA products in *Homo sapiens* (http://www.mirbase.org/index.shtml).

Hepatocellular carcinoma (HCC) is a common cause of cancer-related deaths worldwide. There are more than 250,000 new HCC cases and an estimated 500,000–600,000 HCC deaths annually [4] [5]. The most frequent etiology of HCC is chronic hepatitis B and C (CHB, CHC), or alcoholic liver disease. Although recent advances in functional genomics provide a deeper understanding of viral associated hepatocarcinogenesis (review in [6]), the molecular pathogenesis of HCC remains unclear.

Altered miRNA expression has been observed in a large variety of HCC and a correlation has been found between miRNA expression and histological differentiation [7] [8]. For example, the expression level of miR-26 has been associated with hepatocarcinogenesis and response to interferon therapy [9]. Moreover recently, miR-122 expression was associated with hepatocarcinogenesis, liver homeostasis, and essential liver metabolism [10] [11]. miR-18 has also been highly associated with the occurrence and progression of different types of cancer [12] [13]. In other research, miRNA expression profiles were associated with vascular invasion, the levels of alpha-fetoprotein, and large tumor size [14].

To date, studies exploring the role of miRNAs in hepatocarcinogenesis have relied on microarrays to assay miRNA expression. Deep sequencing, a set of technologies that produce large amounts of sequence data from nucleic acid specimens, is rapidly replacing microarrays as the technology of choice for quantifying and annotating miRNAs [15] [16]. Deep sequencing has the superior ability to capture the scale and complexity of whole transcriptomes [17]. In particular, short read deep sequencing (e.g., the Illumina MiSeq platform) is appropriate for miRNAs because a complete miRNA can be sequenced with a single read. While array design relies on prior knowledge of the miRNAs being investigated, deep sequencing allows for the discovery of novel miRNAs. Furthermore, microarray methods lack the dynamic range to detect and quantify low abundance transcripts, but deep sequencing can identify miRNAs that are expressed at levels that fall below microarray's detectable threshold. In addition, deep sequencing eliminates background problems that result from cross-hybridization in microarrays, thus facilitating interpretation of the signal and obviating the non-linear data manipulation steps required by microarrays. Therefore, the application of deep sequencing to miRNA profiling has the potential to uncover novel miRNAs and to detect expression of rare but functionally significant miRNAs. Recently, deep sequencing was used to analyze non-coding RNAs in HCC, by which miRNAs, PIWI-interacting RNA, and small nucleolar RNAs were identified [18].

In this study, we created miRNA expression profiles for HCC and non-tumorous tissue using NGS. We then compared the miRNA expression profiles obtained by NGA and microarray. Unlike previous studies, we sequenced un-pooled miRNA libraries to a previously unprecedented sequencing depth from multiple replicates and controls across multiple time-points, allowing us to explore the statistically significant temporal changes in miRNA expression in hepatocarcinogenesis.

Materials and Methods

Sample preparation

We isolated total RNA from 14 surgically resected HCC tumors and 6 matched adjacent non-tumor control tissues (Table 1). We confirmed that the 14 samples were accurately diagnosed as HCC by image diagnosis by CT and USTG and pathological findings. All patients or their guardians provided written informed consent, and Osaka City University and Ogaki Municipal Hospital approved all aspects of this study in accordance with the Helsinki Declaration.

RNA preparation, and miRNA deep sequencing and microarray

Total RNA from surgical resection was prepared using mirVana miRNA Isolation kit (Invitrogen), according to the manufacturer's instruction.

Total RNA, containing the small RNA fraction, was reverse transcribed into a cDNA library using the TruSeq Small RNA Sample Prep Kit (Illumina). Briefly, total RNA (1 μg per sample) was ligated overnight with adapters, reverse transcribed, RNase-treated, and PCR-amplified with unique barcode-labeled amplification primers. Then, size-selection was conducted on 6% native polyacrylamide gels. cDNA fragments between 145 and 160 bp corresponding to the miRNA populations were excised from the gel, then eluted and precipitated. The final cDNA pellet was air dried and resuspended in 10 μl of nuclease-free water. The quantity of cDNA in each final miRNA libraries was verified using Qubit fluorometer (Invitrogen). Equimoloar amounts for each final library were pooled at a final concentration of 2 nM cDNA. Barcoded templates were sequenced on a single flowcell of the Illumina MiSeq with 50-bp single-end reads. Eleven of 14 total HCC RNA samples were also assayed by microarray (Agilent human microRNA microarray release 14.0) (Table 1). Hybridization signals were detected with a DNA microarray scanner G2505B (Agilent Technologies) and the scanned images were analyzed using Agilent feature extraction software (v9.5.3.1). Raw data (gProcessedSignal) was normalized so that each expression had a mean of zero and a sample variance of one. The above processes were conducted with various packages and functions implemented in R {http://www.r-project.org}.

The sequence reads obtained in this study have been deposited in the DNA Data Bank of Japan Sequence Read Archive (http://www.ddbj.nig.ac.jp/index-e.html) under accession number DRA001067. All microarray data were deposited in NCBI's Gene Expression Omnibus and are accessible through GEO Series accession number GSE31164.

Bioinformatics

In order to extract the adaptor sequence from each short read obtained by NGS, fastx_clipper from the fastx toolkit {http://hannonlab.cshl.edu/fastx_toolkit/} was used. The adaptor trimmed short reads were then mapped to the human reference genome sequence hg19 by mapper.pl script included in miRDeep2 [19] {http://genomewiki.ucsc.edu/index.php/Hg19_Genome_size_statistics}. miRNA mature and hairpin sequences were obtained from miRBase release 18 {http://www.mirbase.org}. Finally, the resulting fastq files were processed by miRDeep2.pl script. miRNA read counts were extracted from the "read_count" column of the file named"miRNAs_expressed_all_samples_sample_id.csv" file; while sample_id was given automatically by scripts (for sample scripts see Text S1 and for extracted read counts for each miRNA see Table S1). When drawing boxplots, the read count in each sample was normalized such that it had a zero mean and a variance of one. For microarray processing, gProcessedSignal values were extracted from raw data files. gProcessedSignal values were also normalized so that they had a zero mean and a variance of one. Average gProcessedSignal values over probes assigned to common mature miRNA were used to compute the correlation coefficient for NGS and microarray results. The correlation coefficients of logarithmic expression and subtracted expression were computed using only miRNAs with non-negative signals in both NGS and average microarray expression. P-values associated with boxplots were computed using Wilcoxon rank sum test. All bioinformatics computation was performed using functions implemented in R.

To discriminate HCC from non-tumorous tissue when miRNA expression was quantified by NGS, we combined principal components analysis (PCA)-based feature extraction and PCA-based linear discriminant analysis (LDA) [20] [21]. When PCA-based feature extraction was applied, each miRNA was embedded into a two-dimensional space by PCA and M miRNAs located far from the origin (outliers) were selected. Using these selected miRNA, each sample was embedded into a low dimensional space with dimension (M–M'). Samples were then discriminated by LDA using the M' dimensional PC scores. For more details, see Text 2. Novel miRNA candidates were selected from the total set if they satisfied the following criteria: 1) among the novel miRNAs identified by miRDeep2, those with a >80% probability of being a true positive, and 2) the miRNA was reproducibly detected in more than three samples.

Results

Analysis of miRNA sequence reads and reproducibility of NGS analysis

The average number of sequencing reads per sample exceeded 2.2 million, of which approximately 57% mapped to the human reference genome (for more details, see Table S2). A scatter plot of logarithmic miRNA expression measured by NGS and microarray using the first technical replicate of K-177 (K-177_1) is shown in Fig 1.

Table 1. Clinical information of 14 HCC patients analyzed in this study.

code No.	histological differentiation	sex	age	HBsAg	anti-HCV	AFP	PIVKA-II	no tumorous tissue	NGS analysis	microarray analysis
CU-070	moderately	M	53	(−)	(+)	3510	NI	LC	only HCC	only HCC
CU-083	moderately	M	49	(+)	(−)	143830	0.9	LC	both	only HCC
CU-085	moderately	M	55	(−)	(+)	113	0.06	LC	only HCC	only HCC
CU-087	well	M	62	(−)	(+)	NI	NI	NI	both	only HCC
CU-089	moderately	F	61	(−)	(+)	400	0.06	CH	both	only HCC
CU-091	moderately	M	64	(−)	(+)	5	0.06	CH	only HCC	only HCC
K-023	moderately	M	47	(+)	(−)	3500	2.2	LC	only HCC	only HCC
K-147	poorly	M	65	(−)	(+)	NI	NI	NI	only HCC	neither
K-175	moderately	M	67	(−)	(+)	3.4	32	CH	both	neither
K-177	moderately	M	68	(−)	(+)	13	29	NI	both	only HCC
K-181	well	M	LC	(−)	(−)	5.1	19	NI	both	neither
O-086	moderately	F	64	(−)	(+)	218	32	LC	only HCC	only HCC
O-088	moderately	M	74	(+)	(−)	13.4	7991	LC	only HCC	only HCC
O-089	moderately	M	68	(−)	(+)	8	25	LC	only HCC	only HCC

Abbreviations, moderately; moderately differentiated HCC, well; well differentiated HCC, poorly; poorly differentiated HCC, NI; no information, CH; chronic hepatitis, LC; liver cirrhosis, only HCC; only HCC was analyzed by NGS, both; both tumor and non-tumorous tissue were analyzed by NGS, neither; neither HCC nor non-tumorous tissue was not analyzed.

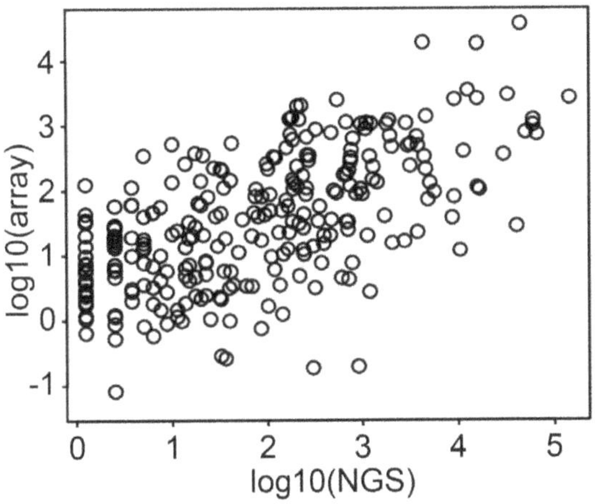

Figure 1. Comparison between logarithmic HCC miRNA expression in NGS (horizontal axis) and microarray (vertical) analysis (K-177_1 means the first technical replicates of code No. K-177). One black circle showed one miRNA. Pearson's correlation coefficient is 0.6059.

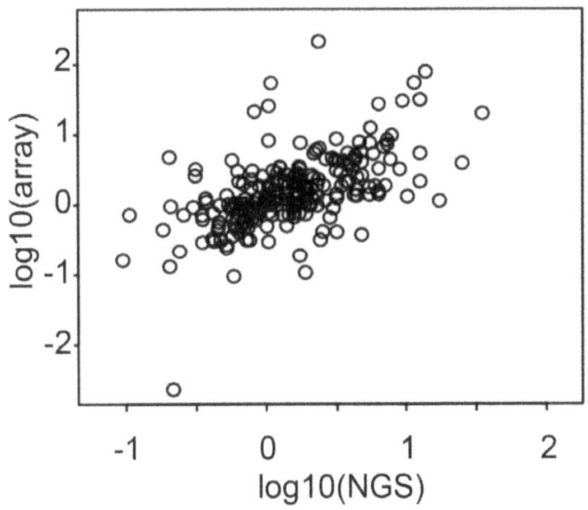

Figure 2. Comparison between differential (K-177 vs. CU-087) logarithmic HCC miRNA expression in NGS (horizontal axis) and microarray (vertical) analysis. Pearson's correlation coefficient is 0.5555.

Although the microarray and NGS expression levels are not perfectly correlated, they are approximately proportional to each other with a positive proportional coefficient. The corresponding scatter plots for the remaining 9 HCC samples are shown in Fig. S1. The similarity in the NGS and microarray miRNA profiling results was relatively independent of the samples considered. The correlation coefficient of logarithmic miRNA expression from 11 HCC miRNA expression profiles as measured by both NGS and microarray was 0.613. This demonstrates that NGS and microarray measurements give similar results.

We next validated the reproducibility of miRNA differential expression across the 11 samples. In general, miRNA expression profiles are not individually evaluated; instead, profiles for distinct samples are analyzed in pairs e.g., compared between tumor and adjacent non-tumorous tissue. Thus, reproducibility between NGS and microarray is more important in differential expression than in any single expression measurement by itself. Fig. 2 shows a scatter plot of differential (K-177 vs. CU-087) logarithmic miRNA expression obtained by NGS and microarray (Fig. S2 shows the full set of scatter plots). Again, we observed that the coincidence between NGS and microarray miRNA profiles was relatively strong irrespective of the sample pair that was considered. The correlation coefficient of differential logarithmic miRNA expression averaged over all pairs of 11 HCC is 0.587. This demonstrates a reasonable level of congruency between miRNA profiling results from NGS and microarray when considering differential logarithmic miRNA expression.

miRNA expression measured by NGS can be applied to diagnosing HCC

In order to discriminate between HCC and non-tumorous tissue, 11 miRNAs quantified by NGS (miR-10a-5p, miR-122-5p, miR-146b-5p, miR-148a-3p, miR-192-5p, miR-22-3p, miR-26a-5p, and miR-27b-3p, miR-10b-5p, miR-143-3p, and miR-21-5p) were chosen by PCA-based feature extraction. The miRNA expression levels in HCC and non-tumorous tissue is shown in Fig 3. The expression level of miR-10a-5p ($p<2.56\times10^{-2}$), miR-122-5p ($p < 1.55\times10^{-3}$), and miR-22-3 ($p<4.64\times10^{-3}$) among the 11 miRNAs differed significantly in the HCC and non-tumorous tissue. miRNA profiling allowed the accurate prediction of HCC with an overall cross-validation accuracy of 90.0% (18/20) by PCA-based feature extraction (Table 2). The p-value and AUC value for diagnostic ability were $<7.22\times10^{-4}$ and 0.92 respectively.

Reproducibility of NGS measurement among technical replicates

We have demonstrated that quantifying miRNA using NGS gives results similar to those obtained by microarray, and that miRNA expression measured by NGS can discriminate HCC from non-tumorous tissue. However, we have found that miRNA profiling using NGS is more accurate in cases where NGS measurement does not vary within multiple technical replicates. For those HCC samples in this study that had more than one technical replicate we validated the reproducibility of NGS miRNA expression between technical replicates. Fig. 4 shows examples of technical replicates (other scatter plots are available in Fig. S3). Among three technical replicates, the correlation coefficients of logarithmic miRNA expression are greater than 0.98. Additionally, the dynamic range is almost 5 digits. This means that technical replicates obtained from NGS measurements are highly reproducible.

Discovery of novel miRNAs in our analysis

NGS detected several miRNA candidates that are not registered in the present miRBase (Rel. 18) (see Materials and Methods for detection criteria, and see Supporting Information for more details about detected miRNAs). We speculate that four precursor miRNAs, hsa-mir-9985, hsa-mir-1843, hsa-mir-548bc, and hsa-mir-9986 and the corresponding four mature miRNAs, hsa-miR-9985, hsa-miR-1843, hsa-miR-548bc, and hsa-miR-9986, were not previously reported because they are not among the miRNAs found at the corresponding genomic coordinates. Fig. 5 shows the sequence of the new miRNA candidates, their alignment with their closest homologous miRNA, and the hairpin structure predicted by RNA-fold with default parameter settings (short reads mapped to these candidate miRNAs are available in Table S3).

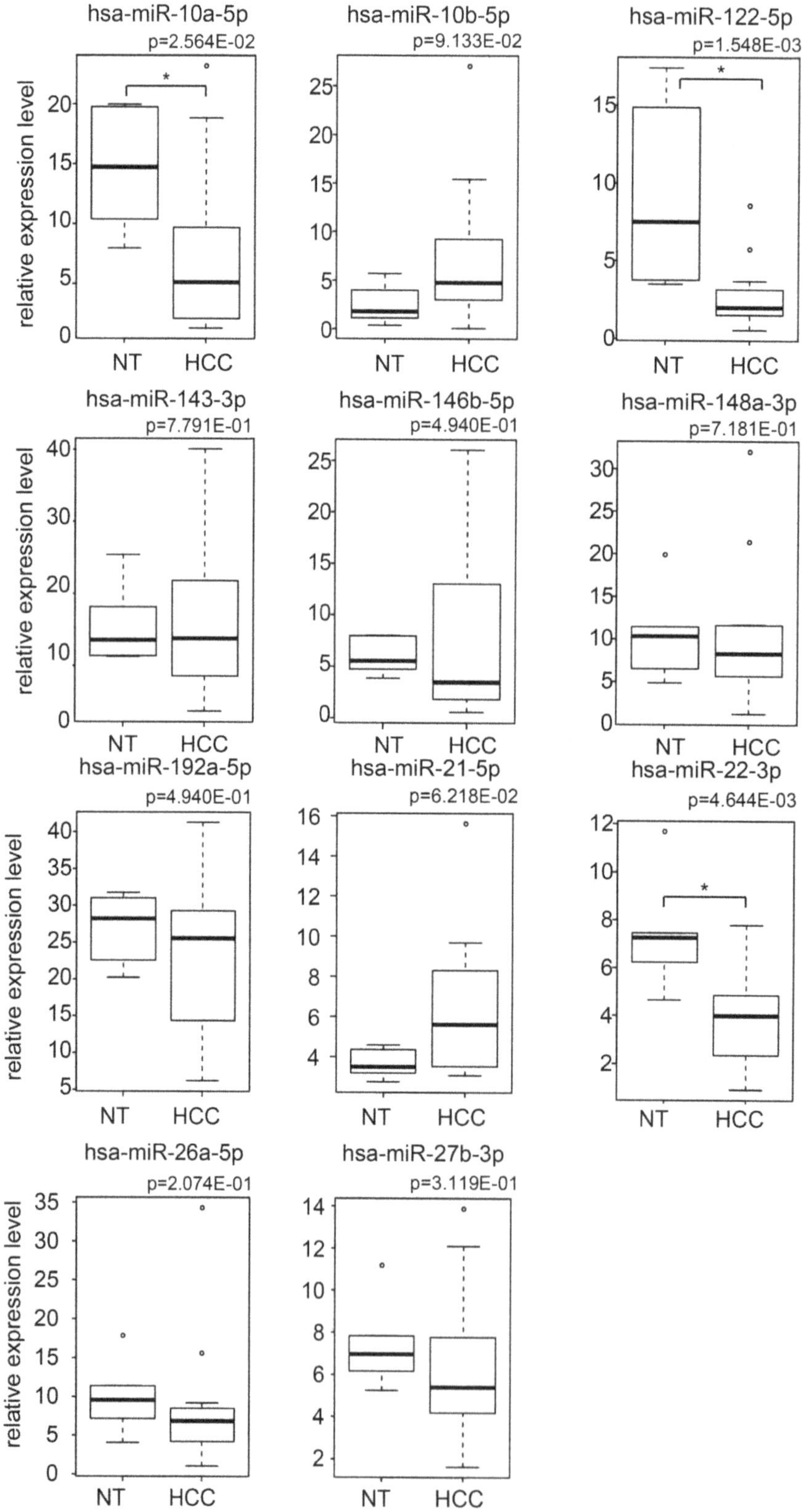

Figure 3. Boxplots of the expression of 11 miRNAs in HCC and non-tumorous tissue obtained by NGS, which were used for the differential analysis. P-values were computed using two-sided Wilcoxon Rank Sum test. Asterisk indicates a significant difference of $p<0.05$ (*).

Table 2. Performance of discrimination between 14 HCC samples and 6 normal tissue samples using miRNA expression obtained by NGS analysis.

		Result	
		Control	**Tumor**
Prediction	Control	12	0
	Tumor	2	6

Discussion

The clinical application of miRNA expression profiling, such as its use as a disease biomarker, has been extensively developed in recent years. This analysis demonstrates that miRNA profiling by NGS has the potential to diagnose HCC with high accuracy. Previous comprehensive analyses of miRNA expression have been performed by microarray; however, the miRBase is currently underdeveloped. An updated miRBase is required to create accurate microarray profiles, and especially because microarray experiments performed using previous version of miRBase are incompatible with microarrays based on the current version. The results from our miRNA expression analysis in HCC suggest that NGS may allow us to overcome this problem. Law et al. has previously reported small RNA transcriptome analysis in HCC by using NGS [18]. However, pre-miRNAs are of a similar length as other more numerous classes of ncRNA, including tRNA and snoRNA, making deep profiling of pre-miRNA sequences difficult [22]. Therefore, this study focused on the analysis on whole miRNA instead of ncRNA.

In order to determine if miRNA expression as measured by NGS technology can discriminate HCC from non-tumorous tissue, we adopted a recently proposed combination of PCA-based feature extraction and PCA-based LDA [20] [21] (for details, see Materials and Methods). Previously, we showed that miRNA expression profiles detected by microarray can accurately discriminate HCC from non-tumorous tissues [7] [23] [24] [25]. Therefore, because NGS produced results similar to those by microarray, and was capable of differentiating HCC from non-tumorous tissues, it is evident that miRNA expression quantified by NGS is as informative as is miRNA expression assessed by microarray. NGS's ability to quantify miRNA expression suggests

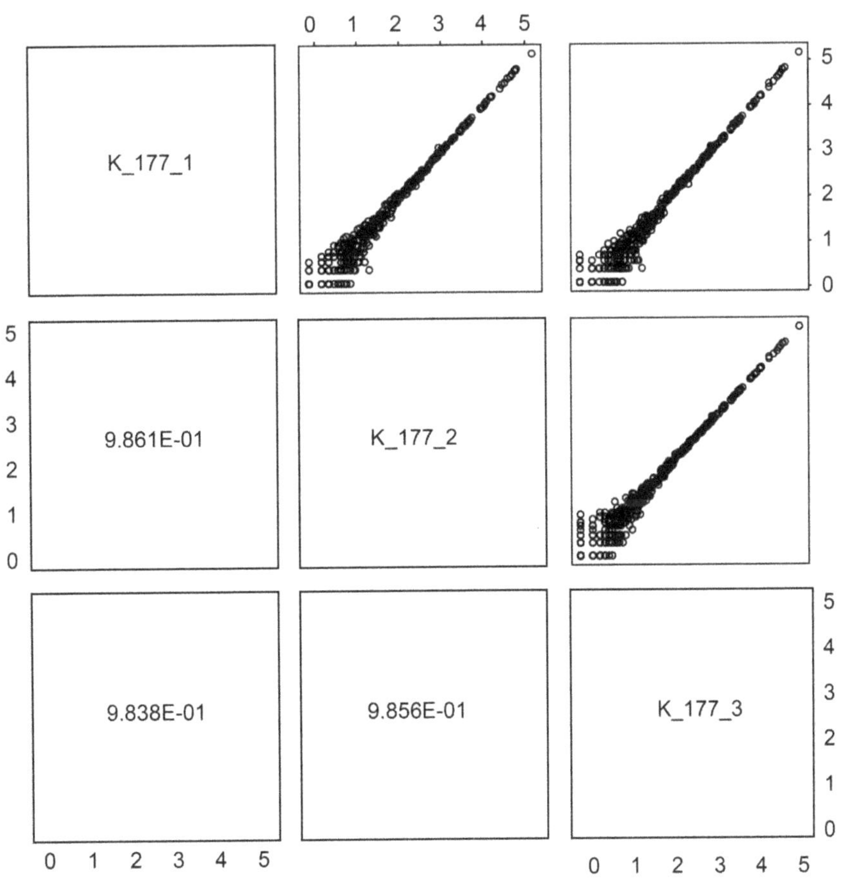

Figure 4. Comparison between logarithmic miRNA expression in HCC and NGS technical replicates (K-177_1 means the first technical replicates of code No. K-177). Pearson's correlation coefficients are greater than 0.9861.

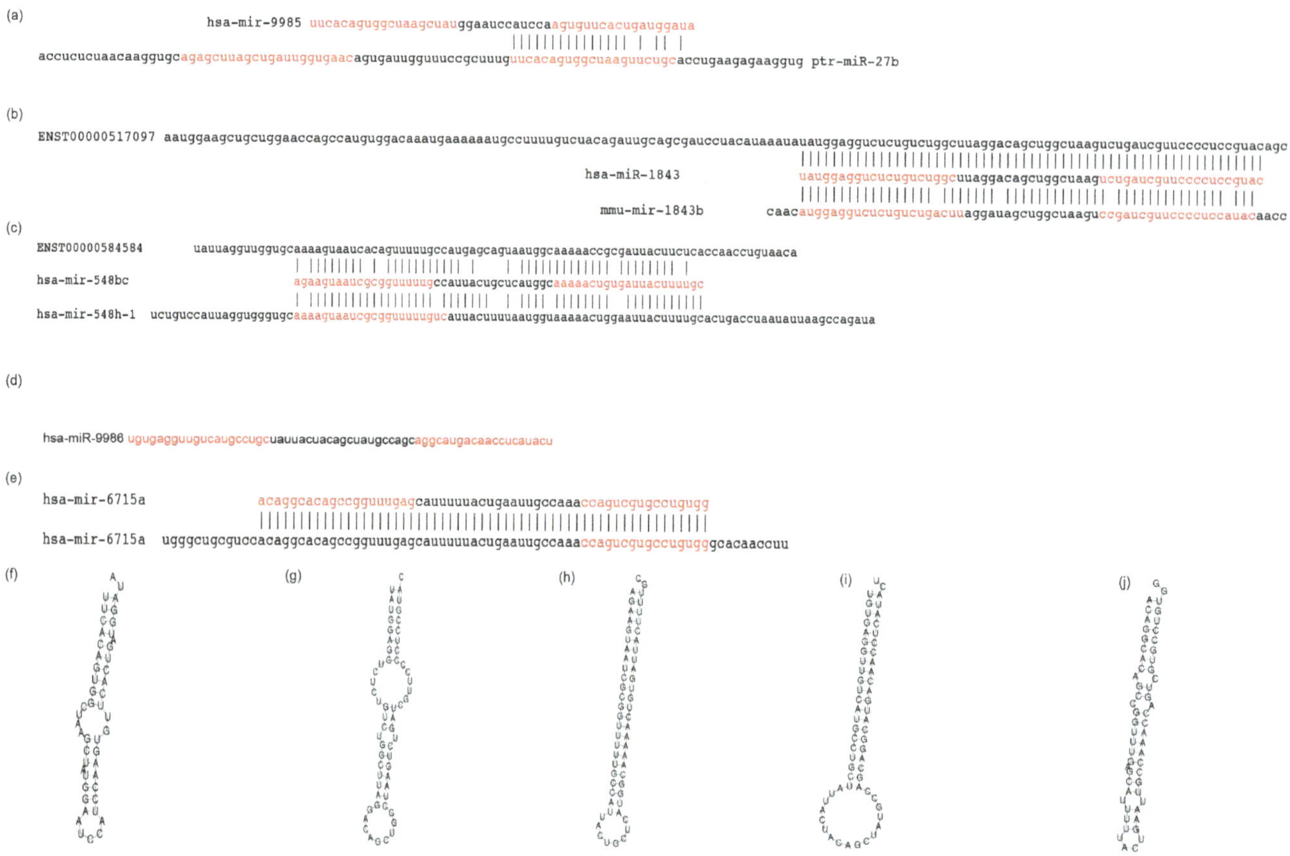

Figure 5. Comparison of novel miRNA candidates ((a) hsa-mir-9985, (b) hsa-mir-1843, (c) hsa-mir-548bc and (d) hsa-mir-9986) with known miRNAs and transcripts. (e) hsa-mir-6715a novel miRNA was not included in miRBase release 18, but was present in later releases. Nucleotides highlighted in red show hairpin constructs. F, g, h, i, and j are constructs of each miRNA and respectively correspond to a, b, c, d, and e.

that the miRNA expression profile measured by NGS can be clinically applicable as a diagnostic tool.

HCC was discriminated from non-tumorous tissues using a linear combination of 11 miRNA expression profiles; however, it may be useful to investigate the expression of individual miRNA in order to understand their biological significance. Fig. 3 shows boxplots of the 11 miRNAs that were used to discriminate between HCC and non-tumorous tissue. Contrary to our expectations, only three (miR-10a-5p, 122-5p and 22-3p) of the 11 miRNAs showed significant differential expression ($p<0.05$) between HCC and non-tumorous tissue. Among these three miRNAs, miR-122-5p and miR-22-3p are well-known to be downregulated in HCC [10] [10] [26] [27]. Among the three miRNAs with significant differential expression between HCC and non-tumorous tissue, miR-10a-5p showed the least difference, with a p-value of 0.03. Recently, it has been reported that miR-10a-5p is involved in HCC metastasis [28]. Thus, the selection of these three miRNAs as potential biomarkers is biologically reasonable. Although the remaining eight miRNAs did not have significant differential expression between HCC and non-tumorous tissues, their inclusion did not reduce the discriminatory performance. This suggests that these eight miRNAs may contribute to diagnosing hepatocarcinogenesis only when combined with other miRNAs. Since controlling the expression of multiple miRNAs simultaneously is experimentally difficult, we were unable to confirm if these miRNAs work together. This may be worth further study in the future.

While investigating novel miRNA candidates, we found that mature miRNAs from hsa-mir-9985 and hsa-miR-9985-5p are almost identical to ptr-miR-27a-3p (Fig 5(a, f)). This may suggest that hsa-mir-9985 has been transposed during its evolution from chimpanzee to human. hsa-miR-1843 was homologous to miR-1843a, which was previously detected in mouse, Chinese hamsters, and brown rats. Near the genomic coordinate where hsa-mir-1843 was detected, Ender reported finding snoRNA (ENSR00000517097), therefore hsa-mir-1843 is likely to be a small nuclear RNA-derived microRNA [29] (Fig, 5(b, g)). It is possible that this explains why researchers have overlooked hsa-mir-1843 despite reports of homologous miRNAs in other animals. While hsa-mir-548bc appears homologous to hsa-mir-548h-1 (Fig. 5(c, h)), hsa-mir-548bc is detected at a distinct genomic coordinate from the original location of hsa-548h-1. Thus, hsa-miR-548bc seems to be a distinct microRNA from hsa-mir-548h-1.

It is interesting to note that the novel miRNA (EST00000584584) not included in the miRBase was reported to be located near the genomic coordinate where hsa-mir-9986 was detected. To our knowledge, this is the first experimental evidence that these predicted novel miRNAs exist. Finally, no homologous miRNA has been reported for hsa-mir-9986 (Fig. 5(d, i)), thus it is possible that hsa-mir-9986 is completely new. In addition to these four new miRNA candidates, hsa-mir-6715a was also detected in our analysis (Fig. 5(e, j)). hsa-miR-6715a was not included in the miRBase release 18, but was included in later releases, which lends support to the reliability and accuracy of our strategy to identify

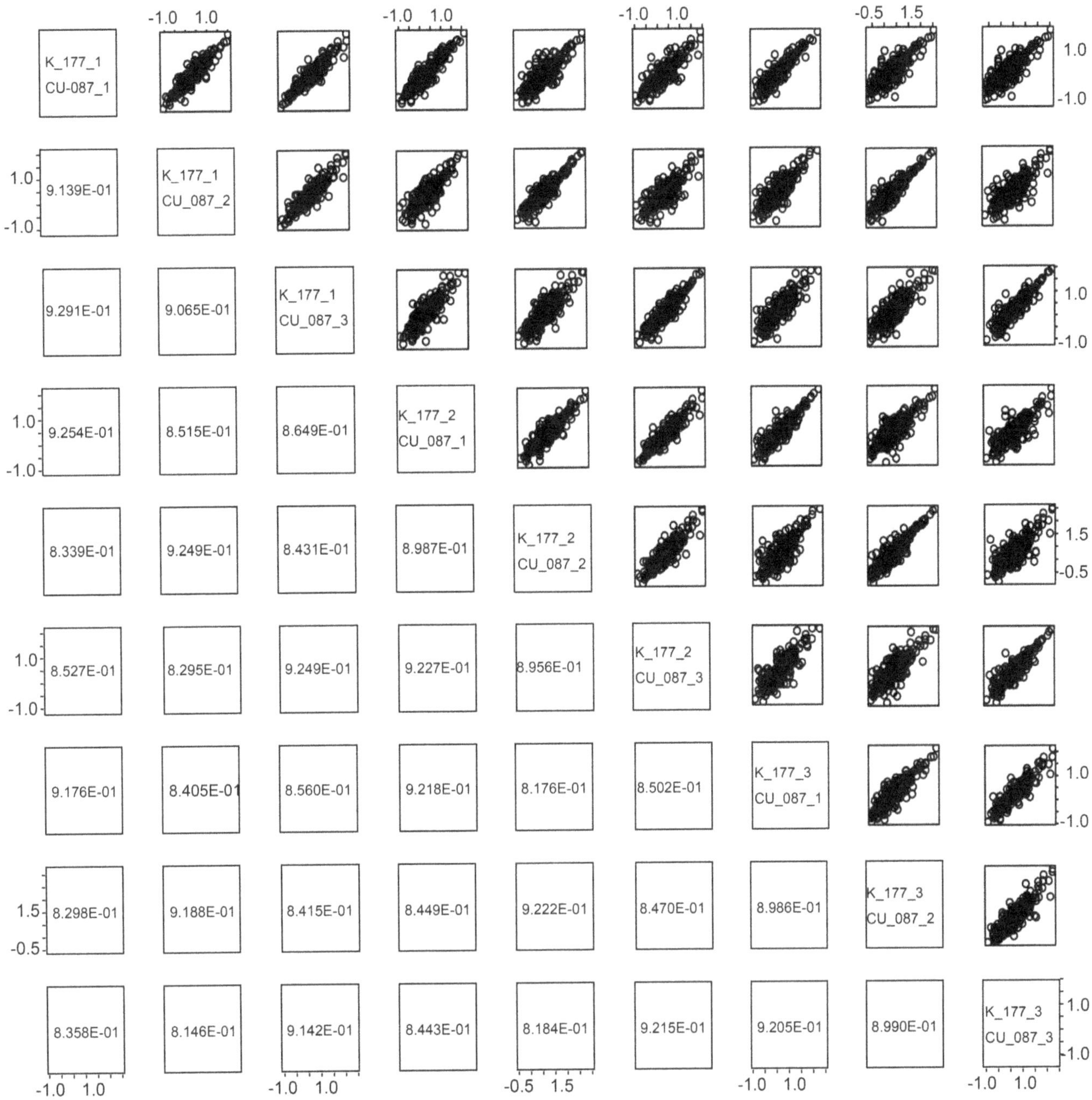

Figure 6. Comparison of differential (K-177 vs. CU-087) logarithmic miRNA expression in HCC among NGS technical replicates. Pearson's correlation coefficients range from 0.80 to 0.93.

novel miRNAs. It is interesting that although hsa-miR-6715a-5p was not reported in the miRBase, it was detected in our analysis although only 10 reads were assigned to the miRNA. The biological significance of these candidate miRNAs requires future examination.

Finally, we also investigated the reproducibility of technical replicates for differential miRNA expression; a full list of scatter plots and correlation coefficients is available in Fig. S4. Fig. 6 shows examples of technical replicates with good correlation. We were unable to identify the specific conditions necessary to achieve highly reproducible technical replicates. However, several of our cross-replicate comparisons were of acceptable quality, leading us to believe that our method has the potential to adequately reproduce differential miRNA expression between technical replicates.

Conclusions

We have shown in this study that miRNA expression profiles obtained from NGS analysis are reproducible and are concordant with that obtained by the standard microarray procedure. Moreover, we have demonstrated that NGS can identify novel miRNAs that are otherwise undetectable by microarray analysis. HCC was distinguished from non-tumorous tissue with high diagnostic accuracy, supporting the clinical application of NGS-based miRNA expression profiling.

Supporting Information

Figure S1 Full set of scatter plots of logarithmic miRNA expression in HCC samples by NGS and microarray analysis. Comparison between logarithmic HCC miRNA expression in NGS (horizontal axis) and microarray (vertical) analysis. One black circle showed one miRNA.

Figure S2 Full set of scatter plots of differential logarithmic miRNA expression in HCC for NGS and microarray analysis. Comparison between differential logarithmic HCC miRNA expression in NGS (horizontal axis) and microarray (vertical) analysis. One black circle showed one miRNA.

Figure S3 Comparison of logarithmic miRNA expression in HCC for NGS technical replicates not included in Fig. 3. Comparison between differential logarithmic HCC miRNA expression in NGS (horizontal axis) and microarray (vertical) analysis. One black circle showed one miRNA.

Figure S4 Comparison of differential logarithmic miRNA expression in HCC for NGS technical replicates not included in Fig. 4. Comparison between differential logarithmic HCC miRNA expression in NGS (horizontal axis) and microarray (vertical) analysis. One black circle showed one miRNA.

Table S1 Extracted read counts of each miRNA obtained by NGS analysis.

Table S2 Detailed NGS analysis of HCC and non-tumorous tissue samples.

Table S3 Detailed mapping of short reads for novel miRNA candidates and hsa-mir-6715a.

Text S1 Sample script that processed short reads using fastx_clipper and miRDeep2.

Text S2 Detailed description of feature extraction and discriminant procedures.

Author Contributions

Conceived and designed the experiments: YM. Performed the experiments: YM TT RO HT. Analyzed the data: TT YT. Contributed reagents/materials/analysis tools: TT RO. Wrote the paper: YM TK ME AT NK YT TA. Read and approved the manuscript: YM TT RO HT TK ME AT NK YT TA.

References

1. Ambros V (2004) The functions of animal microRNAs. Nature 431: 350–355.
2. Bartel DP (2004) MicroRNAs: genomics, biogenesis, mechanism, and function. Cell 116: 281–297.
3. Lee RC, Feinbaum RL, Ambros V (1993) The C. elegans heterochronic gene lin-4 encodes small RNAs with antisense complementarity to lin-14. Cell 75: 843–854.
4. El-Serag HB, Rudolph KL (2007) Hepatocellular carcinoma: epidemiology and molecular carcinogenesis. Gastroenterology 132: 2557–2576.
5. Venook AP, Papandreou C, Furuse J, de Guevara LL (2010) The incidence and epidemiology of hepatocellular carcinoma: a global and regional perspective. Oncologist 15 Suppl 4: 5–13.
6. Arzumanyan A, Reis HM, Feitelson MA (2013) Pathogenic mechanisms in HBV- and HCV-associated hepatocellular carcinoma. Nat Rev Cancer 13: 123–135.
7. Murakami Y, Yasuda T, Saigo K, Urashima T, Toyoda H, et al. (2006) Comprehensive analysis of microRNA expression patterns in hepatocellular carcinoma and non-tumorous tissues. Oncogene 25: 2537–2545.
8. Braconi C, Patel T (2008) MicroRNA expression profiling: a molecular tool for defining the phenotype of hepatocellular tumors. Hepatology 47: 1807–1809.
9. Ji J, Shi J, Budhu A, Yu Z, Forgues M, et al. (2009) MicroRNA expression, survival, and response to interferon in liver cancer. N Engl J Med 361: 1437–1447.
10. Tsai WC, Hsu SD, Hsu CS, Lai TC, Chen SJ, et al. (2012) MicroRNA-122 plays a critical role in liver homeostasis and hepatocarcinogenesis. J Clin Invest 122: 2884–2897.
11. Hsu SH, Wang B, Kota J, Yu J, Costinean S, et al. (2012) Essential metabolic, anti-inflammatory, and anti-tumorigenic functions of miR-122 in liver. J Clin Invest 122: 2871–2883.
12. Bjork JK, Sandqvist A, Elsing AN, Kotaja N, Sistonen L (2010) miR-18, a member of Oncomir-1, targets heat shock transcription factor 2 in spermatogenesis. Development 137: 3177–3184.
13. Murakami Y, Tamori A, Itami S, Tanahashi T, Toyoda H, et al. (2013) The expression level of miR-18b in hepatocellular carcinoma is associated with the grade of malignancy and prognosis. BMC Cancer 13: 99.
14. Toffanin S, Hoshida Y, Lachenmayer A, Villanueva A, Cabellos L, et al. (2011) MicroRNA-based classification of hepatocellular carcinoma and oncogenic role of miR-517a. Gastroenterology 140: 1618–1628 e1616.
15. McCormick KP, Willmann MR, Meyers BC (2011) Experimental design, preprocessing, normalization and differential expression analysis of small RNA sequencing experiments. Silence 2: 2.
16. Wittmann J, Jack HM (2010) New surprises from the deep–the family of small regulatory RNAs increases. ScientificWorldJournal 10: 1239–1243.
17. Costa V, Angelini C, De Feis I, Ciccodicola A (2010) Uncovering the complexity of transcriptomes with RNA-Seq. J Biomed Biotechnol 2010: 853916.
18. Law PT, Qin H, Ching AK, Lai KP, Co NN, et al. (2013) Deep sequencing of small RNA transcriptome reveals novel non-coding RNAs in hepatocellular carcinoma. J Hepatol 58: 1165–1173.
19. Friedlander MR, Mackowiak SD, Li N, Chen W, Rajewsky N (2012) miRDeep2 accurately identifies known and hundreds of novel microRNA genes in seven animal clades. Nucleic Acids Res 40: 37–52.
20. Taguchi YH, Murakami Y (2013) Principal component analysis based feature extraction approach to identify circulating microRNA biomarkers. PLoS One 8: e66714.
21. Murakami Y, Toyoda H, Tanahashi T, Tanaka J, Kumada T, et al. (2012) Comprehensive miRNA expression analysis in peripheral blood can diagnose liver disease. PLoS One 7: e48366.
22. Burroughs AM, Kawano M, Ando Y, Daub CO, Hayashizaki Y (2012) pre-miRNA profiles obtained through application of locked nucleic acids and deep sequencing reveals complex 5'/3' arm variation including concomitant cleavage and polyuridylation patterns. Nucleic Acids Res 40: 1424–1437.
23. Meng F, Henson R, Wehbe-Janek H, Ghoshal K, Jacob ST, et al. (2007) MicroRNA-21 regulates expression of the PTEN tumor suppressor gene in human hepatocellular cancer. Gastroenterology 133: 647–658.
24. Gramantieri L, Ferracin M, Fornari F, Veronese A, Sabbioni S, et al. (2007) Cyclin G1 is a target of miR-122a, a microRNA frequently down-regulated in human hepatocellular carcinoma. Cancer Res 67: 6092–6099.
25. Thorgeirsson SS, Lee JS, Grisham JW (2006) Functional genomics of hepatocellular carcinoma. Hepatology 43: S145–150.
26. Xu J, Zhu X, Wu L, Yang R, Yang Z, et al. (2012) MicroRNA-122 suppresses cell proliferation and induces cell apoptosis in hepatocellular carcinoma by directly targeting Wnt/beta-catenin pathway. Liver Int 32: 752–760.
27. Zhang J, Yang Y, Yang T, Liu Y, Li A, et al. (2010) microRNA-22, downregulated in hepatocellular carcinoma and correlated with prognosis, suppresses cell proliferation and tumourigenicity. Br J Cancer 103: 1215–1220.
28. Yan Y, Luo YC, Wan HY, Wang J, Zhang PP, et al. (2013) MicroRNA-10a is involved in the metastatic process by regulating Eph tyrosine kinase receptor A4-mediated epithelial-mesenchymal transition and adhesion in hepatoma cells. Hepatology 57: 667–677.
29. Ender C, Krek A, Friedlander MR, Beitzinger M, Weinmann L, et al. (2008) A human snoRNA with microRNA-like functions. Mol Cell 32: 519–528.

7

Novel Point and Combo-Mutations in the Genome of Hepatitis B Virus-Genotype D: Characterization and Impact on Liver Disease Progression to Hepatocellular Carcinoma

Somenath Datta[1], Alip Ghosh[1], Debanjali Dasgupta[1], Amit Ghosh[1], Shrabasti Roychoudhury[1], Gaurav Roy[2], Soumyojit Das[1], Kausik Das[1], Subash Gupta[3], Keya Basu[1], Analabha Basu[4], Simanti Datta[1], Abhijit Chowdhury[1], Soma Banerjee[1]*

1 Centre for Liver Research, Institute of Post Graduate Medical Education & Research, Kolkata, India, **2** Molecular Virology Laboratory, Department of Biotechnology, Jamia Millia Islamia, New Delhi, India, **3** Centre for Liver & Biliary Surgery, Indraprastha Apollo Hospital, New Delhi, India, **4** National Institute of Biomedical Genomics, Kalyani, India

Abstract

Background: The contribution of chronic hepatitis B virus (HBV) infection in the pathogenesis of hepatocellular carcinoma (HCC) through progressive stages of liver fibrosis is exacerbated by the acquisition of naturally occurring mutations in its genome. This study has investigated the prevalence of single and combo mutations in the genome of HBV-genotype D from treatment naïve Indian patients of progressive liver disease stages and assessed their impact on the disease progression to HCC.

Methods: The mutation profile was determined from the sequence analysis of the full-length HBV genome and compared with the reference HBV sequences. SPSS 16.0 and R software were used to delineate their statistical significance in predicting HCC occurrence.

Results: Age was identified as associated risk factor for HCC development in chronic hepatitis B (CHB) patients ($p \leq 0.01$). Beyond the classical mutations in basal core promoter (BCP) (A1762T/G1764A) and precore (G1862T), persistence of progressively accumulated mutations in enhancer-I, surface, HBx and core were showed significant association to liver disease progression. BCP_T1753C, core_T147C, surface_L213I had contributed significantly in the disease progression to HCC ($p<0.05$) in HBeAg positive patients whereas precore_T1858C, core_I116L, core_P130Q and preS1_S98T in HBeAg negative patients. Furthermore, the effect of individual mutation was magnified by the combination with A1762T/G1764A in HCC pathogenesis. Multivariate risk analysis had confirmed that core_P130Q [OR 20.71, 95% CI (1.64–261.77), $p = 0.019$] in B cell epitope and core_T147C [OR 14.58, 95% CI (1.17–181.76), $p = 0.037$] in CTL epitope were two independent predictors of HCC in HBeAg positive and negative patients respectively.

Conclusions: Thus distinct pattern of mutations distributed across the entire HBV genome may be useful in predicting HCC in high-risk CHB patients and pattern of mutational combinations may exert greater impact on HCC risk prediction more accurately than point mutations and hence these predictors may support the existing surveillance strategies in proper management of the patients.

Editor: Ranjit Ray, Saint Louis University, United States of America

Funding: Indian Council of Medical Research has funded this study (Project no: 5/13/83/2008-NCD-III). The funder had no role in study design, data collection and analysis, decision to publish, or preparation of the manuscript.

Competing Interests: The authors have declared that no competing interests exist.

* Email: somabanerjee70@gmail.com

Introduction

Chronic infection with hepatitis B virus (HBV) is the commonest cause of hepatocellular carcinoma (HCC) which is fast emerging as a leading cause of cancer related morbidity and mortality globally [1–3]. Decades of successful infection with repetitive cycles of injury and necroinflammation followed by regeneration and repair are the characteristic of chronic hepatitis B (CHB). HCC is the final outcome of CHB and liver fibrosis with or without cirrhosis is the hallmark of progressive CHB. These various clinical outcomes of CHB as a result of complex host–virus immune interplay have a consequential relationship and cirrhosis nearly always precedes HCC development in CHB infection [4]. It is important to note that HBV has tremendous abilities of immune evasion [5] by either acquiring mutations at viral immune dominant epitopes [6,7] or several critically important sites essential for progressive CHB related to liver diseases [8,9]. More intriguingly, it has been demonstrated that viral mutations are accumulated over a period of time and such accumulation of mutations in the viral genome might have pathogenic relevance [9,10].

Viral genetic factors such as genotype and classical mutations at basal core promoter (BCP) and precore (PC) have been shown to correlate with clinical outcomes in HBV related liver diseases [11,12]. Such associations have interesting geographical distribution that has clinical and evolutionary significance. Apart from the classical BCP and PC mutations, several mutations in surface, core, HBx and regulatory regions have been described to occur in CHB over time that might help in defining clinical situations–if studied sequentially [13–15]. India, with an intermediate endemicity of chronic HBV infection [16] and predominant chronic infection with HBV-genotype D [17] presents a unique HCC scenario. Firstly, while the burden of HBV associated cirrhosis is fairly high, the reported prevalence of HCC is relatively low [18,19], although HBV is the most common cause of HCC in India [20]. Secondly, detection of HCC in India is fairly late and hence, the poor prognosis – mandating the need for in depth studies into different aspects of HBV associated HCC in India. Studying the pattern of viral mutations in specific morphological–clinical category of hepatitis B virus infection might provide insights that not only help in elucidating the pathogenesis but also predicting HCC occurrence.

We report here the progressive accumulation of naturally occurring viral mutations in a group of treatment naïve/ineligible HBV infected subjects with different histological subgroups of fibrosis and HCC to seek evidence for any discernible and predictable viral genetic variations that occur in HCC.

Materials and Methods

Ethics statement

Institutional ethical review committee (Institutional Ethics Committee, I.P.G.M.E & R, 244, A.J.C Bose Road, Kolkata-20, India) has approved the study (Inst./IEC/646). Also informed written consent was obtained from each patient who was willing to participate in the study.

Study subjects

A total of 92 Subjects enrolled for detailed virological assessment in current study between the periods of June 2009 to December 2012 form two distinct groups:

A) Those presenting with different clinical manifestations of CHB for evaluation to clinical Hepatology services of the School of Digestive and Liver Diseases, Institute of Post Graduate Medical Education and Research, Kolkata (n = 80).

B) Those undergoing orthotropic liver transplantation for HBV related liver diseases at the centre for liver and biliary diseases, Indraprastha Apollo Hospitals, New Delhi (n = 12).

Detailed history, clinical, biochemical, radiological evaluations and virological examinations were performed on each patient as clinically indicated.

Patients were included into the study only if: (a) treatment naïve/ineligible with chronic HBV infection (b) age above 18 year (c) absence of other co-infections i.e. negative for anti-HCV and anti-HIV (d) no history of alcohol use (e) willingness to comply with study protocol.

Evaluation of liver disease status

For the purpose of categorization of the included patients according to the status of liver diseases focussing on grade of liver fibrosis (LF), presence of liver cirrhosis (LC) and HCC, each patient underwent liver stiffness measurement (LSM) with Fibroscan that uses Transient elastographic technique. LSM less than 7 kPa was taken as normal and more than 12.5 kPa was taken as cut-off for the diagnosis of cirrhosis [21,22]. Liver biopsy was done in non-cirrhotic patients who provided consent for the procedure and the histological status of the explanted liver was used in cases who underwent liver transplantation. All subjects were subsequently sub-classified into four categories: (1) 'no liver fibrosis' (nLF) (n = 22) was diagnosed either by absence of fibrosis in histology or by LSM value less than 7 kPa. (2) 'liver fibrosis less than cirrhosis' (LF) (n = 15) was defined histologically and supplemented with LSM value between 7.1 and 12.5 kPa and endoscopic confirmation of absence of varices and imaging feature of absence of portal hypertension, (3) 'liver cirrhosis' (LC) (n = 23) was diagnosed either by presence of histological feature of cirrhosis or by clinical, endoscopic, radiological parameters and LSM evidences in persons who did not undergo liver biopsy and (4) hepatocellular carcinoma (HCC) (n = 32) was diagnosed as per standard protocol using ultrasound, spiral/triphasic dynamic CT and serum Alfa-fetoprotein (AFP) values, apart from histology of explants. Blood samples were collected from all patients and the separated sera were preserved in −80°C till further use.

Serological parameters tests

Each serum sample was subjected to blood biochemistry such as total protein, albumin, globulin, bilirubin, prothrombin time (INR), ALT/SGPT, AST/SGOT using commercially available kits from Bayer Diagnostics, India. Serological markers such as HBsAg, HBeAg, anti-HBe and anti-HCV were verified using commercially available ELISA kits from General Biologicals, Taiwan and Biomerieux, Boxtel, Netherlands. The normal ranges for AST and ALT are 2–45 IU/L and 2–40 IU/L respectively.

HBV Viral DNA isolation and Quantification

HBV DNA was extracted from serum using QIAamp DNA Mini Kit (Qiagen Inc., Valencia, CA) following manufacturer's instructions. Real-Time PCR was used to quantify viral DNA (Applied Biosystems, Foster city, USA). The lower limit of detection is 250 copies/ml.

Amplification of full-length HBV genome and DNA Sequencing

Full length HBV genome (~3.2 kb) was amplified by one-step PCR method using P1/P2 primers [23] and for samples with low viral load, nested PCR was performed using MP1/R5 and F3/MP2 primers (Table 1). The QIA Quick Gel Extraction Kit (Qiagen, CA) was used to purify PCR products and the sequences were determined using the Big Dye terminator v3.1 cycle sequencing kit (ABI, USA) on an automated DNA Sequencer (ABI Prism 3130). Editing and analysis of the DNA sequences were done using Seqscape V2.5 (ABI, USA) software.

Phylogenetic Tree construction

To construct a Phylogenetic tree, 92 full-length HBV DNA sequences obtained from this study were compared with repre-

Table 1. List of primers used to generate PCR product from HBV genome.

Primer Name	Primer Sequences	Nucleotide Position
P1[a]	5 -CCGGAAAGCTTGAGCTCTTCTTTTTCACCTCTGCCTAATCA- 3′	1821–1841
P2[a]	5′-CGGAAAGCTTGAGCTCTTCAAAAAGTTGCATGGTGCTGG- 3′	1806–1825
MP1[b,c]	5′-GAGCTCTTCTTTTTCACCTCTGCCTAATCA- 3′	1821–1841
MP2[b]	5′-GAGCTCTTCAAAAAGTTGCATGGTGCTGG- 3′	1806–1825
2412F[c]	5′-GCGTCGCAGAAGATCTCAATC-3′	2412–2432
R4[c]	5′ -AGAGGACAAACGGGCAACA- 3′	462–480
R5[b]	5′ -AAAGCCCAAAAGACCCACAAT-3′	997–1017
F3[b,c]	5′ -CGCCTCATTTTGTGGGTCAC- 3′	2801–2820
R3[c]	5′ -AACTGGAGCCACCAGCAG-3′	57–74
F9[c]	5′ -TACCACAAGAGCACATTATACA- 3′	908–929
1482F[c]	5′-CTACCGTCCCCTTCTTCATC-3′	1482–1501

[a]Primers used for one-step full-length PCR,
[b]Primers used for nested PCR,
[c]Primers used for sequencing.

sentative 55 complete HBV sequences of eight different genotypes (A–H) retrieved from GenBank using Clustal W (MEGA 4.1) software. To confirm the reliability of the phylogenetic tree analysis, bootstrap re-sampling and reconstruction were carried out 5000 times. Sequence variability was analysed with the help of multiple sequence alignment.

Accession numbers of submitted Nucleotide sequences

The full genome nucleotide sequences of ninety-two HBV isolates used for analysis in this paper are available in Genbank database http://www.ncbi.nlm.nih.gov/GenBank/index.html by the accession numbers KC875251- KC875342.

Statistical Analysis

All statistical analyses were performed using "R" software version 2.14.1 and SPSS version 16.0. To evaluate the association of a mutation in progression of the disease, ANOVA was performed. Two groups (Non-HCC and HCC) were compared using Mann-Whitney U tests for continuous variables and the $\chi 2$ test or Fisher's exact test for categorical variables. Multivariable analysis applying the method of binary logistic regression was performed to find out the independent risk factors for HCC taking the clinical parameters and HBV genetic mutations, which were found to be significant in univariate analysis as independent variables. Two-tailed p values of <0.05 was considered as statistically significant.

Results

92 treatment naïve patients with chronic HBV infection were screened in the present study at inclusion. The amplified full-length genome or overlapping fragments were sequenced directly and analysed. The phylogenetic tree analysis with complete HBV sequences (n = 92) (Figure S1) showed the presence of HBV-genotype D (n = 68; 74%), HBV-genotype C (n = 14; 15%) and HBV-genotype A (n = 10; 11%). Since we were interested in HBV genotype D, subsequent mutation analysis was pursued exclusively in the sixty-eight HBV-genotype D isolates. During extracting data, we observed escalating trend in several clinical parameters (data not shown) and also in viral mutation rate accompanying with the progression of the disease stages but to identify the risk factor of HCC occurrence, we categorized the four disease stages nLF, LF, LC and HCC into two groups such as HCC and non-HCC which includes nLF, LF and LC.

Demographic profile of the study subjects with chronic HBV-genotype D infection

Table 2 shows the demographic, clinical and biochemical details of sixty-eight patients. 84% (57/68) of the subjects were males and 32% (22/68) had HCC. HCC patients were significantly older than non-HCC group (mean age, 52.8±10.9 yrs. in HCC vs. 38.2±15.2 yrs. in non-HCC; p = 0.0001) and 73% (16/22) of the HCC had underlying cirrhosis. However, neither HBV DNA load (5.02±1.41 and 5.0±1.84 log copies/ml in HCC and non-HCC, respectively; p = 0.97) nor the frequency of HBeAg positivity [40.9% (9/22) vs.45.5% (20/46) in HCC vs. non-HCC; p = 0.79)] was differed significantly between the HCC and non-HCC subjects (Table 2).

Pattern of distribution of mutations across the HBV genome among different stages of liver diseases

The prevalence of mutations, which were showing an increasing trend from nLF (no liver fibrosis) to HCC through LF (liver fibrosis) and LC (liver cirrhosis) is summarized in Table 3. Only those mutations were considered for analysis, which were noted with mutation frequency more than 6% (i.e., present in at least ≥4 samples) among 68 HBV-genotype D subjects.

i. Mutations in the regulatory regions of HBV:

Out of two enhancers and four promoters in the HBV genome, five mutations were noted with rising prevalence through progressive disease stages of nLF-LF-LC and HCC. Two point mutations in enhancer-I region (nt. 1021–1234), T1050G/A and A1053G were noticed first time in HBV-genotype D. Although the prevalence of A1053G was extremely high in both LC (50%) and HCC (50%), it was only 6% in nLF and 11% in LF (p = 0.081) whereas, T1050G/A and their combination T1050G/A+A1053G showed significant escalating trend over the course of infection from nLF (18%, 0%) to HCC (54%, 32%) through LF (22%, 11%) and LC (35%, 25%) (p = 0.035, 0.008 respectively). The most common mutation in BCP (nt.1751–1769) A1762T and G1764A,

Table 2. Clinical, biochemical and demographic profile of sixty-eight patients included in the study.

Parameters	All Patients (n = 68)	Patients without HCC (n = 46)	Patients with HCC (n = 22)	p value
Men; n (%)	57 (84)	37 (80)	20 (91)	NS
Age [year]$^{\Delta}$,	42.9±15.5	38.2±15.2	52.8±10.9	0.0001
HBeAg Positivity; n (%)	29 [43.9]	20 [45.5]	9 [40.9]	0.79
Anti-HBeAg Positivity; n (%)	34 [53.1]	21 [48.8]	13 [61.9]	0.42
HBV DNA [log$_7$ Copies/ml] $^{\Delta}$	5.01±1.7	5.0±1.84	5.02±1.41	0.97
Prevalence of cirrhosis; n (%)	36 [52.9]	20 [43.5]	16 [72.7]	0.01
Total Bilirubin, [mg/dL] $^{\beta}$,	1.5 [0.4–33.3]	1.3 [0.4–20]	2.5 [0.5–33.3]	0.03
ALT [IU/L]$^{\beta}$	65 [19–744]	56 [19–744]	90 [54–254]	0.004
AST [IU/L] $^{\beta}$	86 [22–440]	55 [22–408]	123 [70–440]	0.001
ALP [IU/L] $^{\beta}$	158 [55–702]	136 [55–702]	298 [59–580]	0.005
INR$^{\Delta}$	1.39±0.42	1.36±0.43	1.44±0.42	0.52
Albumin [g/dL] $^{\Delta}$	3.7±0.94	3.8±0.96	3.4±0.84	0.07
Globulin [g/dL] $^{\beta}$	3.3 [0.8–6.3]	3.2 [0.8–6.3]	3.8 [1.2–4.8]	0.09

SD = Standard deviation; NS = Not significant; ALT = Alanine aminotransferase; AST = Aspartate aminotransferase; INR = International normalized ratio; ALP = Alkaline phosphatase; IU = International unit; Δ Parameters presented as Mean±SD; β parameters presented as Median [Range]; δ Mutations with statistically significant difference between the groups are presented.

which reduce the expression of HBeAg were always detected in combination with extremely high frequency in each of the disease stages, 35% in nLF, 44% in LF, 65% in LC and 77% in HCC ($p = 0.01$). Mutation C1653T in enhancer-II and T1753C in BCP, which were reported previously as risk factor for HCC in HBV-genotype C [24], were not observed with significantly enhancing frequencies from nLF to HCC through LF and LC in HBV-genotype D infection ($p = 0.079$, 0.14 respectively).

ii. Mutations in four ORF regions:

Surface ORF. The HBV envelope composed of three forms of Surface antigens: large (encoded by preS1/pre S2/S), middle (coded by pre S2/S) and small (Surface gene). The most notable amino acid substitution observed in overlapping B and T cell epitopes of pre S1 region was S98T, which showed significant association with disease progression from LF (11%) to HCC (32%) through LC (20%) ($p = 0.001$) and was undetected in nLF. In pre S2 and pre S1 regions, few scattered deletions were observed but were not significantly linked to HCC. Interestingly, two mutations in "a determinant region" of surface T125M and T127L were noted inversely correlated with each other. T125M was found with high frequency (>52%) in nLF, LF and LC but low in HCC (32%) whereas T127L was noted only in LC (20%) and HCC (41%). Additionally, a single point mutation L213I in C-terminal region of surface was encountered at a high frequency in LC (45%) and HCC (50%) patients but was statistically insignificant ($p = 0.085$).

HBx ORF. No new amino acid substitution in B cell (aa. 29–48) or T cell (aa. 91–105) immune epitopes of HBx ORF [24] was significantly altered with progression of CHB to HCC, except the changes in BCP region, which induce mutations in overlapping HBx ORF such as T1753C to I127T, A1762T and G1764A to K130M and V131I.

Precore/core ORF. The occurrence of precore mutation, T1858C was noticed with an increasing frequencies of 5.88% in nLF, 11% in LF, 15% in LC and 36% in HCC ($p = 0.08$). Other two precore mutations G1862T and G1896A, which were frequently found in HBeAg negative patients, were noted exclusively in the advanced stages such as LC and HCC (10%, 0% and 18%, 27%; $p = 0.05$ and 0.225 respectively) (Table 3).

Variabilities in T helper (T_h) epitopes (aa. 35–45 and 48–69), B cell epitopes (aa.76–89, 105–116, 130–135) and Cytotoxic T lymphocyte (CTL) epitopes (aa.18–27, 50–69, 74–83, 141–151) of core protein were found important in disease progression to LC and HCC [25]. Overall three mutations in T_h epitope (T12S, S35T, T67N) and one in CTL epitope (T147C) of core showed significant association with HCC ($p < 0.05$) (Table 3). Few other mutations E113Q (36%), I116L (50%) and P130Q (32%) in B cell epitope were observed with high frequency in HCC but the differences were insignificant.

Polymerase ORF. The preS/S ORF is completely overlapped to the polymerase gene. The L213I mutation (TTA to ATG) in surface leads to F221Y and A222T dual mutations in reverse transcriptase (RT) domain of HBV polymerase resulting a change in polymerase activity or viral replication [25] whereas the mutation S98T in pre S1 (L12V in Polymerase) lies in the non-essential spacer region of the polymerase. No other mutations were noticed in the RT domain of the polymerase gene.

Identification of point mutations associated with HCC

The significance of mutations in relation to HCC occurrence was further investigated by univariate logistic regression analysis between two groups' non-HCC (nLF+LF+LC) and HCC. As shown in Figure 1, age was an associated risk factor for HCC development ($p < 0.01$) but the common A1762T/G1764A dual mutation in BCP failed to show significant correlation in both HBeAg positive [89% (8/9)] and negative HCC [69% (9/13)] compared to non-HCC [60% (12/20); $p = 0.2$ and 42% (10/24); $p = 0.17$ in HBeAg positive and negative cases respectively]. Patients harbouring T1753C in BCP, T147C in CTL epitope of core and L213I mutation in surface were found more in HBeAg positive HCC than non-HCC cases (67% vs. 20%; 67% vs. 15% and 67% vs. 20% between HCC and non-HCC respectively). The odds ratios (OR) of these three mutations for HCC risk were significant at 7.3 [95% CI (1.037–67.9), $p = 0.032$] for both T1753C and L213I and 10.1 [95% CI (1.334 106.5), $p = 0.01$] for T147C (Table S1). While the prevalence of T1858C in precore, two mutations in B cell epitopes of core I116L and P130Q and S98T in pre S1 were predominant in HBeAg negative HCC (38%

Table 3. Frequencies of mutations showing escalating trend with the progression of the liver diseases from no liver fibrosis (nLF) or liver fibrosis (LF) to liver cirrhosis (LC) and hepatocellular carcinoma (HCC).

Position of mutations in HBV genome	non-HCC			HCC n [%] n=22	p-value [One way Anova] upto LC	p-value [One way Anova] upto HCC
Regulatory regions (Nucleotide change)	**nLF n[%] n=17**	**LF n[%] n=9**	**LC n[%] n=20**			
Enhancer I/HBx promoter (1021–1373)						
T1050G/A	3 [17.65]	2 [22.22]	7 [35.00]	12 [54.55]	0.17	0.035
A1053G	1 [5.88]	1 [11.11]	10 [50.00]	11 50.00]	0.26	0.081
T1050G/A+A1053G	0 [0.00]	1 [11.11]	5 [25.00]	7 [31.82]	0.04	0.008
Enhancer II (1636–1741)						
C1653T	0 [0.00]	2 [22.22]	5 [25.00]	7 [31.82]	0.26	0.079
BCP (1751–1769)						
T1753C	1[5.88]	2 [22.22]	7 [35.00]	7 [31.82]	0.12	0.14
A1762T/G1764A	6 [35.29]	4 [44.44]	13 [65.00]	17 [77.27]	0.13	0.01
Precore (1814–1900)						
G1862T	0 [0.00]	0 [0.00]	2 [10.00]	4 [18.18]	0.33	0.05
T1858C	1 [5.88]	1 [11.11]	3 [15.00]	8 [36.36]	0.054	0.08
G1896A	0 [0.00]	0 [0.00]	0 [0.00]	6 [27.27]	-	0.225
ORFs (Amino acid change)						
Pre S1						
S98T (T3139A)	0 [0.00]	1 [11.11]	4 [20.00]	7 [31.82]	0.041	0.001
Surface						
T125M (C528T)	9 [52.94]	7 [77.78]	11 [55.00]	7 [31.82]	0.952	0.408
T127L (C534T)	0 [0.00]	0 [0.00]	4 [20.00]	9 [40.91]	0.333	0.057
L213I (T791A)	0 [0.00]	0 [0.00]	9 [45.00]	11 [50.00]	0.333	0.085
HBx						
H94Y (C1653T)	0 [0.00]	2 [22.22]	5 [25.00]	7 [31.82]	0.269	0.079
I127T (T1753C)	1 [5.88]	2 [22.22]	7 [35.00]	7 [31.82]	0.129	0.106
K130M (A1762T)/ V131I (G1764A)	6 [35.29]	4 [44.44]	13 [65.00]	17 [77.27]	0.13	0.01
Core						
T12S (A1934T)	3 [17.65]	3 [33.33]	7 [35.00]	11 [50.00]	0.278	0.036
S35T (T2003A)	0 [0.00]	1 [11.11]	3 [15.00]	6 [27.27]	0.173	0.017
T67N (C2100A)	4 [23.53]	3 [33.33]	7 [35.00]	9 [40.91]	0.247	0.037
E113Q (G2237C)	0 [0.00]	3 [33.33]	5 [25.00]	8 [36.36]	0.212	0.212
I116L (A2246C)	3 [17.65]	4 [44.44]	8 [40.00]	11 [50.00]	0.157	0.157
T147C (A2339T/C2340G)	0 [0.00]	1 [11.11]	5 [25.00]	9 [40.91]	0.041	0.003
P130Q (C2289A)	0 [0.00]	0 [0.00]	3 [15.00]	7 [31.82]	0.333	0.059
Polymerase						
L12V (A2339T/C2340G)	0 [0.00]	1 [11.11]	5 [25.00]	9 [40.91]	0.041	0.003
F221Y (T791A)	0 [0.00]	0 [0.00]	9 [45.00]	11 [50.00]	0.333	0.085

Significant mutations were indicated in bold (p≤0.05) and marginal significant values were represented in italics.

vs. 4%; 62% vs. 25%, 46% vs. 4% and 46% vs. 8% in HCC vs. non-HCC respectively) with significant ORs for HCC risk at 13.2 [95% CI (1.227–705.1), p=0.014], 4.6 [95% CI (0.913–26.2), p=0.039], 17.9[95% CI (1.747–938.7), p=0.004] and 8.7 [95% CI (1.221–107.9), p=0.013] respectively.

Identification of combination of mutations associated with HCC

To evaluate any synergistic effect of HBV mutations on HCC development, the differences in frequencies of mutational combinations were determined using a pattern analysis program in "R" to generate all possible combinations. From a total of more than 100 combination patterns, four patterns (3 in HBeAg positive and 1 in HBeAg negative) were identified which were linked to HCC development. The prevalence of those combinations were

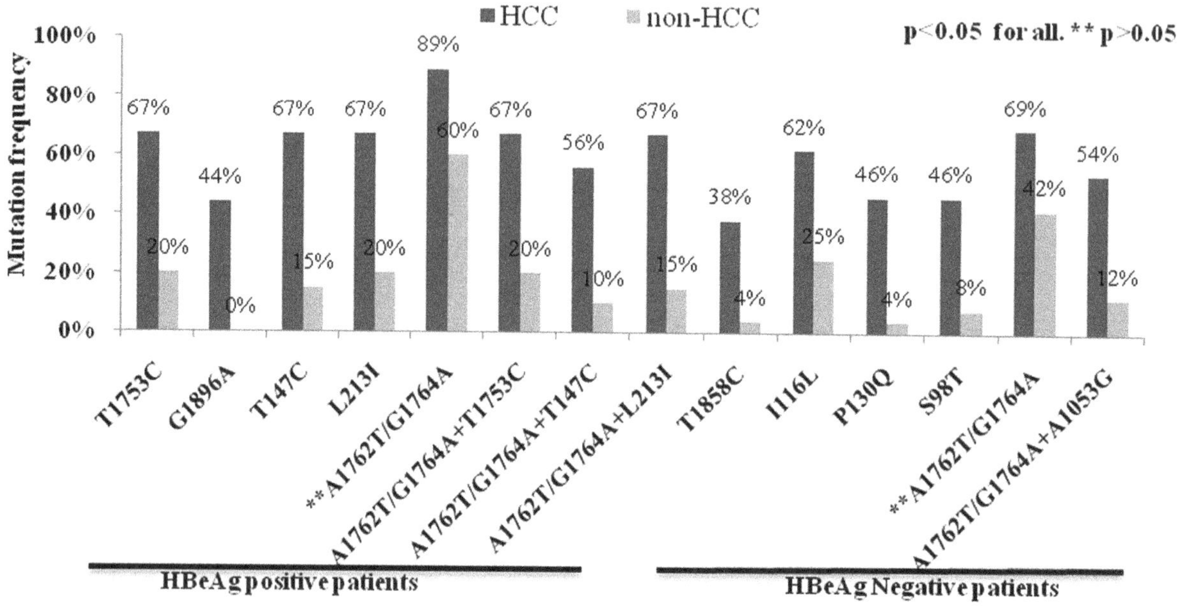

Figure 1. Frequencies of naturally occurring single and combination of mutations accumulated in the HBV genome were found significantly higher in hepatocellular carcinoma (HCC) than non-HCC patients. $p<0.05$ was considered as significant. ** indicates $p>0.05$.

significantly more in HCC than non-HCC, such as A1762T/G1764A with T1753C in enhancer II [67% (6/9) vs. 20% (4/20), p = 0.03], A1762T/G1764A with T147C in core region [56% (5/9) vs. 10% (2/20), p = 0.016)] and A1762T/G1764A with L213I in surface region [67% (6/9) vs. 15% (3/20), p = 0.01)] found in HBeAg positive patients whereas A1762T/G1764A with A1053G in enhancer-I region [54% (7/13) vs. 13% (3/24), p = 0.016] was important in HBeAg negative HCC patients (Figure 1, Table S1). The ORs of all four combinations for HCC prediction were also significant (Table S1).

Multiple logistic regression analysis to determine the risk factors for HCC development

Finally, to identify the independent predictive factor for the development of HCC multiple logistic regression analysis was performed. Older age and the presence of T147C [OR 14.58, 95% CI (1.17–181.76), p = 0.037] in CTL epitope and P130Q [OR 20.71, 95% CI (1.64–261.77), p = 0.019] on B-cell epitope were identified as independent predictor of HCC in HBeAg positive and negative patients respectively (Table 4). No combination of mutations was found as independent risk factor, which might be due to small number of study subjects.

Discussion

We have demonstrated here that progressive accumulation of mutations in HBV genome exert a powerful effect on the occurrence of HCC in HBV infected subjects and such influence of individual mutations are magnified by mutational combinations, indicating synergism rather than an additive effect which is similar to the data suggested from recent meta-analysis studies [26–29]. This is the first study dealing with the full-length genome of HBV and observed mutations in the entire genome of HBV are important for progression of liver diseases. Although, two Indian studies by the same group had delineated several mutations associated with HBV-genotype D related HCC [30,31], but detailed analysis to shape that into a defined predictive group had not been done. Thus this study put into focus several findings at the level of individual genes, beyond the well described classical ones in the precore and basal core promoter regions which are well known to be associated with progressive liver diseases–that are relatively novel and delineate their significance as candidate risk factor of HCC.

According to the previous studies in HBV genotype B, genotype C [32–34] and few studies with genotype D [30,31,35,36], BCP_A1762T/G1764A, precore_G1896A, EnhII_C1653T, BCP_T1753V mutations and pre S2 deletions are frequently associated risk factors of HCC. Our study had also found a significant association of BCP_A1762T/G1764A mutation to the liver disease progression from nLF to HCC (Table 3). This mutation is associated with high viral replication through the removal of nuclear receptor-binding factor and generation of new binding site for hepatocyte nuclear factor (HNF) [37], which is responsible for HCC occurrence and also recurrence after resection [38,39]. Although this dual mutation was highly prevalent in both HBeAg positive and negative HCC (88.88% and 69.23% respectively) compared to non-HCC (60% and 42% respectively), no significant correlation was noted with disease manifestations in binary logistic regression analysis ($P>0.05$, Table S1), which might be because of small study subjects. This combination was also not found associated with HCC in previous study with genotype D [30,31] but showed correlation in HCC with HBV-genotype C [33,26]. The frequency of BCP_C1653T mutation in the enhancer-II region was increasing with disease severity (Table 3) but it did not correlate well with LC or HCC, which was previously documented as an independent risk factor for HCC with HBV-genotype C [40] suggesting its genotype specific role in HCC development.

In a previous study from India BCP_T1753C mutation was reported as risk factor for LC rather than HCC [30,31] which was

Table 4. Multivariate analysis to identify independent risk factors for HCC development in HBeAg positive and negative patients.

Mutations	Multiple logistic regression analysis	
In HBeAg Positive	**OR [95% CI]**	**p value [Fisher's Exact]**
T1753C	11.48 [0.95–139.09]	0.055
T147C	14.58 [1.17–181.76]	**0.037**
L213I	5.61 [0.59–53.05]	0.133
In HBeAg negative		
T1858C	3.08 [0.19–50.44]	0.43
I116L	2.53 [0.37–17.49]	0.348
P130Q	20.71 [1.64–261.77]	**0.019**
S98T	8.91 [0.98–81.08]	0.052

p value <0.05 was considered as significant.

similar to our analysis from frequency distribution (Table 3) but univariate analysis further identified this mutation as risk factor for HCC in HBeAg positive patients. This mutation was also reported as risk factor for HBV-genotype D related HCC from Mongolia [35]. Again, in consistence with the previous report in HBV genotype C, this mutation in combination with BCP_A1762T/G1764A showed significant association with HBeAg positive HCC development (Figure 1). Recently it has been found that this combination of mutations exhibited an enhanced viral replication phenotype like BCP_A1762T/G1764A alone [36] but its exact role in hepatocarcinogenesis is unclear.

The role of HBV enhancer-I region/HBx promoter in HCC has been studied very infrequently, except in one study [41] and almost never in HBV genotype D. However, we observed several sequence heterogeneities in this region. Previously, the G1053A mutation at the p53 factor like binding site was shown to enhance the expression of HBx and it was correlated well with the high replication efficiency of the HBV-genotype C virus [41]. But the clinical relevance of the high prevalence of A1053G and T1050G/A mutation in HBV-genotype D and its association with HCC is not clear (Table 3). These mutations might not affect HBsAg but could alter polymerase activity as another mutation in this region, T1055A has been reported to affect the conformation of two helices and impair HBV DNA-primer interaction [42]. Few new combination of mutations in the enhancer-I region were also noted in LC and HCC such as T1029C/A1032G (>30%), T1059A/A1105C (>25%), and C1249T/T1250C (>15%) indicating their importance in LC and HCC development (data not shown) but not found significant in this study. The B cell (aa. 26–45) and T cell epitope (aa. 116–127) of HBx are frequently altered in HBV-genotype C and B [24], but no significant sequence heterogeneity was noted in the epitopes of HBV–genotype D, except three mutations I127T (T1753C), K130M (A1762T) and V131I (G1764A), though H94Y (T1653C) was present with high frequencies in both LC and HCC (Table 3) as observed in previous study [30].

HBV core region is an important target of immune mediated viral clearance by inducing CTL, T_h cells and B cells response [43]. Mutations in $CD4^+$ T_h epitopes (aa 1–20, 28–47, 50–69, 72–105, 108–165) are usually associated with immune evasion, minimum immune mediated hepatitis and viral persistence than $CD8^+$ CTL epitopes [44]. However association of core gene mutations and HCC has not been well delineated before. Although a large number of mutations in CTL epitopes showed significant association with cirrhosis and HCC [25], no such significant change was observed in the core antigenic CTL region (18–27 amino acids) in this study. While three mutations in T_h epitopes (T12S, S35T, T67N), T147C in CTL epitope and two mutations I116L, P130Q in B cell epitopes showed significant association with disease severity (Table 3). Koschel et al showed that deletion at codon 12 is defective in virion secretion [45] while other two mutations S35T, T67N might be able to evade the host immune response for their persistence at low levels [46,47]. Interestingly, the most frequently observed naturally occurring core protein mutation found in CHB [48,49] and also in HCC patients I97L or F97L [50,51] which is associated with "immature virion secretion" was completely absent in Indian patients with HBV-genotype D while among the "low secretion core variants" such as P5T/A/S, a new variant P5R was noted with high frequency in HBV-genotype D related HCC in previous Indian study [30,31]. This mutation was also not found in our study. But the compensatory mutation of codon 97 at codon 130, P130Q was found as independent risk factor for HCC in HBeAg negative patients. Mutation T147C was not documented as HCC risk factor previously with respect to any genotype. From our multivariate analysis it is obvious that the two core mutations, T147C and P130Q could be potential predictor of HCC in high-risk HBeAg positive and negative CHB patients respectively (Table 4). In addition, T147C with classical BCP mutation A1762T/G1764A was noted significantly high in HCC than non-HCC and hence these mutations in combination could predict the progression of liver diseases more precisely.

We have also studied the naturally occurring mutations in T and B-cell epitopes of pre S1 and pre S2 regions. A recent meta-analysis study has clearly showed the association of pre S deletion with the progression of liver diseases to HCC in HBV genotype C with OR 3.77 [95% CI (2.57–5.52)] [14] whereas point mutations and risk of HCC are rarely studied. To our surprise, few insignificant deletions were identified in pre S1 and pre S2 regions in HCC patients, which are in agreement with two different studies who found deletion in pre S2 might be genotype specific as observed more in HBV-genotype C than genotype B [51,52]. One point mutation L213I observed in the overlapping surface and polymerase gene (F221Y/A222T) in combination with classical BCP mutations A1762T/G1764A showed association with HCC in HBeAg positive patient (Figure 1). This mutation might be associated with immune evasion and active viral replication. The S98T mutation found in the overlapping T and B cell epitope region of pre S1, which is the binding site of heat shock protein 70

(HSP70) (aa74–118) [53] might be an independent predictor for HCC in HBeAg negative patient (Table 4).

The clinical significance of G1896A mutation is ambiguous. In accordance with other studies this mutation was found in advanced form of liver diseases [53] while some studies showed either its occurrence in inactive carrier [54] or it has no association with clinical outcomes [14]. Another precore mutation, T1858C, which makes a pair with G1896A to stabilize the viral encapsidation signal and enhance viral replication, was observed significantly associated with more aggressive course of liver diseases in HBeAg negative HCC (Figure 1) similar to previous study [55].

In accordance to the previously identified risk factors for HCC such as male sex, age>50 yrs, high serum ALT level, HBeAg, high HBV DNA level, HBV genotype C and D and point or combination of mutations in BCP, precore and pre S as powerful contributor in CHB patients [56–58], this study has identified late age, high ALT and several point and combination of mutations in BCP, precore, core and surface as predictors of HCC in HBV genotype D infected CHB patients ($p<0.05$).

Thus in conclusion, comparing the full-length genome sequences of HBV-genotype D isolates from HCC and non-HCC groups, core gene exhibited the most significant alteration in mutation frequency ($p<0.02$). A comparatively larger group of each morphological – Fibrosis phenotype used in the current study might improve the strength of our observations and we are planning that. Despite this limitation in small sample numbers, these findings, depicting a robust correlation of HBV genomic mutational combinations on HCC development in HBV genotype D, are unique and are likely to have connotations as well as relevance for designing downstream studies in this area using high throughput molecular tools. In addition, analogous to the clinical utility that a pattern of combined mutation in somatic genes provide in several cancers [59,60], viral mutational combination patterns may also prove useful in picking up high risk CHB infections at risk for developing HCC and supplement existing surveillance strategies in this group, as a supportive tool.

Supporting Information

Figure S1 Phylogenetic tree analysis of full-length genome of ninety-two HBV isolates from treatment naive patients with different clinical stages along with fifty-five reference sequences of eight different HBV genotypes (A–H), retrieved from Genbank including two HBV sequences of non-primate origin. Reference sequences are indicated by the genotypes followed by accession number and origin of the countries. The tree was constructed using neighbour joining (Nj) method by MEGA 5.10. software and bootstrap re-sampling and re-construction were repeated 5000 times. ◀ and ▶ indicate no liver fibrosis (anti-clockwise) and Liver fibrosis (clockwise) while ■ and ● denote Liver cirrhosis and Hepatocellular carcinoma respectively.

Table S1 Frequencies of single or combination of mutations associated with HBeAg positive and negative HCC patients.

Acknowledgments

We would like to thank to Dr. Saroj K Mahapatra and Dr. Soumalee Basu for their constant support. Somenath Datta, Alip Ghosh, Amit Ghosh and Debanjali Dasgupta have registered their PhD's under West Bengal University of Health Sciences.

Author Contributions

Conceived and designed the experiments: SB. Performed the experiments: Somenath Datta. Analyzed the data: Somenath Datta Alip Ghosh AB AC KD Simanti Datta SB. Contributed reagents/materials/analysis tools: SR DD Amit Ghosh GR SG KB S. Das. Wrote the paper: SB Somenath Datta AC.

References

1. Beasley RP (1988) Hepatitis B virus: the major etiology of hepatocellular carcinoma. Cancer 61: 1942–1956.
2. Nguyen VT, Law MG, Dore GJ (2009) Hepatitis B-related hepatocellular carcinoma: epidemiological characteristics and disease burden. J Viral Hepat 16: 453–63.
3. Perz JF, Armstrong GL, Farrington LA, Hutin YJ, Bell BP (2006) The contributions of hepatitis B virus and hepatitis C virus infections to cirrhosis and primary liver cancer worldwide. J Hepatol 45: 529–538.
4. Llovet JM (2005) Updated treatment approach to hepatocellular carcinoma. J Gastroenterol 40: 225–235.
5. Revill P, Yuan Z (2013) New insights into how HBV manipulates the innate immune response to establish acute and persistent infection. Antivir Ther 18: 1–15.
6. Liu Z, Luo K, He H, Hou J (2005) Hot-spot mutations in hepatitis B virus core gene: eliciting or evading immune clearance? J Viral Hepat 12: 146–153.
7. Torre F, Cramp M, Owsianka A, Dornan E, Marsden H, et al. (2004) Direct evidence that naturally occurring mutations within hepatitis B core epitopes alter CD4+ T-cell reactivity. J Med Virol 72: 370–376.
8. Heriyanto DS, Yano Y, Utsumi T, Anggorowati N, Rinonce HT, et al. (2012) Mutations within enhancer II and BCP regions of hepatitis B virus in relation to advanced liver diseases in patients infected with subgenotype B3 in Indonesia. J Med Virol 84: 44–51.
9. Kao JH, Chen PJ, Lai MY, Chen DS (2003) Basal core promoter mutations of hepatitis B virus increase the risk of hepatocellular carcinoma in hepatitis B carriers. Gastroenterology 124: 327–334.
10. Song BC, Cui XJ, Kim HU, Cho YK (2006) Sequential accumulation of the basal core promoter and the precore mutations in the progression of hepatitis B virus-related chronic liver disease. Intervirology 49: 266–273.
11. Baptista M, Kramvis A, Kew MC (1999) High prevalence of 1762(T) 1764(A) mutations in the basic core promoter of hepatitis B virus isolated from black Africans with hepatocellular carcinoma compared with asymptomatic carriers. Hepatology 29: 946–953.
12. Kao JH (2003) Hepatitis B virus genotypes and hepatocellular carcinoma in Taiwan. Intervirology 46: 400–407.
13. Takahashi K, Akahane Y, Hino K, Ohta Y, Mishiro S (1998) Hepatitis B virus genomic sequence in the circulation of hepatocellular carcinoma patients: comparative analysis of 40 full-length isolates. Arch Virol 143: 2313–2326.
14. Liu S, Zhang H, Gu C, Yin J, He Y, et al. (2009) Associations between hepatitis B virus mutations and the risk of hepatocellular carcinoma: a meta-analysis. J Natl Cancer Inst 101: 1066–1082.
15. Zhu Y, Jin Y, Guo X, Bai X, Chen T, et al. (2010) Comparison study on the complete sequence of hepatitis B virus identifies new mutations in core gene associated with hepatocellular carcinoma. Cancer Epidemiol Biomarkers Prev 19: 2623–2630.
16. Datta S (2008) An overview of molecular epidemiology of hepatitis B virus (HBV) in India. Virol J 5: 156–156.
17. Ismail AM, Puhazhenthi KS, Sivakumar J, Eapen CE, Kannangai R, et al. (2014) Molecular epidemiology and genetic characterization of hepatitis B virus in the Indian subcontinent. Int J Infect Dis 20: 1–10.
18. Dhir V, Mohandas KM (1998) Epidemiology of digestive tract cancers in India. III. Liver. Indian J Gastroenterol 17: 100–103.
19. Paul SB, Sreenivas V, Gulati MS, Madan K, Gupta AK, et al. (2007) Incidence of hepatocellular carcinoma among Indian patients with cirrhosis of liver: an experience from a tertiary care center in northern India. Indian J Gastroenterol 26: 274–278.
20. Asim M, Sarma MP, Kar P (2013) Etiological and molecular profile of hepatocellular cancer from India. Int J Cancer 133: 437–445.
21. Das K, Sarkar R, Ahmed SM, Mridha AR, Mukherjee PS, et al. (2012) "Normal" liver stiffness measure (LSM) values are higher in both lean and obese individuals: a population-based study from a developing country. Hepatology 55: 584–593.
22. Wang JH, Changchien CS, Hung CH, Eng HL, Tung WC, et al. (2009) FibroScan and ultrasonography in the prediction of hepatic fibrosis in patients with chronic viral hepatitis. J Gastroenterol 44: 439–446.

23. Günther S, Li BC, Miska S, Krüger DH, Meisel H, et al. (1995) A novel method for efficient amplification of whole hepatitis B virus genomes permits rapid functional analysis and reveals deletion mutants in immune suppressed patients. J Virol 69: 5437–5444.
24. Hwang GY, Huang CJ, Lin CY, Wu CC (2003) Dominant mutations of hepatitis B virus variants in hepatoma accumulate in B-cell and T-cell epitopes of the HBx antigen. Virus Res 92: 157–164.
25. Kim D, Lyoo KS, Smith D, Hur W, Hong SW, et al. (2011) Number of mutations within CTL-defined epitopes of the hepatitis B Virus (HBV) core region is associated with HBV disease progression. J Med Virol 83: 2082–2087.
26. Yin J, Xie J, Liu S, Zhang H, Han L, et al. (2011) Association between the various mutations in viral core promoter region to different stages of hepatitis B, ranging of asymptomatic carrier state to hepatocellular carcinoma. Am J Gastroenterol 106: 81–92.
27. Liu S, Zhang H, Gu C, Yin J, He Y, et al. (2009) Associations between hepatitis B virus mutations and the risk of hepatocellular carcinoma: a meta-analysis. J Natl Cancer Inst 101: 1066–1082.
28. Park YM, Jang JW, Yoo SH, Kim SH, Oh IM, et al. (2014) Combinations of eight key mutations in the X/preC region and genomic activity of hepatitis B virus are associated with hepatocellular carcinoma. J Viral Hepat 21: 171–177.
29. Qu LS, Zhu J, Liu TT, Shen XZ, Chen TY, et al. (2013) Effect of combined mutations in the enhancer II and basal core promoter of hepatitis B virus on development of hepatocellular carcinoma in Qidong, China. Hepatol Res doi: 10.1111/hepr.12291.
30. Asim M, Malik A, Sarma MP, Polipalli SK, Begum N, et al. (2010) Hepatitis B Virus BCP, Precore/Core, X Gene Mutations/Genotypes and the Risk of Hepatocellular Carcinoma in India. Journal of Medical Virology 82: 1115–1125.
31. Malik A, Singhal DK, Albanyan A, Husain SA, Kar P (2012) Hepatitis B virus gene mutations in liver diseases: a report from New Delhi. PLoS One 7(6): e39028.
32. Tanaka Y, Mukaide M, Orito E, Yuen MF, Ito K, et al. (2006) Specific mutations in enhancer II/core promoter of hepatitis B virus subgenotypes C1/C2 increase the risk of hepatocellular carcinoma. J Hepatol 45: 646–53.
33. Yang HI, Yeh SH, Chen PJ, Iloeje UH, Jen CL, et al. (2008) REVEAL-HBV Study Group. Associations between hepatitis B virus genotype and mutants and the risk of hepatocellular carcinoma. J Natl Cancer Inst 100: 1134–1143.
34. Bai X, Zhu Y, Jin Y, Guo X, Qian G, et al. (2011) Temporal acquisition of sequential mutations in the enhancer II and basal core promoter of HBV in individuals at high risk for hepatocellular carcinoma. Carcinogenesis 32: 63–68.
35. Elkady A, Tanaka Y, Kurbanov F, Oynsuren T, Mizokami M (2008) Virological and clinical implication of core promoter C1752/V1753 and T1764/G1766 mutations in hepatitis B virus genotype D infection in Mongolia. J Gastroenterol Hepatol 23: 474–481.
36. Khan A, Al Balwi MA, Tanaka Y, Hajeer A, Sanai FM, et al. (2013) Novel point mutations and mutational complexes in the enhancer II, core promoter and precore regions of hepatitis B virus genotype D1 associated with hepatocellular carcinoma in Saudi Arabia. Int J Cancer 133: 2864–2871.
37. Long Y, Chen E, Liu C, Huang F, Zhou T, et al. (2009) The correlation of hepatocyte nuclear factor 4 alpha and 3 beta with hepatitis B virus replication in the liver of chronic hepatitis B patients. Viral Hepat 16: 537–546.
38. Chen CJ, Yang HI, Su J, Jen CL, You SL, et al. (2006) REVEAL-HBV Study Group. Risk of hepatocellular carcinoma across a biological gradient of serum hepatitis B virus DNA level. JAMA 295: 65–73.
39. Wu CF, Yu MW, Lin CL, Liu CJ, Shih WL, http://www.ncbi.nlm.nih.gov/pubmed?term=Tsai%20KS%5BAuthor%5D&cauthor=true&cauthor_uid=17999990 et al. (2008) Long-term tracking of hepatitis B viral load and the relationship with risk for hepatocellular carcinoma in men. Carcinogenesis 29: 106–112.
40. Kim JK, Chang HY, Lee JM, Baatarkhuu O, Yoon YJ, et al. (2009) Specific mutations in the enhancer II/core promoter/Precore regions of hepatitis B virus subgenotype C2 in Korean patients with hepatocellular carcinoma. J Med Virol 816: 1002–1008.
41. Cho EY, Kim HC, Choi CS, Shin SR, Park C, et al. (2010) Nucleotide changes related to hepatocellular carcinoma in the enhancer 1/x-promoter of hepatitis B virus subgenotype C2 in cirrhotic patients. Cancer Sci 101: 1905–1912.
42. Wu Y, Gan Y, Gao F, Zhao Z, Jin Y, et al. (2014) Novel natural mutations in the hepatitis B virus reverse transcriptase domain associated with hepatocellular carcinoma. PLoS One 9: e94864.
43. Chisari FV (2000) Rous-Whipple Award Lecture. Viruses, immunity and cancer: lessons from hepatitis B. Am J Pathol 156: 1117–1132.
44. Bertoletti A, Sette A, Chisari FV, Penna A, Levrero M, et al. (1994) Natural variants of cytotoxic epitopesare T-cell receptor antagonists for antiviral cytotoxic T cells. Nature 369: 407–410.
45. Koschel M, Oed D, Gerelsaikhan T, Thomssen R, Bruss V (2000) Hepatitis B virus core gene mutations which block nucleocapsid envelopment. J. Virol 74: 1–7.
46. Assar S, Arababadi MK, Mohit M, Ahmadabadi BN, Pumpens P, et al. (2012) T helper and B cell escape mutations within the HBc gene in patients with asymptomatic HBV infection: a study from the South-Eastern region of Iran. Clin Lab 58: 53–60.
47. Mohebbi SR, Amini-Bavil-Olyaee S, Zali N, Damavand B, Azimzadeh P, et al. (2012) Characterizationof hepatitis B virus genome variability in Iranian patientswith chronic infection, a nationwide study. J Med Virol 84: 414–423.
48. Akarca US, Lok AS (1995) Naturally occurring hepatitis B virus core gene mutations. Hepatology 22: 50–60.
49. Bozkaya H, Ayola B, Lok AS (1996) High rate of mutations in the hepatitis B core gene during the immune clearance phase of chronic hepatitis B virus infection. Hepatology 24: 32–37.
50. Yuan TT, Sahu GK, Whitehead WE, Greenberg R, Shih C (1999) The mechanism of an immature secretion phenotype of a highly frequent naturally occurring missense mutation at codon 97 of human hepatitis B virus core antigen. J Virol 73: 5731–5740.
51. Matsuura K, Tanaka Y, Hige S, Yamada G, Murawaki Y, et al. (2009) Distribution of hepatitis B virus genotypes among patients with chronic infection in Japan shifting toward an increase of genotype A. J Clin Microbiol 47: 1476–1483.
52. Tai PC, Suk FM, Gerlich WH, Neurath AR, Shih C (2002) Hypermodification and immune escape of an internally deleted middle-envelope (M) protein of frequent and predominant hepatitis B virus variants. Virology 292: 44–58.
53. Prange R, Werr M, Löffler-Mary H (1999) Chaperones Involved in Hepatitis B Virus Morphogenesis. Biol Chem 380: 305–14.
54. Tong MJ, Blatt LM, Kao JH, Cheng JT, Corey WG (2007) Basal core promoter T1762/A1764 and precore A1896 gene mutations in hepatitis B surface antigen-positive hepatocellular carcinoma: a comparison with chronic carriers. Liver Int 27: 1356–1363.
55. Tanaka Y, Hasegawa I, Kato T, Orito E, Hirashima N, et al. (2004) A case-control study for differences among hepatitis B virus infections of genotypes A (subtypes Aa and Ae) and D. Hepatology 40: 747–755.
56. Tseng TC, Liu CJ, Yang HC, Su TH, Wang CC, et al. (2012) High levels of hepatitis B surface antigen increase risk of hepatocellular carcinoma in patients with low HBV load. Gastroenterology 142: 1140–1149.
57. Chen CH, Hung CH, Lee CM, Hu TH, Wang JH, et al. (2007) Pre-S deletion and complex mutations of hepatitis B virus related to advanced liver diseases in HBeAg-negative patients. Gastroenterology 133: 1466–1474.
58. Chen CH, Changchien CS, Lee CM, Hung CH, Hu TH, et al. (2008) Combined mutations in pre-s/surface and core promoter/precore regions of hepatitis B virus increase the risk of hepatocellular carcinoma: a case–control study. J. Infect. Dis. 198: 1634–1642.
59. Yeang CH, McCormick F, Levine A (2008) Combinatorial patterns of somatic gene mutations in cancer. FASEB J 22: 2605–2622.
60. Tejpar S, Bertagnolli M, Bosman F, Lenz HJ, Garraway L, et al. (2010) Prognostic and predictive biomarkers in resected colon cancer: current status and future perspectives for integrating genomics into biomarker discovery. Oncologist 15: 390–404.

8

A Serum MicroRNA Panel as Potential Biomarkers for Hepatocellular Carcinoma Related with Hepatitis B Virus

Youwen Tan[1,2]*, Guohong Ge[1], Tengli Pan[1], Danfeng Wen[1], Li Chen[1], Xuejun Yu[1], Xinbei Zhou[1], Jianhe Gan[2]

1 Department of Hepatosis, The Third Hospital of Zhenjiang Affiliated Jiangsu University, Zhenjiang, China, **2** Department of Infectious Diseases, The First Affiliated Hospital of Soochow University, Suzhou, China

Abstract

Background: The identification of new high-sensitivity and high-specificity markers for HCC are essential. We aimed to identify serum microRNAs (miRNAs) as biomarkers to be used in diagnosing hepatitis B virus (HBV) –related hepatocellular carcinoma (HCC).

Methods: We investigated serum miRNA expression in (261 HCC patients, 233 cirrhosis patients, and 173 healthy controls), recruited between August 2010 and June 2013. An initial screening of miRNA expression by Illumina sequencing was performed using serum samples pooled from HCC patients and controls. Quantitative reverse-transcriptase polymerase chain reaction (qRT-PCR) was used to evaluate the expression of selected miRNAs. A logistic regression model was constructed using a training cohort (n = 357) and then validated using an independent cohort (n = 241). The area under the receiver operating characteristic curve (AUC) was used to evaluate the accuracy of the use of the biomarkers for disease diagnosis.

Results: We identified 8 miRNAs (hsa-miR-206, hsa-miR-141-3p, hsa-miR-433-3p, hsa-miR-1228-5p, hsa-miR-199a-5p, hsa-miR-122-5p, hsa-miR-192-5p, and hsa-miR-26a-5p) and constructed an miRNA set that provided high diagnostic accuracy for HCC (AUC = 0.887 and 0.879 for training and validation sets, respectively). The miRNAs could also be used to differentiate HCC patients from healthy (AUC = 0.893) and cirrhosis (AUC = 0.892) patients.

Conclusions: We identified a serum of miRNA panel that has considerable clinical value in HCC diagnosis.

Editor: Xin-Yuan Guan, The University of Hong Kong, China

Funding: This work was supported by the Natural Science Foundation of Jiangsu Province, China (BK2011151) (http://www.jstd.gov.cn/), Medical Project of Health Department, Jiangsu Province (H201248) (http://www.jswst.gov.cn/), and the Social Development Project of Zhenjiang City (SH201346) (http://kjj.zhenjiang.gov.cn/). The funders played no role in the study design, data collection and analysis, decision to publish, or preparation of the manuscript.

Competing Interests: The authors have declared that no competing interests exist.

* Email: tyw915@sina.com

Introduction

Hepatocellular carcinoma (HCC) is currently the third leading cause of cancer-related deaths in the world, with mortality rates reaching up to 500,000 deaths per annum. Patients with HCC show the shortest survival time among patients with different forms of cancer, with most patients dying within 12 months of developing the tumour [1]. A previous study has suggested that early diagnosis of HCC and effective treatment are likely to prolong the lifetime of liver cancer patients [2]. Current methods for the diagnosis of HCC fall into two main categories: imaging and biomarker tests. However, the diagnostic performance of these methodsis unsatisfactory, particularly for the diagnosis of early-stage HCC. Currently, only 30% to 40% of patients with HCC are found eligible for potentially curative intervention at diagnosis, due to late clinical presentation and the lack of effective early-detection measures. Therefore, the identification of new markers with high sensitivity and specificity for HCC is the need of the hour.

MicroRNAs (miRNAs) are an emerging class of highly conserved, non-coding small RNAs that regulate gene expression at the post-transcriptional level. It is now clear that miRNAs can potentially regulate every aspect of cellular activity, including differentiation and development, metabolism and proliferation; they also play a role in regulating apoptotic cell death, cellular responses to viral infection, and tumorigenesis [3]. Recent studies provide clear evidence that miRNAs are abundant in the liver and modulate a diverse spectrum of liver functions [4]. Circulating miRNAs are extremely stable and protected from RNAase-mediated degradation in body fluids; they, therefore, have emerged as candidate biomarkers for many diseases [5,6,7]. The use of miRNAs as noninvasive biomarkers is of particular interest in diagnosis of liver diseases [8,9,10].

Many studies have demonstrated that miRNA expression profiles in HCC and non-tumor tissue are significantly different [11,12,13,14,15]. In fact, differential expression of several microRNAs in the serum, including miR-16, miR-122, miR-21, miR-223, miR-25, miR-375, and let-7f in patients with HCC, patients with hepatitis B, and healthy individuals has been reported recently [16,17]. However, those studies had one or more of the following limitations: Limited number of screened miRNAs, small sample size, failure to differentiate HCC from hepatitis B virus (HBV) infection, and lack of independent validation.

In our study, we investigated miRNA expression profiles with independent validation in a large cohort of participants, in order to identify a set of miRNAs for the diagnosis of HCC. The cohort included healthy individuals and patients with cirrhosisand HCC related to HBV.

Materials and Methods

Ethics statement

The study was approved by the Medical Ethics Committee of The First Affiliated Hospital of Soochow University and The Third Hospital Affiliated to Jiangsu University (No. 2012046 and No. 272), and written informed consent was obtained from each patient prior to participation. The study was conducted in accordance with the Declaration of Helsinki.

Study design, patients, and healthy controls

A multistage, case-control study was designed to identify a serum miRNA profile as a surrogate marker for HCC (Fig. 1). A total of 261 HCC patients, 233 cirrhosi patients and 173 healthy controls were enrolled in our study. In the discovery biomarker stage, 9 serum samples pooled from 3 healthy control donors, 3 HCC patients and 3 cirrhosi patients treated at The First Affiliated Hospital of Soochow University were subjected to Illumina Hiseq 2000 deep sequencing to identify the miRNAs that were significantly differentially expressed. In the biomarker selection stagedifferent expression miRNAs were validated by qRT-PCR in 20 HCC patients, 20 cirrhosis patients and 20 healthy controls. Subsequently, 135 HCC patients, 132 cirrhosis patients and 90 healthy controls (from The First Affiliated Hospital of Soochow University and The Third Hospital of Zhenjiang Affiliated Jiangsu University) formed a training set. Sequential validation was performed using a hydrolysis probe-based qRT-PCR assay to refine the number of serum miRNAs as an HCC signature. Whereas an additional 103 HCC patients, 78 cirrhosis patients and 60 healthy controls serum samples (from The Third Hospital of Zhenjiang Affiliated Jiangsu University) formed an independent validation set. All patients were diagnosed with HCC and cirrhosis between August 2010 and June 2013, and blood samples were collected prior to any therapeutic procedure.

Chronic HBV infection was defined as positivity for HBV surface antigen for at least 6 months, positivity for HBV DNA by PCR analysis, and HBV infection-compatible results in a liver biopsy. All patients were positive for HBsAg and did not have any other types of liver diseases such as chronic hepatitis C, alcoholic liver diseases, autoimmune liver diseases, or metabolic liver diseases. The diagnosis of HCC and cirrhosis was histopathologically confirmed. Data on all subjects were obtained from medical records, pathology reports and personal interviews with the subjects. Tumor-free healthy control subjects were recruited from a large pool of individuals seeking a routine health check-up at the Healthy Physical Examination Centre of The First Affiliated Hospital of Soochow University who showed no evidence of disease. The demographics and clinical features of the patients arelisted in Table. 1.

RNA isolation and library preparation

About 5 mL of venous blood was collected from each participant. The whole blood was separated into serum and cellular fractions by centrifugation at 4,000 rpm for 10 min, followed by 5 min centrifugation at 13,000 rpm for complete removal of cell debris. The supernatant serum was stored at −80°C until analysis. Total RNA was isolated using LCS TRK1001 miRNeasy kit (LC Sciences, Hangzhou, China). The libraries were constructed from total RNA using the Illumina Truseq Small RNA Sample Preparation Kit (Illumina, San Diego, CA, USA) according to the manufacturer's protocol. Briefly, RNA 3′ (P-UCGUAUGCCGUCUUCUGCUUG-UidT) and 5′ (GUUCAGAGUU CUACAGUCCGACGAUC) adapters were ligated to target miRNAs in two separate steps. Reverse transcription reaction was applied to the ligation products to create single stranded cDNA. The cDNA was amplified by PCR using a common primer and a primer containing the index sequence (CAAGCAGAAGACGGCATACGA). The quantity and purity of total RNAs were monitored using a NanoDrop

Overview of the design strategy

Discovery phase: Illumina Hiseq 2000 deep sequencing on pooled samples (3 HCC vs 3 cirrhosis, 3 HCC vs 3 healthy controls.)

↓ Threshold: miRNAs have at least 20 counts, fold change>2 and P value<0.05

Selection phase: qRT-PCR detected Ct and $2^{-\Delta\Delta Ct}$ in screening set samples (20 HCC vs 20 cirrhosis and 20HCC vs. 20 healthy controls)

↓ Threshold: miRNA Ct value<35 and detection rate>75%;*p*<0.05

Training phase: qRT-PCR detected Ct in training set samples (135 HCC vs 132 cirrhosis and 135 HCC vs. 90 healthy controls)

↓ Threshold: Established miRNA panel based on the logistic regression model

Validation phase: validated on independent validation set samples (103 HCC,78 cirrhosis and 60 healthy controls)

↓ Threshold: comparison ROC curves between miRNA panel and AFP

The profile of serum base 8 miRNAs provides an unique non-invasive biomarker for HCC diagnosis

Figure 1. A flow-chart of the experimental design.

Table 1. Characteristics of study subjects in the three datasets.

Variable	screening set		training set		validation set		statistics	p
	No.	%	No.	%	No.	%		
healthy count	n = 20		n = 90		n = 60			
age								
mean	40.25		40.2		41.43		$F = 0.569$	0.567[a]
SD	7.57		6.61		7.76			
sex								
male	15	75	64	71.1	42	70	$x^2 = 0.183$	0.912[b]
female	5	25	26	28.9	18	30		
ALT								
<40 U/L	20	100	90	100	60	100	match	
AFP								
<400 ng/ml	20	100	90	100	60	100	match	
cirrhosis count	n = 20		n = 132		n = 78			
age								
mean	44.4		40.8		43.97		$F = 2.907$	0.057[a]
SD	12.03		9.44		10.81			
sex								
male	14	70	88	66.7	46	59	$x^2 = 1.57$	0.456[b]
female	6	30	44	33.3	32	41		
ALT								
<40 U/L	14	70	66	50	47	60.3	$x^2 = 4.021$	0.134[b]
≥40 U/L	6	30	66	50	31	39.7		
AFP								
<400 ng/ml	20	100	131	99.2	77	99.1	$x^2 = 0.913$	1[c]
≥400 ng/mL	0	0	1	0.8	1	0.9		
HCC count	n = 20		n = 135		n = 103			
age								
mean	49.8		53.57		52.01		$F = 1.311$	0.271[a]
SD	10.85		11.59		10.21			
sex								
male	16	80	112	83	76	73.8	$x^2 = 2.984$	0.225[b]
female	4	20	23	17	27	26.2		
ALT								

Table 1. Cont.

Variable	screening set		training set		validation set		statistics	p
	No.	%	No.	%	No.	%		
<40 U/L	11	55	47	34.8	44	42.7	$x^2 = 3.696$	0.158[b]
≥40 U/L	9	45	88	65.2	59	57.3		
AFP								
<400 ng/ml	15	75	84	62.2	62	60.2	$x^2 = 1.569$	0.456[b]
≥400 ng/mL	5	25	51	37.8	41	39.8		

[a]One-Way ANOVA,
[b]Pearson Chi-Square,
[c]Fisher's Exact Test.

ND-1000 spectrophotometer (NanoDrop Inc, Wilmington, DE, USA) at a 260/280 ratio >2.0. The integrity of total RNAs was analyzed using an Agilent 2100 Bioanalyzer system and RNA 6000 Nano LabChip Kit (Agilent Tech, Santa Clara, CA, USA) with RNA integrity number >8.0. Finally, Illumina sequencing technology was employed to sequence these prepared samples.

Illumina sequencing and data analysis

The raw sequences were processed using the Illumina pipeline program. After masking of adaptor sequences and removal of contaminated reads, the clean reads were filtered for miRNA prediction with the software package ACGT101-miR-v4.2 (LC Sciences, Houston, Texas, USA) and subsequently analyzed according to report [18]. Secondary structure prediction of individual miRNAs was performed by Mfold software (Version 2.38; http://mfold.rna.albany.edu/?q=mfold/RNA-Folding-Form) using the default folding conditions. The raw dates were reduced to cleaned sequences by removal of the following sequences: (1) 3ADT&length filter: reads were removed due to 3ADT not being found, and reads with length <18 and >26 were removed. (2) Junk reads: Junk: ≥2N, ≥7A, ≥8C, ≥6G, ≥7T, ≥10 Dimer, ≥6 Trimer, or ≥5 Tetramer. (3) Rfam: Collection of many common non-coding RNA families except miRNAs (http://rfam.janelia.org). (4) Repeats: Prototypic sequences representing repetitive DNA from different eukaryotic species (http://www.girinst.org/repbase). (5) Notes: There was overlap in mapping of reads with mRNA, rRNA, tRNA, snRNA, snoRNA, and repeats. (6) mRNA Database: (http://www.ncbi.nlm.nih.gov/). The clean sequence reads were mapped with miRBase 20.0, allowing a mismatch of one or two nucleotide bases. More detailed description of the computational pipeline employed for data handling is reported in a flow-chart outline of study procedures (Figure. S1). All data were transformed to log base 2. Differences between the samples were calculated using chi-square and fisher's exact test. Only miRNAs with fold difference >2.0 and $P<0.05$ were considered statistically significant.

qRT-PCR validation study and data analysis

qRT-PCR-based relative quantification of miRNAs (300 μL of serum from each participant) was performed with SYBR Premix Ex Taq (TaKaLa) according to the manufacturer's instructions using a Rotor-Gene 3000 Real-time PCR machine (Corbett Life Science, Sydney, Australia). According to the results obtained, miRNA-24 has been reported to be consistently present in human serum [19,20]. Moreover, our previous experience is that miRNA-24 maintains a stable expression, and that the level of miRNA-24 served as an internal control in serum miRNA relative quantitative analysis. The specificity of each PCR product was validated by melting curve analysis at the end of PCR cycles. All samples were analyzed in triplicate, and the cycle threshold (Ct) value was defined as the number of cycles required for the fluorescent signal to reach the threshold. The relative expression levels of miRNAs in serum were calculated using the formula $2^{-\Delta\Delta Ct}$ where $\Delta\Delta Ct = [Ct\ (target, test) - Ct\ (ref, test)] - [Ct\ (target, calibrator) - Ct\ (ref, calibrator)]$. All primers used were obtained from Invitrogen company (Shanghai, China).

Statistical analysis

All Illumina sequencing data were transformed to log base2. Differences between the samples were calculated using chi-square and fisher's exact test. Only miRNAs with fold difference >2.0 and $P<0.05$ were considered statistically significant. Data were presented as median ± SD. The data of demographic and clinical features of the HCC patients and healthy controls were analyzed using the statistical Package for the Social Sciences(SPSS) version

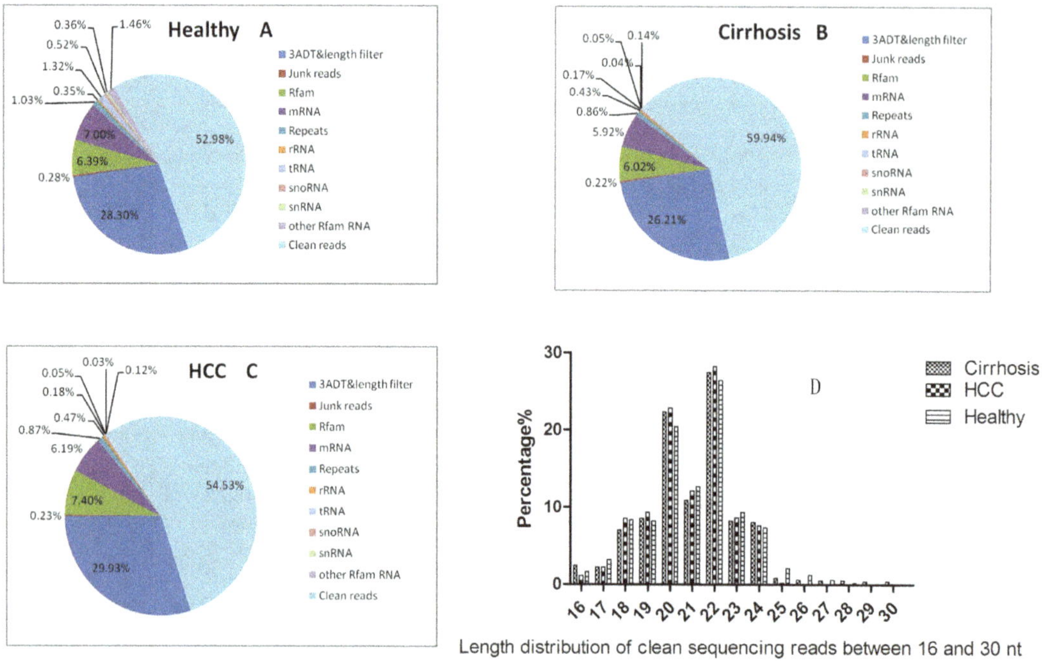

Figure 2. Sequenced reads and the distribution of reads. The Illumina Hiseq 2000 sequencing of the microRNAs obtained from the sera of patients in the control group, carrier group, and CHB group, produced 9,364,754,10,491,694, and 7,896,608 raw-reads, respectively, which, after extensive preprocessing and quality control, were reduced to 459,890,859,216, and 494,523 clean reads (Fig. 2A–C). All the distribution of reads of 16–30 nt length is presented in Fig. 2D.

21.0 software (SPSS Inc, Chicago, IL, USA). For the data $2^{-\Delta\Delta Ct}$ of miRNAs obtained by qRT-PCR, Mann-Whitney unpaired test was used to compare between HCC patients and controls. A stepwise logistic regression model was used to select diagnostic miRNA markers based on the training dataset. The predicted probability of being diagnosed with HCC was used as a surrogate marker to construct the receiver operating characteristic (ROC) curve. Area under the ROC curve (AUC) was used as an accuracy index for evaluating the diagnostic performance of the selected miRNA panel. The ROC and regression analysis was performed using the software 21 MedCalc (Version 10.4.7.0; MedCalc, Mariakerke, Belgium). All P-values were two-sided.

Table 2. Differentially expressed miRNAs in HCC and healthy groups.

no.	miR_name	fold change	fold change (log2)	up/down	miR_seq
1	hsa-miR-190b_R+1	12.4564	3.6388	up	UGAUAUGUUUGAUAUUGGGUUU
2	hsa-miR-141-3p	6.8951	2.7856	up	UAACACUGUCUGGUAAAGAUGG
3	hsa-miR-4532_R+2	6.6370	2.7305	up	CCCCGGGGAGCCCGGCGCG
4	hsa-mir-6127-p3	4.6459	2.2160	up	UGAGGGAGUGGGUGGGAGG
5	hsa-miR-99b-3p_R−2	4.5838	2.1965	up	CACCCGUAGAACCGACCUUG
6	hsa-miR-1228-5p	4.4131	2.1418	up	GUGGGCGGGGGCAGGUGUGUG
7	hsa-miR-30a-3p	0.4634	−1.1098	down	UGUAAACAUCCUCGACUGGAAG
8	hsa-miR-199a-5p	0.4452	−1.1673	down	ACAGUAGUCUGCACAUUGGUUA
9	hsa-let-7f-5p	0.3459	−1.5315	down	UGAGGUAGUAGAUUGUAUAGUU
10	hsa-miR-122-5p	0.3405	−1.5541	down	UGGAGUGUGACAAUGGUGUUUG
11	hsa-miR-192-5p	0.2755	−1.8601	down	CUGACCUAUGAAUUGACAGCC
12	hsa-miR-98-5p	0.2603	−1.9419	down	UGAGGUAGUAAGUUGUAUUGUU
13	hsa-miR-574-3p	0.1954	−2.3556	down	UGAGUGUGUGUGUGUGAGUGUGU
14	hsa-miR-30e-3p	0.1895	−2.3999	down	CUUUCAGUCGGAUGUUUACAGC
15	hsa-miR-6852-5p	0.0739	−3.7583	down	CCCUGGGGUUCUGAGGACAUG

Table 3. Differentially expressed miRNAs in HCC and cirrhosis groups.

no.	miR_name	fold change	fold change (log2)	up/down	miR_seq
1	hsa-miR-206	12.1198	3.5993	up	UGGAAUGUAAGGAAGUGUGUGG
2	hsa-mir-1285-1-p5	7.2943	2.8668	up	GAUCUCACUUUGUUGCCCAGG
3	hsa-miR-10a-5p	6.2059	2.6336	up	UACCCUGUAGAUCCGAAUUUGUG
4	hsa-miR-511-5p	5.8074	2.5379	up	GUGUCUUUUGCUCUGCAGUCA
5	hsa-miR-433-3p	5.6166	2.4897	up	AUCAUGAUGGGCUCCUCGGUGU
6	hsa-miR-100-5p_R−1	0.4026	−1.3125	down	AACCCGUAGAUCCGAACUUGUG
7	hsa-miR-483-5p_R−1	0.4002	−1.3213	down	AAGACGGGAGGAAAGAAGGGAG
8	hsa-miR-584-5p_R−1	0.3461	−1.5308	down	UUAUGGUUUGCCUGGGACUGG
9	hsa-miR-28-5p_R−2	0.2386	−2.0672	down	AAGGAGCUCACAGUCUUGAG
10	hsa-miR-30b-5p	0.2379	−2.0716	down	UGUAAACAUCCUACACUCAGCU
11	hsa-miR-30c-5p	0.1856	−2.4300	down	UGUAAACAUCCUACACUCUCAGC
12	hsa-miR-26a-5p	0.1677	−2.5757	down	UUCAAGUAAUCCAGGAUAGGCU
13	hsa-miR-4454_L-2	0.1593	−2.6498	down	GGAUCCGAGUCACGGCACCA
14	hsa-let-7e-5p	0.1351	−2.8884	down	UGAGGUAGGAGGUUGUAUAGUU
15	hsa-let-7c-5p	0.1275	−2.9709	down	UGAGGUAGUAGGUUGUAUGGUU
16	hsa-miR-4433b-5p	0.0891	−3.4882	down	AUGUCCCACCCCCACUCCUGU
17	hsa-miR-455-5p	0.0681	−3.8764	down	UAUGUGCCUUUGGACUACAUCG

Results

Description and clinical features of patients

The characteristics of the study participants are presented in Table. 1. There was no significant difference in the distribution of age, sex, and alanine aminotransferase (ALT) expression among the three groups (healthy, cirrhosis, and HCC).

Global analysis of miRNAs by deep sequencing

Illumina HiSeq 2000 sequencing of the miRNAs obtained from the sera of patients in the healthy control group, cirrhosis group and HCC group produced 9,364,754, 10,491,694, and 7,896,608 raw-reads, respectively, which, after extensive preprocessing and quality control, were reduced to 459,890, 859,216, and 494,523 clean reads (Fig. 2A–C, Table. S1). Distribution of reads of 16–30 nt length is presented in (Fig. 2D). In our study, we found that the length of miRNA is generally 20 to 22 nt. Clean reads were mapped to human miRNA (miRs) database v20.0 (ftp://mirbase.org/pub/mirbase/CURRENT/), pre-miRNA (mirs) database v20.0 (ftp://mirbase.org/pub/mirbase/CURRENT/), and genome database (ftp.ncbi.nih.gov/genomes/H sapiens/Assembled chromosomes/seq/). A total of 2,754 unique reads map to human miRNAs or pre-miRNAs in miRbase and the pre-miRNAs further map to the human genome and expressed sequence tags.

Analysis of differentially expressed miRNAs

We normalized the differential expression of miRNA count data, and the number of individual miRNA reads was standardized by the total numbers of 1,000,000 reads in each sample. Comparing the HCC and healthy control groups, the differential expression levels of 143 miRNAs have significant differences. Among them, 6 miRNAs were up-regulated (fold change >4-fold, $P<0.05$) in the control group, 9 down-regulated (fold change > 2-fold, $P<0.05$), shown in Table. 2. Comparing the HCC and cirrhosis groups, differential expression levels of 84 miRNAs have significant differences. Among them, 5 miRNAs were up-regulated (fold change >4-fold, $P<0.05$) in cirrhosis group, 12 down-regulated (fold change >2-fold, $P<0.05$), shown in Table. 3.

Differential Expression Profile of Eight Selected miRNAs

We used qRT-PCR assay to confirm the expression of 32 candidate miRNAs that were selected from the previous step from an independent cohort of 60 serum samples. Threshold levels were found to be as follows: MiRNA Ct<35 and detection rate >75%. We determined the $2^{-\Delta\Delta Ct}$ of 32 candidate miRNAs in three groups, Mann-Whitney unpaired test was used to compare between HCC patients and controls. Eight of the 32 miRNAs had significantly different expression levels between the HCC and control groups (healthy + cirrhosis group), as shown in Table. 4. These were hsa-miR-206, hsa-miR-141-3p, hsa-miR-433-3p, hsa-miR-1228-5p, hsa-miR-199a-5p, hsa-miR-122-5p, hsa-miR-192-5p, and hsa-miR-26a-5p.

MiRNA expression profile for HCC patients versus control patients in the training cohort

We used qRT-PCR assay to confirm the expression of 8 candidate miRNAs that were selected from the previous step. There were 6 miRNAs with significantly different expression between HCC and healthy groups, as shown in (Fig. 3A and Table. 5), and 6 other miRNAs showed significantly different expression between HCC and cirrhosis groups (Fig. 3B and Table. 5). We identified 8 of these miRNAs that showed significantly different expression when compared with the control group (Fig. 3C and Table. 5); These were then selected for the next validation. These were hsa-miR-206, hsa-miR-141-3p, hsa-miR-433-3p, hsa-miR-1228-5p, hsa-miR-199a-5p, hsa-miR-122-5p, hsa-miR-192-5p, and hsa-miR-26a-5p. Compared to Ct of their levels in the control samples, the diagnostic accuracy using these miRNAs, as measured by AUC, was 0.665,0.68, 0.607,

Table 4. Expression profiles of 32 candidate miRNA on qRT-PCR in screening set.

no.	miR_name	HCC versus control	HCC versus healthy		HCC versus cirrhosis	
		p value	p value	fold change	p value	fold change
1	hsa-miR-190b_R+1	0.2900	0.3500	0.9800	0.108	3.6709
2	**hsa-miR-206**	0.0030	0.0060	9.9350	0.03	3.5094
3	hsa-mir-1285-1-p5	0.0530	1.0000	1.1356	0.108	1.7391
4	**hsa-miR-141-3p**	0.0000	0.0000	11.0410	0.0000	5.8240
5	hsa-miR-4532_R+2	ND	ND	ND	ND	ND
6	hsa-miR-10a-5p	0.2600	0.2890	1.9650	0.602	1.3910
7	hsa-miR-511-5p	0.1010	0.2890	3.6600	0.108	2.8090
8	**hsa-miR-433-3p**	0.0000	0.0060	3.1180	0.004	4.1835
9	hsa-mir-6127-p3	ND	ND	ND	ND	ND
10	**hsa-miR-1228-5p**	0.0140	0.6020	3.1970	0.782	1.8180
11	hsa-miR-99b-3p_R−2	0.1000	1.0000	1.7900	0.031	2.0200
12	hsa-miR-30a-3p	ND	ND	ND	ND	ND
13	**hsa-miR-199a-5p**	0.0000	0.0000	0.5818	0.0001	0.8745
14	hsa-miR-100-5p_R−1	0.0950	0.0300	0.9230	0.108	1.0251
15	hsa-miR-483-5p_R−1	ND	ND	ND	ND	ND
16	hsa-miR-584-5p_R−1	0.0970	0.0900	0.7550	0.723	0.7840
17	hsa-let-7f-5p	0.1430	0.1080	0.8180	0.602	0.9250
18	**hsa-miR-122-5p**	0.0000	0.0000	0.2735	0.0000	0.5409
19	**hsa-miR-192-5p**	0.0010	0.0060	0.7650	0.012	0.8460
20	hsa-miR-98-5p	0.2643	0.2890	0.7714	0.122	0.8330
21	hsa-miR-28-5p_R−2	0.2386	0.1080	0.9360	0.289	0.9260
22	hsa-miR-30b-5p	0.0970	0.0300	0.9020	0.125	0.8740
23	hsa-miR-574-3p	0.1954	0.6020	1.2540	0.268	0.9190
24	hsa-miR-30e-3p	ND	ND	ND	ND	ND
25	hsa-miR-30c-5p	ND	ND	ND	ND	ND
26	**hsa-miR-26a-5p**	0.0010	0.0060	0.6530	0.0008	0.5370
27	hsa-miR-4454_L-2	ND	ND	ND	ND	ND
28	hsa-let-7e-5p	0.0980	0.1830	1.0130	0.0734	0.8360
29	hsa-let-7c-5p	0.2690	0.2470	0.8530	0.0772	0.7630
30	hsa-miR-4433b-5p	0.0891	0.1320	0.7640	0.112	0.7780
31	hsa-miR-6852-5p	ND	ND	ND	ND	ND
32	hsa-miR-455-5p	0.2250	0.3520	0.9740	0.074	0.6840

ND:not determined, miRNA Ct value >35 and detection rate <75%.

0.534,0.609,0.729,0.69 and 0.677, respectively (Table. S2–4, Fig. 4A–H).

Establishing the predictive miRNA panel for HCC versus control

A stepwise logistic regression model was applied on the training data set to estimate the chances of being diagnosed with HCC. All of the 8 miRNAs turned out to be significant predictors. The predicted probability of being diagnosed with HCC from the logit model based on the 8-miRNA panel (Table S5), logitP = −11.8472 + 0.52147miR122 − 0.22949miR1228 − 0.27621miR141 + 0.34063miR192 + 0.33325mi199a − 0.30556miR206 + 0.40777miR26a − 0.38006miR433, was used to construct the ROC curve. The diagnostic performance for the established miRNA panel was evaluated using ROC analysis. The AUC for the miRNA panel was 0.887 (95% CI = 0.850 to 0.918), sensitivity = 85.55%, specificity = 73.3%, Fig. 5A).

Validating the miRNA panel

The parameters estimated from the training data set were used to predict the probability of being diagnosed with HCC for the independent validation data set (251 serum samples). Similarly, the predicted probability was used to construct the ROC curve. The AUC of the miRNA panel was 0. 879 (95% CI = 0.842–0.941; sensitivity = 90.3%, specificity = 76.2%, Fig. 5B).

The performance of the miRNA panel in differentiating the HCC group from the healthy as well as the cirrhosis groups was also evaluated. The analysis demonstrated that the miRNAs had a high accuracy in distinguishing HCC patients from healthy patients (AUC = 0.893; 95% CI, 0.849 to 0.94; sensitivity

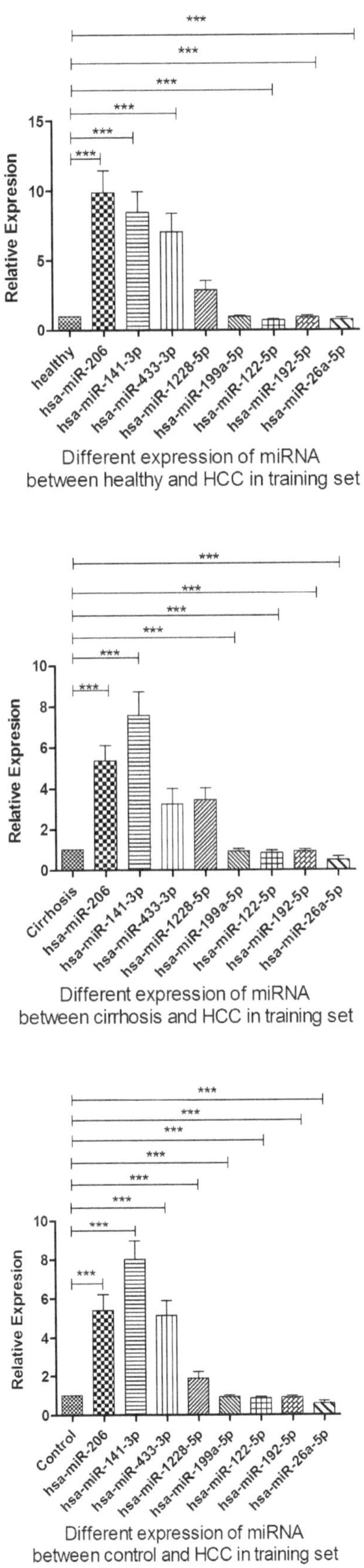

Figure 3. Differential expression of microRNAs in the training set.

82.8%; specificity 83.3%, Fig. 5C) and cirrhosis patients (AUC = 0.892; 95% CI, 0.844 to 0.939; sensitivity 81.6%; specificity 84.6%. Fig. 5D).

Comparison of the AUC of the miRNA panel with that of AFP in the validation set

Using the same serum samples, we evaluated the AUC of the AFP in different groups. The analysis demonstrated that the AFP also had a high accuracy in distinguishing HCC from healthy patients (AUC = 0.844; 95% CI, 0.785 to 0.902; sensitivity 60.2%; specificity 100%), cirrhosis patients (AUC = 0.708; 95% CI, 0.632 to 0.783; sensitivity 57.3%, specificity 79.5%) and control subjects (AUC = 0.766; 95% CI, 0.703 to 0.829; sensitivity 59.2%, specificity 87%).

We also compared the AUC of the miRNA panel with that of AFP. There was no difference between the AUC values of the miRNA panel and those of AFP (difference between areas = 0.0735, 95% CI = 0.000145 to 0.148, $P = 0.514$, Fig. 6A) in the healthy group. However, there were significant differences between the AUC values of the miRNA panel and those of AFP in the cirrhosis group (difference between areas = 0.184, 95% CI = 0.0925 to 0.276, $P = 0.0001$, Fig. 6B) and control group (difference between areas = 0.113, 95% CI = 0.0344 to 0.192, $P = 0.0049$, Fig. 6C).

Discussion

Sensitive and specific cancer biomarkers are essential for early detection and diagnosis of HCC, as well as for developing preventive screening. However, current methods are insufficient to detect HCC in the early stages. Advances in magnetic resonance imaging and computed tomography have greatly improved imaging of focal hypervascular masses consistent with HCC, but these procedures are costly and not readily available in developing countries. Laboratory data including serum alfa-fetoprotein (AFP) and des-gamma carboxyprothrombin (DCP) levels have been used as HCC biomarkers for a long time. However, the accuracy of AFP is modest (sensitivity: 39–65%; specificity: 76–94%). One-third of cases of early-stage HCC (tumors <3 cm) are missed using AFP analysis [21], and serum AFP levels are also elevated in patients with benign liver diseases, such as hepatitis and cirrhosis [22,23].

Many miRNAs are dysregulated in HCC; thus, it is to be expected that circulating miRNA levels are also affected by HCC progression. The high stability of miRNAs in circulation makes them perfect biomarkers, especially for detection of early stage, presymptomatic disease [24]. It is interesting that circulating miR-21 [16,25], miR-222 [25], and miR-223 [26] were found to be upregulated in the serum/plasma of HCC patients associated with HBV or HCV.

Downregulation of subsets of miRNAs is a common finding in HCC, suggesting that some of these miRNAs may act as putative tumor suppressor genes. Restoration of tumor suppressive miRNAs leads to cell cycle block, increased apoptosis, and reduced tumor angiogenesis and metastasis by inhibiting migration and invasion. Of these miRNAs, miR-122 and miR-199 appear to be particularly important in HCC [27,28,29]. Liver-specific miR-122 is the most abundant miRNA in the liver and it plays an important role in regulating hepatocyte development and differentiation [30,31]. The expression of miR-122 is downregulated in HCC tumor tissues and cancer cell lines, while its overexpression has been found to induce apoptosis and suppress proliferation in HepG2 and Hep3B cells [32]. The role of miR-122 in liver cancer

Table 5. Expression profiles of 8 candidate miRNA from qRT-PCR in training set.

no.	miR_name	HCC versus control	HCC versus healthy		HCC versus cirrhosis	
		p value	**p value**	**fold change**	**p value**	**fold change**
1	**hsa-miR-206**	0.0010	0.0000	9.8846	0.0000	4.7465
2	**hsa-miR-141-3p**	0.0000	0.0000	8.4126	0.0000	7.5844
3	**hsa-miR-433-3p**	0.0000	0.0060	7.0355	0.737	3.2273
4	**hsa-miR-1228-5p**	0.0245	0.1452	2.8560	0.315	3.4431
5	**hsa-miR-199a-5p**	0.0000	0.2450	0.9462	0.0000	0.9104
6	**hsa-miR-122-5p**	0.0000	0.0001	0.6942	0.0000	0.8349
7	**hsa-miR-192-5p**	0.0001	0.0006	0.9218	0.0000	0.8958
8	**hsa-miR-26a-5p**	0.0000	0.0001	0.7231	0.0000	0.4831

ND:not determined, miRNA Ct value >35 and detection rate <75%.

has been demonstrated directly by the generation of miR-122 knockout mice [33,34].

Our study revealed that serum hsa-miR-206, hsa-miR-141-3p, hsa-miR-433-3p, hsa-miR-1228-5p, hsa-miR-199a-5p, hsa-miR-122-5p, hsa-miR-192-5p, and hsa-miR-26a-5p were potential circulating markers for HCC diagnosis. The miRNA panel with eight miRNAs from the multivariate logistic regression model demonstrated high accuracy in HCC diagnosis. The association at the tissue level between HCC and four ofthe eight miRNAs (miR-122, miR-199, miR-192, and miR-26a) in our study has been reported previously [17,35,36].

At the circulating blood level, the diagnostic performance of miR-21, miR-122, and miR-223 in discriminating patients with HCC from the healthy group was reported by Xu et al [16]. However, their study failed to distinguish HCC from chronic hepatitis. Qu et al [37] found miR-16 to have moderate diagnostic accuracy of HCC, with sensitivity of 72.1% and specificity of 88.8%. In our study, miR-16 did show significant down-regulation in HCC as compared to control, but it did not meet our candidate microRNA selection criteria at the microarray level. Li et al [13] reported an extraordinarily high diagnostic accuracy of serum microRNA profiles for the diagnosis of HCC (AUC = 0.97–1.00) with miRNAs10a, 125b, 223, 23a, 23b, 342-3p, 375, 423, 92a, and 99a. However, the need for different markers for different group comparisons with different critical values in their study (HCC versus healthy, HCC versus HBV, healthy versus HBV, healthy versus HCV, and HBV versus HCV) raised concerns about the robustness of these markers. Furthermore, these results were not validated either internally or externally.

AFP is the most widely used tumor biomarker currently available for the early detection of HCC. Findings of a previous clinical study demonstrated that serum AFP had a sensitivity of 41–65% and specificity of 80–100% [38]. We found that AFP showed high accuracy in discriminating HCC patients from healthy subjects. At present, AFP measurement and ultrasound at 6-month intervals are the standard tools to screen for HCC in China. AFP is considered to be a useful and feasible tool for screening and early diagnosis in China due to its convenience,

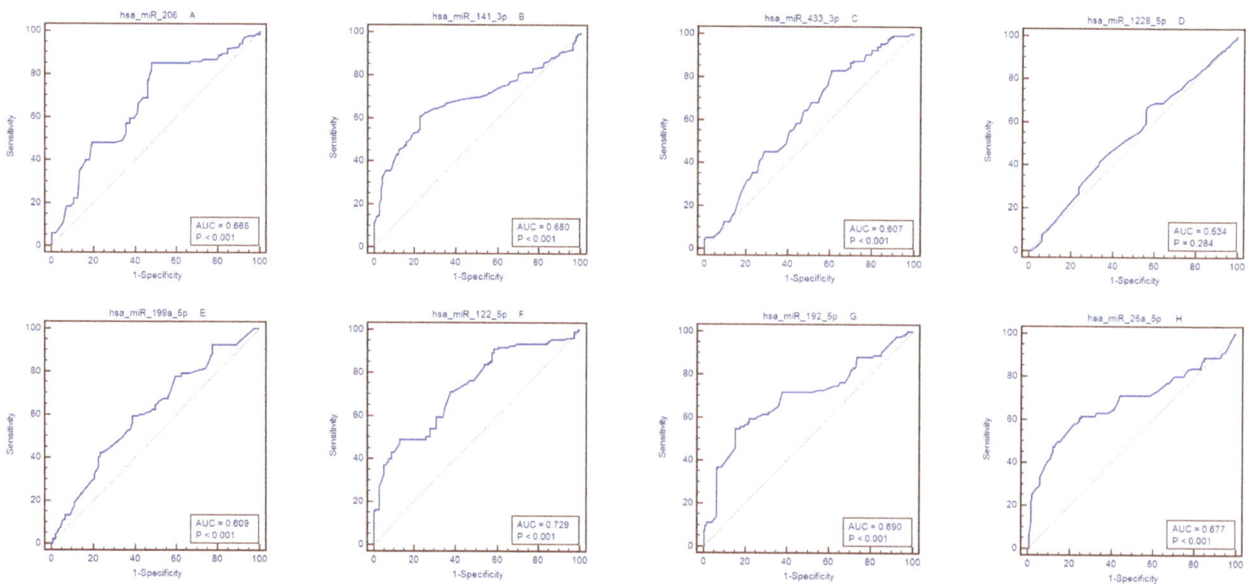

Figure 4. AUC of microRNAs for control subjects and HCC patients. Area under the curve (AUC) for the microRNAs (miRs). A:hsa-miR-206,B:hsa-miR-141-3p,C:hsa-miR-433-3p,D:hsa-miR-1228-5p,E:hsa-miR-199a-5p,F:hsa-miR-122-5p,G:hsa-miR-192-5p, and H:hsa-miR-26a-5p.

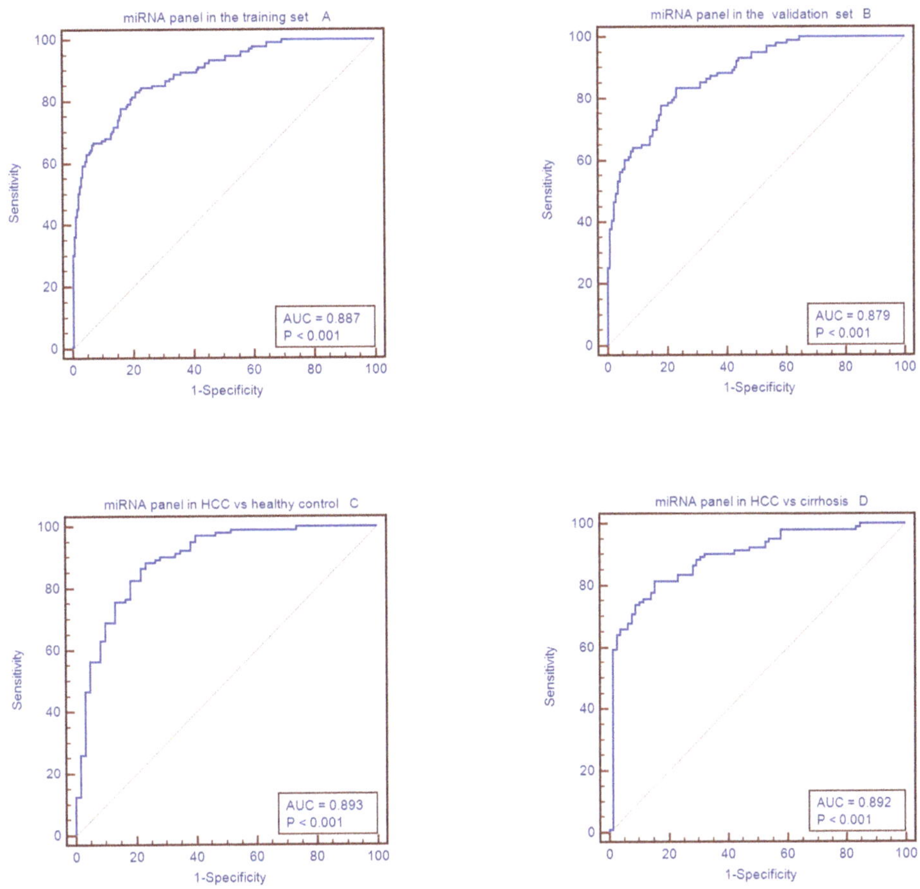

Figure 5. The diagnosis value of miRNA panel. A:The AUC for the microRNAs panel in the training set; B: the AUC of the microRNAs panel in the validation set; C: is AUC of the microRNAs panel used to distinguish HCC patients from healthy patients, and D is AUC of the microRNAs panel used to distinguish HCC patients from cirrhosis patients.

especially due to the fact that more than 60% of patients with HCC have an AFP level of >400 ng/ml [39]. However, the widely used marker AFP does not yield satisfactory results for early diagnosis of HCC, particularly AFP-negative HCC. AFP results are positive during pregnancy, as well as for active liver disease, embryonic tumor and certain gastrointestinal tumors; Furthermore, false-negative results and limitations in terms of sensitivity in different detection methods add to the limitations of this biomarker. For example, a small hepatic tumor results in AFP expression being lower than the limit of detection, whereas AFP expression is delayed or higher than the limit of detection when the tumor is large, yielding AFP-negative HCC. We compared the AUC of the miRNA panel with that of AFP. There were significant differences between the AUC values of the miRNA panel and those of AFP in the cirrhosis group. Compared with other studies of circulating miRNA in HCC diagnosis [13,17,23,26], our study is unique for the following reasons: first, we screened a large number of serum miRNAs via the Illumina

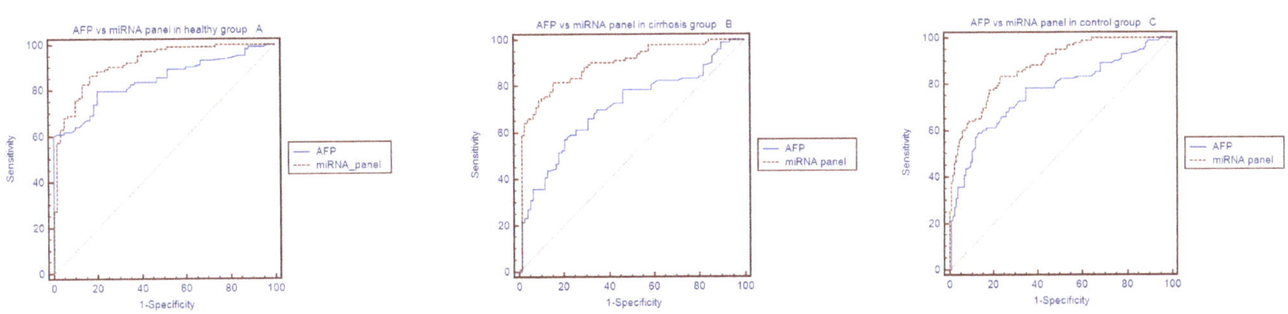

Figure 6. Comparison of AUC of the microRNA panel with that of AFP in the validation set. A:In healthy group;B:In cirrhosis group, and C:In control group.

Hiseq 2000 sequencing method, which gave us a better chance to identify potential diagnostic markers. Secondly, we included not only HCC and healthy groups, but a cirrhosis group as well. It is well-known that the pathogenesis of HCC is heterogenous and that multiple mechanisms of tumorigenesis could be involved (tumor suppressor gene, oncogene, viral effects, angiogenesis, etc). Nonetheless, we hypothesized that, similar to the adenoma-carcinomasequence in colorectal cancer, the clinical pathway of most HBV-related HCC may follow the four stages of healthy, hepatitis, cirrhosis, and HCC. Because of the long incubation time, miRNA disturbance might occur during any of these stages (hepatitis, cirrhosis, or HCC) before the clinical/pathophysiological manifestationof HCC. Thus, all the representative differential miRNAs, namely HCC versus healthy, HCC versus hepatitis, and HCC versus cirrhosis should be considered. Failure to do so might be the source of the unsatisfactory differentiation of HCC from hepatitis or cirrhosis in other studies. Finally, the microRNA panel identified in our study was validated by a large, independent cohort from two independent medical centers.

In summary, we identified a serum microRNA panel that differentiates HCC from healthy and cirrhosis with a high degree of accuracy and validated it in a large number of subjects. Our study demonstrates that this serum microRNA panel has considerable clinical value for early diagnosis of HCC, so that more patients, who would have otherwise missed the curative treatment window, can benefit from therapy.

Supporting Information

Figure S1 A flow-chart of study procedures.

Table S1 Overview of reads from raw data to cleaned sequences.

Table S2 AUC of ROC curves between HCC and healthy controls in the training set.

Table S3 AUC of ROC curves between HCC and cirrhosis in the training set.

Table S4 AUC of ROC curves between HCC and control in the training set.

Table S5 Logistic regression of miRNAs between HCC patients and control subjects in the training set.

Author Contributions

Conceived and designed the experiments: YWT GHG. Performed the experiments: YWT TLP XJY DFW. Analyzed the data: LC XBZ. Contributed reagents/materials/analysis tools: XJY JHG. Contributed to the writing of the manuscript: YWT.

References

1. Flores A, Marrero JA (2014) Emerging Trends in Hepatocellular Carcinoma: Focus on Diagnosis and Therapeutics. Clin Med Insights Oncol 8: 71–76.
2. Zhao YJ, Ju Q, Li GC (2013) Tumor markers for hepatocellular carcinoma. Mol Clin Oncol 1: 593–598.
3. Giordano S, Columbano A (2013) MicroRNAs: new tools for diagnosis, prognosis, and therapy in hepatocellular carcinoma? Hepatology 57: 840–847.
4. Bala S, Petrasek J, Mundkur S, Catalano D, Levin I, et al. (2012) Circulating microRNAs in exosomes indicate hepatocyte injury and inflammation in alcoholic, drug-induced, and inflammatory liver diseases. Hepatology 56: 1946–1957.
5. Blanco-Calvo M, Calvo L, Figueroa A, Haz-Conde M, Anton-Aparicio L, et al. (2012) Circulating microRNAs: molecular microsensors in gastrointestinal cancer. Sensors (Basel) 12: 9349–9362.
6. Ge Y, Chen G, Sun L, Liu F (2011) [MicroRNA-29 and fibrosis diseases]. Zhong Nan Da Xue Xue Bao Yi Xue Ban 36: 908–912.
7. He Y, Huang C, Zhang SP, Sun X, Long XR, et al. (2012) The potential of microRNAs in liver fibrosis. Cell Signal 24: 2268–2272.
8. Cermelli S, Ruggieri A, Marrero JA, Ioannou GN, Beretta L (2011) Circulating microRNAs in patients with chronic hepatitis C and non-alcoholic fatty liver disease. PLoS One 6: e23937.
9. Chen YP, Jin X, Xiang Z, Chen SH, Li YM (2013) Circulating MicroRNAs as potential biomarkers for alcoholic steatohepatitis. Liver Int 33: 1257–1265.
10. Chen YJ, Zhu JM, Wu H, Fan J, Zhou J, et al. (2013) Circulating microRNAs as a Fingerprint for Liver Cirrhosis. PLoS One 8: e66577.
11. Kutay H, Bai S, Datta J, Motiwala T, Pogribny I, et al. (2006) Downregulation of miR-122 in the rodent and human hepatocellular carcinomas. J Cell Biochem 99: 671–678.
12. Ladeiro Y, Couchy G, Balabaud C, Bioulac-Sage P, Pelletier L, et al. (2008) MicroRNA profiling in hepatocellular tumors is associated with clinical features and oncogene/tumor suppressor gene mutations. Hepatology 47: 1955–1963.
13. Li LM, Hu ZB, Zhou ZX, Chen X, Liu FY, et al. (2010) Serum microRNA profiles serve as novel biomarkers for HBV infection and diagnosis of HBV-positive hepatocarcinoma. Cancer Res 70: 9798–9807.
14. Meng F, Henson R, Wehbe-Janek H, Ghoshal K, Jacob ST, et al. (2007) MicroRNA-21 regulates expression of the PTEN tumor suppressor gene in human hepatocellular cancer. Gastroenterology 133: 647–658.
15. Pineau P, Volinia S, McJunkin K, Marchio A, Battiston C, et al. (2010) miR-221 overexpression contributes to liver tumorigenesis. Proc Natl Acad Sci U S A 107: 264–269.
16. Xu J, Wu C, Che X, Wang L, Yu D, et al. (2011) Circulating microRNAs, miR-21, miR-122, and miR-223, in patients with hepatocellular carcinoma or chronic hepatitis. Mol Carcinog 50: 136–142.
17. Zhou J, Yu L, Gao X, Hu J, Wang J, et al. (2011) Plasma microRNA panel to diagnose hepatitis B virus-related hepatocellular carcinoma. J Clin Oncol 29: 4781–4788.
18. Zhou Q, Li M, Wang X, Li Q, Wang T, et al. (2012) Immune-related microRNAs are abundant in breast milk exosomes. Int J Biol Sci 8: 118–123.
19. Peltier HJ, Latham GJ (2008) Normalization of microRNA expression levels in quantitative RT-PCR assays: identification of suitable reference RNA targets in normal and cancerous human solid tissues. RNA 14: 844–852.
20. Zhang H, Li QY, Guo ZZ, Guan Y, Du J, et al. (2012) Serum levels of microRNAs can specifically predict liver injury of chronic hepatitis B. World J Gastroenterol 18: 5188–5196.
21. Collier J, Sherman M (1998) Screening for hepatocellular carcinoma. Hepatology 27: 273–278.
22. Oka H, Tamori A, Kuroki T, Kobayashi K, Yamamoto S (1994) Prospective study of alpha-fetoprotein in cirrhotic patients monitored for development of hepatocellular carcinoma. Hepatology 19: 61–66.
23. Abdalla MA, Haj-Ahmad Y (2012) Promising Candidate Urinary MicroRNA Biomarkers for the Early Detection of Hepatocellular Carcinoma among High-Risk Hepatitis C Virus Egyptian Patients. J Cancer 3: 19–31.
24. Petrelli A, Perra A, Cora D, Sulas P, Menegon S, et al. (2014) MicroRNA/gene profiling unveils early molecular changes and nuclear factor erythroid related factor 2 (NRF2) activation in a rat model recapitulating human hepatocellular carcinoma (HCC). Hepatology 59: 228–241.
25. Li J, Wang Y, Yu W, Chen J, Luo J (2011) Expression of serum miR-221 in human hepatocellular carcinoma and its prognostic significance. Biochem Biophys Res Commun 406: 70–73.
26. Tomimaru Y, Eguchi H, Nagano H, Wada H, Kobayashi S, et al. (2012) Circulating microRNA-21 as a novel biomarker for hepatocellular carcinoma. J Hepatol 56: 167–175.
27. Murakami Y, Yasuda T, Saigo K, Urashima T, Toyoda H, et al. (2006) Comprehensive analysis of microRNA expression patterns in hepatocellular carcinoma and non-tumorous tissues. Oncogene 25: 2537–2545.
28. Jiang J, Gusev Y, Aderca I, Mettler TA, Nagorney DM, et al. (2008) Association of MicroRNA expression in hepatocellular carcinomas with hepatitis infection, cirrhosis, and patient survival. Clin Cancer Res 14: 419–427.
29. Hou J, Lin L, Zhou W, Wang Z, Ding G, et al. (2011) Identification of miRNomes in human liver and hepatocellular carcinoma reveals miR-199a/b-3p as therapeutic target for hepatocellular carcinoma. Cancer Cell 19: 232–243.
30. Morita K, Taketomi A, Shirabe K, Umeda K, Kayashima H, et al. (2011) Clinical significance and potential of hepatic microRNA-122 expression in hepatitis C. Liver Int 31: 474–484.
31. Chang J, Nicolas E, Marks D, Sander C, Lerro A, et al. (2004) miR-122, a mammalian liver-specific microRNA, is processed from hcr mRNA and may downregulate the high affinity cationic amino acid transporter CAT-1. RNA Biol 1: 106–113.

32. Datta J, Kutay H, Nasser MW, Nuovo GJ, Wang B, et al. (2008) Methylation mediated silencing of MicroRNA-1 gene and its role in hepatocellular carcinogenesis. Cancer Res 68: 5049–5058.
33. Hsu SH, Wang B, Kota J, Yu J, Costinean S, et al. (2012) Essential metabolic, anti-inflammatory, and anti-tumorigenic functions of miR-122 in liver. J Clin Invest 122: 2871–2883.
34. Tsai WC, Hsu SD, Hsu CS, Lai TC, Chen SJ, et al. (2012) MicroRNA-122 plays a critical role in liver homeostasis and hepatocarcinogenesis. J Clin Invest 122: 2884–2897.
35. Kota J, Chivukula RR, O'Donnell KA, Wentzel EA, Montgomery CL, et al. (2009) Therapeutic microRNA delivery suppresses tumorigenesis in a murine liver cancer model. Cell 137: 1005–1017.
36. Ji J, Shi J, Budhu A, Yu Z, Forgues M, et al. (2009) MicroRNA expression, survival, and response to interferon in liver cancer. N Engl J Med 361: 1437–1447.
37. Qu KZ, Zhang K, Li H, Afdhal NH, Albitar M (2011) Circulating microRNAs as biomarkers for hepatocellular carcinoma. J Clin Gastroenterol 45: 355–360.
38. Debruyne EN, Delanghe JR (2008) Diagnosing and monitoring hepatocellular carcinoma with alpha-fetoprotein: new aspects and applications. Clin Chim Acta 395: 19–26.
39. Song P, Tobe RG, Inagaki Y, Kokudo N, Hasegawa K, et al. (2012) The management of hepatocellular carcinoma around the world: a comparison of guidelines from 2001 to 2011. Liver Int 32: 1053–1063.

9

Factors Associated with Alcohol Consumption in Hepatitis B Carriers

Boyoung Park, Kyu-Won Jung, Chang-Mo Oh, Kui Son Choi, Mina Suh, Jae Kwan Jun*

National Cancer Control Institute, National Cancer Center, Goyang-si, Korea

Abstract

This study was conducted to investigate the prevalence of alcohol consumption and identify the sociodemographic factors associated with alcohol consumption among individuals with hepatitis B virus(HBV) infection. We used data from the Korean National Health and Nutrition Examination Surveys, a nationwide survey conducted between 2007 and 2011. "Monthly alcohol consumption" was defined as having consumed alcohol at least once per month during the past year, and "high-risk alcohol consumption" was defined as having consumed alcohol twice or more per week and, for males, having consumed at least 60 g of alcohol on one occasion or, for females, having consumed at least 40 g of alcohol on more than one occasion. The prevalence of monthly alcohol consumption was 53.2%, and that of high-risk alcohol consumption was 11.8% among HBV carriers. Less education was associated with both monthly and high-risk alcohol consumption(OR = 1.75 [95% CI = 1.02−3.02] for monthly alcohol consumption among those with less than a high school education; OR = 2.48 [95% CI = 1.19−5.17] for high-risk alcohol consumption among those with less than a high school education and OR = 2.02 [95% CI = 1.12−3.64] among those with a high school education). Additionally, smoking and being male increased the risk of alcohol consumption, and older age and having a normal body mass index decreased the risk. HBV carriers who were less educated, overweight, and smokers were more likely to consume alcohol or meet criteria for high-risk drinking. Health policies and intervention programs aimed at promoting a generally healthy lifestyle in HBV carriers should consider educational inequalities and alcohol consumption.

Editor: Sang Hoon Ahn, Yonsei University College of Medicine, Korea, Republic Of

Funding: This study was supported by a Grant-in-Aid for Cancer Research and Control from the National Cancer Center of Korea (#1310232). The funders had no role in study design, data collection and analysis, decision to publish, or preparation of the manuscript.

Competing Interests: The authors have declared that no competing interests exist.

* Email: jkjun@ncc.re.kr

Introduction

Hepatitis B virus (HBV) infection is a major global public health issue. It is estimated that, worldwide, more than 2 billion people are infected with HBV and that 378 million are chronic carriers. Additionally, about 4.5 million new HBV infections develop worldwide each year; about one-quarter of these progress to further liver disease and approximately 600,000 individuals die of HBV-related causes each year [1]. The disease burden of HBV infection is especially high in Asian countries. Indeed, about 75% of chronic HBV carriers reside in the Asia–Pacific region, and 15–25% die of HBV-related liver diseases [2]. People who are chronically infected with HBV are at high risk of developing life-threatening chronic diseases, such as liver cirrhosis and hepatocellular carcinoma (HCC) [3]. HCC accounts for 70–85% of primary liver cancer cases [4], which is the sixth most common cancer and the third leading cause of death from cancer worldwide [5].

The outcome of HBV infection is influenced by several viral and host factors, and alcohol consumption is one of the host factors that affects the progress of HBV infection [6]. Alcohol consumption itself is also a major cause of chronic liver diseases, such as liver cirrhosis and HCC, and it contributes to the progression of liver damage when other risk factors exist [7]. Alcohol intake independently increases the risk of liver cirrhosis and HCC in HBV carriers [8]. Some researchers have even suggested a multiplicative interactive effect between HBV infection and heavy alcohol consumption on the risk of liver cirrhosis [7]. In terms of HCC development, compared with non-viral-induced cirrhosis, cirrhosis related to viral infection, especially chronic HBV infection, is associated with a higher risk of developing HCC [9]. Several previous studies have shown that alcohol consumption and HBV infection operate synergistically [10–12] and share mechanisms of action in the development of HCC [13].

The Republic of Korea is among the regions with a high prevalence (≥8%) of HBV infection [14]. Although the prevalence of HBV infection has decreased because of the nationwide vaccination program implemented in 1995, HBV infection is still considered endemic in the Republic of Korea, which is now classified as intermediate in this regard [15].

The prevalence of drinkers and the amount of alcohol consumed per capita in the Republic of Korea is among the highest worldwide and the prevalence of alcohol consumption in the population has been increasing [16]. Considering the disease burden of HBV infection, efforts to combat the development of liver disease must focus not only on the primary prevention of HBV infection through HBV vaccination but also on the modification of risk factors, such as reducing alcohol consumption in HBV carriers.

Thus, in this study, we investigated the prevalence of alcohol consumption, a major factor that operates synergistically with other factors in the development of liver disease, among HBV carriers and compared it with that among HBV non-carriers. We also identified the sociodemographic factors associated with alcohol consumption in individuals with HBV infection using a nationally representative sample of the population of the Republic of Korea.

Materials and Methods

Study population

This study used data from the Korean National Health and Nutrition Examination Surveys (KNHANES), a series of cross-sectional, population-based nationally representative surveys that relied on independent rolling survey sampling based on a complex survey design. This survey had been implemented every 3 years between 1998 and 2005; since 2007, it has been conducted annually. KNHANES uses a standardized questionnaire to examine health behavior, a health examination survey, and a nutrition survey using a food-frequency questionnaire. Details of the survey have been described fully on the KNHANES official website, and the survey data are publicly available (http://knhanes.cdc.go.kr/). The study protocol was approved by the Institutional Review Board of the Korean Centers for Disease Control and Prevention.

Our analysis included data from the KNHANES conducted between 2007 and 2011. During the period, 53,232 individuals were sampled, and 42,347 participated in the survey (response rate: 71.2% in 2007, 77.8% in 2008, 82.8% in 2009, 81.9% in 2010, and 80.4% in 2011). Individual HBV surface antigen (HBsAg) values were measured in serum with an electrochemiluminescence immunoassay (Roche Diagnostics, Switzerland) in those aged 10 years or older. Of these, we selected 28,340 individuals aged 20 years or older with complete HBsAg test results; 27,318 of this group were negative for HBsAg, and 1,022 were positive. Thus, 3.7% of the population aged 20 years or older was infected with HBV, and the weighted prevalence was 3.5%. We defined those whose serum was HBsAg-positive as HBV carriers and those whose serum was HBsAg-negative as HBV non-carriers.

Data collection

Participants' drinking patterns, including alcohol consumption, frequency of alcohol consumption during the previous year, and amount of alcohol consumed on one occasion, were accessed by questionnaire. The World Health Organization (WHO) defines high-risk drinking as drinking 60 g of alcohol or more for males and 40 g of alcohol or more for females on a single day [17]. We defined "monthly alcohol consumption" as having consumed alcohol once or more per month during the past year, and "high-risk alcohol consumption" as having consumed alcohol twice or more per week and, for males, having consumed at least 60 g of alcohol on one occasion or, for females, having consumed at least 40 g of alcohol on one occasion [18].

Demographic data (sex, age, area of residence), socioeconomic factors (monthly household income, educational level), life style-related factors (subjective health status, recognition of HBV infection status, smoking) were collected using a standardized questionnaire. We defined "recognition of HBV infection" as being serum HBsAg-positive and diagnosed with HBV infection by a physician. Body mass index (BMI) was calculated based on the height and weight data collected during the health examination.

Statistical analyses

All analyses incorporated sampling weights, stratification, and clustering. The total proportions of baseline characteristics among HBV carriers and non-carriers were compared with the *chi*-square test. In addition, the annual prevalence of the monthly alcohol consumption and high-risk alcohol consumption for 2007 and 2011 was analyzed. We performed multiple logistic regression to estimate the odds ratios (ORs) and 95% confidence intervals (CIs) for the association between sociodemographic factors and monthly alcohol consumption and high-risk alcohol consumption among HBV carriers to control for the effects of other sociodemographic variables and showed the frequency and percent of each sociodemographic factor. A p-value of <0.05 was considered to indicate statistical significance. All statistical analyses were performed using the SAS software (ver. 9.1; SAS, Inc., Cary, NC, USA).

Results

Among HBV carriers, 53.2% consumed alcohol at least once per month during the previous year, but this figure did not differ significantly from that for non-carriers (56.0% for non-carriers, $P = 0.168$). The prevalence of high-risk alcohol consumption was 11.8% in HBV carriers and 12.0% in HBV non-carriers. The prevalence of high-risk alcohol consumption also did not significantly differ between HBV carriers and non-carriers ($P = 0.867$). Figure 1 and 2 shows the annual prevalence of the monthly alcohol consumption and high-risk alcohol consumption for the years 2007 and 2011 among HBV carriers and non-carriers age 20 years or older.

Table 1 compares the baseline characteristics of HBV carriers and non-carriers in 2007–2011 in the Republic of Korea. Among HBV carriers, 52.4% were males and 47.6% were females. Most HBV carriers (79.1%) in Korea did not recognize their infection status, nearly 50% of HBV carriers considered their health status to be moderate, and 44% of HBV carriers were smokers. Compared with non-carriers, more HBV carriers tended to be male, in their 40s and 50s, and to consider their health status bad or moderate. Other baseline characteristics were not significantly different.

Table 2 presents the sociodemographic factors associated with monthly alcohol consumption in HBV carriers. Being male, smoking, and less education were significantly associated with higher rates of monthly alcohol consumption (OR = 2.56 [95% CI = 1.62−4.03, $P<0.001$] for males; OR = 2.28 [95% CI = 1.47−3.54, $P<0.001$] for smokers; and OR = 1.75 [95% CI = 1.02−3.02, $P = 0.044$] for those with less than a high school education vs. those with at least some college). People older than 50 drank less than did people younger than 40 ($P<0.001$), and low household income and normal BMI (18.5–24.9) were significantly associated with less monthly drinking (OR = 0.43 [95% CI = 0.24−0.80, $P = 0.008$] for the those in the first quartile of household income vs. those in the fourth quartile, and OR = 0.69 [95% CI = 0.48−0.99, $P = 0.045$] for normal BMI vs. those with BMI ≥25 m/Kg^2). Area of residence, recognition of HBV infection, and subjective health status were not associated with monthly drinking.

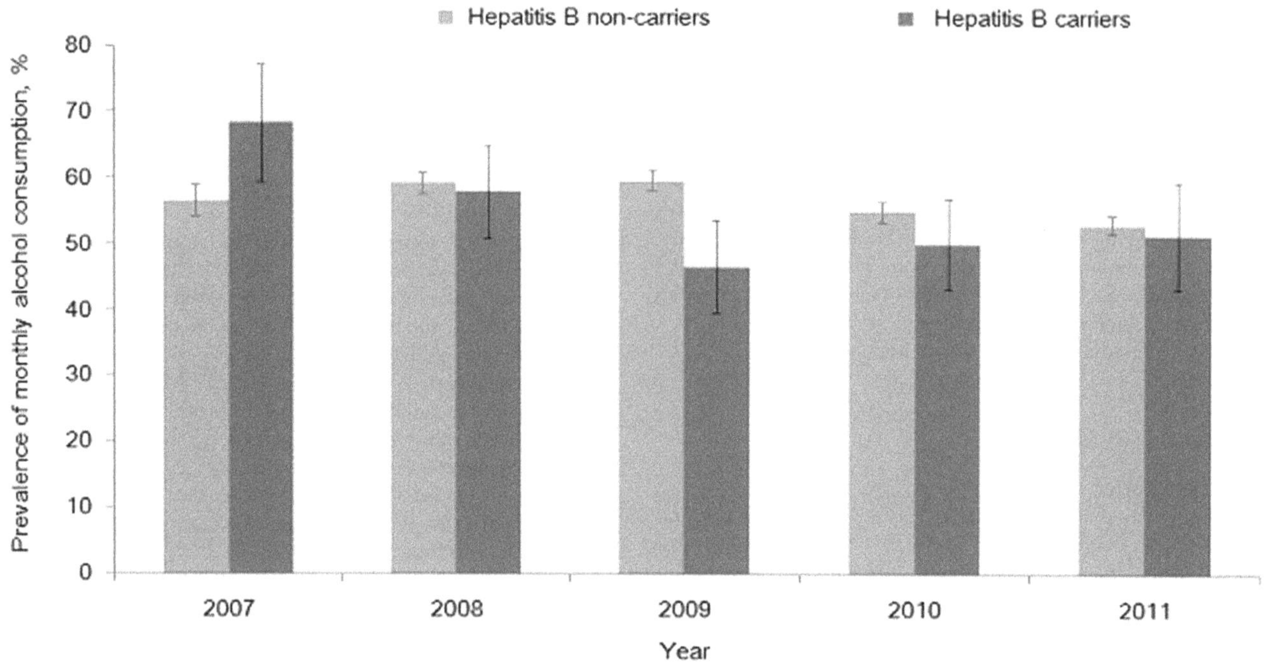

Figure 1. The annual prevalence of monthly alcohol consumption and high-risk alcohol consumption during the year of 2007–2011 among HBV carriers and non-carriers aged 20 or older.

Table 3 shows the associations between individual sociodemographic factors and high-risk alcohol consumption in HBV carriers. Similar to the association with monthly alcohol consumption, being male, smoking, and less education were significantly associated with a higher prevalence of high-risk alcohol consumption (OR = 3.46 [95% CI = 1.33−9.00, $P<$ 0.011] for males; OR = 4.15 [95% CI = 1.75−9.85, $P = 0.001$] for smokers; and OR = 2.48 [95% CI = 1.19−5.17, $P = 0.016$] for those with less than high school education and OR = 2.02 [95% CI = 1.12−3.64, $P = 0.020$] for those with a high school education

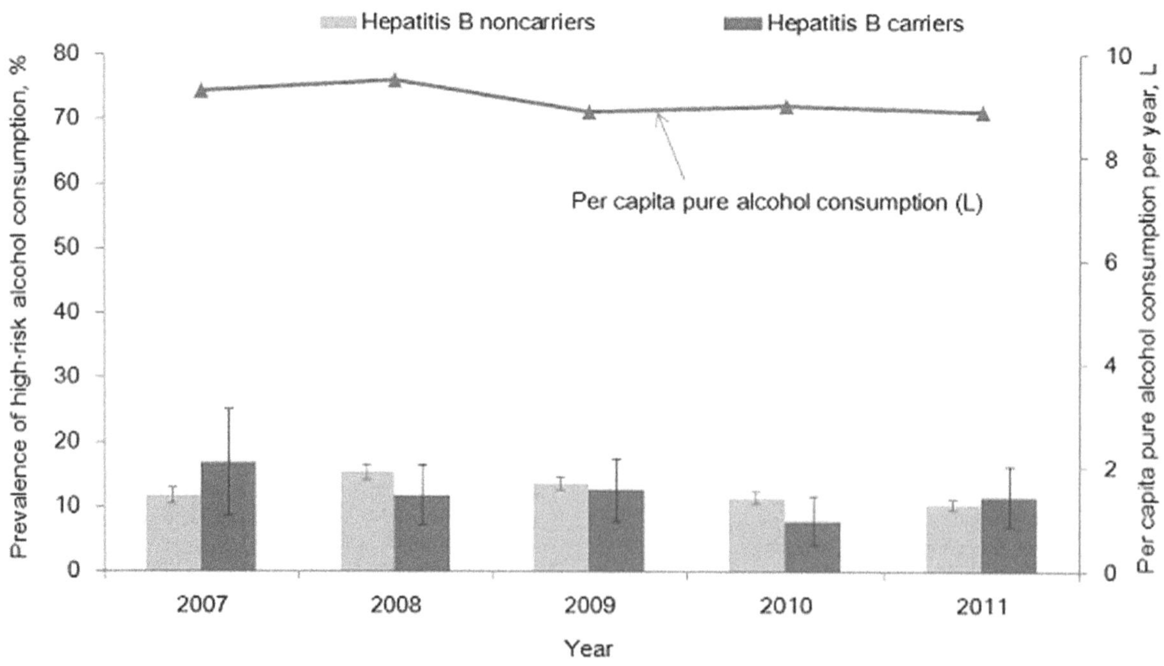

Figure 2. Trends in annual prevalence of high-risk alcohol consumption during the year of 2007–2011 among hepatitis B carriers and non-carriers aged 20 or older and per capita pure alcohol consumption per year in general population. The prevalence of high-risk alcohol consumption was calculated from Korean National Health and Nutrition Examination Surveys and Korean Statistical Information Service data was applied for per capita pure alcohol consumption.

Table 1. Weighted prevalence of baseline characteristics of participants aged 20 years and older with hepatitis B virus surface antigen and non-carriers (KNHANES 2007–2011).

	Hepatitis B carriers			Hepatitis B non-carriers			P-value
	Sample size	Prevalence (%)	95% CI	Sample size	Prevalence (%)	95% CI	
Overall	1022			27318			
Sex							
Male	492	52.4	(48.9–56.0)	11676	46.0	(45.5–46.6)	0.001
Female	530	47.6	(44.0–51.1)	15642	54.0	(53.4–54.5)	
Age							
<40	300	31.2	(18.5–24.4)	8748	35.6	(34.4–36.8)	<0.001
40–49	252	25.1	(19.1–25.4)	5298	20.3	(19.5–21.1)	
50–59	224	22.7	(21.8–28.4)	4935	18.3	(17.5–19.0)	
≥60	246	21.4	(27.8–34.6)	8337	25.9	(24.8–27.0)	
Area of residence							
Urban	768	79.3	(75.4–83.2)	20719	80.1	(77.5–82.8)	0.610
Rural	254	20.7	(16.8–24.6)	6599	19.9	(17.2–22.5)	
Household income							
Low	166	14.3	(11.8–16.9)	5446	17.5	(16.5–18.4)	0.161
Mid–low	264	26.3	(23.0–29.6)	6757	25.0	(23.9–26.0)	
Mid–high	260	26.9	(23.3–30.6)	7317	27.8	(26.8–28.9)	
High	310	30.5	(26.9–34.0)	7243	27.8	(26.4–29.2)	
Missing	22	1.9	(1.0–2.9)	555	1.9	(1.6–2.2)	
Education							
Less than high school	376	33.3	(29.7–36.8)	10378	33.1	(31.8–34.3)	0.319
High school	328	32.7	(29.1–36.3)	9067	35.6	(34.6–36.5)	
College or more	306	32.0	(28.2–35.8)	7543	29.9	(28.7–31.0)	
Missing	12	2.1	(0.9–3.3)	330	1.5	(1.3–1.8)	
Body mass index							0.170
<18.5	31	3.2	(1.9–4.4)	1221	4.6	(4.3–5.0)	
18.5–24.9	640	61.8	(58.4–65.2)	17312	63.1	(62.4–63.8)	
≥25.0	347	34.5	(31.1–37.8)	8659	31.8	(31.1–32.5)	
Missing	4	0.5	(−0.1–1.1)	126	0.4	(0.3–0.6)	
Subjective health status							
Bad	246	20.9	(17.9–23.8)	5975	19.2	(18.6–19.9)	<0.001
Moderate	469	49.6	(45.9–53.4)	10785	42.3	(41.4–43.2)	
Good	295	27.4	(24.1–30.7)	10243	37.0	(36.1–37.9)	
Missing	12	2.1	(0.9–3.3)	315	1.5	(1.2–1.7)	
Smoking							

Table 1. Cont.

	Hepatitis B carriers			Hepatitis B non-carriers			P-value
	Sample size	Prevalence (%)	95% CI	Sample size	Prevalence (%)	95% CI	
Smoker	414	43.7	(40.1–47.3)	10624	41.0	(40.4–41.7)	0.278
Non-smoker	597	54.5	(50.9–58.1)	16384	57.5	(56.9–58.1)	
Missing	11	1.8	(0.7–2.9)	310	1.5	(1.2–1.7)	
Awareness of HBV infection							
Unaware	809	79.1	(76.0–82.2)	-			
Aware	213	20.9	(17.8–24.0)	-			

vs. those with at least some college). Being older, having a normal BMI, and moderate self-rated health status were associated with less high–risk alcohol consumption. Area of residence, household income, and recognition of HBV infection were unrelated to high–risk alcohol consumption.

Discussion

This study found that 53.2% of HBV carriers consumed alcohol on a monthly basis and that 11.8% of this group met criteria for high-risk alcohol consumption, but these figures did not significantly differ from those for HBV non-carriers. Less education, smoking, and being overweight were associated with monthly drinking and high-risk drinking in HBV carriers, and we confirmed the existence of educational inequalities in the alcohol consumption of HBV carriers. To our knowledge, this is the first published study to investigate the prevalence of alcohol consumption among HBV carriers who are at high risk for chronic liver disease.

The proportion of Korean adults who drink alcohol is among the highest in the world and is increasing [19]. The proportion of high-risk alcohol drinkers has also been increasing [18], and both the prevalence of high-risk alcohol consumption and total alcohol consumption per capita are high in the Republic of Korea compared with most other countries [16].

In the Republic of Korea, the prevalence of those with serum HBsAg-positive status has been decreasing rapidly, from 8.6% in 1980 [15] to 3.2% in 2009, due to a nationwide HBV vaccination program implemented in 1995 [20]. However, the decrease in the disease burden related to chronic liver diseases, including liver cancers, is not as dramatic as is the decrease in the prevalence of HBsAg. To further decrease the risk for developing liver disease, it has been recommended that HBV carriers stop drinking [6]. Indeed, the treatment guidelines for chronic hepatitis B developed by the Korean Association for the Study of the Liver recommend that HBV carriers avoid drinking [21]. However, more than 50% of HBV carriers drank alcohol and more than 10% were heavy drinkers. Thus, in addition to current efforts that focus on reducing high-risk groups, such as HBV carriers, through vaccination, more efforts are needed to prevent the gradual development of liver disease in general, especially in high-risk groups.

Educational attainment and alcohol use have been associated with each other in several previous studies. Several studies have suggested that *less* education is associated with alcohol dependence [22–24], whereas others have proposed that *more* education is associated with *increased* daily alcohol consumption or problematic drinking [25] or that there is *no* association between these factors [26]. In this study, we showed that lower educational levels were associated with increased monthly alcohol consumption and high-risk alcohol consumption in HBV carriers. The odds ratios of educational attainment were more significant for high-risk alcohol consumption than for monthly alcohol consumption, showing educational disparities in both alcohol consumption, in general, and heavy drinking patterns, in particular. In Korea, there are differences in mortality due to liver cancer and liver diseases according to educational attainment, and these differences reflect major inequalities [27]. Our results showing differences in drinking according to educational level in HBV carriers may, at least in part, explain the inequalities in liver cancer and liver disease mortality.

Our results showed that smokers who were HBV carriers were more likely to drink alcohol on a monthly basis and to be heavy drinkers, which is similar to previous results indicating that

Table 2. Multivariate analysis of association between monthly alcohol consumption[a] and sociodemographic factors in HBV carriers.

	Monthly alcohol consumers		Non-consumers		Odds ratio	95% CI	*P-value*
	N	%[b] (95% CI)	N	%[b] (95% CI)			
Sex							
Male	327	68.1(63.8–72.4)	157	34.4(29.4–39.4)	2.56	(1.62–4.03)	<0.01
Female	175	31.9(27.6–36.2)	349	65.6(60.6–70.6)	1		
Age							
<40	179	36.9(32.3–41.4)	166	29.9(25.3–34.5)	1		
40–49	143	29.6(24.8–34.3)	117	24.8(20.1–29.6)	0.68	(0.43–1.06)	0.09
50–59	104	20.0(15.9–24.1)	108	20.8(16.7–24.8)	0.31	(0.19–0.50)	<0.01
≥60	76	13.5(10.2–16.9)	115	24.5(20.3–28.6)	0.23	(0.13–0.42)	<0.01
Area of residence							
Urban	383	79.3(74.7–83.8)	373	79.3(74.8–83.9)	0.76	(0.50–1.18)	0.22
Rural	119	20.7(16.2–25.3)	133	20.7(16.1–25.2)	1		
Household income							
Low	55	8.6(6.0–11.1)	108	20.6(16.3–24.8)	0.43	(0.24–0.80)	0.01
Mid–low	138	28.7(24.0–33.5)	124	24.2(19.6–28.7)	1.02	(0.66–1.59)	0.93
Mid–high	133	27.4(22.6–32.3)	123	26.5(21.7–31.4)	0.65	(0.42–1.01)	0.06
High	167	33.9(29.2–38.6)	141	27.1(22.7–31.6)	1		
Education							
Less than high school	148	27.3(23.0–31.6)	228	41.6(36.3–46.8)	1.75	(1.02–3.02)	0.04
High school	184	36.0(30.9–41.2)	142	29.8(25.0–34.6)	1.34	(0.88–2.05)	0.18
College or more	169	36.3(31.3–41.3)	135	28.3(23.6–33.0)	1		
Body mass index							
<18.5	15	3.4(1.6–5.2)	15	2.9(1.2–4.7)	1.12	(0.49–2.58)	0.79
18.5–24.9	302	58.2(53.3–63.1)	326	64.8(59.8–69.7)	0.69	(0.48–0.99)	0.04
≥25.0	182	37.5(32.6–42.3)	164	32.3(27.6–37.0)	1		
Awareness of HBV infection							
Unaware	394	77.1(72.4–81.7)	401	80.4(76.3–84.5)	1.02	(0.67–1.55)	0.92
Aware	108	22.9(18.3–27.6)	105	19.6(15.5–23.7)	1		
Subjective health status							
Bad	94	17.5(13.8–21.1)	151	25.6(21.0–30.2)	0.75	(0.48–1.18)	0.21
Moderate	249	53.3(48.4–58.1)	219	47.6(42.4–52.9)	0.96	(0.66–1.39)	0.81
Good	158	28.9(24.4–33.4)	135	26.4(21.8–31.0)	1		
Smoking							
Smoker	284	58.7(54.0–63.4)	130	28.6(23.8–33.5)	2.28	(1.47–3.54)	<0.01
Non–smoker	218	41.3(36.6–46.0)	375	71.2(66.4–76.0)	1		

[a] "Monthly alcohol consumption" was defined as having consumed alcohol at least once per month during the past year.
[b] The sum of the percentage may not be 100 because the number of missing values were not presented. Missing values were treated as dummy variables in the analysis.

Table 3. Multivariate analysis of association between high-risk alcohol consumption[a] and sociodemographic factors in HBV carriers.

	High-risk alcohol consumers		Non-high-risk consumers		Odds ratio	95% CI	*P-value*
	N	%[b] (95% CI)	N	%[b] (95% CI)			
Sex							
Male	95	87.0(80.9–93.0)	397	47.8(44.1–51.6)	3.46	(1.33–9.00)	0.01
Female	12	13.0(7.0–19.1)	518	52.2(48.4–55.9)	1		
Age							
<40	9	8.0(3.2–12.8)	237	23.2(20.1–26.4)	1		
40–49	17	15.7(8.4–23.0)	207	23.1(19.7–26.6)	0.92	(0.50–1.70)	0.79
50–59	41	38.7(29.7–47.6)	211	23.3(20.0–26.6)	0.29	(0.13–0.64)	<0.01
≥60	40	37.6(28.0–47.2)	260	30.3(26.7–34.0)	0.19	(0.06–0.60)	<0.01
Area of residence							
Urban	78	81.5(75.4–87.6)	690	79.0(75.0–83.1)	1.09	(0.61–1.93)	0.78
Rural	29	18.5(12.4–24.6)	225	21.0(16.9–25.0)	1		
Household income							
Low	9	6.1(1.3–10.8)	157	15.4(12.7–18.2)	0.49	(0.17–1.42)	0.19
Mid–low	33	29.7(21.5–37.9)	231	25.8(22.4–29.3)	1.28	(0.67–2.44)	0.45
Mid–high	31	29.4(21.3–37.5)	229	26.6(22.9–30.3)	0.84	(0.44–1.63)	0.61
High	33	34.4(25.6–43.3)	277	29.9(26.3–33.6)	1		
Education							
Less than high school	26	23.4(15.7–31.1)	14	2.4(1.1–3.7)	2.48	(1.19–5.17)	0.01
High school	44	42.8(33.4–52.2)	395	45.7(41.6–49.7)	2.02	(1.12–3.64)	0.02
College or more	37	33.8(24.6–42.9)	506	51.9(47.9–55.9)	1		
Body mass index							
<18.5	3	4.2(1.5–7.0)	28	3.0(1.8–4.2)	1.23	(0.31–4.91)	0.77
18.5–24.9	55	49.1(40.3–57.8)	585	63.5(60.0–67.0)	0.51	(0.31–0.82)	0.01
≥25.0	49	46.7(38.0–55.4)	298	32.8(29.4–36.3)	1		
Awareness of HBV infection							
Unaware	85	76.4(67.6–85.2)	724	79.4(76.3–82.6)	1.16	(0.63–2.13)	0.64
Aware	22	23.6(14.8–32.4)	191	20.6(17.4–23.7)	1		
Subjective health status							
Bad	19	18.6(11.0–26.2)	227	21.2(18.0–24.3)	0.62	(0.32–1.22)	0.16
Moderate	47	44.1(35.2–53.1)	422	50.4(46.5–54.2)	0.49	(0.28–0.84)	0.01
Good	41	37.3(28.2–46.4)	254	26.1(22.8–29.4)	1		
Smoking							
Smoker	88	81.1(73.5–88.7)	326	38.7(34.9–42.5)	4.15	(1.75–9.85)	<0.01
Non–smoker	19	18.9(11.3–26.5)	578	59.3(55.5–63.0)	1		

[a]"High-risk alcohol consumption" was defined as having consumed alcohol twice or more per week and, for males, having consumed at least 60 g of alcohol on one occasion or, for females, having consumed at least 40 g of alcohol on more than one occasion.
[b]The sum of the percentage may not be 100 because the number of missing values were not presented. Missing values were treated as dummy variables in the analysis.

smoking and drinking are related in the general population [28]. Similar to previous studies that showed an association between obesity and alcohol consumption [29,30], the odds that individuals who were of normal weight (18.5≤ BMI <25 kg/m^2) consumed alcohol were significantly lower than were those that overweight or obese people (BMI ≥25 kg/m^2) did so. Additionally, our results showed no statistically significant differences in monthly drinking or high-risk drinking between obese people (BMI ≥25 kg/m^2) and people with BMI <18.5 kg/m^2. Considering the synergistic effects of smoking and HBV infection and of obesity and HBV infection on the risk of HCC [12,29], the higher prevalence of smokers or overweight/obese people with HBV infection may further increase the risk of developing HCC.

To reduce the disease burden related to the morbidity and mortality of liver cancer, which is end-stage liver disease [13], Korea implemented nationwide liver cancer screening in 2003 as part of the National Cancer Screening Program for secondary prevention. Alpha-fetoprotein and ultrasonography tests are provided for men and women aged 40 years or older with chronic HBV or hepatitis C virus (HCV) infection, liver cirrhosis, or chronic liver disease of any cause [30,31]. However, there is no specific national program for the primary prevention of liver diseases that targets high-risk populations. A previous study conducted by our team suggested that sex, age, awareness of infection status, and monthly household income are associated with liver cancer screening among HBV carriers [32]. Another study also showed that HBV or HCV carriers who knew their infection status sought liver cancer screening more often than carriers unknown infection status during their lifetime [33]. Although awareness of infection status was the most important factor related to undergoing liver cancer screening among HBV carriers, we found that it was not associated with alcohol consumption among HBV carriers, suggesting that we may need a different approach to the primary and secondary prevention of liver diseases in HBV carriers.

This study has several limitations. First, the information related to demographic, socioeconomic, and life style-related factors was self-reported in health surveys, and thus might be subject to information bias and/or recall bias. Although the alcohol consumption measured in household surveys might be underreported [34], it is possible to use such questions in epidemiological studies [35]. In addition, studies have shown that self-reported information regarding risk factors, including alcohol consumption and smoking, was reasonably reproducible, suggesting reasonable reliability [36,37]. Therefore, although the questions used in KNHANES might not be validated, the bias was expected to be minimal. Second, because hepatitis B surface antibodies and total hepatitis B core antibodies were not assessed in the KNHANES, only current HBV infections could be examined, and we could not be certain whether the individuals with HBsAg were acutely infected or chronic carriers. Third, these results are based on cross-sectional study data, and we did not assess the order of the association between sociodemographic factors and drinking. Despite these limitations, a major strength of the study is that the KNHANES data are representative of the Korean population and, by applying sampling weights in the analysis, the results can be applied to all HBV carriers in Korea. Second, the prevalence of alcohol consumption and its associated factors among HBV carriers may provide opportunities for the primary prevention of liver cirrhosis or HCC in a high-risk population.

HBV infection is endemic in Korea, and the burden of liver diseases related to HBV infection is substantial [14,15]. Efforts, from primary prevention to tertiary prevention, are necessary across the natural history of disease to decrease the burden related to the morbidity and mortality associated with HBV infection. Previous studies focusing on secondary prevention through liver cancer screening found that the awareness of infection status was an important contributor to undergoing liver cancer screening [32,33]. However, sociodemographic factors, especially education, were important in terms of primary prevention via healthy lifestyle choices (e.g., abstaining from alcohol consumption). Thus, our findings indicate that efforts to reduce the disease burden caused by HBV infection need to focus on less educated socioeconomic groups to achieve more effective primary prevention. Additionally, other health-related behaviors, such as smoking and obesity, affect alcohol consumption in the population at high risk for HCC. Considering these are other independent and synergistic contributors to the development of HCC in HBV carriers [12,29], efforts should focus not only on abstinence but also on promoting a generally healthy lifestyle. The difference in alcohol consumption according to educational level among HBV carriers should be considered by health policies or intervention programs that are aimed at HBV carriers and at promoting generally healthy lifestyles.

Author Contributions

Conceived and designed the experiments: BP JKJ. Performed the experiments: BP KSC MS. Analyzed the data: KWJ CMO. Contributed reagents/materials/analysis tools: KWJ. Wrote the paper: BP JKJ.

References

1. WHO (2009) Weekly epidemiological record. World Health Organization 84: 405–420.
2. Liaw YF (2009) Antiviral therapy of chronic hepatitis B: opportunities and challenges in Asia. J Hepatol 51: 403–410.
3. Zanetti AR, Van Damme P, Shouval D (2008) The global impact of vaccination against hepatitis B: a historical overview. Vaccine 26: 6266–6273.
4. Venook AP, Papandreou C, Furuse J, de Guevara LL (2010) The incidence and epidemiology of hepatocellular carcinoma: a global and regional perspective. Oncologist 15 Suppl 4: 5–13.
5. Ferlay J, Shin HR, Bray F, Forman D, Mathers C, et al. (2010) Estimates of worldwide burden of cancer in 2008: GLOBOCAN 2008. Int J Cancer 127: 2893–2917.
6. Aggarwal R, Ranjan P (2004) Preventing and treating hepatitis B infection. BMJ 329: 1080–1086.
7. Stroffolini T, Cotticelli G, Medda E, Niosi M, Del Vecchio-Blanco C, et al. (2010) Interaction of alcohol intake and cofactors on the risk of cirrhosis. Liver Int 30: 867–870.
8. Fattovich G, Bortolotti F, Donato F (2008) Natural history of chronic hepatitis B: special emphasis on disease progression and prognostic factors. J Hepatol 48: 335–352.
9. Bialecki ES, Di Bisceglie AM (2005) Clinical presentation and natural course of hepatocellular carcinoma. Eur J Gastroenterol Hepatol 17: 485–489.
10. Donato F, Tagger A, Gelatti U, Parrinello G, Boffetta P, et al. (2002) Alcohol and hepatocellular carcinoma: the effect of lifetime intake and hepatitis virus infections in men and women. Am J Epidemiol 155: 323–331.
11. Hassan MM, Hwang LY, Hatten CJ, Swaim M, Li D, et al. (2002) Risk factors for hepatocellular carcinoma: synergism of alcohol with viral hepatitis and diabetes mellitus. Hepatology 36: 1206–1213.
12. Yuan JM, Govindarajan S, Arakawa K, Yu MC (2004) Synergism of alcohol, diabetes, and viral hepatitis on the risk of hepatocellular carcinoma in blacks and whites in the U.S. Cancer 101: 1009–1017.
13. Zakhari S (2013) Bermuda Triangle for the liver: alcohol, obesity, and viral hepatitis. J Gastroenterol Hepatol 28 Suppl 1: 18–25.
14. Chan HL, Jia J (2011) Chronic hepatitis B in Asia-new insights from the past decade. J Gastroenterol Hepatol 26 Suppl 1: 131–137.
15. Chae HB, Kim JH, Kim JK, Yim HJ (2009) Current status of liver diseases in Korea: hepatitis B. Korean J Hepatol 15 Suppl 6: S13–24.
16. WHO (2014) Global status report on alcohol and health. Switzerland: World Health Organization.
17. WHO (2000) International guide for monitoring alcohol consumption and related harm. Switzerland: World Health Organization.
18. KCDC (2005) Ministry of Health and Welfare. The Fourth Korea National Health and Nutrition Examination Survey (KNHANES IV), 2007–2009–Summary. Seoul: Korea Centers for Disease Control and Prevention.

19. Koh K (2000) Estimates of alcohol consumption based on pure alcohol content and their comparison with data of other countries. Health and Welfare Policy Forum 6: 77–86.
20. Park B, Choi KS, Lee HY, Jun JK, Park EC (2012) Socioeconomic inequalities in completion of hepatitis B vaccine series among Korean women: results from a nationwide interview survey. Vaccine 30: 5844–5848.
21. (2011) Korean Association for the Study of Liver. The treatment guideline of chronic hepatitis B Seoul: Korean Association for the Study of Liver.
22. Tenconi MT, Romanelli C, Gigli F, Sottocornola F, Laddomada MS, et al. (1992) The relationship between education and risk factors for coronary heart disease. Epidemiological analysis from the nine communities study. The Research Group ATS-OB43 of CNR. Eur J Epidemiol 8: 763–769.
23. Fong CW, Bhalla V, Heng D, Chua AV, Chan ML, et al. (2007) Educational inequalities associated with health-related behaviours in the adult population of Singapore. Singapore Med J 48: 1091–1099.
24. Grant JD, Scherrer JF, Lynskey MT, Agrawal A, Duncan AE, et al. (2012) Associations of alcohol, nicotine, cannabis, and drug use/dependence with educational attainment: evidence from cotwin-control analyses. Alcohol Clin Exp Res 36: 1412–1420.
25. Huerta MC, Borgonovi F (2010) Education, alcohol use and abuse among young adults in Britain. Soc Sci Med 71: 143–151.
26. Schroder H, Rohlfs I, Schmelz EM, Marrugat J (2004) Relationship of socioeconomic status with cardiovascular risk factors and lifestyle in a Mediterranean population. Eur J Nutr 43: 77–85.
27. Khang YH, Lynch JW, Kaplan GA (2004) Health inequalities in Korea: age- and sex-specific educational differences in the 10 leading causes of death. Int J Epidemiol 33: 299–308.
28. Woitas-Slubowska D, Hurnik E, Skarpanska-Stejnborn A (2010) Correlates of smoking with socioeconomic status, leisure time physical activity and alcohol consumption among Polish adults from randomly selected regions. Cent Eur J Public Health 18: 179–185.
29. Chuang SC, Lee YC, Hashibe M, Dai M, Zheng T, et al. (2010) Interaction between cigarette smoking and hepatitis B and C virus infection on the risk of liver cancer: a meta-analysis. Cancer Epidemiol Biomarkers Prev 19: 1261–1268.
30. Noh DK, Choi KS, Jun JK, Lee HY, Park EC (2012) Factors associated with attending the National Cancer Screening Program for liver cancer in Korea. Asian Pac J Cancer Prev 13: 731–736.
31. Lee EH, Han MA, Lee HY, Jun JK, Choi KS, et al. (2010) Liver cancer screening in Korea: a report on the 2008 National Cancer Screening Programme. Asian Pac J Cancer Prev 11: 1305–1310.
32. Park B, Choi KS, Suh M, Shin JY, Jun JK (2013) Factors associated with compliance with recommendations for liver cancer screening in Korea: a nationwide survey in Korea. PLoS One 8: e68315.
33. Cho ER, Shin A, Choi KS, Lee HY, Kim J (2010) Factors associated with use of ultrasonography screening for hepatocellular carcinoma among hepatitis B or C carriers. Cancer Epidemiol 34: 713–716.
34. Stockwell T, Donath S, Cooper-Stanbury M, Chikritzhs T, Catalano P, et al. (2004) Under-reporting of alcohol consumption in household surveys: a comparison of quantity-frequency, graduated-frequency and recent recall. Addiction 99: 1024–1033.
35. Ekholm O, Strandberg-Larsen K, Christensen K, Gronbaek M (2008) Comparison of assessment methods for self-reported alcohol consumption in health interview surveys. Eur J Clin Nutr 62: 286–291.
36. Brownson RC, Jackson-Thompson J, Wilkerson JC, Kiani F (1994) Reliability of information on chronic disease risk factors collected in the Missouri Behavioral Risk Factor Surveillance System. Epidemiology 5: 545–549.
37. Bowlin SJ, Morrill BD, Nafziger AN, Lewis C, Pearson TA (1996) Reliability and changes in validity of self-reported cardiovascular disease risk factors using dual response: the behavioral risk factor survey. J Clin Epidemiol 49: 511–517.

10

Comparing Outcomes of Two Vascular Inflow Occlusion Techniques and Treatment without Vascular Occlusion during Major Hepatectomy in Patients with Hepatitis B-Related Hepatocellular Carcinoma

Zhiping Huang[1], Peng Zhang[2], Haiqing Wang[2], Lunan Yan[2], Wentao Wang[2]*

1 Department of hepatopancreatobiliary Surgery, Yongchuan Hospital, Chongqing Medical University, Yongchuan, Chongqing, China, **2** Department of Liver Surgery, Liver Transplantation Center, West China Hospital of Sichuan University, Chengdu, Sichuan Province, China

Abstract

Background: Significant hemorrhage together with blood transfusion has negative impact on postoperative morbidity, mortality, and long-term survival of liver resection. Various techniques of vascular occlusion have been developed to reduce intraoperative blood loss. The objective of this study was to compare the outcomes of Pringle maneuver, hemi-hepatic vascular occlusion, and treatment without vascular occlusion used during liver resection.

Method: Data of 574 patients with Hepatitis B virus (HBV)-related hepatocellular carcinoma (HCC), who underwent major hepatectomy between January 2009 to March 2013 by Pringle maneuver (N = 158), hemi-hepatic vascular inflow occlusion (N = 216), or without any vascular occlusion (N = 200), were included in this retrospective study. Perioperative blood transfusion, intraoperative blood loss, and postoperative liver function, and surgical complications were analyzed and compared between the three groups.

Result: There were no significant difference observed in postoperative bilirubin, liver enzyme, and albumin levels between three groups ($P>0.05$). 5 patients (2.5%) in no occlusion group, 2 (1.3%) in Pringle group, and 8 (3.7%) in hemi-hepatic group had liver failure; but, there were no differences ($P>0.05$). The overall postoperative complications rate between three groups did not reach significant differences (33.5% vs 34.2% vs 42.6%, respectively; $P>0.05$). However, significant differences in intraoperative blood loss between no occlusion group (638.2±426.8 ml) and Pringle group (518.0±451.0 ml) or hemi-hepatic group (513.0±366.7 ml) ($P<0.01$).

Conclusion: Although there were no differences found between three groups regarding postoperative complications rate, no vascular occlusion group had more blood loss than the other two groups during liver resection.

Editor: Helge Bruns, University Hospital Heidelberg, Germany

Funding: This study is supported by a grant from the National Sciences and Technology Major Project of China (2012ZX10002-016) and (2012ZX10002-017). The funders had no role in study design, data collection and analysis, decision to publish, or preparation of the manuscript.

Competing Interests: The authors have declared that no competing interests exist.

* Email: wwthzhp@163.com

Introduction

Hepatocellular Carcinoma (HCC) is one of the most prevalent and deadly cancers [1]; it is the sixth most common cancer worldwide with 749,000 new cases yearly, and the third leading cause of cancer deaths with 692,000 deaths yearly. In China, a high incidence of HCC with cirrhosis is largely due to hepatitis B infections, which is in marked contrast to the West, where the main causes of cirrhosis are hepatitis C or alcohol related[2–4]. Currently, there are various effective treatments available for HCC such as liver resection, liver transplantation, radiofrequency ablation, and transcatheter hepatic arterial chemoembolization. However, partial hepatectomy is still the most commonly used technique [5], and Barcelona Clinic Liver Cancer (BCLC) staging system recommends it as the primary therapeutic method for patients with early stage HCC [6].

Liver resection has experienced more than 100 years of development as the primary treatment for HCC. To the end of 19th century, the animal experiments had shown the feasibility of liver parenchyma incision. William keen (1899) was considered as the first American surgeon to perform liver resection; he reported three successful surgical cases. However, the perioperative mortality (70%–90%) of liver resection was very high during that period [7]. One of main reasons was that intraoperative blood loss in the surgery could not be effectively controlled. Significant hemorrhage together with blood transfusion increases postoperative morbidity and mortality of hepatic resection [8–10]. Various techniques of vascular occlusion have been developed to reduce intraoperative blood loss.

The Pringle maneuver, a technique of transient hepatic vascular inflow occlusion, was described by J.H.Pringle, a British surgeon in

1908 [11]. It is performed encircling the hepatoduodenal ligament with a tape and then applying a tourniquet or vascular clamp until the hepatic arterial pulse disappears distally. The validity of this technique in reducing hemorrhage in liver resection had been proved by Man et al [12]. However, the Pringle maneuver can induce ischemia-reperfusion injury to the remnant liver [13,14], and some surgeons even claimed that the Pringle maneuver should be avoided in the partial hepatectomy because of its induction of tumor recurrence and worse prognosis [15,16].

To avoid ischemia-reperfusion injury to the remnant liver, Makuuchi [17] et al proposed a hemi-hepatic inflow vascular occlusion technique, which could only block the blood supply of right or left hemi-hepatic at tumor location, allowing normal blood supply at contralateral hemi-liver. The advantage of this technique is especially seen in patients with cancer who need right or left hemi-liver resection, because no liver tissues would subject to ischemia-reperfusion. However, the adverse effect of hemi-hepatic vascular occlusion includes more bleeding from the raw surface of the other hemi-liver. Liver surgeons should be experienced in dissecting and lowering hilar plate to avoid any injury to bile ducts and vessels. Although the Pringle maneuver and hemi-hepatic vascular occlusion are the most commonly used techniques in clinical practice, no consensus has still arrived among surgeons on choosing an optimal method during liver.

This retrospective cohort study was designed to compare the outcomes of Pringle maneuver, hemi-hepatic vascular occlusion, and treatment without vascular occlusion used during liver resection in patients with HCC.

Patients and Methods

Trail design

This study was approved by Institutional Review Board of the West China Hospital of Sichuan University. Although written or verbal informed consent given by participants could not be obtained, patient records/information was anonymized and de-identified. All the data were collected retrospectively from the HCC database of the hospital.

From January 2009 to March 2013, 574 patients with Hepatitis B virus (HBV)-related HCC who underwent major hepatectomy [18] (defined as the resection of liver, at least, three Couianud's segments), formed this study set. The diagnosis of HCC was based on American Association for the Study of Liver Diseases (AASLD) and European Association for the Study of the Liver (EASL) guidelines [1,19,20] and proved by cytological/histological after resection. All patients were operated only when Child-Turcotte-Pugh (CTP) score was A, or CTP class A was reached by the treatment that adopted for patients with CTP class B. Patients who met the following criteria were excluded from the study: (1) diagnosis was not HCC; (2) no requirement for major hepatectomy; (3) a history of previous partial hepatectomy; and (4) having major concomitant surgery including adrenal resection, esophageal devascularization, and gastrostomy. All surgical procedures were guided by the same team of liver surgeons who had experience in liver resections. The main endpoints were the intraoperative blood loss, postoperative liver function, postoperative morbidity and mortality rate.

All patients were divided into 3 groups according to the technique of vascular occlusion used in hepatic resection: no vascular occlusion, Pringle maneuver, and hemi-hepatic vascular inflow occlusion groups.

Preoperative examination

All patients had a chest x-ray, electrocardiogram, ultrasonography, and contrast computed tomography or magnetic resonance imaging of abdomen. Laboratory blood tests included blood routine, antigen of hepatitis B (HBsAg), antibody of hepatitis C (HCVAb), aspartate aminotransferase (AST), alanine aminotransferase (ALT), serum total bilirubin (TB), alpha-fetoprotein (AFP), and prothrombin time (PT). The Anesthesia grade [21] (American Society of Anesthesiologists), Charlson index [22] (used to quantify preoperative comorbidities), and CTP score were determined.

Surgical procedure

Right subcostal oblique incision was chosen to perform surgery. When the abdominal cavity was opened, intraoperative ultrasonography was used routinely to check the extent of tumor and its position and to assess whether there were any extra-hepatic metastases. The liver was mobilized as soon as the resectability of the tumor was determined. After that, the technique of vascular occlusion was selected or not, according to the surgeon's preference and patient's intraoperative condition.

The Pringle maneuver was performed by encircling the hepatoduodenal ligament with a catheter and then applying a vascular clamp until the hepatic arterial pulse disappeared distally. Tightening or loosening the catheter resulted in blocking or not blocking the vascular inflow to the liver. In this method, intermittent vascular occlusion was applied. The circulation of blocking and not blocking vascular inflow was 15/5 min.

A special technique called lowering the liver hilar plate, which was put forward by Hepp and Couinaud in 1956, was adopted [23], when performing hemi-hepatic vascular occlusion. However, this technique had a potential risk to injure the bile ducts and vessels. Procedures of hemi-hepatic vascular occlusion from our center had been described in previous published works [24,25] (Figure 1).

For liver parenchymal division, hooking with ligation or Cavitron ultrasonic surgical aspirator (CUSA) was used. Hooking with ligation is a simple and effective technique for liver resection, introduced by Yan in 1994 [24,25] (Figure 2). When no vascular occlusion or hemi-occlusion technique was used in the liver surgery, CUSA was selected for liver parenchymal transection. However, when the Pringle maneuver was used in the surgery, hooking with ligation was chosen, because only a short time (always less than 30 min) was needed for liver resection.

Postoperative evaluation

The measurements of blood loss were made before, during, and after liver resection. The volume of blood loss was measured from the weight of the soaked gauze and blood collected from the containers of the suction apparatus and ultrasonic dissector. The volume of irrigation fluid was deduced accordingly. Generally speaking, whole blood was not transfused unless the hematocrit value became less than 30% during surgery. All patients were carefully observed after operation. Admission at the intensive care unit (ICU) was determined by patients' intraoperative condition. Routine tests of liver function were performed after operation. Mortality (defined as death within 90 days after surgery or death during the same hospital admission of surgery), morbidity, postoperative hospitalization duration, and ICU stay were record in detail.

Statistical analysis

Statistical analysis was performed using SPSS (Version 17.0). The results of continuous variables were expressed as means ±

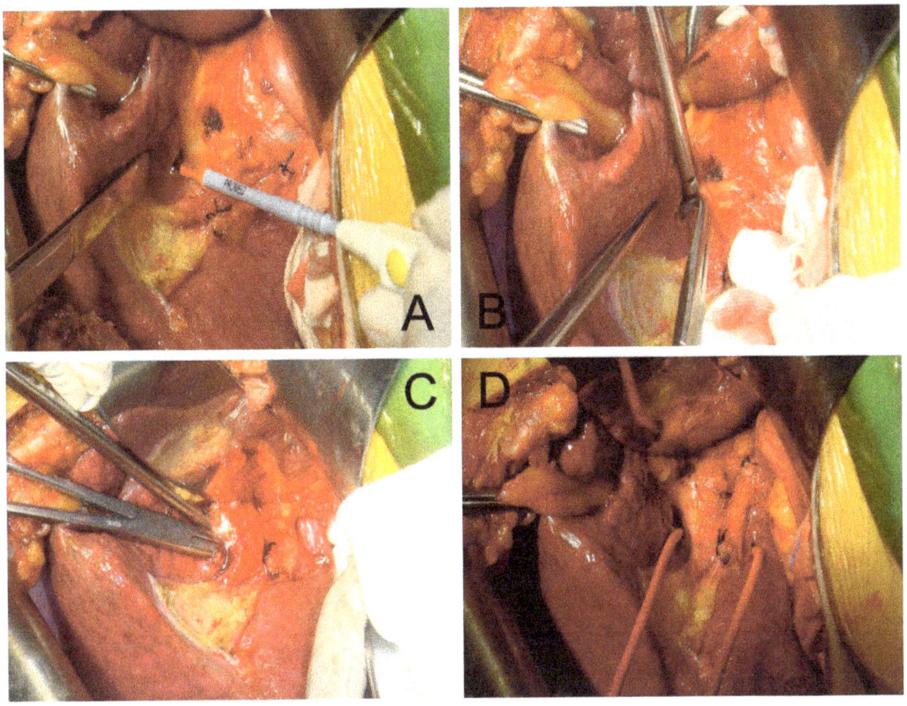

Figure 1. Simple hemi-occlusion. A: On the visceral envelope overlying the confluence, a small hole was made using a sharp blade; **B:** A right-angle forceps was inserted to gently mobilize the liver parenchyma outside Glisson's sheath; **C:** The right-angle forceps should mobilize in the liver parenchyma towards the caudate lobe; **D:** A catheter was introduced.

standard deviation or median with interquartile range. The variables were compared using one-way analysis of variance. Non-parametric variables used the Mann-Whitney U test or Kruskal-wallis test. Chi-square test was used to compare categorical variables. P<0.05 was considered statistically significant.

Result

In this retrospective study, data of 574 patients with HBV-related HCC were analyzed. The preoperative demographic and baseline data are described in Table 1. There were no significant differences between three groups regarding age, sex, Charlson score, portal hypertension (defined as esophageal varices detected by endoscopy or a splenomegaly (major diameter >12 cm) with a platelet count <100 000/mm3 according to the BCLC group criteria [19,20]), anesthesia grade, and laboratory blood tests related to liver function. However, most patients in three groups had different degree of liver cirrhosis during liver resection.

Result of occlusion time, intraoperative blood loss, blood transfusion requirement

The intraoperative data are listed in Table 2. 141 patients (24.6%) had perioperative blood transfusion. Occlusion time in the Pringle group was 41.9±12.3 min vs 44.3±18.7 min in the hemi-hepatic group (P>0.05).

There were significant differences between three groups in intraoperative blood loss (P<0.01). The median blood loss in the Pringle group was 518.0±451.0 ml vs 513.0±366.7 ml in the hemi-hepatic group (P>0.05). There were significant differences between no occlusion group (638.2±426.8 ml) and Pringle or hemi-hepatic groups in intraoperative blood loss (P<0.01). There were also no difference in blood transfusion requirements (P>0.05).

About 45.5% had three segments of liver resection in no occlusion group vs 43.0% in Pringle group and 52.8% in hemi-hepatic group (P>0.05). The percentage of patients who had four segments of liver resection included 50.5%, 48.1%, and 42.1%, respectively in no occlusion group, Pringle group, and hemi-hepatic group (P>0.05). There were also no significant differences between three groups of patients who had five segments of liver resection (4.0% vs 9.9% vs 5.1%, respectively, P>0.05).

Result of postoperative liver function

The postoperative liver function data are listed in Table 3. Serum total bilirubin and liver enzymes were increased in three groups on days 1, 3, and 5. The elevated bilirubin and liver enzymes had a tendency to return to the baseline value on 5th postoperative day. However, there were no significant difference observed between three groups in bilirubin, liver enzymes, and albumin (P>0.05).

Five patients (2.5%) in no occlusion group, 2 (1.3%) in Pringle group, and 8 (3.7%) in hemi-hepatic group had liver failure (defined as prothrombin time<50% and serum bilirubin level> 50 μmol/L on the on day 5 after liver resection [28]) and they did not reach significant difference (P>0.05, Table 4).

Result of postoperative surgical complications, ICU stays, and hospital mortality

The postoperative data are shown in Table 4 and Table 5. The Clavien-Dindo Classification of surgical complications [26,27] was used to evaluation the postoperative complications. The overall postoperative morbidity rate was 34.8% (200/574). However, there were no significant differences between three groups in postoperative complications: 33.5% in no occlusion group vs 34.2% in Pringle group vs 42.6% in hemi-hepatic group (P>0.05). The most common postoperative complications with grade III–V

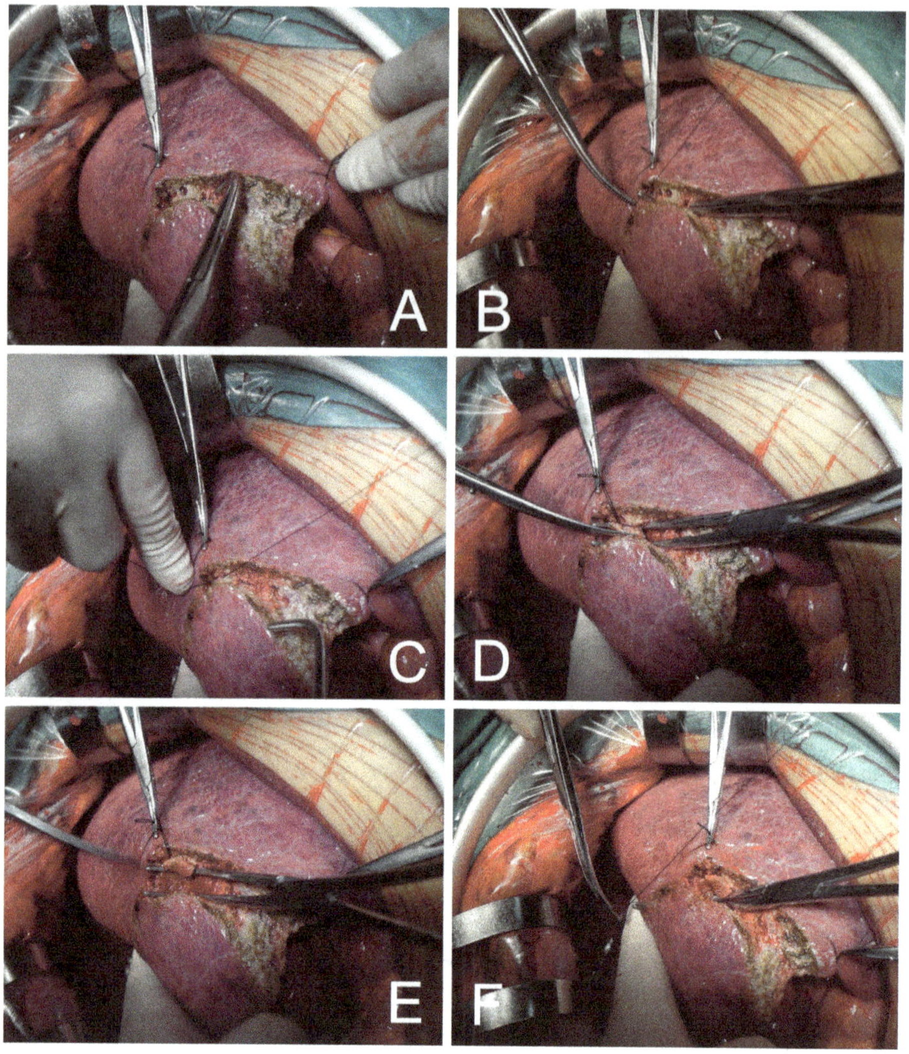

Figure 2. Hooking with ligation. A: The resection line was marked by electrocautery on the hepatic surface, B: The liver was dissected by rightangle forceps hooking the hepatic tissue; C, D, and E: Cannular structures were ligated and cut; F: Right-angle forceps hooked the hepatic tissue forward one by one.

were bile leakage, pleural effusion, and liver failure. Only 1 patient in Pringle group and 1 in hemi-hepatic group need reoperation due to intra-abdominal hemorrhage.

The overall hospital mortality was 2.3% (13/574) in this study: two in no occlusion group, six in Pringle group, and five in hemi-hepatic group. There were no significant differences between three groups in hospital mortality ($P>0.05$; 1% vs 3.8% vs 2.3% in no occlusion group, Pringle group, hemi-hepatic group, respectively). Among these patients, nine died of liver failure, two died of sudden cardiac arrest, and two died of perioperative intra-abdominal hemorrhage. The time of stay in the ICU did not reach significant differences between three groups ($P>0.05$).

Discussion

Controlling blood loss in an effective, safe, and quick manner is the primary goal of liver surgeons when performing hepatectomy. The amount of intraoperative blood loss and perioperative transfusion requirements will markedly affect the postoperative liver function, postoperative morbidity and mortality, and long-term survival [8–10]. To decrease blood loss during hepatectomy, various hepatic vascular occlusion techniques have been developed such as total vascular exclusion [29], Pringle maneuver, hemi-hepatic vascular occlusion, hepatic vascular exclusion [30], and hepatic vascular exclusion with veno-venous bypass [31].

However, Pringle maneuver is most commonly used in clinical practice because of its simplicity, but it can induce ischemia-reperfusion injury to liver, which can result in metabolic, immunological, and microvascular changes [32]. Ischemia-reperfusion could even promote liver metastasis [15]. In addition, Pringle maneuver can induce visceral congestion and instability in hemodynamic status, and it can increase the mean arterial pressure by 10%, decrease in pulmonary artery pressure by 5% and cardiac index by 10% [33].

To avoid ischemia-reperfusion injury to the remnant liver and visceral congestion, some surgeons put forward ischemic preconditioning, which involves a brief period of ischemia and reperfusion to liver prior to Pringel vascular occlusion. However, the best time of ischemic preconditioning still remains to be study [34–36]. Because of this the technique of hemi-hepatic vascular inflow occlusion was suggested. It can block the blood supply of right or left hemi-hepatic portions at tumor location, allowing

Table 1. Preoperative characteristic of patients.

	No occlusion group (n = 200)	The Pringle group (n = 158)	The hemi-hepatic group (n = 126)	P value
Age(years)	50.4±12.6	48.5±12.0	49.3±12.8	0.358
Sex(M/F)	175/25	129/29	187/29	0.253
Charlson score Median(IQR)	1(1–3)	1(1–3)	1(1–3)	0.573
Portal hypertension	24(12.0%)	31(19.6%)	31(14.4%)	0.127
Anesthesia grade (I+II/III+IV)	169/31	137/21	187/29	0.783
HBsAg(+)	155(77.5%)	134(84.8%)	169(78.2%)	0.179
ALT (u/l)	56.8±52.6	55.9±45.8	58.0±49.4	0.918
AST (u/l)	63.1±70.6	62.8±50.6	57.5±47.7	0.545
Albumin(g/l)	40.6±4.6	39.4±5.3	39.9±4.6	0.063
Hemoglobin(g/l)	138.5±20.0	138.5±22.2	140.5±20.0	0.516
Plate(10x9/l)	167.5±80.6	163.9±79.8	175.3±83.6	0.378
Leukocyte(10x9/l)	6.5±2.4	6.1±2.7	6.3±2.2	0.301

IQR: interquartile range; **ALT:** alanine aminotransferase; **AST:** aspartate aminotransferase; **HBsAg:** antigen of hepatitis B.

normal blood supply at the contralateral hemi-liver. However, one of concerns of the hemi-hepatic vascular occlusion is that there is a risk of bleeding from the contralateral hemi-liver. Liver surgeons should have experience in dissecting the hilar plate and lowering hilar plate to avoid injury to bile ducts and vessels.

Generally speaking, The Pringle group should have a higher postoperative serum albumin level. However, in this retrospective study, we found that there were no significant difference observed between three groups in bilirubin, liver enzymes, and albumin (P> 0.05). There were two possible reasons: one was that intermittent vascular occlusion which could decrease ischemia-reperfusion injury to liver was applied when perform Pringle vascular occlusion; the other was that we use hooking with ligation to perform liver resection when Pringle maneuver was chosen. On the other hand, CUSA was used to perform liver parenchyma division when hemi-hepatic vascular occlusion or no vascular occlusion was selected. Hooking with ligation is a simple and quick method of liver resection, and the ischemia-reperfusion time of liver will be significantly reduced. On the contrary, the time of ischemia-reperfusion was prolonged when CUSA was used.

As all the patients were suffering from hepatocellular carcinomas with hepatitis B, most of them had postoperative hypoproteinemia. Ascites were the most common postoperative complications which usually required diuretic treatment or peritoneocentesis.

To the best of our knowledge, in a prospective random controlled study by Ni et al [37], it was reported that although there were no significance differences in blood loss between two groups such as Pringle maneuver and hemi-hepatic vascular occlusion, the complication rate after liver resection was higher in the Pringle maneuver group. Fu et al [38] reported that the two techniques were safe and efficacious, but the hemi-hepatic group had an earlier recovery of liver function than Pringle maneuver group. Chau et al [39] reported that hemi-hepatic group could

Table 2. Intraoperative data.

	No occlusion group (n = 200)	The Pringle group (n = 158)	The hemi-hepatic group (n = 216)	P value
Types of resection				
3 segments of liver	91(45.5%)	68(43.0%)	114(52.8%)	0.136
4 segments of liver	101(50.5%)	76(48.1%)	91(42.1%)	0.213
5 segments of liver	8(4.0%)	14(9.9%)	11(5.1%)	0.127
Occlusion time(min)	0	41.9±12.3	44.3±18.7	0.150
Intraoperative Blood loss(ml)	638.2±426.8	518.0±451.0	513.0±366.7	0.03 I vs II = 0.906 I vs III = 0.001 II vs III = 0.01
Blood transfusion YES/NO	45/155(22.5%)	42/166(26.6%)	54/162(25.0%)	0.661

I: Hemi-hepatic group, **II:** Pringle group, **III:** No occlusion group.

Table 3. The postoperative liver function data.

	No occlusion group (n = 200)	The Pringle group (n = 158)	The hemi-hepatic group (n = 216)	P value
Day 1				
TBIL(umol/l)	28.0±16.4	28.2±15.2	30.8±20.0	0.209
ALT(u/l)	413.9±415.8	409.7±319.8	432.5±574.5	0.873
AST(u/l)	392.2±389.7	417.5±390.5	438.7±623.2	0.627
Albumin(g/l)	28.4±5.1	28.3±5.4	28.8±5.6	0.560
Day 3				
TBIL(umol/l)	33.3±20.4	33.5±19.8	37.1±31.5	0.229
ALT(u/l)	282.1±262.0	296.9±243.2	281.8±266.9	0.827
AST(u/l)	139.7±123.7	151.6±140.6	147.0±129.0	0.681
Albumin(g/l)	31.7±4.1	31.2±4.6	31.4±5.1	0.578
Day 5				
TBIL(umol/l)	28.0±24.1	28.0±20.8	32.1±32.0	0.196
ALT(u/l)	127.7±106.1	133.2±104.4	129.4±111.8	0.885
AST(u/l)	56.4±37.3	60.8±40.8	66.4±68.3	0.141
Albumin(g/l)	34.1±4.8	34.5±5.6	34.8±5.0	0.422

TBIL: total serum bilirubin; **ALT:** alanine aminotransferase; **AST:** aspartate aminotransferase;

respond better than Pringle maneuver group. When vascular occlusion time was ≥45 min, hemi-hepatic group had an earlier recovery of liver function. On the contrast, Tanaka et al [40] reported there were no differences between two groups in the perioperative data. Taniguchi et al [41] reported that though there were no significant difference in blood loss and operative time between Pringle maneuver group and no vascular occlusion group, and the liver enzymes and total bilirubin were elevated in Pringle group.

There are other known factors that affect the amount of blood loss and transfusion in the liver surgery. Various new surgical devices are used when performing hepatic resection such as water jet dissector, CUSA, and LigaSure (a vessel sealing system). A report by Une et al [42] indicated that although there were no differences in blood loss and operative time, water jet could show the surgical field more clearly. In our center, there is no strict standard for choosing the tools to perform hepatectomy. The choice is made according to the selection of vascular occlusion technique. Another known factor is the central venous pressure (CVP) during liver resection. A retrospective study by Smyrniotis reported that elevated CVP during major liver resections could result in greater blood loss and longer hospital stay [43]. However, a consensus was reached by liver surgeons that maintenance of a low CVP was always associated with less intraoperative blood loss and better postoperative outcomes. In our institution, a low central venous pressure in a range of 5 cm H_2O is usually maintained.

At present, the two vascular occlusion techniques are selectively used in our center. When tumors limit within hemi-liver, hemi-

Table 4. Postoperative data.

	No occlusion group (n = 200)	The Pringle group (n = 158)	The hemi-hepatic group (n = 216)	P value
The days of staying in ICU (IQR)	0(0–1)	0(0–1)	0(0–1)	0.604
Hospital mortality (%)	2(1%)	6(3.8%)	5(2.3%)	0.210
Complication rate (%)	67(33.5)	54(34.2%)	92(42.6%)	0.103
Grade I	20	13	19	
Grade II	23	19	40	
Grade III	14	11	18	
Grade IIIa	14	8	15	
Grade IIIb	0	3	3	
Grade IV	8	5	10	
Grade IVa	7	5	9	
Grade IVb	1	0	1	
Grade V	2	6	5	

IQR: interquartile range.

Table 5. The main Types of complications.

	No occlusion group (n = 200)	The Pringle group (n = 158)	The hemi-hepatic group (n = 216)
Bile leakage	9	8	0
Liver failure	5	2	8
Abdominal abscess	1	5	1
Lung infection	15	12	17
Wound infection	5	2	6
Pleural effusion	4	5	6
Intra-abdominal hemorrhage	3	3	3

hepatic vascular occlusion is usually chosen. If tumors are beyond the scope of hemi-liver, Pringle maneuver is preferred. If there is a massive hemorrhage in hepatic vein or injury to inferior vena cava, hepatic vascular exclusion is immediately applied.

In summary, this retrospective study showed that either Pringle maneuver or simple hemi-occlusion technique could be used safely and effectively to reduce complications during major hepatectomy. Although the overall complications rate between three groups did not reach significant differences, no vascular occlusion group had more blood loss than the other two groups during liver resection.

Author Contributions

Conceived and designed the experiments: ZH LY WW. Performed the experiments: ZH. Analyzed the data: ZH HW. Contributed reagents/ materials/analysis tools: PZ. Wrote the paper: ZH. Revised the manuscript: WW.

References

1. (2012) EASL-EORTC clinical practice guidelines: management of hepatocellular carcinoma. European journal of cancer (Oxford, England : 1990) 48: 599–641.
2. El-Serag HB, Rudolph KL (2007) Hepatocellular carcinoma: epidemiology and molecular carcinogenesis. Gastroenterology 132: 2557–2576.
3. McGlynn KA, Tsao L, Hsing AW, Devesa SS, Fraumeni JF Jr (2001) International trends and patterns of primary liver cancer. International journal of cancer Journal international du cancer 94: 290–296.
4. Parkin DM (2001) Global cancer statistics in the year 2000. The lancet oncology 2: 533–543.
5. (2012) EASL-EORTC clinical practice guidelines: management of hepatocellular carcinoma. Journal of hepatology 56: 908–943.
6. Llovet JM, Bru C, Bruix J (1999) Prognosis of hepatocellular carcinoma: the BCLC staging classification. Seminars in liver disease 19: 329–338.
7. Lai EC, Fan ST, Lo CM, Chu KM, Liu CL, et al. (1995) Hepatic resection for hepatocellular carcinoma. An audit of 343 patients. Annals of surgery 221: 291–298.
8. Chikamoto A, Beppu T, Masuda T, Otao R, Okabe H, et al. (2012) Amount of operative blood loss affects the long-term outcome after liver resection for hepatocellular carcinoma. Hepato-gastroenterology 59: 1213–1216.
9. Katz SC, Shia J, Liau KH, Gonen M, Ruo L, et al. (2009) Operative blood loss independently predicts recurrence and survival after resection of hepatocellular carcinoma. Annals of surgery 249: 617–623.
10. Kusano T, Sasaki A, Kai S, Endo Y, Iwaki K, et al. (2009) Predictors and prognostic significance of operative complications in patients with hepatocellular carcinoma who underwent hepatic resection. European journal of surgical oncology : the journal of the European Society of Surgical Oncology and the British Association of Surgical Oncology 35: 1179–1185.
11. Pringle JH (1908) V. Notes on the Arrest of Hepatic Hemorrhage Due to Trauma. Annals of surgery 48: 541–549.
12. Man K, Fan ST, Ng IO, Lo CM, Liu CL, et al. (1997) Prospective evaluation of Pringle maneuver in hepatectomy for liver tumors by a randomized study. Annals of surgery 226: 704–711; discussion 711–703.
13. Weigand K, Brost S, Steinebrunner N, Buchler M, Schemmer P, et al. (2012) Ischemia/Reperfusion injury in liver surgery and transplantation: pathophysiology. HPB surgery : a world journal of hepatic, pancreatic and biliary surgery 2012: 176723.
14. Serracino-Inglott F, Habib NA, Mathie RT (2001) Hepatic ischemia-reperfusion injury. American journal of surgery 181: 160–166.
15. Xiaobin F, Zipei L, Shuguo Z, Jiahong D, Xiaowu L (2009) The Pringle manoeuvre should be avoided in hepatectomy for cancer patients due to its side effects on tumor recurrence and worse prognosis. Medical hypotheses 72: 398–401.
16. van der Bilt JD, Kranenburg O, Nijkamp MW, Smakman N, Veenendaal LM, et al. (2005) Ischemia/reperfusion accelerates the outgrowth of hepatic micrometastases in a highly standardized murine model. Hepatology (Baltimore, Md) 42: 165–175.
17. Makuuchi M, Mori T, Gunven P, Yamazaki S, Hasegawa H (1987) Safety of hemihepatic vascular occlusion during resection of the liver. Surgery, gynecology & obstetrics 164: 155–158.
18. Pol B, Campan P, Hardwigsen J, Botti G, Pons J, et al. (1999) Morbidity of major hepatic resections: a 100-case prospective study. The European journal of surgery = Acta chirurgica 165: 446–453.
19. Bruix J, Sherman M (2005) Management of hepatocellular carcinoma. Hepatology (Baltimore, Md) 42: 1208–1236.
20. Bruix J, Sherman M (2011) Management of hepatocellular carcinoma: an update. Hepatology (Baltimore, Md) 53: 1020–1022.
21. Owens WD, Felts JA, Spitznagel EL Jr (1978) ASA physical status classifications: a study of consistency of ratings. Anesthesiology 49: 239–243.
22. Charlson ME, Pompei P, Ales KL, MacKenzie CR (1987) A new method of classifying prognostic comorbidity in longitudinal studies: development and validation. Journal of chronic diseases 40: 373–383.
23. Hepp J, Couinaud C (1956) [Approach to and use of the left hepatic duct in reparation of the common bile duct]. La Presse medicale 64: 947–948.
24. Wen T, Chen Z, Yan L, Li B, Zeng Y, et al. (2007) Continuous normothermic hemihepatic vascular inflow occlusion over 60 min for hepatectomy in patients with cirrhosis caused by hepatitis B virus. Hepatology research : the official journal of the Japan Society of Hepatology 37: 346–352.
25. Yan LN, Yuan CX, Zhang ZD (1994) [Hepatopetal blood occlusion of half liver during hepatectomy in 29 patients]. Zhonghua wai ke za zhi [Chinese journal of surgery] 32: 35–36.
26. Clavien PA, Barkun J, de Oliveira ML, Vauthey JN, Dindo D, et al. (2009) The Clavien-Dindo classification of surgical complications: five-year experience. Annals of surgery 250: 187–196.
27. Dindo D, Demartines N, Clavien PA (2004) Classification of surgical complications: a new proposal with evaluation in a cohort of 6336 patients and results of a survey. Annals of surgery 240: 205–213.
28. Balzan S, Belghiti J, Farges O, Ogata S, Sauvanet A, et al. (2005) The "50–50 criteria" on postoperative day 5: an accurate predictor of liver failure and death after hepatectomy. Annals of surgery 242: 824–828, discussion 828–829.
29. Heaney JP, Stanton WK, Halbert DS, Seidel J, Vice T (1966) An improved technic for vascular isolation of the liver: experimental study and case reports. Annals of surgery 163: 237–241.
30. Huguet C, Nordlinger B, Galopin JJ, Bloch P, Gallot D (1978) Normothermic hepatic vascular exclusion for extensive hepatectomy. Surgery, gynecology & obstetrics 147: 689–693.
31. Yamaoka Y, Ozawa K, Kumada K, Shimahara Y, Tanaka K, et al. (1992) Total vascular exclusion for hepatic resection in cirrhotic patients. Application of venovenous bypass. Archives of surgery (Chicago, Ill : 1960) 127: 276–280.
32. Jaeschke H (2003) Molecular mechanisms of hepatic ischemia-reperfusion injury and preconditioning. American journal of physiology Gastrointestinal and liver physiology 284: G15–26.
33. Belghiti J, Noun R, Malafosse R, Jagot P, Sauvanet A, et al. (1999) Continuous versus intermittent portal triad clamping for liver resection: a controlled study. Annals of surgery 229: 369–375.

34. Clavien PA, Yadav S, Sindram D, Bentley RC (2000) Protective effects of ischemic preconditioning for liver resection performed under inflow occlusion in humans. Annals of surgery 232: 155–162.
35. Clavien PA, Selzner M, Rudiger HA, Graf R, Kadry Z, et al. (2003) A prospective randomized study in 100 consecutive patients undergoing major liver resection with versus without ischemic preconditioning. Annals of surgery 238: 843–850; discussion 851–842.
36. Carini R, Albano E (2003) Recent insights on the mechanisms of liver preconditioning. Gastroenterology 125: 1480–1491.
37. Ni JS, Lau WY, Yang Y, Pan ZY, Wang ZG, et al. (2013) A prospective randomized controlled trial to compare pringle manoeuvre with hemi-hepatic vascular inflow occlusion in liver resection for hepatocellular carcinoma with cirrhosis. Journal of gastrointestinal surgery : official journal of the Society for Surgery of the Alimentary Tract 17: 1414–1421.
38. Fu SY, Lau WY, Li GG, Tang QH, Li AJ, et al. (2011) A prospective randomized controlled trial to compare Pringle maneuver, hemihepatic vascular inflow occlusion, and main portal vein inflow occlusion in partial hepatectomy. American journal of surgery 201: 62–69.
39. Chau GY, Lui WY, King KL, Wu CW (2005) Evaluation of effect of hemihepatic vascular occlusion and the Pringle maneuver during hepatic resection for patients with hepatocellular carcinoma and impaired liver function. World journal of surgery 29: 1374–1383.
40. Tanaka K, Shimada H, Togo S, Nagano Y, Endo I, et al. (2006) Outcome using hemihepatic vascular occlusion versus the pringle maneuver in resections limited to one hepatic section or less. Journal of gastrointestinal surgery : official journal of the Society for Surgery of the Alimentary Tract 10: 980–986.
41. Taniguchi H, Takahashi T, Shioaki Y, Itoh A, Oguro A (1992) Vascular inflow exclusion and hepatic resection. The British journal of surgery 79: 672–675.
42. Une Y, Uchino J, Sato N (1998) Clinical comparison of water jet dissector and ultrasonic surgical aspirator in hepatic resection. Asian journal of surgery 21: 219–226.
43. Smyrniotis V, Kostopanagiotou G, Theodoraki K, Tsantoulas D, Contis JC (2004) The role of central venous pressure and type of vascular control in blood loss during major liver resections. American journal of surgery 187: 398–402.

11

The Histone Deacetylase Inhibitor, Vorinostat, Represses Hypoxia Inducible Factor 1 Alpha Expression through Translational Inhibition

Darren M. Hutt[1,¶], Daniela Martino Roth[1,¶], Hélène Vignaud[2], Christophe Cullin[2], Marion Bouchecareilh[2]*

1 Department of Cell and Molecular Biology, The Scripps Research Institute, La Jolla, California, United States of America, **2** Institut de Biochimie et Génétique Cellulaires, CNRS UMR 5095, Université de Bordeaux, Bordeaux, France

Abstract

Hypoxia inducible factor 1α (HIF-1α) is a master regulator of tumor angiogenesis being one of the major targets for cancer therapy. Previous studies have shown that Histone Deacetylase Inhibitors (HDACi) block tumor angiogenesis through the inhibition of HIF-1α expression. As such, Vorinostat (Suberoylanilide Hydroxamic Acid/SAHA) and Romidepsin, two HDACis, were recently approved by the Food and Drug Administration (FDA) for the treatment of cutaneous T cell lymphoma. Although HDACis have been shown to affect HIF-1α expression by modulating its interactions with the Hsp70/Hsp90 chaperone axis or its acetylation status, the molecular mechanisms by which HDACis inhibit HIF-1α expression need to be further characterized. Here, we report that the FDA-approved HDACi Vorinostat/SAHA inhibits HIF-1α expression in liver cancer-derived cell lines, by a new mechanism independent of p53, prolyl-hydroxylases, autophagy and proteasome degradation. We found that SAHA or silencing of HDAC9 mechanism of action is due to inhibition of HIF-1α translation, which in turn, is mediated by the eukaryotic translation initiation factor - eIF3G. We also highlighted that HIF-1α translation is dramatically inhibited when SAHA is combined with eIF3H silencing. Taken together, we show that HDAC activity regulates HIF-1α translation, with HDACis such as SAHA representing a potential novel approach for the treatment of hepatocellular carcinoma.

Editor: Sonia Rocha, University of Dundee, United Kingdom

Funding: MB was supported by a fellowship from the Foundation pour la Recherche Médicale (FRM), SPF20130526734. The funder had no role in study design, data collection and analysis, decision to publish, or preparation of the manuscript.

Competing Interests: The authors have declared that no competing interests exist.

* Email: mbouchecareilh@gmail.com

¶ These authors contributed equally to this work.

Introduction

Hepatocellular carcinoma (HCC) is the most common of all primary liver tumors and represents the third leading cause of cancer related death worldwide [1,2]. One of the most critical risk factors is cirrhosis, with 90% of HCC cases occurring in cirrhotic livers [3–5]. HCC has been linked to dysregulation of diverse signaling pathways affecting cell proliferation, invasion, metastasis and angiogenesis, thereby limiting the development of therapeutic strategies. Currently, the multi-kinase inhibitor Sorafenib is the only treatment approved by the Food and Drug Administration (FDA) for patients with advanced disease, but resection and transplantation remain the only curative treatment available, therefore highlighting the need for identifying novel therapeutic targets [6–8].

Histone deacetylase inhibitors (HDACi) are some of the most promising anti-cancer drugs currently being developed [9] with Vorinostat (Suberoylanilide Hydroxamic Acid (SAHA)) and Romidepsin, being recently approved for the treatment of cutaneous T cell lymphoma (CTCL) [10]. A recent study has provided evidence for the therapeutic benefit of HDACi in the treatment of HCC, where the pan-HDACi, panobinostat, improved the efficacy of Sorafenib, resulting in a significant decrease in tumor volume and vessel density, leading to increased survival in HCC xenografts [11]. Furthermore, a phase I clinical trial is underway for the combination treatment of Vorinostat and Sorafenib for patients with advanced renal cell carcinoma and non-small cell lung cancer [12], supporting the use of such combinatorial therapies. Recent evidence has shown that Vorinostat can modulate the IGF-IR signaling pathway and IGF-I promoter activity in endometrial type-I and –II cancers [13], however, the pro-apoptotic activity of this HDACi proved insensitive to a blocking anti-IGF-IR monoclonal antibody. Despite numerous such studies, which provide insight into Vorinostat-responsive signaling pathways, the mechanism of action for the therapeutic benefit of Vorinostat and other HDACi in the treatment of various cancers remains elusive.

Histone deacetylases mediate the removal of acetyl groups from target proteins, which include histones, transcription factors and other cellular proteins, thereby regulating their function. Therefore, HDACi treatment would results in the hyperacetylation of histones and other proteins such as the chaperone Hsp90 [14,15] involved in regulating the expression and stability of several genes, including those involved in cell-cycle arrest, death and/or apoptosis of cancer cells. In support of this proposed mechanism of action, HDACi have been shown to negatively regulate the expression and function of VEGF, p53 and Hypoxia Inductible Factor-1α (HIF1α), angiogenic factors that promote tumor proliferation and metastasis [16,17].

HIF-1 is a heterodimeric complex composed of the HIF-1α and HIF-1β subunits and a central regulator of angiogenesis and energy metabolism in tumors [18–20]. HIF-1α is regulated by oxygen levels, thereby providing a means of regulating the transcriptional activity of HIF-1 [21]. Under normoxic conditions, proline residues in HIF-1α are hydroxylated by prolyl hydroxylase domain (PHD) containing oxygenases, which serve as a recognition signal for the E3 ubiquitin ligase, Von Hipple-Lindau (VHL) complex, which targets HIF-1α for degradation by the ubiquitin proteosomal system (UPS). Conversely, under hypoxic conditions, the oxygen-dependent PHD-containing oxygenases have reduced activity [22], resulting in stabilization of HIF-1α [23,24], which dimerizes with the constitutively expressed HIF-1β to activate the transcription of genes involved in angiogenesis, cell proliferation and survival [18,21,24]. Cellular HIF-1α levels are also regulated by p53, which promotes MDM2-mediated ubiquitination [21,25,26], as well as by autophagy [21,25,26]. HIF-1α can also be activated under normoxic conditions by growth factors, oncogenic mutation or inactivation of tumor suppressors [27–29]. It is overexpressed in many different types of tumors and mediates resistance to chemo and radiation therapy [20,21,30–32], making it a primary target for cancer therapy [18,19].

Previous studies have shown that the HDACi, Trichostatin A (TSA), reduces cellular levels of HIF-1α in a UPS-dependent manner [33]. In support of this observation, Kong *et al* have shown that the silencing of HDAC6 disrupts the Hsp90-mediated folding of HIF-1α, leading to its degradation by the UPS [33]. Conversely, the silencing of HDAC4, which also promotes a down-regulation of this pro-angiogenic factor is dependent on N-terminal lysine residues of HIF-1α [34], suggesting a direct acetylation as a possible regulatory mechanism for HIF-1α. These data suggest that there are multiple HDAC-regulated pathways by which to regulate HIF-1α, suggesting that more evidence is required to better understand the mechanism of action mediating the therapeutic benefit of these HDACi.

Herein, we present evidence that SAHA drastically decreases HIF-1α expression in HCC cell lines by a pathway independent of p53- or prolyl-hydroxylases/VHL-mediated proteasomal degradation and autophagy. Rather, SAHA acts through HDAC9 to alter HIF-1α translation in an eIF3G-dependent manner. We also observed that HIF-1α translation is dramatically inhibited when SAHA is combined with eIF3H silencing. These data provide insight into the mechanism of action of the FDA-approved HDACi, SAHA, which has led us to identify HDAC9, eIF3G and eIF3H as new targets for therapeutic development in hepatocellular carcinoma and possibly other cancers.

Results

SAHA down regulates HIF-1α protein levels independent of protein degradation

HDAC inhibitors have garnered a lot of attention in recent years for their therapeutic benefit in treating cancer, with Romidepsin (FK-228) and Vorinostat (SAHA) having been FDA-approved for the treatment of CTCL [10]. In light of the recent clinical trial combining SAHA with Sorafenib for the treatment of patients with advanced cancers [12], we focused our attention on defining the mechanism of action of this HDACi. We first examined the effect of SAHA on HIF-1α protein expression in HuH7 and Hep3B cells, commonly used HCC cell culture models. As mentioned above, HIF-1α protein levels are inversely correlated with the activity of prolyl hydroxylases and therefore the treatment of cells with prolyl hydroxylase inhibitors, such as cobalt chloride ($CoCl_2$), desferrioxamine (DFO) or dimethyloxallyl glycine (DMOG) lead to a stabilization in the cellular levels of HIF-1α (Figure 1A–C). We observed that this stabilization in HIF-1α could be abrogated by co-treating cells with SAHA (Figure 1A–C), a result consistent with previously published data showing that HDACi can mitigate the increased expression of this angiogenic factor [33]. We next sought to determine the optimal concentration of SAHA required for reducing HIF-1α protein levels. Here, HuH7 cells were treated with increasing concentrations of SAHA for 24 h and then analyzed for HIF-1α expression. We found that HIF-1α protein levels in HuH7 cells were maximally decreased at a dose of 5 μM (Figure 1D), which coincided with a significant decrease of HDAC7 expression, a result consistent with previous reports on the effect of SAHA on HDAC7 expression [35,36] (Figure 1D).

To investigate the mechanism underlying the SAHA-mediated repression of HIF-1α protein expression, we used the proteosome inhibitor, MG132, to determine if the UPS was contributing to the SAHA effect, as previously reported for the HDACi, TSA [33]. The treatment of HuH7 and Hep3B cells with MG132 resulted in increased cellular levels of HIF-1α, similar to the effect seen with $CoCl_2$, DFO and DMOG, but it failed to block the SAHA effect on decreasing HIF-1α expression (Figure 1E–F), suggesting that the SAHA-mediated reduction in HIF-1α is not occurring by promoting increased proteosomal degradation. We also observed a reduction in p53 levels in response to SAHA treatment of HuH7 and Hep3B cell lines (Figure 1E–F), a result consistent with previously published observations [37]. This reduction was observed whether SAHA was used alone or in combination with $CoCl_2$, DFO, DMOG or MG132 (Figure 1A–F). This reduction in p53 protein expression in response to SAHA would have been predicted to reduce the MDM2-dependent ubiquitination of HIF-1α, thereby increasing its expression level and/or activity in HCC cells. These data therefore further support the conclusion that the SAHA-mediated reduction in HIF-1α acts independently of p53 and does not occur by promoting its proteosomal degradation.

In addition to the UPS degradation to clear HIF-1α, the lysosomal pathway has also been described as a clearance pathway for HIF-1α [26]. Therefore to address the contribution of autophagy in the SAHA-mediated reduction in cellular HIF-1α, we monitored the cleavage of LC3-I to its lipidated LC3-II state, a marker of autophagy induction. We did not observe any changes in LC3-I cleavage in response to SAHA treatment, either alone or in combination with MG132 (Figure 1F), suggesting that the SAHA-mediated reduction in cellular HIF-1α levels is not acting through activation of the autophagic pathway. This result was confirmed by our observation that ammonium chloride-mediated inhibition of the lysosome, which alone mediates an increase in HIF1α levels (Figure 1G), failed to block the SAHA-mediated decrease in HIF-1α protein levels (Figure 1G), further suggesting that SAHA does not act through the autophagic pathways to reduce HIF-1α expression.

Taken together the above data suggests that the suppressive effect of SAHA on HIF-1α protein levels is not increasing the activity of HIF-1α clearance pathways.

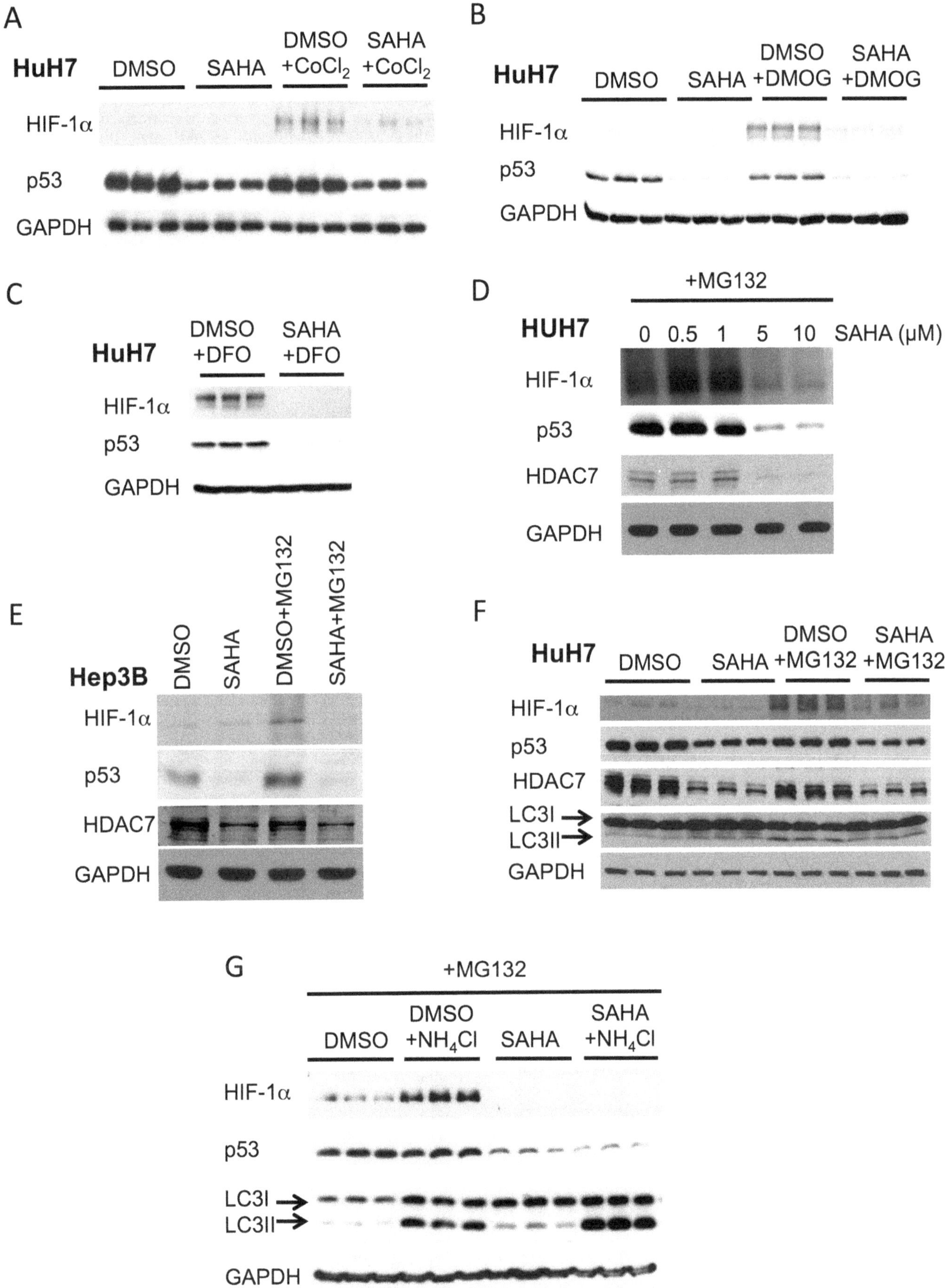
A
HuH7
DMSO
SAHA
DMSO +CoCl2
SAHA +CoCl2
HIF-1α
p53
GAPDH
B
HuH7
DMSO
SAHA
DMSO +DMOG
SAHA +DMOG
HIF-1α
p53
GAPDH
C
HuH7
DMSO +DFO
SAHA +DFO
HIF-1α
p53
GAPDH
D
+MG132
HUH7
0 0.5 1 5 10 SAHA (μM)
HIF-1α
p53
HDAC7
GAPDH
E
Hep3B
DMSO
SAHA
DMSO+MG132
SAHA+MG132
HIF-1α
p53
HDAC7
GAPDH
F
HuH7
DMSO
SAHA
DMSO +MG132
SAHA +MG132
HIF-1α
p53
HDAC7
LC3I
LC3II
GAPDH
G
+MG132
DMSO
DMSO +NH4Cl
SAHA
SAHA +NH4Cl
HIF-1α
p53
LC3I
LC3II
GAPDH

Figure 1. SAHA represses HIF-1α induction in response to hypoxic mimics. (**A**) Immunoblot analysis of HIF-1α, p53 and GAPDH protein expression from cell lysates following treatment of HuH7 cells with 5 μM SAHA, DMSO, DMSO+150 μM cobalt chloride ($CoCl_2$) or SAHA+150 μM cobalt chloride ($CoCl_2$) for 24 h. (**B**) Immunoblot analysis of HIF-1α, p53 and GAPDH protein expression from cell lysates following treatment of HuH7 cells with 5 μM SAHA, DMSO, DMSO+500 μM dimethyloxallyl glycine (DMOG) or SAHA+500 μM dimethyloxallyl glycine (DMOG) for 24 h. (**C**) Immunoblot analysis of HIF-1α, p53 and GAPDH protein expression from cell lysates following treatment of HuH7 cells with 5 μM SAHA or DMSO for 24 h in the presence or absence of 100 μM desferrioxamine (DFO) for 18 h. (**D**) Immunoblot analysis of HIF-1α, p53, HDAC7 and GAPDH protein expression from cell lysates following treatment of HuH7 cells after SAHA treatment at the indicate concentration is shown in combination with 50 μM MG132 for 4 h. (**E**) and Hep3B cells with 5 μM SAHA or DMSO for 24 h in the presence or absence of 50 μM MG132 for 4 h. (**F**) Immunoblot analysis of HIF-1α, p53, HDAC7 and GAPDH protein expression as well as the splicing of LC3 following treatment of HuH7 cells with 5 μM SAHA or DMSO for 24 h in the presence or absence of 50 μM MG132 for 4 h. (**G**) Immunoblot analyses of HIF-1α, p53 as well as the splicing of LC3 following treatment of HuH7 cells with 50 μM MG132+5 μM SAHA or DMSO in presence or absence of 10 mM ammonium chloride (NH_4Cl) for 8 h. In all panels GAPDH is used as loading control and HDAC7 is used as control to SAHA treatment.

SAHA decreases HIF-1α protein expression through HDAC9 inhibition

Previous reports have shown that HDAC4 and HDAC6 co-immunoprecipitate with HIF-1α and their inhibition by the HDACi, TSA and LAQ824, compromised the stability and transcriptional activity of HIF-1α [33,34,38]. To address the role of individual HDACs in the SAHA-mediated reduction of HIF-1α protein levels, we used siRNA-mediated silencing of individual HDAC family members in HuH7 cells (Figure 2A). There are 18 human HDACs that cluster into five classes by sequence homology [39,40]: the Zn2+-dependent class I (HDACs 1, 2, 3 and 8), class IIa (HDACs 4, 5, 7 and 9), class IIb (HDACs 6 and 10) and class IV (HDAC11) enzymes, and the NAD+-dependent class III enzymes (sirtuins). The latter are not inhibited by SAHA [41] and are therefore not examined herein. Following an analysis of the HIF-1α protein levels in response to MG132 treatment combined with the siRNA-mediated silencing of HDACs 1–11, we noted that the silencing of HDAC9 (Figure S1A) exhibited the most pronounced reduction of the MG132-induced HIF-1α up-regulation (Figure 2A), resulting in a 4.3-fold decrease in cellular HIF-1α protein levels relative to control (siScramble (siScr) + MG132). We observed that the silencing of HDAC9 also resulted in a reduction of the DFO-induced HIF-1α up-regulation (Figure S1B). The silencing of numerous other HDACs also led to a partial reduction in HIF-1α (Figure 2A), with HDACs 1, 2 and 6 having the most notable effect. These data suggest that the inhibition of several HDACs could explain the robust SAHA-mediated reduction in HIF-1α protein levels, which failed to be recapitulated by any individual siHDAC. Interestingly, the silencing of HDAC10 (Figure S1A) resulted in the most efficient reduction of p53 (Figure 2B), exhibiting a 25% decrease in protein expression, suggesting that the observed SAHA-mediated reduction of HIF-1α and p53 is occurring through inhibition of different HDAC family members.

To provide additional support for our interpretation that the observed SAHA-mediated reduction in HIF-1α protein levels is acting primarily through inhibition of HDAC9, we compared the effect of SAHA alone (Scr - Figure 2C) or in combination with siHDAC9 on HIF-1α protein levels (Figure 2C). The SAHA+ siHDAC9 combination did not result in a further reduction of HIF-1α protein levels compared to SAHA alone (Figure 2C), supporting the conclusion that the observed SAHA-mediated HIF-1α repression is acting primarily through a HDAC9-dependent mechanism.

SAHA and HDAC9 silencing do not affect transcription of HIF-1α

Previous reports have shown that SAHA treatment can lead to a reduction in p53 mRNA levels in human keratinocyte and colorectal adenocarcinoma cell lines [37], a result consistent with the role of HDACs in epigenetic regulation. To determine whether the level of HIF-1α mRNA is also regulated by SAHA, we measured the levels of HIF-1α and p53 mRNA using real time quantitative PCR (qRT-PCR). Consistent with the previous report discussed above, we observed a dose dependent reduction in p53 mRNA levels in response to SAHA treatment (Figure 3A). Conversely, we did not observe any SAHA-mediated changes in HIF-1α mRNA levels (Figure 3B) at the 5 μM dose where the maximal HIF1α protein reduction is observed, suggesting that transcriptional changes are not responsible for the SAHA-mediated reduction in HIF-1α protein levels.

In light of our observations described above, that the SAHA-mediated effect on HIF-1α and p53 are in part mediated by inhibition of HDAC9 and HDAC10 respectively, we analyzed whether their silencing altered the mRNA levels of HIF-1α or p53. Consistent with the observations reported above for SAHA treatment, the silencing of HDAC9 (Figure S1A) did not alter the cellular mRNA levels of HIF-1α (Figure 3C). Conversely, we did observe that the silencing of HDAC10 led to a significant reduction of p53 mRNA levels (Figure 3D), consistent with the conclusion that the SAHA-mediated reduction in p53 is acting in part through inhibition of HDAC10. Since we did not see any SAHA-mediated changes in HIF-1α transcription or protein degradation, we hypothesized that the SAHA-mediated reduction in cellular levels of HIF-1α could be acting through translational regulation.

SAHA decreases HIF-1α protein levels by an eIF3G-dependent translation mechanism

Cap-dependent translation is initiated and regulated by the eukaryote Initiation Factor (eIF) family. Recent work has shed light on the role of some of these family members in regulating HIF-1α translation, including eIF2α [42,43], eIF3E [44] and eIF4E [45–47]. It has been shown that the mammalian Target Of Rapamycin Complex 1 (mTORC1) signalling pathway regulates HIF-1α translation by mediating the phosphorylation of eIF4E binding protein 1 (4E-BP1) [45–47], which disrupts its binding to eIF4E thereby stimulating cap-dependent translation [48,49]. Despite this latter observation, we observed a statistically significant decrease in HIF-1α protein expression when we combined mTOR silencing with the MG132 and SAHA treatments (Figure S2A), ruling out a role for mTORC1 in the SAHA-mediated reduction in cellular HIF-1α protein levels.

To address the role of eIF family members in the SAHA-mediated suppression of HIF-1α, we examined the effect of siRNA-mediated silencing of individual eIFs in HuH7 cells following treatment with SAHA and MG132 (Figure 4 and S2B). eIF2 is a heterotrimer composed of α, β and γ subunits where the silencing of the α and γ subunits result in toxicity in HuH7 cells. We therefore targeted the eIF2β subunit to monitor the role of eIF2. We observed that the silencing of eIF3 subunits B, C, G and M, eIF4 subunits E and G1 as well as eIF2β blocked the

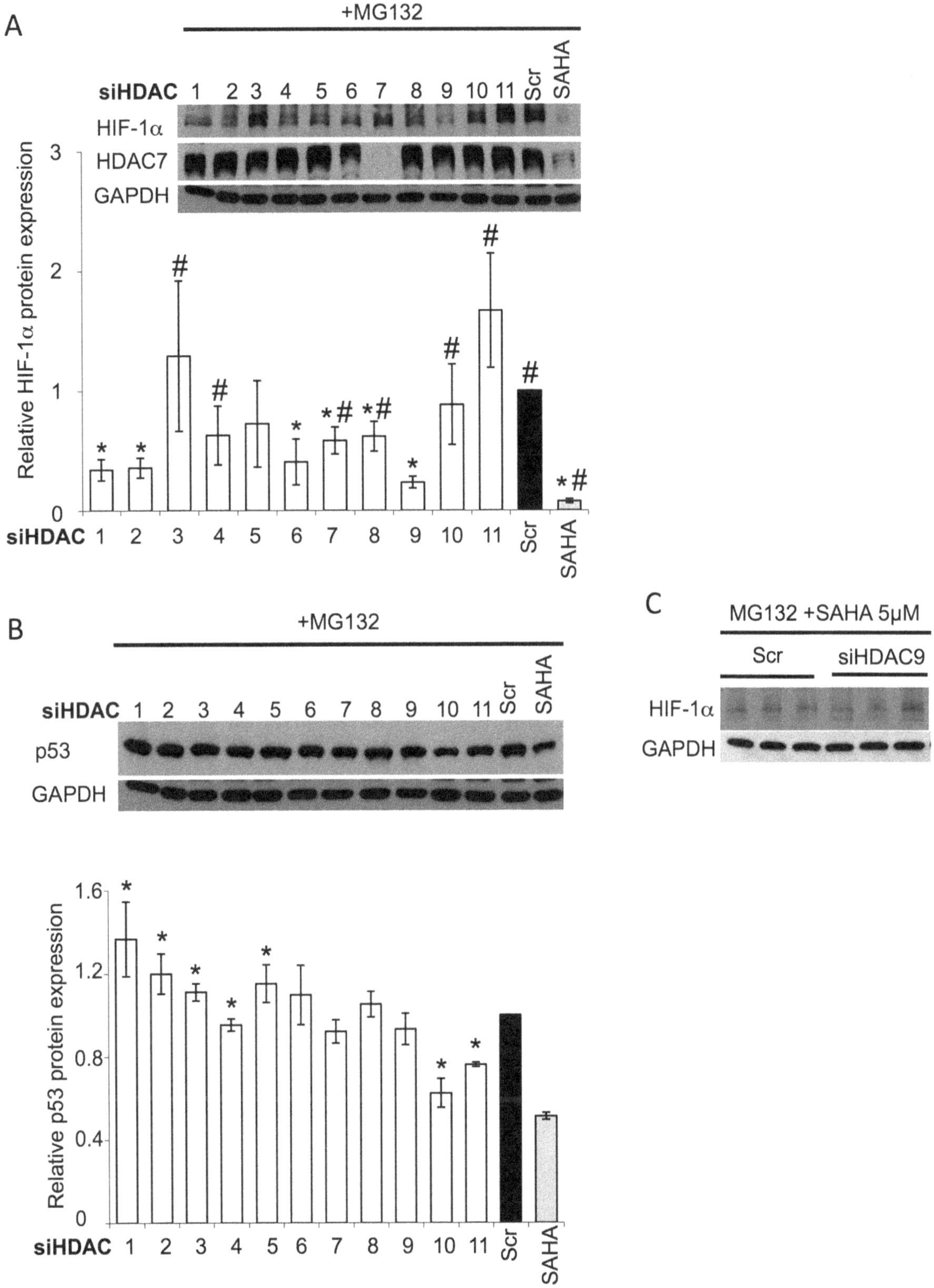

Figure 2. Silencing of HDAC9 represses HIF-1α induction. (**A**) Immunoblot analysis of HIF-1α, HDAC7 and GAPDH protein expression in cell lysates following siRNA-mediated silencing of HDACs 1–11 in HuH7 cells. Quantitative analysis (lower) of the level of HIF-1α in response to silencing of the indicated HDAC in HuH7 cells. Data shown denote the fold change in HIF-1α protein expression relative to scramble (Scr) control (black bar) (mean ± SD, n = 3). Asterisks indicates $p<0.05$ as determined by two-tailed t-test using Scr control (black bar) as the reference and # indicates $p<0.05$ as determined by two-tailed t-test using HDAC9 siRNA as the reference. (**B**) Immunoblot analysis of p53 and GAPDH protein expression in cell lysates following siRNA-mediated silencing of HDACs 1–11 in HuH7 cells. Quantitative analysis (lower) of the level of p53 in response to silencing of the indicated HDAC in HuH7 cells. Data shown denote the fold change in p53 protein expression relative to scramble (Scr) control (black bar) (mean ± SD, n = 3). Asterisks indicates $p<0.05$ as determined by two-tailed t-test using Scr control as the reference. (**C**) Immunoblot analysis of HIF-1α and

GAPDH protein expression in cell lysates following siRNA-mediated silencing of HDAC9 (siHDAC9) in the presence of 5 μM SAHA+50 μM MG132 in HuH7 cells. In all panels GAPDH is used as loading control and HDAC7 is used as control to SAHA treatment.

SAHA-mediated decrease in HIF-1α protein expression, with sieIF3G and sieIF2β having the most pronounced effect (Figure 4 and S2B). We noted a significant increase in toxicity in response to eIF2β silencing, an effect not observed with optimal SAHA dosing, therefore we focused our analysis on the contribution of eIF3G in the SAHA-mediated decrease of HIF-1α. The silencing of eIF3G was also able to block the SAHA-mediated reduction of HIF1α, restoring a partial DFO-induced up-regulation of HIF1α (Figure S2C). We also noted that the silencing of eIF3A, D, E, F, I, J and K were able to partially block the SAHA-mediated decrease in HIF-1α (Figure 4), suggesting a central role for the eIF3

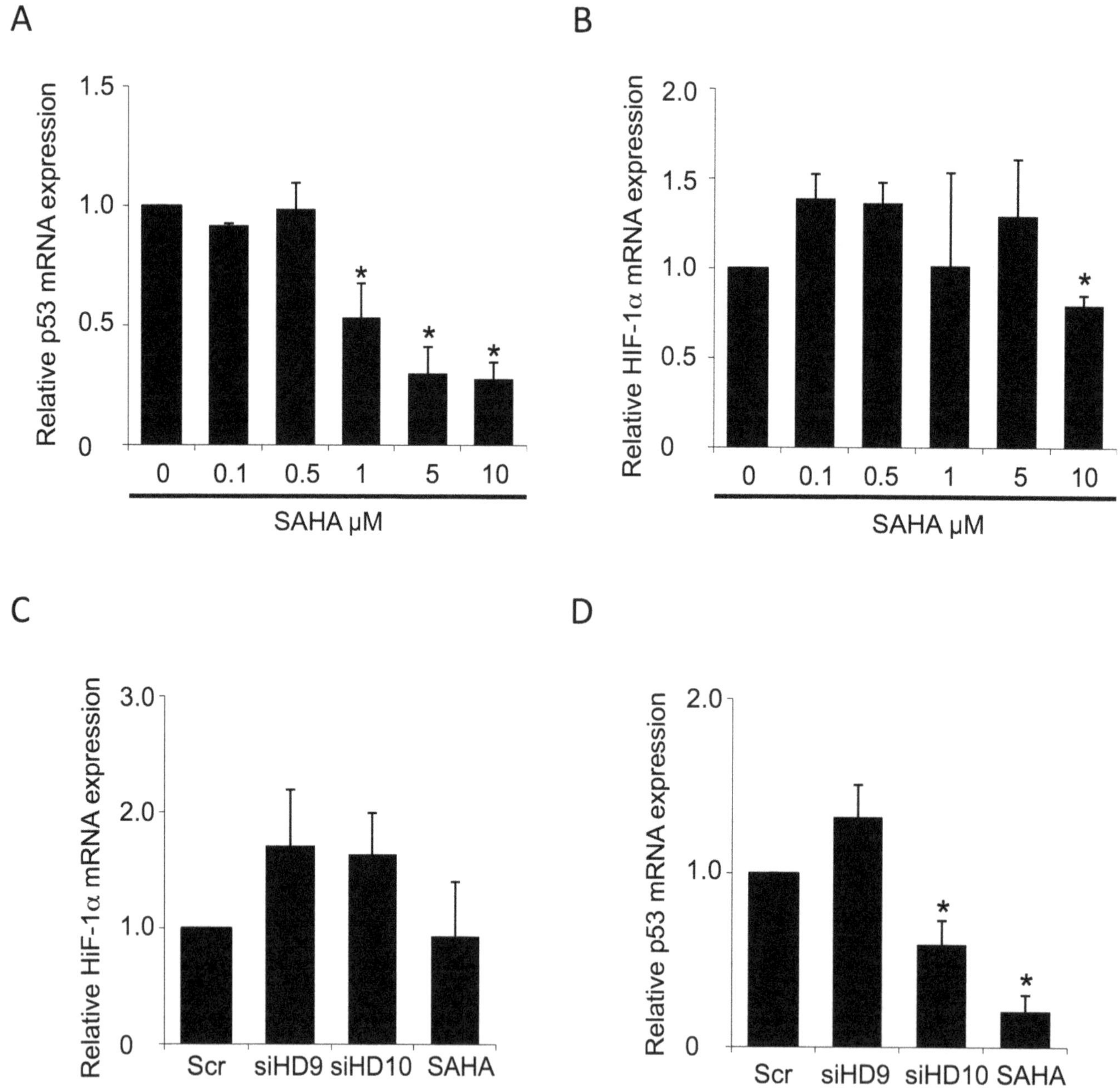

Figure 3. SAHA did not affect the level of HIF-1α mRNA. (**A and D**) qRT-PCR analysis of p53 mRNA level in HuH7 cell line following the indicated concentration of SAHA (**A**) or HDAC9 and HDAC10 silencing (**D**). Data is shown as the fold change of the ratio of p53 to GAPDH mRNA relative to that seen for DMSO (0 μM) (**A**) or scrambled (Scr) siRNA control (**D**) (mean ± SD, n = 3). In all panels, asterisk indicates $p<0.05$, as determined by two-tailed t-test using scrambled siRNA (Scr) (**D**) or DMSO (0 mM) (**A**) as the reference. (**B–C**) qRT-PCR analysis of HIF-1α mRNA level in HuH7 cell line following the indicated concentration of SAHA (**B**) or HDAC9 and HDAC10 silencing (**C**). Data is shown as the fold change of the ratio of HIF-1α to GAPDH mRNA relative to that seen for DMSO (0 μM) (**B**) or scrambled (Scr) siRNA control (**C**) (mean ± SD, n = 3). In all panels, asterisk indicates $p<0.05$, as determined by two-tailed t-test using scrambled siRNA (Scr) (**C**) or DMSO (0 μM) (**B**) as the reference.

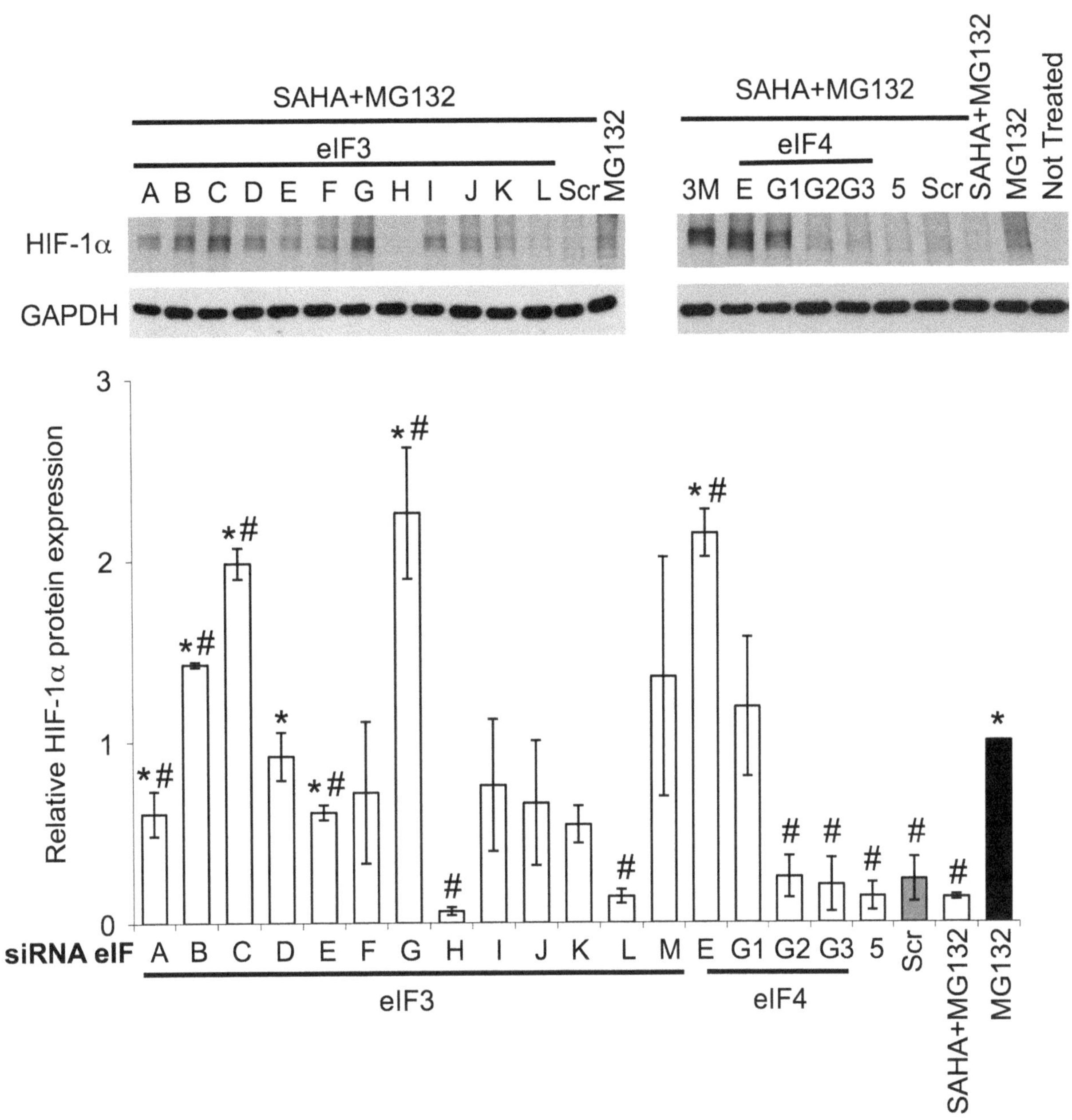

Figure 4. eIF3G silencing reversed SAHA effect on HIF-1α repression in response to hypoxic mimic. Immunoblot analysis of HIF-1α and GAPDH protein expression in cell lysates following siRNA-mediated silencing of eIF3 A-M, eIF4 E, G1–3 and eIF5 in HuH7 cells in presence or absence of SAHA+MG132. Quantitative analysis of the level of HIF-1α in response to silencing of the indicated eIF in HuH7 cells. Data shown denote the fold change in HIF-1α protein expression relative to MG132 treatment alone (black bar) (mean ± SD, n = 3). Asterisks indicates $p<0.05$ as determined by two-tailed t-test using Scr control (grey bar) as the reference and # indicates $p<0.05$ as determined by two-tailed t-test using MG132 (black bar) as the reference. In all panels GAPDH is used as loading control.

machinery in mediating the action of SAHA on HIF-1α expression.

Conversely, we observed that the silencing of eIF3H in combination with SAHA was able to further decrease HIF-1α protein levels (Figure 4). To further address the role of eIF3H in the SAHA mediated decrease in HIF-1α expression, we examined the effect of eIF3H silencing (sieIF3H) on HIF-1α expression (Figure 5A–B). We noted that the silencing of eIF3H alone was able to reverse the DFO- and MG132-mediated HIF-1α up-regulation (Figure 5A–B), resulting in a ~2-fold decrease in cellular HIF-1α protein levels relative to control (siScramble (siScr) + MG132 or DFO). Moreover, when eIF3H-silenced cells were treated with SAHA, we observed a further reduction in HIF-1α expression relative to that seen with either treatment alone (Figure 5A–B), suggesting that SAHA and sieIF3H target HIF-1α via parallel pathways.

We also observed that the silencing of eIFs were additive to the SAHA-mediated decrease in p53 expression (Figure S3), a result consistent with our data above that SAHA mediates a reduction in p53 mRNA level and that inhibition of the translational machinery provides a second level of regulation to reduce the expression of p53. These results support the conclusion that the

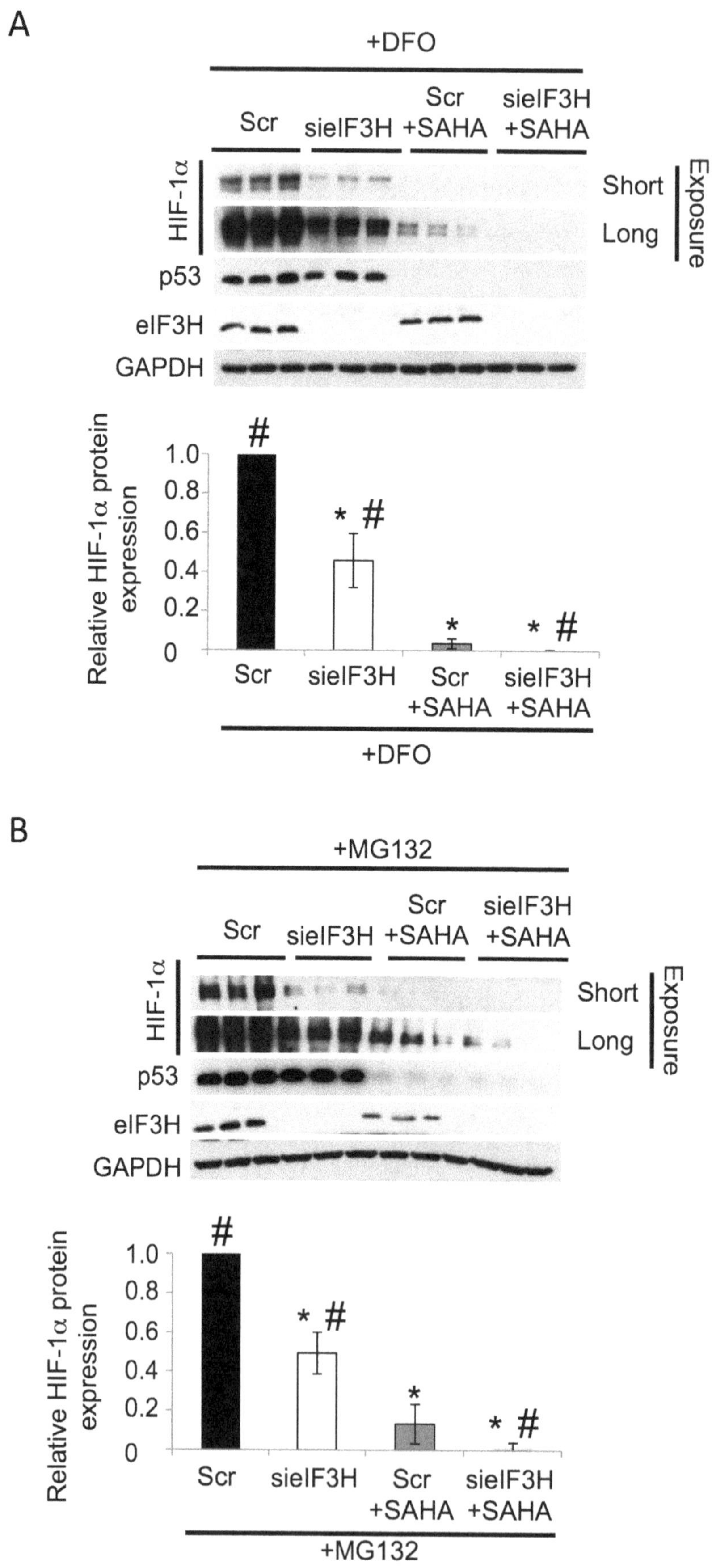
A
+DFO
Scr
sieIF3H
Scr +SAHA
sieIF3H +SAHA
HIF-1α
p53
eIF3H
GAPDH
Short
Long
Exposure
Relative HIF-1α protein expression
1.0
0.8
0.6
0.4
0.2
0
#
* #
*
* #
B
+MG132

Figure 5. Combined effect of eIF3H silencing and SAHA treament. (**A–B**) Immunoblot analysis of HIF-1α, p53, eIF3H and GAPDH protein expression in cell lysates following siRNA-mediated silencing of eIF3H (sieIF3H) in presence or absence of SAHA+DFO (**A**) or SAHA+MG132 (**B**) in HuH7 cells. Quantitative analysis of the level of HIF-1α in response to silencing of the indicated eIF3H in HuH7 cells. Data shown denote the fold change in HIF-1α protein expression relative to DFO treatment+Scr control (**A**) MG132 treatment+Scr control (**B**) (black bar) (mean ± SD, n = 3). Asterisks indicates $p<0.05$ as determined by two-tailed t-test using Scr control+DFO (**A**) or Scr control+MG132 (**B**) (black bar) as the reference and # indicates $p<0.05$ as determined by two-tailed t-test using SAHA+MG132 (**B**) or SAHA+DFO (grey bar) as the reference. In all panels GAPDH is used as loading control.

translational machinery in general and eIF3G specifically provide a point of regulation for the HDACi, SAHA in regulating the expression of HIF-1α.

SAHA does not regulate eIF3G directly

Given that the silencing of eIF3G can inhibit the SAHA-mediated decrease in HIF-1α protein levels, we sought to address its mechanism of action. We first addressed whether eIF3G is directly affected by SAHA treatment. Our analysis revealed that SAHA did not alter the subcellular localization of eIF3G or its protein expression level nor did it change its acetylation state (Figure S4A–C), suggesting that the SAHA-mediated effect on HIF-1α translation is not the result of directly targeting eIF3G. Next, we addressed whether SAHA altered the assembly of the eIF3 complex or its association with the ribosome. Our analysis revealed that SAHA did not alter the interaction of eIF3G with eIF3B or ribosomal protein S6 (Figure S4D) [50].

The eIF3 family activates a number of biological pathways, including the formation of stress granules, which are also regulated by HDACs [51]. Stress granules contain non-translating mRNAs, translation initiation components, and many additional proteins affecting mRNA translation [52]. To explore the possible role of stress granules in the observed effect of SAHA on HIF-1α, we performed an immunofluorescence analysis of the stress granule associated proteins, TIA-1 (T-cell intracellular antigen-1) and TIAR (TIA-1 related protein) [53]. Neither SAHA (Figure S4E) nor SAHA+MG132 (data not shown) treatments induced the formation of stress granules (Figure S4E), a phenomenon that was observed in response to Tunicamycin treatment (positive control) (Figure S4E). These data suggest that changes in stress granules formation or regulation are not involved in the SAHA-mediated changes in HIF-1α protein levels.

Although we noted that the silencing eIF3G alone did not impact the expression level of HIF-1α (Figure S5A), the overexpression of Myc-tagged eIF3G, in the absence of SAHA treatment, induced a statistically significant increase in HIF-1α and p53 protein levels (Figure S5B). Combining the overexpression of eIF3G with the SAHA treatment did not further alter the SAHA-mediated reduction in HIF-1α, further supporting the conclusion that eIF3G is required for the SAHA-mediated impediment of HIF-1α translation.

Discussion

HIF-1α is a master regulator in angiogenesis, metabolic reprogramming, epithelial-mesenchymal transition, stem cell maintenance, invasion, metastasis and resistance to several therapies making it a major target for therapeutic development in cancer [18,19], however development of small-molecule HIF-1α inhibitors has been a major challenge. The HDACi, SAHA, has been reported to provide therapeutic benefit in a number of oncogenic conditions, including pancreatic, breast, prostate, colon, liver and hematological cancers. SAHA is well tolerated when administrated either intravenously or orally, and has been found to have antitumor activity in advanced solid tumors refractory to other therapeutic interventions. By consequence, SAHA represents a promising anti-tumor drug in both preclinical and clinical development. Interestingly, HDACi have been reported to be potent HIF-1α inhibitors [16,17], however, the mechanism of action for this inhibition remains to be elucidated. Here, we found that SAHA was able to repress the expression of the angiogenic factor, HIF-1α without altering its transcription or degradation. Rather we report that the HDAC inhibitor, SAHA, regulates HIF-1α translation in HCC cell lines, in a mechanism dependent on the eukaryotic translation initiation machinery.

Under normoxic conditions and in the absence of growth factor stimulation, the HIF-1α protein is targeted for degradation [23,24]. The accumulation of HIF-1α can therefore be altered through increased protein synthesis or inhibition of protein degradation. Herein, we observe that SAHA can reverse the aberrant accumulation of HIF-1α seen in response to inhibition of HIF-1α degradation such as treatment with the prolyl hydroxylase inhibitors, $CoCl_2$, desferrioxamine (DFO) and dimethyloxallyl glycine (DMOG) or the proteasome inhibitor, MG132. Additionally, SAHA mediates a transcriptional block of p53, which would be predicted to reduce the MDM2-mediated ubiquitination and subsequent proteosomal degradation of HIF-1α [21,25,26]. These data clearly demonstrate that the SAHA effect on HIF-1α is occurring at the level of protein expression rather than by promoting the degradation of this angiogenic factor, however no changes in HIF-1α mRNA levels were observed in response to SAHA treatment.

The role of SAHA in protein translation has already been demonstrated for other proteins. Indeed, SAHA has been shown to exhibit a regulatory function on the mTOR pathway to suppress the translation of cyclin D1 [56], a pathway previously shown to also regulate HIF-1α translation [45–47]. Additionally, Sorafenib, the only drug clinically approved for patients with advanced HCC, has been shown to induce suppression of mTOR/p70S6K/4E-BP1 pathway [54], which could account for its therapeutic benefit in HCC. However, we failed to detect a dependence on the mTOR pathway for the SAHA-mediated reduction in HIF-1α (Figure S2A). These data could account for the synergistic effect of the combined SAHA and Sorafenib treatment currently under clinical investigation for a number of cancers, including HCC.

More generally, protein translation is subject to a number or regulatory steps, the first of which involves the eukaryotic initiation factors (eIF), which are involved in mRNA cap binding, ribosome recruitment and start codon scanning. Here the eIF4F complex, which is composed of the cap binding protein eIF4E, the ATP-dependent RNA helicase, eIF4A and the scaffolding protein eIF4G1, binds to the mRNA molecule and recruits the eIF3-bound ribosome through interaction with eIF4G1. The eIF3 complex is composed of 13 subunits (A through M) with eIF3A, B, C, E, F & H composing the essential core of the initiation complex [55] and the remaining subunits providing poorly defined regulatory functions. Herein, we report a clear dependence on the presence of a functional translational initiation complex for the SAHA-mediated reduction in HIF-1α protein level, with the eIF4E, 4G1 and 3G subunits providing the most dramatic block of the SAHA-mediated inhibition of HIF-1α. Unlike eIF4E and 4G1, which are critical components of translation initiation, eIF3G has been shown to provide a more regulatory role [55] by promoting mRNA circularization [56]. Nonetheless, these data provide evidence that the impact of SAHA on HIF-1α expression is occurring at the level of translational regulation. Furthermore, our data shows that these factors must be present at endogenous expression levels for the SAHA-mediated effect be observed and that their silencing mediate sustained or increased HIF-1α expression.

The translation initiation factor eIF3G has never been demonstrated to play an important role in tumor development. Here, our results further support the conclusion that eIF3G is a target for the anti-cancer properties of SAHA for the treatment of HCC and possibly other types of cancers and that its therapeutic benefit would be independent of a potential increased expression level of eIF3G (Figure S5B). Additionally, increased expression of eIF3 subunits have been reported in cancer [51]. Among those subunits, the overexpression of eIF3H has been found to be increased in several types of cancer [57,58], where it has been speculated to regulate translation of mRNAs specifically involved in cell growth or apoptosis [59] and consequently may favor oncogenic transformation. Our results are in agreement with these ideas and suggest an eIF3H-mediated control of HIF-1α translation that could explain in part its oncogenic properties. Interestingly, combining eIF3H silencing with SAHA treatment had an additive effect on HIF-1α repression. This observation could open a new avenue in therapeutic development in cancer by screening for small molecule inhibitors of eIF3H activity or expression.

Our characterization of the mechanism of action for the SAHA-mediated HIF-1α protein repression indicates that SAHA acts through HDAC9 silencing. Previous reports have highlighted the role of HDAC family members, namely 1, 3, 4, 6 and 7, on HIF-1α protein stability and activity [34; 35; 36; 53;5 4]. However, only the silencing of HDAC4 and 6 were shown to regulate the protein expression level of HIF-1α, by altering its post-translational acetylation and its subsequent interaction with the Hsp70/Hsp90 chaperone machinery [34;35;36]. Our experimental data demonstrates that HDAC9 is a prominent target for the SAHA-mediated reduction in HIF-1α protein expression. Recently, a study using high-resolution copy-number analysis and whole-exome sequencing of HCC tumors [60] identified 135 homozygous deletions and 994 somatic mutations of genes with predicted functional consequences, including a missense mutation in the HDAC9 gene (Leu1043Gln) [60]. The functional consequences of this mutation are unclear, but in light of our recent data, a deregulation of HDAC9 activity could impact the expression and function of HIF-1α and possibly other oncogenes. Furthermore, there are 9 variants of HDAC9 differing in their 3′, 5′ UTR regions as well as in the coding sequence. In light of this information, future studies addressing which variants of HDAC9 are targeted by SAHA to account for the reduction in HIF-1α protein expression are warranted.

Our combined results lead us to suggest a model where in absence of treatment, HIF-1α translation is enhanced by HDAC9 activity (Left panel-Figure 6). In this condition, HIF-1α translation is regulated by cellular oxygen levels, being either degraded or imported to the nucleus (Left panel-Figure 6A). Upon SAHA treatment, HDAC9 is inhibited and HIF-1α translation is repressed (Middle panel-Figure 6B). SAHA may induce the expression of other, yet identified, key protein(s) (referred as X in Figure 6) that negatively modulate HIF-1α translation. Upon eIF3G silencing, these other HIF-1α modulators are differentially expressed thereby blocking the SAHA-mediated repression of HIF-1α (Right panel-Figure 6C).

In summary, we report that the HDAC inhibitor, SAHA, regulates HIF-1α translation in HCC cell lines, in a mechanism dependent on the eukaryotic translation initiation machinery. Our results highlight the importance of further investigating the functional relationship between eIFs and HIF-1α for the possible therapeutic development of anti-cancer compounds.

Materials and Methods

Materials

HDACi (suberoylanilide hydroxamic acid; SAHA) was purchased from Cayman Chemical (Ann Arbor, MI, USA). Ammonium chloride, cobalt chloride (II), desferrioxamine (DFO), dimethyloxallyl glycine (DMOG) and MG132 (Z-leu-leu-leu-al) were purchased from Sigma (StLouis, MO, USA). Tunicamycin was purchased from Calbiochem (Merck Bioscience, Darmstadt, Germany) and was dissolved in DMSO to a final stock concentration of 10 mg/ml. SiRNA were obtained from Ambion (Austin, TX, USA). RNA extraction kits were from Qiagen (Valencia, CA, USA). Rabbit anti-human HDAC7 and anti-Myc tag antibodies were purchased from Abcam (Cambridge, MA, USA). Anti-human H3 acetylated antibody was purchased from Millipore (Billerica, MA, USA). Rabbit anti-human eIF3G antibody was purchased from Novus Biologicals (Littleton, CO, USA). Mouse anti-human Hsp90, TIA-1/TIAR and goat anti-human eIF3B antibodies were purchased from Santa Cruz Biotechnology (Santa Cruz, CA, USA). Mouse anti-human GAPDH was purchased from Genetex (Irvine, CA, USA). Mouse anti-human HIF-1α antibody was purchased from BD biosciences (Franklin Lakes, NJ, USA). Rabbit anti-human LC3 antibody was purchased from Sigma (St Louis, MO, USA). Mouse anti-human p53 was purchased from Calbiochem (Merck Bioscience, Darmstadt, Germany). Rabbit anti-human Total acetyl antibody, rabbit anti-human eIF3H and mouse anti-human ribosomal protein S6 antibody were purchased from Cell Signaling (Danvers, MA, USA).

DNA Constructs

eIF3G cDNA was cloned from human liver cDNA using the Gateway technology (Invitrogen-Carlsbad, CA, USA) in pRK5-Myc expression plasmid. Primers used for cloning are 5′-ggggacaagtttgtacaaaaaagcaggcttgcctactggagactttgattcgaa-3′ and 5′-ggggaccactttgtacaagaaagctgggtattagttggtggacggcttg-3′. eIF3G cDNA devoid of ATG, were amplified by PCR using the Platinium *Taq* DNA Polymerase High Fidelity (Invitrogen-Carlsbad, CA, USA). These PCR products were purified using PCR Clean-Up System Promega (Wisconsin, USA) and recombined into pDONR221 using the Gateway BP clonase (Invitrogen-Carlsbad, CA, USA). These plasmids were then transformed into competent DH5α cells and positive clones selected and sequenced. These clones were then recombined into destination vectors (pRK5-Myc) from Eric Chevet Lab (Bordeaux, France) using LR clonase (Invitrogen-Carlsbad, CA, USA).

Cell culture, transfections and treatments

HuH7 and Hep3B cells were obtained from Eric Chevet Lab (Bordeaux, France). These cells were cultured in DMEM containing 10% (v/v) fetal bovine serum (FBS). Cells were treated with the indicated concentrations of SAHA, MG132, desferrioxamine (DFO), dimethyloxallyl glycine (DMOG), ammonium chloride, cobalt chloride (II) and tunicamycin or vehicle (DMSO, water) in complete growth media (above). HDACs silencing and

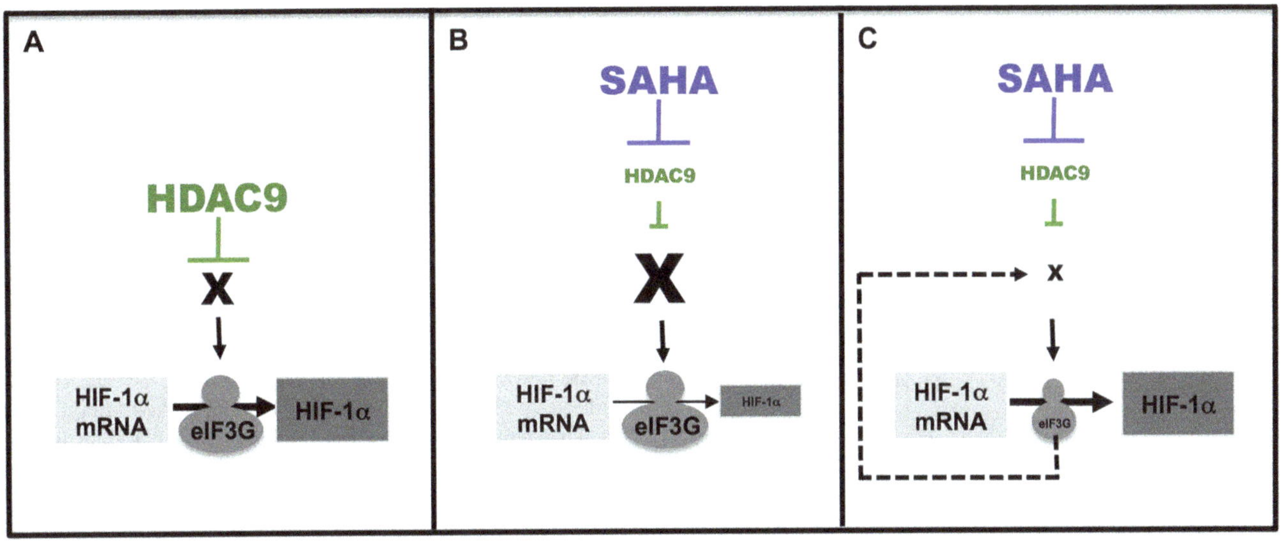

Figure 6. A model for SAHA mediated effects on HIF-1α translation. In non-treated conditions (left panel-A), HIF-1α translation is controlled by HDAC9 and then HIF-1α mRNA is translated in protein. Following SAHA treatment (middle panel-B), HDAC9 is inhibited and we suggest that SAHA could promote mRNA and protein expression of an unknown protein (referred as X) that controls HIF-1α translation. As a result of this, the unknown protein could repress specifically HIF-1α translation. Upon the combined treatment SAHA and eIF3G silencing (right panel-C), we suggest that eIF3G may play a regulatory role in translation of the mRNA coding the unknown protein. By consequence, the silencing of eIF3G results in the inhibition of the unknown protein translation. As the expression of this unknown protein is down regulated, HIF-1α translation is not repressed anymore and could be translated *de novo*.

eIFs silencing were performed with RNAiMax (Invitrogen, Carlsbad, CA, USA) as per the manufacturer's protocol using 50 nM of the indicated siRNA. HuH7 cells were transiently transfected with the pRK5-Myc eIF3G plasmid. Transfection were done using PromoFectine-hepatocyte (PromoCell, Heidelberg, Germany) according to the manufacturer's recommendations.

siRNA-mediated silencing of HDACs and eIFs

HuH7 cells were plated in 12-wells plates and grown to 30–40% confluence. Silencing of individual HDACs and eIFs were performed as indicated above and as described previously [35].

qRT-PCR

Quantitative PCR was performed as described previously [61] and using the following primers and using the following primers for HIF-1α: 5′-gaacaaaacacacagcgaag-3′ and 5′-acaaatcagcaccaagcag-3′; p53: 5′-tctccacttcttgttcccc-3′ and 5′-ctccccacaacaaaacacc-3′; qRT-PCR for HDAC9 and HDAC10 were performed as described previously [35]. RNA was standardized by quantification of GAPDH mRNA using primers 5′-AAGGTGAAGGTCGGAGTCAA-3′ and 5′-CATGGGTGGAATCATATTGG-3′, and all values are expressed relative to GAPDH.

Immunoblotting

Cell lysates were prepared in 50 mM Tris-HCl, 150 mM NaCl, 1% (v/v) Triton X-100 and protease inhibitors and protein concentrations determined by Bradford protein assay (Thermo Scientific, Rockford, IL, USA). Total protein were resuspended in 1X SDS sample buffer containing DTT and incubated at 95°C for 5 min. The samples 10–25 µg of total protein are then separated on a 10% (v/v) SDS-PAGE, transferred to nitrocellulose and immunoblotted with anti-human HIF-1α antibody (BD biosciences, Franklin Lakes, NJ, USA) or indicated primary antibodies. Detection was performed using chemiluminescence and the appropriate horseradish peroxidase (HRP)-conjugated secondary antibodies.

Immunoprecipitation

Cell lysates were prepared as described in Immunoblotting section and 1 mg of pre-cleared (1 h at 4°C with Protein G Sepharose) cell lysate was incubated overnight at 4°C with the indicated antibody (anti-Myc tag). Immunoprecipitations with non-coupled antibodies were incubated for 1 h at 4°C with Protein G Sepharose beads. Beads and bound proteins are washed with three changes of lysis buffer without protease inhibitor and resuspended in 1X SDS sample buffer containing DTT and incubated at 95°C for 5 min. Input and bound material were separated on a 10% (v/v) SDS-PAGE, transferred to nitrocellulose and immunoblotted with anti-human total acetylated antibody. Detection was performed as described in Immunoblotting section.

ImmunoFluorescence

For staining of eIF3G protein and stress granules, HuH7 cells were grown in 24-well plates, fixed with 4% paraformaldehyde for 10 min, and permeabilized with 0.1% Triton X-100 for 1 min at room temperature. Cells were then incubated with anti-Myc Tag and anti-TIA-1/TIAR antibodies for 1 h at room temperature followed by incubation with fluorescently labeled secondary antibodies. Protein subcellular localization was performed using an epifluorescence microscope with a Zeiss 63 1.4 oil immersion objective, recorded with a digital camera, and analyzed with Northern Eclipse software (Emprix Imaging, Mississauga, Ontario, Canada). The percentage of stress granules per cells was performed as described previously [62].

Supporting Information

Figure S1 Silencing of HDAC9 represses HIF-1α protein expression. (**A**) qRT-PCR analysis of mRNA levels of HDAC 9 (Left) and 10 (Right) in HuH7 cell line following their respective silencing. Data are shown as the fractional recovery of the indicated HDAC mRNA, normalized to GAPDH mRNA, relative to the level seen with scrambled (Scr) siRNA (mean ± SD, n = 3). (**B**) Immunoblot analysis of HIF-1α, p53 and GAPDH protein expression in cell lysates following siRNA-mediated silencing of HDAC9 or Scr (Scramble control)+100 μM desferrioxamine (DFO) for 18 h in HuH7 cells and following treatment of HuH7 cells with 5 μM SAHA for 24 h+100 μM desferrioxamine (DFO) for 18 h. In all panels GAPDH is used as loading control.

Figure S2 Effects of eIF2β, eIF3G and mTOR silencing on HIF-1α protein level. (**A**) Immunoblot analysis of HIF-1α and GAPDH protein expression in cell lysates following siRNA-mediated silencing of mTOR in HuH7 cells in presence of SAHA+MG132 or following Scr (Scramble control) in presence of MG132. Quantitative analysis (lower) of the level of HIF-1α following siRNA-mediated silencing of mTOR in HuH7 cells in presence of SAHA+MG132. Data shown denote the fold change in HIF-1α protein expression relative to scramble (Scr)+MG132 control (black bar) (mean ± SD, n = 6). Asterisks indicates $p<0.05$ as determined by two-tailed t-test using Scr+MG132 as the reference, # indicates $p<0.05$ as determined by two-tailed t-test using Scr+SAHA+MG132 as the reference. (**B**) Immunoblot analysis of HIF-1α and GAPDH protein expression in cell lysates following siRNA-mediated silencing of eIF2β in HuH7 cells in presence of SAHA+MG132. (**C**) Immunoblot analysis of HIF-1α, eIF3G and GAPDH protein expression in cell lysates following siRNA-mediated silencing of eIF3G in HuH7 cells in presence of SAHA+DFO or DFO. In all panels GAPDH is used as loading control.

Figure S3 eIF silencing did not reverse SAHA effect on p53 protein level. Immunoblot analysis of p53, HDAC7 and GAPDH protein expression in cell lysates following siRNA-mediated silencing of eIF3 A-M, eIF4 E, G1–3 and eIF5 in HuH7 cells in presence or absence of SAHA+MG132. Quantitative analysis (lower) of the level of p53 in response to silencing of the indicated eIF in HuH7 cells. Data shown denote the fold change in p53 protein expression relative to Scrambled (Scr) siRNA control (black bar) (mean ± SD, n = 3). Asterisks indicates $p<0.05$ as determined by two-tailed t-test using Scr control (black bar) as the reference. In all panels GAPDH is used as loading control and HDAC7 is used as control to SAHA treatment.

Figure S4 SAHA does not target eIF3G directly. (**A**) Immunofluorescence analysis of Myc tag protein expression following DMSO and SAHA+MG132. (**B**) Immunoblot analysis of eIF3G, acetylated histone H3 (Acetyl H3) and GAPDH protein expression in cell lysates following DMSO or SAHA treatment in HuH7 cells. (**C**) Immunoblot analysis of eIF3G, acetylated histone H3, acetylated lysine and Hsp90 before (input/upper) and after immunoprecipitation of Myc tag (IP Myc/lower) in HuH7 cells following DMSO or SAHA (5 μM) treatment. (**D**) Immunoblot analysis of Myc-eIF3G, ribosomal protein S6 and eIF3B before (input/left) and after immunoprecipitation of Myc tag (IP Myc/right) in HuH7 cells following DMSO or SAHA (5 μM) treatment. (**E**) Immunofluorescence analysis of TIA-1/TIAR protein expression following DMSO, SAHA (5 μM) or Tunicamycin (2 μg/ml) treatments for 24 h. Quantitative analysis (lower) of TIA-1/TIAR stress granules in HuH7 cells in response to DMSO, SAHA or tunicamycin (TUN) treatments. The percentage of stress granules per cells was obtained as described previously [62]. Data shown denote the fold change in TIA-1/TIAR stress granules relative to DMSO (white bar) treatment (mean ± SD, n = 6). Asterisks indicates $p<0.05$ as determined by two-tailed t-test using DMSO as the reference. In all panels Hsp90 and GAPDG are used as loading control and acetylated histone H3 is used as control to SAHA treatment.

Figure S5 eIF3G is required for SAHA-mediated repress of HIF-1α translation. (**A**) Immunoblot analysis of HIF-1α, eIF3G and GAPDH protein expression in cell lysates following siRNA-mediated silencing of eIF3G in HuH7 cells in presence of MG132. (**B**) Immunoblot analysis (left) of HIF-1α, p53, Myc tag, acetylated histone H3 (Acetyl H3) and GAPDH protein expression in cell lysates following Myc tag or Myc-eIF3G overexpression in HuH7 cells in presence or absence of SAHA+MG132. Quantitative analysis (right) of the level of HIF-1α and p53 in response to Myc-eIF3G overexpression in HuH7 cells in presence or absence of SAHA+MG132. Data shown denote the fold change in HIF-1α (black bar) and p53 (grey bar) protein expression relative to Myc tag overexpression (Myc) (mean ± SD, n = 6). Asterisks indicates $p<0.05$ as determined by two-tailed t-test using Myc tag overexpression in presence of DMSO+MG132 as the reference. In all panels GAPDH is used as loading control and acetylated histone H3 is used as control to SAHA treatment.

Acknowledgments

We thank Dr. E. Chevet (INSERM U1053, Université de Bordeaux, Bordeaux, France) for his gift of HuH7 and Hep3B cells and plasmids and his helpful discussions. We are grateful to Dr. B. Drogat (Université Libre de Bruxelles, IRIBHM, Brussels B-1070, Belgium) for his help and fruitful discussions.

Author Contributions

Conceived and designed the experiments: DMH DMR HV CC MB. Performed the experiments: MB. Analyzed the data: DMH DMR HV CC MB. Contributed reagents/materials/analysis tools: DMH DMR MB. Contributed to the writing of the manuscript: DMH DMR CC MB.

References

1. El-Serag HB (2011) Hepatocellular carcinoma. N Engl J Med 365: 1118–1127.
2. Sherman M (2005) Hepatocellular carcinoma: epidemiology, risk factors, and screening. Semin Liver Dis 25: 143–154.
3. Schlaeger C, Longerich T, Schiller C, Bewerunge P, Mehrabi A, et al. (2008) Etiology-dependent molecular mechanisms in human hepatocarcinogenesis. Hepatology 47: 511–520.
4. Velazquez RF, Rodriguez M, Navascues CA, Linares A, Perez R, et al. (2003) Prospective analysis of risk factors for hepatocellular carcinoma in patients with liver cirrhosis. Hepatology 37: 520–527.
5. Kumar M, Kumar R, Hissar SS, Saraswat MK, Sharma BC, et al. (2007) Risk factors analysis for hepatocellular carcinoma in patients with and without cirrhosis: a case-control study of 213 hepatocellular carcinoma patients from India. J Gastroenterol Hepatol 22: 1104–1111.
6. Llovet JM, Ricci S, Mazzaferro V, Hilgard P, Gane E, et al. (2008) Sorafenib in advanced hepatocellular carcinoma. N Engl J Med 359: 378–390.
7. Llovet JM, Burroughs A, Bruix J (2003) Hepatocellular carcinoma. Lancet 362: 1907–1917.
8. Villanueva A, Llovet JM (2011) Targeted therapies for hepatocellular carcinoma. Gastroenterology 140: 1410–1426.
9. Moeini A, Cornella H, Villanueva A (2012) Emerging Signaling Pathways in Hepatocellular Carcinoma. Liver Cancer 1: 83–93.
10. Boumber Y, Issa JP (2011) Epigenetics in cancer: what's the future? Oncology (Williston Park) 25: 220–226, 228.
11. Lachenmayer A, Toffanin S, Cabellos L, Alsinet C, Hoshida Y, et al. (2012) Combination therapy for hepatocellular carcinoma: additive preclinical efficacy of the HDAC inhibitor panobinostat with sorafenib. J Hepatol 56: 1343–1350.

12. Dasari A, Gore L, Messersmith WA, Diab S, Jimeno A, et al. (2013) A phase I study of sorafenib and vorinostat in patients with advanced solid tumors with expanded cohorts in renal cell carcinoma and non-small cell lung cancer. Invest New Drugs 31: 115–125.
13. Sarfstein R, Bruchim I, Fishman A, Werner H (2011) The mechanism of action of the histone deacetylase inhibitor vorinostat involves interaction with the insulin-like growth factor signaling pathway. PLoS One 6: e24468.
14. Scroggins BT, Robzyk K, Wang D, Marcu MG, Tsutsumi S, et al. (2007) An acetylation site in the middle domain of Hsp90 regulates chaperone function. Mol Cell 25: 151–159.
15. Siegel D, Hussein M, Belani C, Robert F, Galanis E, et al. (2009) Vorinostat in solid and hematologic malignancies. J Hematol Oncol 2: 31.
16. Ellis L, Hammers H, Pili R (2009) Targeting tumor angiogenesis with histone deacetylase inhibitors. Cancer Lett 280: 145–153.
17. Liang D, Kong X, Sang N (2006) Effects of histone deacetylase inhibitors on HIF-1. Cell Cycle 5: 2430–2435.
18. Semenza GL (2003) Targeting HIF-1 for cancer therapy. Nat Rev Cancer 3: 721–732.
19. Brown JM, Wilson WR (2004) Exploiting tumour hypoxia in cancer treatment. Nat Rev Cancer 4: 437–447.
20. Semenza GL (2012) Hypoxia-inducible factors: mediators of cancer progression and targets for cancer therapy. Trends Pharmacol Sci 33: 207–214.
21. Schmid T, Zhou J, Brune B (2004) HIF-1 and p53: communication of transcription factors under hypoxia. J Cell Mol Med 8: 423–431.
22. Stiehl DP, Wirthner R, Koditz J, Spielmann P, Camenisch G, et al. (2006) Increased prolyl 4-hydroxylase domain proteins compensate for decreased oxygen levels. Evidence for an autoregulatory oxygen-sensing system. J Biol Chem 281: 23482–23491.
23. Ke Q, Costa M (2006) Hypoxia-inducible factor-1 (HIF-1). Mol Pharmacol 70: 1469–1480.
24. Powis G, Kirkpatrick L (2004) Hypoxia inducible factor-1alpha as a cancer drug target. Mol Cancer Ther 3: 647–654.
25. Ravi R, Mookerjee B, Bhujwalla ZM, Sutter CH, Artemov D, et al. (2000) Regulation of tumor angiogenesis by p53-induced degradation of hypoxia-inducible factor 1alpha. Genes Dev 14: 34–44.
26. Hubbi ME, Hu H, Kshitiz, Ahmed I, Levchenko A, et al. (2013) Chaperone-mediated autophagy targets hypoxia-inducible factor-1alpha (HIF-1alpha) for lysosomal degradation. J Biol Chem 288: 10703–10714.
27. Thornton RD, Lane P, Borghaei RC, Pease EA, Caro J, et al. (2000) Interleukin 1 induces hypoxia-inducible factor 1 in human gingival and synovial fibroblasts. Biochem J 350 Pt 1: 307–312.
28. Fukuda R, Hirota K, Fan F, Jung YD, Ellis LM, et al. (2002) Insulin-like growth factor 1 induces hypoxia-inducible factor 1-mediated vascular endothelial growth factor expression, which is dependent on MAP kinase and phosphatidylinositol 3-kinase signaling in colon cancer cells. J Biol Chem 277: 38205–38211.
29. Zundel W, Schindler C, Haas-Kogan D, Koong A, Kaper F, et al. (2000) Loss of PTEN facilitates HIF-1-mediated gene expression. Genes Dev 14: 391–396.
30. Semenza GL (2013) HIF-1 mediates metabolic responses to intratumoral hypoxia and oncogenic mutations. J Clin Invest 123: 3664–3671.
31. Moeller BJ, Richardson RA, Dewhirst MW (2007) Hypoxia and radiotherapy: opportunities for improved outcomes in cancer treatment. Cancer Metastasis Rev 26: 241–248.
32. Rohwer N, Cramer T (2011) Hypoxia-mediated drug resistance: novel insights on the functional interaction of HIFs and cell death pathways. Drug Resist Updat 14: 191–201.
33. Kong X, Lin Z, Liang D, Fath D, Sang N, et al. (2006) Histone deacetylase inhibitors induce VHL and ubiquitin-independent proteasomal degradation of hypoxia-inducible factor 1alpha. Mol Cell Biol 26: 2019–2028.
34. Geng H, Harvey CT, Pittsenbarger J, Liu Q, Beer TM, et al. (2011) HDAC4 protein regulates HIF1alpha protein lysine acetylation and cancer cell response to hypoxia. J Biol Chem 286: 38095–38102.
35. Bouchecareilh M, Hutt DM, Szajner P, Flotte TR, Balch WE (2012) Histone deacetylase inhibitor (HDACi) suberoylanilide hydroxamic acid (SAHA)-mediated correction of alpha1-antitrypsin deficiency. J Biol Chem 287: 38265–38278.
36. Hutt DM, Herman D, Rodrigues AP, Noel S, Pilewski JM, et al. (2010) Reduced histone deacetylase 7 activity restores function to misfolded CFTR in cystic fibrosis. Nat Chem Biol 6: 25–33.
37. Yan W, Liu S, Xu E, Zhang J, Zhang Y, et al. (2013) Histone deacetylase inhibitors suppress mutant p53 transcription via histone deacetylase 8. Oncogene 32: 599–609.
38. Qian DZ, Kachhap SK, Collis SJ, Verheul HM, Carducci MA, et al. (2006) Class II histone deacetylases are associated with VHL-independent regulation of hypoxia-inducible factor 1 alpha. Cancer Res 66: 8814–8821.
39. Marks PA, Dokmanovic M (2005) Histone deacetylase inhibitors: discovery and development as anticancer agents. Expert Opin Investig Drugs 14: 1497–1511.
40. Blander G, Guarente L (2004) The Sir2 family of protein deacetylases. Annu Rev Biochem 73: 417–435.
41. Liu T, Liu PY, Marshall GM (2009) The critical role of the class III histone deacetylase SIRT1 in cancer. Cancer Res 69: 1702–1705.
42. Zhang J, Cao J, Weng Q, Wu R, Yan Y, et al. (2010) Suppression of hypoxia-inducible factor 1alpha (HIF-1alpha) by tirapazamine is dependent on eIF2alpha phosphorylation rather than the mTORC1/4E-BP1 pathway. PLoS One 5: e13910.
43. Zhu K, Chan W, Heymach J, Wilkinson M, McConkey DJ (2009) Control of HIF-1alpha expression by eIF2 alpha phosphorylation-mediated translational repression. Cancer Res 69: 1836–1843.
44. Sesen J, Cammas A, Scotland SJ, Elefterion B, Lemarie A, et al. (2014) Int6/eIF3e is essential for proliferation and survival of human glioblastoma cells. Int J Mol Sci 15: 2172–2190.
45. Bernardi R, Guernah I, Jin D, Grisendi S, Alimonti A, et al. (2006) PML inhibits HIF-1alpha translation and neoangiogenesis through repression of mTOR. Nature 442: 779–785.
46. Thomas GV, Tran C, Mellinghoff IK, Welsbie DS, Chan E, et al. (2006) Hypoxia-inducible factor determines sensitivity to inhibitors of mTOR in kidney cancer. Nat Med 12: 122–127.
47. Toschi A, Lee E, Gadir N, Ohh M, Foster DA (2008) Differential dependence of hypoxia-inducible factors 1 alpha and 2 alpha on mTORC1 and mTORC2. J Biol Chem 283: 34495–34499.
48. Dunlop EA, Tee AR (2009) Mammalian target of rapamycin complex 1: signalling inputs, substrates and feedback mechanisms. Cell Signal 21: 827–835.
49. Magagnin MG, van den Beucken T, Sergeant K, Lambin P, Koritzinsky M, et al. (2008) The mTOR target 4E-BP1 contributes to differential protein expression during normoxia and hypoxia through changes in mRNA translation efficiency. Proteomics 8: 1019–1028.
50. Martineau Y, Wang X, Alain T, Petroulakis E, Shahbazian D, et al. (2014) Control of Paip1-eukayrotic translation initiation factor 3 interaction by amino acids through S6 kinase. Mol Cell Biol 34: 1046–1053.
51. Dong Z, Zhang JT (2006) Initiation factor eIF3 and regulation of mRNA translation, cell growth, and cancer. Crit Rev Oncol Hematol 59: 169–180.
52. Buchan JR, Parker R (2009) Eukaryotic stress granules: the ins and outs of translation. Mol Cell 36: 932–941.
53. Gottschald OR, Malec V, Krasteva G, Hasan D, Kamlah F, et al. (2010) TIAR and TIA-1 mRNA-binding proteins co-aggregate under conditions of rapid oxygen decline and extreme hypoxia and suppress the HIF-1alpha pathway. J Mol Cell Biol 2: 345–356.
54. Schult C, Dahlhaus M, Ruck S, Sawitzky M, Amoroso F, et al. (2010) The multikinase inhibitor Sorafenib displays significant antiproliferative effects and induces apoptosis via caspase 3, 7 and PARP in B- and T-lymphoblastic cells. BMC Cancer 10: 560.
55. Masutani M, Sonenberg N, Yokoyama S, Imataka H (2007) Reconstitution reveals the functional core of mammalian eIF3. EMBO J 26: 3373–3383.
56. Martineau Y, Derry MC, Wang X, Yanagiya A, Berlanga JJ, et al. (2008) Poly(A)-binding protein-interacting protein 1 binds to eukaryotic translation initiation factor 3 to stimulate translation. Mol Cell Biol 28: 6658–6667.
57. Okamoto H, Yasui K, Zhao C, Arii S, Inazawa J (2003) PTK2 and EIF3S3 genes may be amplification targets at 8q23-q24 and are associated with large hepatocellular carcinomas. Hepatology 38: 1242–1249.
58. Nupponen NN, Porkka K, Kakkola L, Tanner M, Persson K, et al. (1999) Amplification and overexpression of p40 subunit of eukaryotic translation initiation factor 3 in breast and prostate cancer. Am J Pathol 154: 1777–1783.
59. Kim TH, Kim BH, Yahalom A, Chamovitz DA, von Arnim AG (2004) Translational regulation via 5′ mRNA leader sequences revealed by mutational analysis of the Arabidopsis translation initiation factor subunit eIF3h. Plant Cell 16: 3341–3356.
60. Guichard C, Amaddeo G, Imbeaud S, Ladeiro Y, Pelletier L, et al. (2012) Integrated analysis of somatic mutations and focal copy-number changes identifies key genes and pathways in hepatocellular carcinoma. Nat Genet 44: 694–698.
61. Bouchecareilh M, Higa A, Fribourg S, Moenner M, Chevet E (2011) Peptides derived from the bifunctional kinase/RNase enzyme IRE1alpha modulate IRE1alpha activity and protect cells from endoplasmic reticulum stress. FASEB J 25: 3115–3129.
62. Dewey CM, Cenik B, Sephton CF, Dries DR, Mayer P 3rd, et al. (2011) TDP-43 is directed to stress granules by sorbitol, a novel physiological osmotic and oxidative stressor. Mol Cell Biol 31: 1098–1108.

12

Measurement of Glycosylated Alpha-Fetoprotein Improves Diagnostic Power over the Native Form in Hepatocellular Carcinoma

Hyunsoo Kim[1]⁹, Kyunggon Kim[2]⁹, Jonghwa Jin[2], Jiyoung Park[1], Su Jong Yu[3], Jung-Hwan Yoon[3], Youngsoo Kim[1,2*]

1 Department of Biomedical Sciences, Seoul National University College of Medicine, Seoul, Republic of Korea, **2** Department of Biomedical Engineering, Seoul National University College of Medicine, Seoul, Republic of Korea, **3** Department of Internal Medicine, Seoul National University College of Medicine, Seoul, Republic of Korea

Abstract

Serum alpha-fetoprotein (AFP) has long been used as a diagnostic marker for hepatocellular carcinoma (HCC), albeit controversially. Although it remains widely used in clinics, the value of AFP in HCC diagnosis has recently been challenged due to its significant rates of false positive and false negative findings. To improve the efficacy of AFP as HCC diagnostic marker, we developed a method of measuring total and glycosylated AFP by multiple reaction monitoring (MRM)-MS. In this study, we verified the total amount of AFP (nonglycopeptide levels) and the degree of glycosylated AFP (deglycopeptide levels) in 60 normal (41 men and 19 women; mean age 53 years; range 32–74 years), 35 LC (23 men and 12 women; mean age 56 years; range 43–78 years; HBV-related), and 60 HCC subjects (42 men and 18 women; mean age 58 years; range 38–76 years; HBV-related; 30 stage I, 15 stage II, and 10 stage III). By MRM-MS analysis, the nonglycopeptide had 56.7% sensitivity, 68.3% specificity, and an AUC of 0.687 [cutoff value: ≥0.02 (light/heavy ratio)], comparing the normal and HCC group, whereas the deglycopeptide had 93.3% sensitivity, 68.3% specificity, and an AUC of 0.859 [cutoff value: ≥0.02 (light/heavy ratio)]. In comparing the stage I HCC subgroup with the LC group, the nonglycopeptide had a sensitivity of 66.7%, specificity of 80.0%, and an AUC of 0.712 [cutoff value: ≥0.02 (light/heavy ratio)], whereas the deglycopeptide had a sensitivity of 96.7%, specificity of 80.0%, and an AUC of 0.918 [cutoff value: ≥0.02 (light/heavy ratio)]. These data demonstrate that the discriminatory power of the deglycopeptide is greater than that of the nonglycopeptide. We conclude that deglycopeptide can distinguish cancer status between normal subjects and HCC patients better than nonglycopeptide.

Editor: Lian-Yue Yang, Xiangya Hospital of Central South University, China

Funding: This work was supported by a National Research Foundation of Korea grant (No. 2011-0030740) and the Proteogenomic Research Program, funded by the Korea government [MISP]. This work was also supported by the Industrial Strategic Technology Development Program (#10045352), funded by the Ministry of Knowledge Economy (MKE, Korea). The funders had no role in study design, data collection and analysis, decision to publish, or preparation of the manuscript.

Competing Interests: The authors have declared that no competing interests exist.

* Email: biolab@snu.ac.kr

⁹ These authors contributed equally to this work.

Introduction

Glycosylation is one of the most important and common post-translational modifications (PTMs) of proteins that are secreted into serum. Glycosylation influences many functional aspects of proteins, including their structure and functions [1]. The expression and degree of glycosylation is significantly altered by various diseases, such as cancer, and thus, glycoproteins are associated with abnormal phenomena in patients with cancer [2–4]. To this end, quantitative measurements of glycoproteins might be useful in discovering biomarkers for cancer.

The carbohydrates on glycosylated protein biomarkers undergo modifications in cancer. For example, the carbohydrate moieties of AFP are altered in cancer, and such changes are considered to be more useful markers of HCC [5]. Studies from the past several decades have demonstrated that total AFP is a collection of heterogeneous glycoproteins that can be fractionated by affinity electrophoresis into 3 glycoforms–AFP-L1, AFP-L2, and AFP-L3–based on their reactivity with the lectin Lens culinaris agglutinin (LCA). AFP-L3 binds strongly to LCA through an α1-6 bond between its additional fucose and the reducing terminus of N-acetylglucosamine, in contrast to AFP-L1 [6–8].

AFP levels are sometimes elevated in patients with chronic hepatitis and cirrhosis who have no evidence of HCC [9]. AFP has a reported sensitivity of 39% to 65% and a specificity of 65% to 94%; approximately one-third of early-stage HCC patients with small tumors (<3 cm) have normal AFP levels [10,11]. Thus, clinicians are dissatisfied with AFP as a marker due to its high false-positive and false-negative rates [12].

Multiple reaction monitoring (MRM)-based quantification using triple quadrupole mass spectrometry (MS) is especially useful for measuring glycosylated biomarkers. MRM-MS, a multiplexed, targeted proteomic platform, is a rapid and cost-effective approach for measuring protein biomarkers for preclinical verification [13]. Nonglycopeptides (unmodified native peptides) and glycopeptides (glycosylated peptides) of glycoprotein markers are valuable biomarkers for the diagnosis and prediction of diseases, because their expression levels and degree of glycosylation reflect quantitative differences of disease states, as in cancer.

In this study, we measured total AFP and glycosylated AFP by MRM-MS. Total AFP was represented by common nonglycopeptides among all forms of AFP, and glycosylated AFP comprised the portion of deglycosylated peptides after treatment of glycosylated peptides with PNGase F. Measurement of the deglycopeptide fraction from the glycosylated AFP yielded better AUC values than the nonglycopeptides of total AFP. Consequently, on measuring AFP concentrations in serum from HCC patients versus normal healthy controls and early-stage HCC versus liver cirrhosis by MRM-MS, AFP deglycopeptides had greater power in distinguishing, compared with nonglycopeptides.

Notably, total AFP and glycosylated AFP were measured effectively by MRM-MS in the form of nonglycopeptides and deglycopeptides, respectively, improving our diagnosis of HCC versus normal and early-stage HCC versus LC serum. In addition, MRM-MS is a platform that improves the measurement of total AFP and glycosylated AFP in glycoprotein biomarker assays, which is more advantageous compared with conventional methods, such as antibody-based measurements by lectin affinity electrophoresis and liquid-phase binding assays.

Materials and Methods

Materials

Standard glycoprotein (origin: yeast) was purchased from Sigma-Aldrich (St. Louis, MO). Trypsin was obtained from Promega (Madison, WI). Peptide-N-glycosidase F (PNGase F) was purchased from New England Biolabs (NEB, Beverly, MA). HPLC-grade water and acetonitrile were obtained from Thermo Fisher Scientific (Bremen, Germany). Serum depletion was performed for the 6 most abundant proteins using a multiple affinity removal system (MARS), consisting of an LC column (Agilent, 5185–5984); buffer A for sample loading, washes, and equilibration (Agilent, 5185–5987); and buffer B for elution (Agilent, 5185–5988). Stable isotope-labeled peptides [isotopically labeled (^{13}C and ^{15}N) amino acids] were obtained from JPT (Berlin, Germany).

Clinical sample information

The institutional review board (IRB) of Seoul National University Hospital (approval No. H-1103-056-355) approved the study protocol, and written informed consent was obtained from each patient or legally authorized representative. The clinical characteristics of the patients are shown in Table 1.

The clinical sample set comprised healthy controls (n = 60), patients with liver cirrhosis (n = 35), and patients with hepatocellular carcinoma (n = 60). The healthy control group (normal group) comprised sixty healthy volunteers who visited the Healthcare Center of Seoul National University Hospital. All control subjects were confirmed, based on normal liver function test results, including serum alanine and aspartate aminotransferases, and were negative for hepatitis B virus surface antigen and anti-hepatitis C virus. Liver ultrasonography was performed to screen for fatty liver disease, and all healthy controls had normal findings.

The liver cirrhosis group (LC group) included 35 patients with compensated HBV cirrhosis and no HCC. The cirrhosis group had at least 1 year of follow-up from the time that serum was obtained for these studies. Patients were diagnosed with cirrhosis, based on established clinical, laboratory, and imaging criteria with ultrasound examination.

Sixty patients before HCC treatment who were infected with hepatitis B virus (HBV) were also enrolled, from whom serum samples were collected and defined as the HCC group. The diagnosis of HCC was made per the American Association for the Study of Liver Diseases by a hepatologist with more than 20 years of experience [14]. To reduce causal heterogeneity, HCC patients who had other types of chronic liver disease, except chronic hepatitis B, such as chronic hepatitis C and alcoholic hepatitis, were excluded.

HCC stage was classified per the tumor-node-metastasis (TNM) staging system (7th edition, 2010, the American Joint Committee on Cancer staging system). TNM staging of the 55 cases demonstrated stage I in 30 cases, stage II in 15 cases, stage III in 10 cases, and stage IV in 0 cases. Insufficient information was available to assign stage in 5 HCC cases.

All subjects (n = 155) were recruited during the study period from September 2005 to August 2012 and collected by the Liver Research Institute, Seoul National University College of Medicine. Blood samples were centrifuged immediately at 3000 rpm for 10 min at 4°C to fractionate the serum. The resulting supernatant was aliquoted (100 μL) and stored at −80°C until analysis.

Sample size calculations

We calculate the sample size that was needed for clinical MRM verification with reference to previous studies using AUC (area under the curve) [15]. The sample size was calculated, based on an AUC with a type I error rate α of 0.05 and type II error rate β of 0.10 (90% power). To anticipate similar AUC values as in previous studies, we needed a sample size of 29 each in the normal and HCC groups, each totaling 58, and 24 each in the HCC and recovery groups, totaling 48. A minimum sample size of 29 per group was necessary for the MRM assays to determine a significant difference between groups (Table S1).

Standard glycoprotein preparation

Standard glycoprotein (INV1) was prepared to 100 μg/μL. Standard glycoprotein samples were denatured with 6 M urea, 100 mM Tris, pH 8.0, and 20 mM dithiothreitol (DTT) at 37°C for 60 min and alkylated with 50 mM iodoacetamide (IAA) at room temperature in the dark for 30 min. The urea was diluted 15-fold with 100 mM Tris, pH 8.0. One INV1 sample was deglycosylated with 2 μL of PNGase F (500,000 units/mL) at 37°C for 12 h and incubated and digested in a solution of 1:50 trypsin (w/w) at 37°C for 16 h. The other INV1 sample was incubated in 2 μL 100 mM Tris, pH 8.0 (untreated PNGase F) at 37°C for 12 h and digested as described above. The 2 INV1 digests were dried on a speed vacuum, diluted in mobile phase A, and spiked with stable isotope-labeled standard (SIS) peptide, as needed.

Clinical serum sample preparation

The 6 most abundant proteins in human serum (albumin, transferrin, IgG, IgA, haptoglobin, and α1-antitrypsin) were depleted on an HPLC system (Shimadzu Co., Kyoto, Japan) that was equipped with a multiple affinity removal system LC column (Agilent Technologies, Santa Clara, CA). Crude human serum samples were diluted by a factor of 5 with buffer A and passed through 0.22-μm filters by centrifugation (12,000 g, room temperature, 2–3 min). Diluted crude serum was injected at 0.25 mL/min, and flowthrough fractions were collected and stored at −80°C. Depleted serum samples were concentrated by

Table 1. Characteristics of clinical subjects for MRM-MS analysis.

	Normal group	LC group	HCC group
Total patient number	60	35	60
Gender (Male/Female)	41/19	23/12	42/18
Age (Mean, Range)	53 (32–74)	56 (43–78)	58 (38–76)
Etiology of liver disease		HBV, 35 (100%)	HBV, 60 (100%)
AFP value (mean, range)			
<20 ng/ml	60	35	26
20–400 ng/ml	0	0	18
>400 ng/ml	0	0	16
Albumin (g/dL)	4.3±0.18	4.2±0.3	3.6±0.5
Bilirubin (mg/dL)	1.3±0.4	1.4±0.7	1.3±0.8
AST (IU/L)	22.5±6.0	32.3±24.3	89.1±142.3
ALT (IU/L)	20.2±8.3	37.6±35.0	97.1±249.9
ALP (IU/L)	41.7±19.2	78.4±20.6	123.5±77.6
HBV DNA levels (IU/mL)[a]			
Not detected		11	1
Detected (<10^3/units)		9	3
Detected (≥10^3/units)		6	25
Antiviral therapy[b]			
Yes (%)		23 (65.7%)	17 (28.3%)
No (%)		12 (34.3%)	43 (71.7%)
Treatment type			
Surgical resection			1
RFA			3
PEIT			22
TACE			30
TACE & PEIT			4
Tumor size (cm)[c]			
<2			21
2~5			16
>5			3
Tumor stage[d]			
I			30
II			15
III			10
IV			0
Target lesion response			
CR			38
PR			19
SD			3
PD			0

Abbreviations
TACE: Transcatheter arterial chemoembolization.
PEIT: Percutaneous ethanol injection therapy.
RFA: Radiofrequency ablation.
AFP: Alpha-fetoprotein.
ALT: Alanine aminotransferase; AST: Aspartate aminotransferase; ALP: Alkaline phosphatase.
CR: Complete Response; PR: Partial Response; SD: Stable disease; PD: Progressive disease.
Albumin, Bilirubin, AST, ALT, ALP, and HBV DNA levels data are presented as mean ± SD.
[a]HBV DNA levels were provided for 26 among a total of 35 liver cirrhosis patients, and 29 among the 60 HCC patients.
[b]Antiviral therapy was treatment with Entecavir, Tenofovir, Zeffix, Hepsera and Revovir.
[c]Tumor size was provided for 40 among a total of 60 HCC patients.
[d]According to American Joint Committee on Cancer (AJCC) staging system (7th edition, 2010).

centrifugal filtration using a 3000-Da molecular weight cutoff (MWCO) (Millipore, Bedford, MA). Concentrated serum protein was quantified by bicinchoninic acid (BCA) assay.

Aliquots of serum samples (100 µg) were denatured and digested as described above. Tryptic digestion was stopped with formic acid (FA) at a final concentration of 1% and desalted on OASIS HLB 1-cc (30 mg) extraction cartridges (Waters Corp., Milford, MA). The cartridges were equilibrated sequentially with 3 mL acetonitrile (ACN) and 5 mL water/0.1% FA prior to loading of the tryptic digestions. The cartridges were washed with 3 mL water/0.1% FA and eluted with 1 mL of 60% ACN/0.1% FA. The eluted samples were frozen and lyophilized on a speed vacuum. Before MRM-MS analysis, the samples were reconstituted in mobile phase A to 1 µg/µL.

MRM-MS transition (Q1/Q3) selection

Skyline software was used to generate a list of all possible b-, y-series fragment ions for 2^+ precursor ion charge states, spanning the m/z range from 300 to 1400. In brief, full-length protein sequences were imported into Skyline in FASTA format and designed into peptides, each with a list of product ions for monitoring by MRM-MS. In selecting transitions through Skyline, the peptide filter condition was as follows: maximum length of peptide of 24, including at least 6 amino acids.

Peptides with repeat arginines (Arg, R) or lysines (Lys, K) were discarded. If methionine (Met, M) was included in the peptide, it was discarded to avoid the risk of modification. If proline (Pro, P) was next to arginine (Arg, R) or lysine (Lys, K), the peptide was discarded. If a peptide contained histidine (His, H), it was discarded to avoid the risk of charge alterations. Peptides that satisfied these conditions were used as Q1 transitions. Next, we selected a maximum of 10 Q3 transitions from the fragmentation ions that were derived from the Q1 transitions in descending order.

For glycopeptides, theoretical transition values were selected, based on the original FASTA sequences after changing asparagine (Asn, N) in the NxS/T motif into aspartic acid (Asp, D), using Skyline. In addition, to verify that the measured peptides originated from the endogenous peptide that was tested, a stable isotope-labeled standard (SIS) peptide was used. The sequence of the SIS peptide is identical to that of the measured peptide but has ^{13}C and ^{15}N in the C-terminal arginine (Arg, R) and lysine (Lys, K). This result is described in Table S2.

Quantification by multiple reaction monitoring

An Agilent 1260 Infinity HPLC system was used to inject 5 µL of digestion samples directly into a reversed phase analytical column (150 mm×0.5 mm i.d., Agilent Zorbax SB-C18, 3.5-µm particle size) that was maintained at 40°C. Mobile phase A consisted of water/0.1% FA, and mobile phase B comprised ACN/0.1% FA. The peptides were separated and eluted at 20 µL/min on a linear gradient of mobile phase B from 3% to 40% B in 45 min. The gradient was ramped to 70% B for 5 min and 3% B for 10 min to equilibrate the column for the next run. The total LC run time was 60 min.

The MRM-MS data were analyzed using ESI on an Agilent 6490 triple quadrupole (QQQ) mass spectrometer (Agilent Technologies, Santa Clara, CA) that was equipped with an iFunnel Technology source and controlled by MassHunter Workstation software (Agilent, B.06.00). The MRM-MS analysis was conducted in the positive ion mode with the ion spray capillary voltage and nozzle voltage set to 2500 and 2000 V, respectively. The drying gas temperature was set to 250°C at 15 L/min, and the sheath gas temperature was 350°C at 12 L/min. The nebulizer was set to 30 psi, the fragmentor voltage was 380 V, and the cell accelerator voltage was 5 V. For the MRM-MS acquisition, delta EMV was set to 200 V. Quadrupoles 1 and 3 were maintained at unit (0.7 FWHM) resolution.

Collision energy optimization

The initial collision energy (CE) linear equation was derived from our optimized experiments, prior to the Skyline CE optimization step, using 600 stable isotope-labeled standard (SIS) peptides that were measured (data not shown). In the CE optimization module in Skyline, "Step count" was set to 5 on either side of the equation-predicted value, and "Step size" was set to 2V. The b and y ions for 2^+ precursor ion charge states were used, and in total, 11 collision energy voltage values were considered for each fragment ion. The maximum number of concurrent measurements was set to 132. The data were acquired and imported into Skyline for peak area integration, which was reviewed manually and finalized by a single investigator.

Study design for blocking and randomization

Blocking and randomization can prevent the negative impacts of nonbiologic effects on molecular biomarker discovery [16]. In our experiments, nonbiologic effects could have been introduced during the sample preparation (order of MARS depletion and order of tryptic digestion) and MRM-MS analysis (order of injection). Three step where the experimenter's subjectivity could have led to bias of sample groups was negated by blocked randomization method.

We applied the blocked randomization design when assigning the sample group to remove confounding nonbiologic effects. There were equal numbers of cases (HCC group) and controls (normal group) in every block, with random block size. We then assigned each group of order to a random permutation of the samples in the corresponding group (Table S3). Blocked randomization was performed using Excel (2013, Microsoft) and Random Allocation (version 1.00, University of Medical Sciences).

Statistical analysis of MRM-MS data

To analyze the MRM-MS data, raw MRM-MS data files were processed in Skyline. To increase the accuracy of the peak area integration, we manually confirmed and corrected the wrong automatic assignments for each targeted peak area. In our peak integration step, we used the Savitzky-Golay smoothing algorithm. Differences were analyzed by *T*-test between the normal versus HCC group and the LC versus stage I HCC subgroup. To evaluate the discriminatory power of the serum biomarkers between groups, we analyzed the receiver operator characteristic (ROC) curves and generated interactive plots. ROC curves were compared using DeLong's method [17]. All statistical analyses were performed using MedCalc (Mariakerke, Belgium, version 12.2.1).

Results

Overall scheme

We performed a combined measurement in a single run of the total AFP concentration and glycosylated AFP fraction after PNGase F treatment. There are 3 glycosylated forms of AFP–AFP-L1, L2, and L3–based on its reactivity to Lens culinaris agglutinin (LCA) by affinity electrophoresis (Figure S1A). The concentration of total AFP and the N-linked glycosylated AFP fraction (AFP-L1, L2 and L3) that can be cleaved by PNGase F (Figure S1B) could be measured by MRM-MS in the same MRM run.

To develop an MRM-MS method for measuring glycoprotein concentration, such as AFP, we measured a standard glycoprotein of INV1 to determine whether MRM-MS was suitable for measuring glycoprotein concentrations and applied MRM-MS to measure AFP concentrations (Figure 1). The total AFP concentration was measured, based on nonglycopeptides, whereas the glycosyated AFP fraction was represented by the corresponding deglycopeptide that was generated by PNGase F treatment. Consequently, the discriminatory power was examined for total AFP and glycosylated AFP in serum samples from normal healthy controls versus HCC patients and liver cirrhosis versus early-stage HCC patients.

Establishment of MRM-MS measurement using standard glycoprotein

We first determine whether MRM-MS is suitable for measuring glycoproteins using standard glycoproteins, such as yeast INV1. Four peptides were examined in developing and assessing the MRM-MS method (Figure S2A and Table S2): 2 peptides (IEIYSSDDLK and VVDFGK) were nonglycopeptides, and 2 were glycopeptides (NPVLAA*N*STQFR and FAT*N*TTLTK).

In examining their ability to be detected, all nonglycopeptides and deglycopeptides (SIS standard: Asn to Asp) coeluted with the corresponding SIS heavy peptides, whereas glycopeptides did not coelute with its SIS heavy peptide form (SIS standard: Asn with no

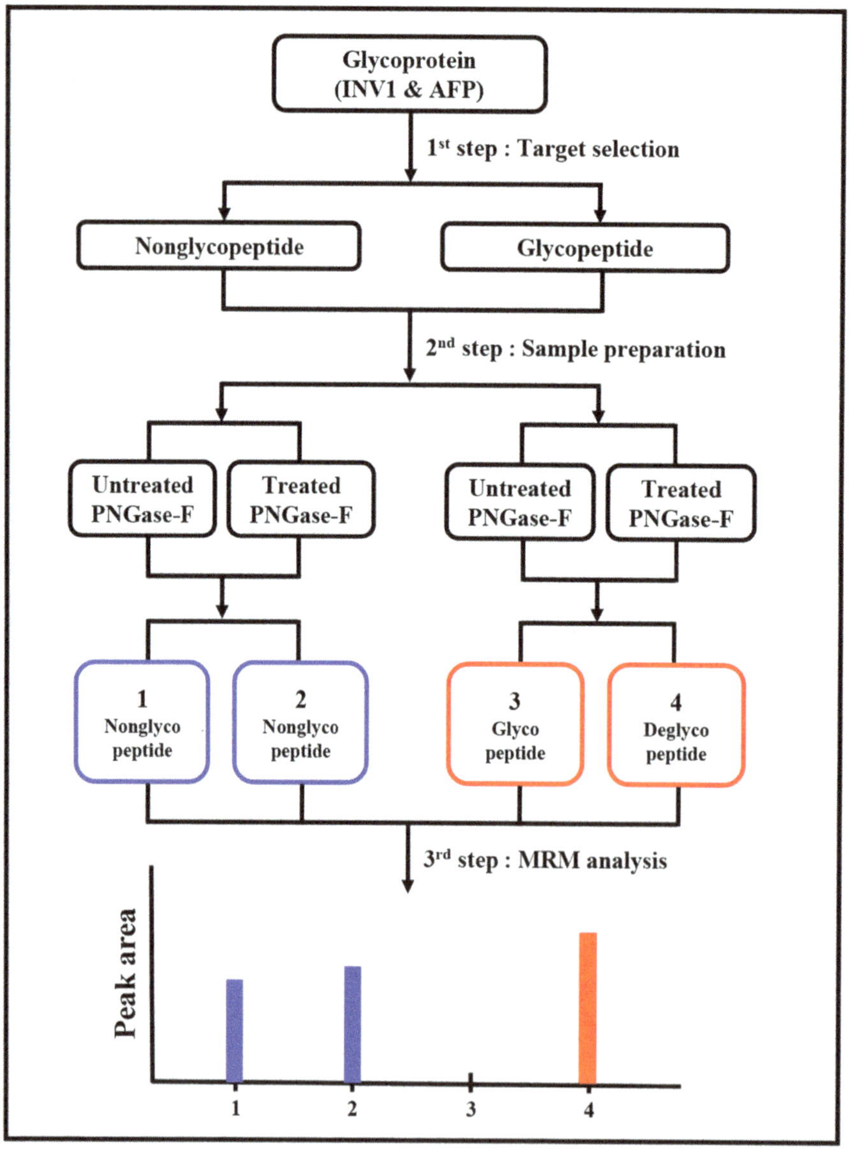

Figure 1. Development of MRM-MS method for measuring glycoproteins. To develop the MRM-MS method for measuring nonglycopeptides, glycopeptides, and deglycopeptides, we determined whether our MRM-MS approach was suitable for measuring glycoproteins using a standard glycoprotein, such as yeast invertase 1 (INV1), and applied the MRM-MS method to measure the alpha-fetoprotein (AFP) in human serum samples.

glycan). Because the SIS heavy peptides were synthesized only using Asn with no glycan, the SIS heavy peptide that represents the glycopeptide comprises only amino acid residues; thus, the existence of a glycopeptide is measured alternatively in the form as in the MRM-MS (eg, glycosylated Asn is measured as Asn or Asp). We measured the 4 peptides using the corresponding SIS heavy peptides, as detailed in Figure S3A–H. Because we could not use glycosylated SIS heavy peptides for the 2 glycopeptides, we measured the SIS heavy peptides NPVLAA*D*STQFR and FAT*D*TTLTK indirectly as substitutes for the glycopeptides NPVLAA*N*STQFR and FAT*N*TTLTK (Figure S3E & S3G).

Two nonglycopeptides (IEIYSSDDLK; Figure S3A & S3B, and VVDFGK; Figure S3C & S3D) were detected in the PNGase F-untreated (S3A, S3C) and PNGase F-treated (S3B, S3D) samples; the 2 nonglycopeptides had slightly greater intensity with PNGase F treatment (Figure S4). It is possible that PNGase F removes the glycan of a peptide, which may effect the absence of steric hindrance due to the glycan, allowing trypsin approach to a target peptide more easily. Consequently this accessibility might increase digestion and affect the peak intensity of MS/MS spectra [18].

The 2 glycopeptides (NPVLAA*N*STQFR and FAT*N*TTLTK) were detected only with PNGage F treatment as peaks of the corresponding deglycopeptides (NPVLAA*D*STQFR; Figure S3F, and FAT*D*TTLTK; Figure S3H). In the PNGase F-untreated, no extracted ion chromatogram (XIC) was detected for the endogenous glycopeptide forms, whereas SIS heavy peptides were detected with unglycosylated Asn (NPVLAA*N*STQFR; Figure S3E, and FAT*N*TTLTK; Figure S3G). In the MRM-MS analysis, glycopeptides could not be detected, because they were measured, based on the original sequence–ie, NPVLAA*N*STQFR and FAT*N*TTLTK, respectively. Conversely, the corresponding deglycosylated sequences for PNGage F-treated glycopeptides–NPVLAA*D*STQFR and FAT*D*TTLTK–were detected as MRM peaks for the glycosylated peptides of NPVLAA*N*STQFR and FAT*N*TTLTK, respectively.

To develop the quantitative method, we evaluated the linearity of nonglycopeptides, glycopeptides, and deglycopeptides that originated from INV1 by analyzing the standard curves of serial dilutions for known concentrations of SIS heavy peptides. To generate calibration curves for the 3 types of peptides, SIS heavy peptides were serially diluted (0, 4, 13, 40, 120, and 370 fmol), with the light peptides as internal standards. Digested light yeast peptide (370 nmol) was added to each diluted sample. Each experiment was repeated in triplicate to generate coefficients of variation (%CV) and calibration curve values (R^2).

The calibration curves demonstrated linearity over more than 2 orders of magnitude for the concentration ranges and strong linear correlation (R^2>0.99) in all 3 peptide forms (Figure S5A–D). By MRM-MS analysis using the standard peptides, we developed the MRM-MS method for measuring glycoprotein concentrations. Notably, the PNGase F-untreated endogenous light glycopeptides (NPVLAA*N*STQFR and FAT*N*TTLTK, filled downward arrows) did not generate peaks from MRM, as shown in Figure S5C–D.

Preliminary MRM-MS using pooled serum samples

Prior to MRM-MS of AFP using individual samples, we first selected predictable transitions using Skyline, in which the N-linked glycopeptide included the NxS/T motif, whereas the nonglycopeptide did not. Table 2 shows 3 AFP peptides that were used in the MRM-MS; the sequences of the nonglycopeptide, glycopeptide, and deglycopeptide of AFP were GYQELLEK, V*N*FTEIQK, and V*D*FTEIQK, respectively. For MRM-MS of the 3 AFP peptides, we determined their detectability in the preliminary MRM-MS run.

Nonglycopeptides (GYQELLEK) and deglycopeptide (V*D*FTEIQK) of AFP coeluted with the endogenous light and SIS heavy peptides at the same retention time. In brief, the nonglycopeptide (GYQELLEK) was coeluted in the PNGase F-untreated (Figure S6A) and PNGase F-treated (Figure S6B) conditions. However, the glycopeptide was not detected (Figure S6C) when the PNGase F-untreated glycosylated peptide was analyzed by the glycopeptide form with the no-glycan form (V*N*FTEIQK). The PNGage F-treated glycosylated peptide coeluted (Figure S6D) with the deglycopeptide form (V*D*FTEIQK).

Serum AFP concentrations rise in HCC patients versus normal subjects [19–22]; thus, we examined this difference between the normal healthy and HCC group using MRM-MS measurements. 20 normal samples and 20 HCC samples were pooled separately and analyzed by MRM-MS using the nonglycopeptide (GYQELLEK). The MS/MS intensity for the nonglycopeptide increased in the normal versus HCC group (Figure 2).

With regard to measuring glycopeptide concentrations, because the glycosylated glycopeptide form (V*N*FTEIQK) could not be detected directly using MRM-MS, we analyzed the deglycopeptide form (V*D*FTEIQK), which was generated by treating V*N*FTEIQK with PNGase F. The normalized peak area for the nonglycopeptide and deglycopeptide increased in HCC patients versus the normal group (Figure 2). Particularly, the peak area ratio of HCC to the normal group was 6.5 and 66.5 for the nonglycopeptide and deglycopeptide, respectively, indicating that total AFP concentration is a useful index for liver cancer diagnostics and that measuring the fraction of glycosylated AFP that has been treated by PNGase F is a more important element in HCC diagnosis.

Linearity of calibration curve for SIS AFP peptide

In the quantitative MRM-MS analysis, we determined the linearity of the nonglycopeptide (GYQELLEK) and deglycopeptide (V*D*FTEIQK) with regard to AFP, which was performed by generating a standard curve for the nonglycopeptide and deglycopeptide, composed of serial dilutions for known concentrations of SIS heavy peptides. SIS heavy peptides were serially diluted (9 concentrations: 0.0, 0.8, 1.6, 3.1, 6.3, 12.5, 25.0, 50.0, and 100.0 fmol) with the endogenous light peptide as an internal standard (pooled serum: 5 µg), added to each serially diluted sample. Each experiment was repeated in triplicate to generate coefficients of variation (%CV) and calibration curve values (R^2). The calibration curves were linear over more than 2 orders of magnitude in concentration, wherein the nonglycopeptide (GYQELLEK) and deglycopeptide (V*D*FTEIQ) showed strong linearity (R^2>0.99) (Figure 3).

MRM-MS measurements of AFP peptides using individual serum samples

To measure the nonglycopeptide (GYQELLEK) and deglycopeptide (V*D*FTEIQK) of AFP using MRM-MS in individual normal and HCC serum samples, we determined the optimal spiking concentrations for SIS heavy peptides that minimized the measurement errors for the peak area ratio between endogenous light peptide and SIS heavy peptide. By MRM analysis using pooled samples, which comprised endogenous light (pooled serum: 5 µg) and serially diluted SIS heavy peptides (0–200 fmol), we determined the optimal range of SIS heavy peptide for spiking (peak area ratio of light peptide to heavy peptide = 1). The concentrations of SIS heavy peptides for the nonglycopeptide (GYQELLEK) and deglycopeptide (V*D*FTEIQK) that were used to spike were 10.3 and 7.3 fmol, respectively.

Table 2. AFP peptides and their parameters for MRM-MS.

Peptide type	Peptide sequence	Q1 (m/z)	Q1 ion charge	Q3 (m/z)	Q3 ion charge	Q3 ion type	Retention time (min)	Isotope	Fragmentor (volt)	Initial CE (volt)	Optimized CE (volt)
Nonglycopeptide	GYQELLEK	490.3	2	759.4	1	y6	23.6	light	380	17.3	11.3
				631.4	1	y5	23.6	light	380	17.3	13.3
				502.3	1	y4	23.6	light	380	17.3	15.3
				389.2	1	y3	23.6	light	380	17.3	17.3
				276.2	1	y2	23.6	light	380	17.3	21.3
				221.1	1	b2	23.6	light	380	17.3	11.3
				349.2	1	b3	23.6	light	380	17.3	9.3
				591.3	1	b5	23.6	light	380	17.3	11.3
				704.4	1	b6	23.6	light	380	17.3	7.3
				833.4	1	b7	23.6	light	380	17.3	9.3
	GYQELLEK	494.3	2	767.4	1	y6	23.6	heavy	380	17.3	11.3
				639.4	1	y5	23.6	heavy	380	17.3	13.3
				510.3	1	y4	23.6	heavy	380	17.3	15.3
				397.3	1	y3	23.6	heavy	380	17.3	17.3
				284.2	1	y2	23.6	heavy	380	17.3	21.3
				221.1	1	b2	23.6	heavy	380	17.3	11.3
				349.2	1	b3	23.6	heavy	380	17.3	9.3
				591.3	1	b5	23.6	heavy	380	17.3	11.3
				704.4	1	b6	23.6	heavy	380	17.3	7.3
				833.4	1	b7	23.6	heavy	380	17.3	9.3
Glycopeptide[a]	VNFTEIQK	489.8	2	879.5	1	y7	22.0	light	380	17.3	13.3
				765.4	1	y6	22.0	light	380	17.3	13.3
				618.3	1	y5	22.0	light	380	17.3	15.3
				517.3	1	y4	22.0	light	380	17.3	11.3
				388.3	1	y3	22.0	light	380	17.3	21.3
				275.2	1	y2	22.0	light	380	17.3	21.3
				361.2	1	b3	22.0	light	380	17.3	9.3
				462.2	1	b4	22.0	light	380	17.3	9.3
				591.3	1	b5	22.0	light	380	17.3	11.3
				704.4	1	b6	22.0	light	380	17.3	9.3
				832.4	1	b7	22.0	light	380	17.3	7.3
	VNFTEIQK	493.8	2	887.5	1	y7	22.0	heavy	380	17.3	13.3
				773.4	1	y6	22.0	heavy	380	17.3	13.3
				626.4	1	y5	22.0	heavy	380	17.3	15.3
				525.3	1	y4	22.0	heavy	380	17.3	11.3
				396.3	1	y3	22.0	heavy	380	17.3	21.3

Table 2. Cont.

Peptide type	Peptide sequence	Q1 (m/z)	Q1 ion charge	Q3 (m/z)	Q3 ion charge	Q3 ion type	Retention time (min)	Isotope	Fragmentor (volt)	Initial CE (volt)	Optimized CE (volt)
				283.2	1	y2	22.0	heavy	380	17.3	21.3
				361.2	1	b3	22.0	heavy	380	17.3	9.3
				462.2	1	b4	22.0	heavy	380	17.3	9.3
				591.3	1	b5	22.0	heavy	380	17.3	11.3
				704.4	1	b6	22.0	heavy	380	17.3	9.3
				832.4	1	b7	22.0	heavy	380	17.3	7.3
Deglycopeptide	VDFTEIQK	490.3	2	880.4	1	y7	22.7	light	380	17.3	13.3
				765.4	1	y6	22.7	light	380	17.3	13.3
				618.3	1	y5	22.7	light	380	17.3	15.3
				517.3	1	y4	22.7	light	380	17.3	11.3
				388.3	1	y3	22.7	light	380	17.3	21.3
				275.2	1	y2	22.7	light	380	17.3	21.3
				362.2	1	b3	22.7	light	380	17.3	9.3
				463.2	1	b4	22.7	light	380	17.3	9.3
				592.3	1	b5	22.7	light	380	17.3	11.3
				705.3	1	b6	22.7	light	380	17.3	9.3
				833.4	1	b7	22.7	light	380	17.3	7.3
	VDFTEIQK	494.3	2	888.5	1	y7	22.7	heavy	380	17.3	13.3
				773.4	1	y6	22.7	heavy	380	17.3	13.3
				626.4	1	y5	22.7	heavy	380	17.3	15.3
				525.3	1	y4	22.7	heavy	380	17.3	11.3
				396.3	1	y3	22.7	heavy	380	17.3	21.3
				283.2	1	y2	22.7	heavy	380	17.3	21.3
				362.2	1	b3	22.7	heavy	380	17.3	9.3
				463.2	1	b4	22.7	heavy	380	17.3	9.3
				592.3	1	b5	22.7	heavy	380	17.3	11.3
				705.3	1	b6	22.7	heavy	380	17.3	9.3
				833.4	1	b7	22.7	heavy	380	17.3	7.3

[a]The molecular mass of glycopeptide is estimated based on Asn with no glycan moiety.

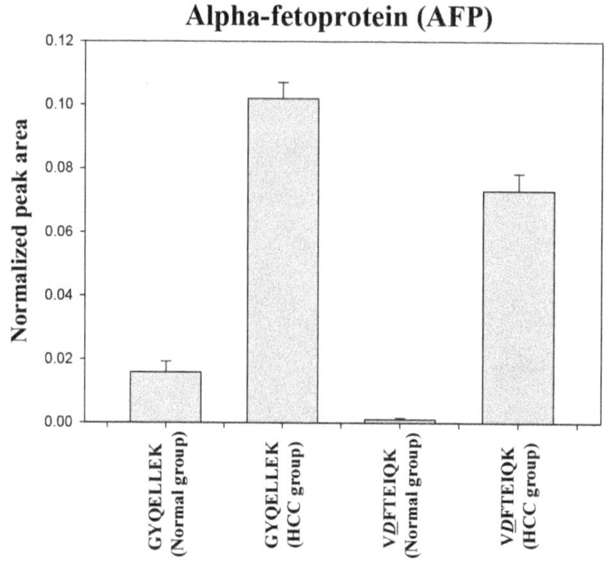

	Nonglycopeptide (GYQELLEK)		Deglycopeptide (VDFTEIQK)	
	Normal group	HCC group	Normal group	HCC group
1 set	0.0183	0.1064	0.0016	0.0675
2 set	0.0118	0.0963	0.0010	0.0782
3 set	0.0173	0.1032	0.0008	0.0734
Average	0.0158	0.1020	0.0011	0.0731
STDEV	0.0035	0.0051	0.0004	0.0054
CV (%)	22.3	5.0	38.5	7.3
Fold-change (HCC / Normal)		**6.5**		**66.1**

Figure 2. Preliminary MRM-MS analysis using pooled serum samples. Normal samples (n = 20) and HCC samples (n = 20) were pooled separately and analyzed by MRM-MS using the nonglycopeptide (GYQELLEK) and deglycopeptide (VDFTEIQK).

Individual serum samples were analyzed using the MRM-MS measurements with the spiked SIS heavy peptide mixture of nonglycopeptide (GYQELLEK) and deglycopeptide (VDFT EIQK) as the internal standard. Based on the MRM measurements using 155 individual serum samples, we measured the concentrations of the nonglycopeptide (GYQELLEK) and deglycopeptide (VDFTEIQK) of AFP in the normal (n = 60), LC group (n = 35) and HCC group (n = 60). The MRM measurements were imported into Skyline, and the peak areas of each transition were calculated, after normalization by the peak area of the spiked SIS heavy peptide (Figure S7). Next, the relative quantities of each transition were compared between the nonglycopeptide (GYQELLEK) and deglycopeptide (VDFTEIQK) in the normal versus HCC group and the LC versus stage I HCC subgroup.

To determine the efficacy of serum biomarkers in distinguishing HCC versus normal controls and the stage I HCC subgroup versus LC group, we drew receiver operator characteristic (ROC) curves and interactive plots, and the MRM-MS data on the nonglycopeptide (GYQELLEK) and deglycopeptide (VDF TEIQK) from both groups were analyzed. (Figure 4).

HCC group was compared to normal control group, the nonglycopeptide had a sensitivity of 56.7%, specificity of 68.3%, AUC of 0.687 [cutoff value: ≥0.02 (light/heavy ratio)] whereas the deglycopeptide had sensitivity of 93.3%, specificity of 68.3%, AUC of 0.859 [cutoff value: ≥0.02 (light/heavy ratio)] (Figure 4A).

In comparing the stage I HCC subgroup with the LC group, the nonglycopeptide had a sensitivity of 66.7%, specificity of 80.0%, and AUC of 0.712 [cutoff value: ≥0.02 (light/heavy ratio)], whereas the deglycopeptide had a sensitivity of 96.7%, specificity of 80.0%, and AUC of 0.918 [cutoff value: ≥0.02 (light/heavy ratio)] (Figure 4B). Thus, the discriminatory power of the deglycopeptide was greater versus the nonglycopeptide.

Pairwise differences in AUC values between nonglycopeptide and deglycopeptide estimations were analyzed by DeLong test [17]–the difference in AUC values was significant (normal vs HCC: P-value = 0.0010; LC vs stage I HCC: P-value = 0.0042) (Table S4).

Notably, considering that the nonglycopeptide (GYQELLEK) is measuring total AFP, it would be more advantageous to measure the deglycopeptide (VDFTEIQK) or take a combined measurement of nonglycopeptide (GYQELLEK) and deglycopeptide (VDFTEIQK), which could improve the diagnostic power in HCC.

Discussion

Most protein biomarkers are based on the premise that native proteins are differentially expressed in normal versus disease states. Recent studies have also demonstrated that protein biomarkers can discriminate such states according to the degree of glycosylation of native proteins [23–28].

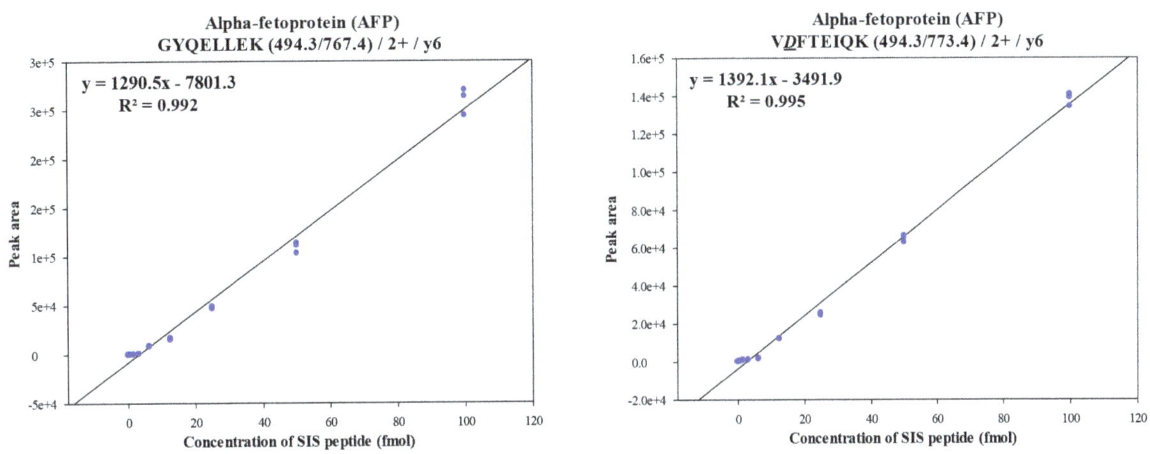

GYQELLEK (494.3/767.4) / 2+ / y6

Conc. (fmol)	Blank	0.0	0.8	1.6	3.1	6.3	12.5	25.0	50.0	100.0
Mean Area	7.33	70.67	441.00	524.33	1064.33	8809.33	16086.33	48325.33	109508.67	259150.09
STDEV	2.31	48.60	9.64	28.45	121.23	277.69	809.40	1110.34	5383.50	13769.43
CV (%)	31.49	68.78	2.19	5.43	11.39	3.15	5.03	2.30	4.92	5.31

VDFTEIQK (494.3/773.4) / 2+ / y6

Conc. (fmol)	Blank	0.0	0.8	1.6	3.1	6.3	12.5	25.0	50.0	100.0
Mean Area	7.00	307.00	640.00	1109.33	1296.67	1900.33	12319.33	25216.00	64973.00	138138.00
STDEV	5.57	14.11	61.59	83.20	12.90	194.20	76.85	669.63	1838.58	3336.99
CV (%)	79.54	4.60	9.62	7.50	0.99	10.22	0.62	2.66	2.83	2.42

Figure 3. Generation of calibration curve for nonglycopeptide (GYQELLEK) and deglycopeptide (VDFTEIQK) of AFP. To generate a calibration curve for the nonglycopeptide and deglycopeptide, SIS heavy peptides were serially diluted (9 concentration points: 0.0, 0.8, 1.6, 3.1, 6.3, 12.5, 25.0, 50.0, and 100.0 fmol) with the endogenous light peptide as an internal standard (pooled serum: 5 μg), added to each serially diluted sample. Each experiment was performed in triplicate to generate coefficients of variation (%CV) and calibration curve values (R^2).

In this study, we performed MRM measurements for 2 types of peptides (nonglycopeptide and deglycopeptide) that target a glycoprotein and serum AFP, wherein the amount of nonglycopeptide represents the total glycoprotein concentration and the deglycopeptide represents the glycosylated fraction of the glycoprotein. Based on our hypothesis, we compared the total AFP

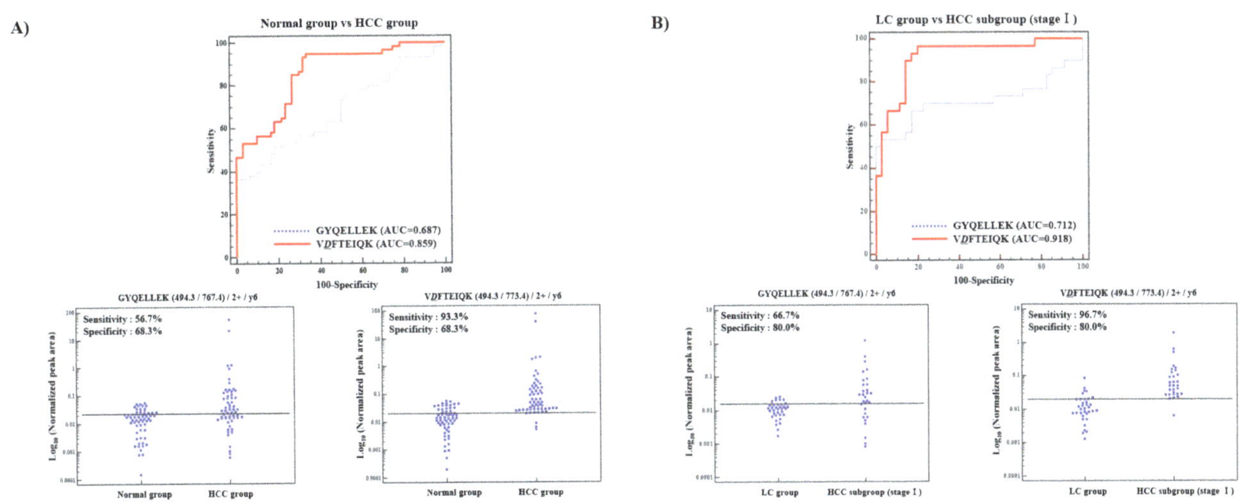

Figure 4. Receiver operating characteristic (ROC) curves and interactive plots for the nonglycopeptide (GYQELLEK) and deglycopeptide (VDFTEIQK) of AFP, respectively. The normalized peak areas of transitions were compared between normal and HCC group. In the interactive plots, sensitivity was calculated based on a specificity of 68.3%, which was calculated per an AFP cutoff value of 20 ng/mL (56.7% sensitivity), representing significant prognostic impact for HCC (A) LC was compared to Stage I HCC subgroup, in the interactive plots, sensitivity was calculated based on a specificity of 80.0% which was calculated with optimal deglycopeptide level (B).

concentration (represented as nonglycopeptide: GYQELLEK) with the glycosylated AFP fraction (represented as deglycopeptide: VDFTEIQK) between the normal, LC, and HCC groups.

To quantitatively analyze the total AFP and glycosylated AFP, respectively, we established an MRM-MS method for measuring the nonglycopeptide and deglycopeptide that corresponded to the glycosylated glycopeptide in serum samples. In developing this method, we first assessed whether the MRM-MS approach was suitable for measuring glycoprotein levels. We observed that MRM-MS measured the nonglycopeptide and deglycopeptide as alternatives to total AFP concentration and the glycosylated AFP fraction that was cleaved by PNGase F, respectively. Then, we performed MRM measurements for the endogenous light peptides and the SIS heavy peptides that coeluted with them as internal standards.

The nonglycopeptide was detected in the PNGase F-untreated and PNGase F-treated conditions, whereas the glycosylated glycopeptide was seen only after PNGase F treatment in the deglycopeptide form, because the original amino acid sequence with glycan could not be detected by MRM-MS. Specifically, although the PNGase F-treated deglycosylated state could be measured based on the deglycopeptide sequence (Asn changed to Asp), no glycopeptide could be detected by MRM in the glycosylated state (PNGase F-untreated). Thus, this sequence-based approach to the MRM measurements is useful in measuring the glycoprotein concentrations.

AFP is a significant marker for the clinical diagnosis and evaluation of suspected HCC patients. As a diagnostic tool for HCC, AFP level is determined by immunoenzymatic chemiluminescence; the cutoff of serum AFP levels for significant prognostic impact for HCC is 20 ng/mL (AFP-negative: <20 ng/mL and AFP-positive: ≥20 ng/mL) [22].

However, some reports have demonstrated that AFP level (cutoff value: ≥20 ng/mL) is a poor diagnostic tool in HCC, with a sensitivity of 54%. For example, 46%, 36%, and 18% of 1158 HCC patients had normal (<20 ng/mL), elevated (20–400 ng/mL), and diagnostic AFP levels (>400 ng/mL), respectively [29,30]. We noted the similar trend in AFP level in our HCC patients–as shown in Table 1, 43%, 30%, and 27% of 60 HCC patients had normal (<20 ng/mL), elevated (20–400 ng/mL), and diagnostic levels of AFP (>400 ng/mL), respectively (yielding a sensitivity of 56.7%). This result suggests that solely using total AFP level is not an effective method for distinguishing HCC from healthy subjects.

There are other biomarkers besides AFP that can be used to screen for HCC, such as DCP, also known as prothrombin induced by vitamin K absence II (PIVKA II). DCP is an abnormal product of liver carboxylation during thrombogen formation. The serum level of DCP in patients with HCC is significantly higher than in healthy adults and patients with nonmalignant hepatopathy (chronic hepatitis and cirrhosis) [31,32].

DCP can be used as a prognostic indicator for patients with small HCC tumors. High serum levels of DCP are also associated with a greater risk of HCC recurrence and worse overall survival in patients with an HCC tumor under 3 cm [33,34]. DCP can be used to evaluate the prognosis of patients with small HCC tumors but remains insufficient in the primary screening of HCC patients [35].

Recently, AFP-L3 (%) has been used as an additional indicator of total AFP in the diagnosis of HCC, demonstrating superior performance compared with measuring total AFP alone [36–41]. Similarly, we developed a MRM-based measurement approach using a deglycopeptide of AFP as an alternative to the glycosylated AFP fraction (AFP-L1, L2 and L3). By MRM-MS, the nonglycopeptide had a sensitivity of 56.7%, specificity of 68.3%, and AUC of 0.687 in distinguishing normal and HCC subjects versus 93.3%, 68.3%, and 0.859, respectively with the deglycopeptide. Also, the nonglycopeptide had a sensitivity of 66.7%, specificity of 80.0%, and AUC of 0.712 in distinguishing LC and the stage I HCC subgroup versus 96.7%, 80.0%, and 0.918, respectively, with the deglycopeptide. Thus, the discriminatory power of the deglycopeptide was better than that of the nonglycopeptide (Figure 4). To compare the nonglycopeptide and deglycopeptide of AFP accurately, we fixed their specificity in calculating the sensitivity.

In total, 30 HCC patients were primarily TNM stage I–ie, the early stage of HCC–suggesting that these findings can be applied to clinical settings in discriminating early-stage HCC from LC. Thus, deglycopeptide levels can differentiate small tumors from cirrhotic liver, which is significant, because other markers can not distinguish between early-stage HCC and LC. Our data indicate that upregulated deglycopeptide levels in early-stage HCC patients function in tumorigenesis and can be used as a marker for the early detection of a cirrhotic liver that progresses to HCC.

Our MRM-MS-based method has benefits in verifying glycoprotein biomarkers in human samples, because it does not require any complex or irreproducible glycoprotein enrichment steps. Further, determining the amount and extent of glycosylation in glycoproteins is difficult through conventional methods. Specifically, the differences in expression and degree of glycosylation of AFP have not been compared using antibody-based assays, such as western blot and ELISA (enzyme-linked immunosorbent assay).

Ultimately, 2 types of peptide markers–a nonglycopeptide and deglycopeptide–were used to distinguish HCC from normal controls and early-stage HCC from the LC group. Further verification of their value in larger samples should facilitate the development of better biomarkers for HCC.

Author Contributions

Conceived and designed the experiments: J-HY YK. Performed the experiments: HK KK. Analyzed the data: JJ SJY JP. Contributed reagents/materials/analysis tools: J-HY YK. Contributed to the writing of the manuscript: HK KK. Modified the manuscript: J-HY YK.

References

1. Bertozzi CR, Sasisekharan R (2009) Glycomics. In: Varki A, Cummings RD, Esko JD, Freeze HH, Stanley P, et al., editors. Essentials of Glycobiology. Cold Spring Harbor NY: The Consortium of Glycobiology Editors, La Jolla, California.
2. Durand G, Seta N (2000) Protein glycosylation and diseases: blood and urinary oligosaccharides as markers for diagnosis and therapeutic monitoring. Clin Chem 46: 795–805.
3. Spiro RG (2002) Protein glycosylation: nature, distribution, enzymatic formation, and disease implications of glycopeptide bonds. Glycobiology 12: 43R-56R.
4. Anderson NL, Anderson NG (2002) The human plasma proteome: history, character, and diagnostic prospects. Mol Cell Proteomics 1: 845–867.
5. Miyoshi E, Noda K, Yamaguchi Y, Inoue S, Ikeda Y, et al. (1999) The alpha1-6-fucosyltransferase gene and its biological significance. Biochim Biophys Acta 1473: 9–20.
6. Kamoto T, Satomura S, Yoshiki T, Okada Y, Henmi F, et al. (2002) Lectin-reactive alpha-fetoprotein (AFP-L3%) curability and prediction of clinical course after treatment of non-seminomatous germ cell tumors. Jpn J Clin Oncol 32: 472–476.
7. Li D, Mallory T, Satomura S (2001) AFP-L3: a new generation of tumor marker for hepatocellular carcinoma. Clin Chim Acta 313: 15–19.
8. Khien VV, Mao HV, Chinh TT, Ha PT, Bang MH, et al. (2001) Clinical evaluation of lentil lectin-reactive alpha-fetoprotein-L3 in histology-proven hepatocellular carcinoma. Int J Biol Markers 16: 105–111.

9. Chu CW, Hwang SJ, Luo JC, Lai CR, Tsay SH, et al. (2001) Clinical, virologic, and pathologic significance of elevated serum alpha-fetoprotein levels in patients with chronic hepatitis C. J Clin Gastroenterol 32: 240–244.
10. Wang B, Chen D, Chen Y, Hu Z, Cao M, et al. (2012) Metabonomic profiles discriminate hepatocellular carcinoma from liver cirrhosis by ultraperformance liquid chromatography-mass spectrometry. J Proteome Res 11: 1217–1227.
11. Daniele B, Bencivenga A, Megna AS, Tinessa V (2004) Alpha-fetoprotein and ultrasonography screening for hepatocellular carcinoma. Gastroenterology 127: S108–112.
12. Colli A, Fraquelli M, Casazza G, Massironi S, Colucci A, et al. (2006) Accuracy of ultrasonography, spiral CT, magnetic resonance, and alpha-fetoprotein in diagnosing hepatocellular carcinoma: a systematic review. Am J Gastroenterol 101: 513–523.
13. Boja E, Rivers R, Kinsinger C, Mesri M, Hiltke T, et al. (2010) Restructuring proteomics through verification. Biomark Med 4: 799–803.
14. Bruix J, Sherman M (2011) Management of hepatocellular carcinoma: an update. Hepatology 53: 1020–1022.
15. Kim H, Kim K, Yu SJ, Jang ES, Yu J, et al. (2013) Development of biomarkers for screening hepatocellular carcinoma using global data mining and multiple reaction monitoring. PLoS One 8: e63468.
16. Qin LX, Zhou Q, Bogomolniy F, Villafania L, Olvera N, et al. (2014) Blocking and randomization to improve molecular biomarker discovery. Clin Cancer Res 20: 3371–3378.
17. DeLong ER, DeLong DM, Clarke-Pearson DL (1988) Comparing the areas under two or more correlated receiver operating characteristic curves: a nonparametric approach. Biometrics 44: 837–845.
18. Lee JY, Kim JY, Park GW, Cheon MH, Kwon KH, et al. (2011) Targeted mass spectrometric approach for biomarker discovery and validation with nonglycosylated tryptic peptides from N-linked glycoproteins in human plasma. Mol Cell Proteomics 10: M111 009290.
19. Malaguarnera G, Giordano M, Paladina I, Berretta M, Cappellani A, et al. (2010) Serum markers of hepatocellular carcinoma. Dig Dis Sci 55: 2744–2755.
20. Witjes CD, van Aalten SM, Steyerberg EW, Borsboom GJ, de Man RA, et al. (2013) Recently introduced biomarkers for screening of hepatocellular carcinoma: a systematic review and meta-analysis. Hepatol Int 7: 59–64.
21. Lai Q, Melandro F, Pinheiro RS, Donfrancesco A, Fadel BA, et al. (2012) Alpha-fetoprotein and novel tumor biomarkers as predictors of hepatocellular carcinoma recurrence after surgery: a brilliant star raises again. Int J Hepatol 2012: 893103.
22. Zhou L, Rui JA, Wang SB, Chen SG, Qu Q (2012) The significance of serum AFP cut-off values, 20 and 400 ng/mL in curatively resected patients with hepatocellular carcinoma and cirrhosis might be of difference. Hepatogastroenterology 59: 840–843.
23. Alavi A, Axford JS (2008) Glyco-biomarkers: potential determinants of cellular physiology and pathology. Dis Markers 25: 193–205.
24. Peracaula R, Barrabes S, Sarrats A, Rudd PM, de Llorens R (2008) Altered glycosylation in tumours focused to cancer diagnosis. Dis Markers 25: 207–218.
25. An HJ, Kronewitter SR, de Leoz ML, Lebrilla CB (2009) Glycomics and disease markers. Curr Opin Chem Biol 13: 601–607.
26. Drake PM, Cho W, Li B, Prakobphol A, Johansen E, et al. (2010) Sweetening the pot: adding glycosylation to the biomarker discovery equation. Clin Chem 56: 223–236.
27. Hua S, An HJ (2012) Glycoscience aids in biomarker discovery. BMB Rep 45: 323–330.
28. Reis CA, Osorio H, Silva L, Gomes C, David L (2010) Alterations in glycosylation as biomarkers for cancer detection. J Clin Pathol 63: 322–329.
29. Farinati F, Marino D, De Giorgio M, Baldan A, Cantarini M, et al. (2006) Diagnostic and prognostic role of alpha-fetoprotein in hepatocellular carcinoma: both or neither? Am J Gastroenterol 101: 524–532.
30. Kulik LM (2007) Advancements in hepatocellular carcinoma. Curr Opin Gastroenterol 23: 268–274.
31. Cui R, Wang B, Ding H, Shen H, Li Y, et al. (2002) Usefulness of determining a protein induced by vitamin K absence in detection of hepatocellular carcinoma. Chin Med J (Engl) 115: 42–45.
32. Marrero JA, Su GL, Wei W, Emick D, Conjeevaram HS, et al. (2003) Des-gamma carboxyprothrombin can differentiate hepatocellular carcinoma from nonmalignant chronic liver disease in american patients. Hepatology 37: 1114–1121.
33. Khan KN, Yatsuhashi H, Yamasaki K, Yamasaki M, Inoue O, et al. (2000) Prospective analysis of risk factors for early intrahepatic recurrence of hepatocellular carcinoma following ethanol injection. J Hepatol 32: 269–278.
34. Nagaoka S, Yatsuhashi H, Hamada H, Yano K, Matsumoto T, et al. (2003) The des-gamma-carboxy prothrombin index is a new prognostic indicator for hepatocellular carcinoma. Cancer 98: 2671–2677.
35. Koike Y, Shiratori Y, Sato S, Obi S, Teratani T, et al. (2001) Des-gamma-carboxy prothrombin as a useful predisposing factor for the development of portal venous invasion in patients with hepatocellular carcinoma: a prospective analysis of 227 patients. Cancer 91: 561–569.
36. Taketa K, Endo Y, Sekiya C, Tanikawa K, Koji T, et al. (1993) A collaborative study for the evaluation of lectin-reactive alpha-fetoproteins in early detection of hepatocellular carcinoma. Cancer Res 53: 5419–5423.
37. Aoyagi Y, Suzuki Y, Isemura M, Nomoto M, Sekine C, et al. (1988) The fucosylation index of alpha-fetoprotein and its usefulness in the early diagnosis of hepatocellular carcinoma. Cancer 61: 769–774.
38. Aoyagi Y, Saitoh A, Suzuki Y, Igarashi K, Oguro M, et al. (1993) Fucosylation index of alpha-fetoprotein, a possible aid in the early recognition of hepatocellular carcinoma in patients with cirrhosis. Hepatology 17: 50–52.
39. Oda K, Ido A, Tamai T, Matsushita M, Kumagai K, et al. (2011) Highly sensitive lens culinaris agglutinin-reactive alpha-fetoprotein is useful for early detection of hepatocellular carcinoma in patients with chronic liver disease. Oncol Rep 26: 1227–1233.
40. Yamashiki N, Seki T, Wakabayashi M, Nakagawa T, Imamura M, et al. (1999) Usefulness of Lens culinaris agglutinin A-reactive fraction of alpha-fetoprotein (AFP-L3) as a marker of distant metastasis from hepatocellular carcinoma. Oncol Rep 6: 1229–1232.
41. Hayashi K, Kumada T, Nakano S, Takeda I, Sugiyama K, et al. (1999) Usefulness of measurement of Lens culinaris agglutinin-reactive fraction of alpha-fetoprotein as a marker of prognosis and recurrence of small hepatocellular carcinoma. Am J Gastroenterol 94: 3028–3033.

ROCK is Involved in Vasculogenic Mimicry Formation in Hepatocellular Carcinoma Cell Line

Ji-Gang Zhang[1], Xiao-Yu Li[1], Yu-Zhu Wang[1], Qi-Di Zhang[2], Sheng-Ying Gu[1], Xin Wu[1], Guan-Hua Zhu[1], Qin Li[1]*, Gao-Lin Liu[1]***

1 Department of Pharmacy, Shanghai First People's Hospital, School of medicine, Shanghai Jiao Tong University, Shanghai, P.R. China, **2** Department of Gastroenterology, Shanghai First People's Hospital, School of medicine, Shanghai Jiao Tong University, Shanghai, P.R. China

Abstract

Ras homolog family member A (RhoA) and Rho-associated coiled coil-containing protein kinases 1 and 2 (ROCK1 and 2) are key regulators of focal adhesion, actomyosin contraction and cell motility. RhoA/ROCK signaling has emerged as an attractive target for the development of new cancer therapeutics. Whether RhoA/ROCK is involved in regulating the formation of tumor cell vasculogenic mimicry (VM) is largely unknown. To confirm this hypothesis, we performed *in vitro* experiments using hepatocellular carcinoma (HCC) cell lines. Firstly, we demonstrated that HCC cells with higher active RhoA/ROCK expression were prone to form VM channels, as compared with RhoA/ROCK low-expressing cells. Furthermore, Y27632 (a specific inhibitor of ROCK) rather than exoenzyme C3 (a specific inhibitor of RhoA) effectively inhibited the formation of tubular network structures in a dose-dependent manner. To elucidate the possible mechanism of ROCK on VM formation, real-time qPCR, western blot and immunofluorescence were used to detect changes of the key VM-related factors, including VE-cadherin, erythropoietin-producing hepatocellular carcinoma-A2 (EphA2), phosphoinositide 3-kinase (PI3K), matrix metalloproteinase (MMP)14, MMP2, MMP9 and laminin 5γ2-chain (LAMC2), and epithelial-mesenchymal-transition (EMT) markers: E-cadherin and Vimentin. The results showed that all the expression profiles were attenuated by blockage of ROCK. In addition, *in vitro* cell migration and invasion assays showed that Y27632 inhibited the migration and invasion capacity of HCC cell lines in a dose-dependent manner markedly. These data indicate that ROCK is an important mediator in the formation of tumor cell VM, and suggest that ROCK inhibition may prove useful in the treatment of VM in HCC.

Editor: Hidayatullah G. Munshi, Northwestern University, United States of America

Funding: This work was supported by grants from the National Natural Science Foundation of China (NSFC, No.81372310) and (NSFC, No.81100800). The funders had no role in study design, data collection and analysis, decision to publish, or preparation of the manuscript.

Competing Interests: The authors have declared that no competing interests exist.

* Email: gaolinliu@aliyun.com (GLL); liqin0626@hotmail.com (QL)

These authors contributed equally to this work.

Introduction

Vasculogenic mimicry (VM) was first described by Maniotis et al. [1] as a new blood supply system independent of endothelial vessels in malignant melanoma. It reflects the plasticity of aggressive tumor cells that express vascular cell markers and line tumor vasculature as has been demonstrated in many malignant tumors including HCC, the third most common cause of cancer mortality worldwide [2–5]. As extensive signaling pathways involved in the pathogenesis of HCC reflect the heterogeneity and complexity of liver carcinogenesis, understanding the roles of these pathways in the pathogenesis of HCC is essential for the effective prevention and treatment of HCC. Recently, a growing number of *in vitro* and *in vivo* studies using tumor-derived cell lines, primary tumors and animal cancer models strongly suggest that altered Rho GTPase signaling plays an important role in the development and progression of HCC. The overexpression or repression of GTPases or some upstream or downstream elements of Rho signaling has been reported to be associated with many human tumors [6].

The presence of VM was reported to be associated with a high tumor grade, short survival, and invasion and metastasis [7,8]. Metastasis is the biggest threat to survival of patients with solid tumors, and cell migration is a pivotal step in metastasis [9]. Indeed, loss of polarity, disruption of cell-cell contacts and increase in cell motility are key events in the acquisition of the pro-invasive and metastatic phenotypes [10]. Interestingly, the RhoA small GTPase and its serine/threonine kinase downstream effector (ROCK1 and 2) control a wide variety of ubiquitous biological processes including the acquisition of unlimited proliferation potential, survival and evasion from apoptosis, tissue invasion differentiation, gene expression, and in particular, regulation of cell detachment, cell movement and establishment of metastasis [6,11]. In addition, VM formation involving tumor cells mimics endothelial cells consisting of a type of mesenchymal cells, which is similar to epithelial to EMT, a process whereby fully differentiated epithelial cells lose epithelial characteristics and acquire mesenchymal ones. EMT is proposed to be a crucial mechanism regulating the initial steps in metastatic progression [12]. It has been demonstrated that Rho activity is required to induce EMT in a number of cell typesm [13,14]. However, RhoA/ROCK as a therapeutic target for VM has not been documented.

Since the introduction of VM, a plethora of studies have attributed mechanistic insights into the induction, formation and targeting of VM across a variety of cancers. However, the pathogenesis of VM is a complex process involving extensive signaling pathways. The first two proteins identified to play a role in mediating melanoma VM are VE-cadherin, a cell-cell adhesion molecule associated with endothelial cells, and EphA2, an epithelial cell associated kinase involved in ephrin-A1-induced angiogenesis [15]. VE-cadherin regulates EphA2 activity by mediating its ability to get phosphorylated through interactions with its membrane-bound ligand ephrin-A1, thus activating the expression of PI3K, MMP14 and MMP2. Both MMP14 and MMP2 promote the cleavage of LAMC2 into promigratory $\gamma 2'$ and $\gamma 2\times$ fragments, which in turn stimulates migration, invasion, and VM in melanoma cells [16]. The MMPs family, especially MMP2, MMP9 and MMP14, together with LAMC2, PI3K, VE-cadherin and EphA2, participate in the key signaling pathway of VM formation [17]. Interestingly, Rho GTPases can also regulate the production of MMPs, affecting matrix remodeling and tumor cell invasion. Rho can induce the expression or secretion of MMPs [18]. The purpose of this study was to determine whether RhoA/ROCK signaling was involved in HCC cell VM formation *in vitro*, and explore the possible mechanism.

In this study, we sought to characterize the ability of RhoA/ROCK signaling to act as a mediator in the process of VM formation. It was found that the expression of RhoA, ROCK1 and ROCK2 proteins varied in HCC cell lines, indicating different VM formation potentials. Furthermore, we examined the ROCK paralog-specific roles in EMT to investigate the possible mechanism of its contribution to VM formation. Finally, we blocked the RhoA/ROCK pathway with the pharmacological inhibitor exoenzyme C3 and Y27632 and analyzed the biological effects using *in vitro* angiogenic assays to monitor tube formation, the key VM-related factors expression, migration and survival.

Results

Correlations between the expression level of RhoA/ROCK and the capacity of VM formation

To examine the involvement of RhoA/ROCK signaling in VM formation, VM capacity and expression of RhoA, ROCK1 and ROCK2 were investigated in five HCC cell lines with different metastasis potentials and one hepatocyte cell line. Human umbilical vein endothelial cells (HUVEC) were used as positive controls. Test of formation of tubular network structures on Matrigel was used to determine the capacity of VM *in vitro*. It was found that MHCC97H and HUVEC had the capacity of VM formation (Figure. 1A). However, the other HCC cell lines failed to form any tube or network. As shown in (Figure. 1B), both RhoA and ROCK were present at detectable levels. Statistical analysis showed that the expression level of RhoA, ROCK1 and ROCK2 in HUVEC and MHCC97H was significantly higher than that in other HCC cell lines (Figure. 1C, $^{*}P<0.05$ and $^{**}P<0.01$ *vs.* HUVEC and $^{\#}P<0.05$ and $^{\#\#}P<0.01$ *vs.* MHCC97H). However, there were no statistically significant differences between MHCC97H and HUVEC ($P>0.05$ *vs.* HUVEC). These data indicate that compared with the low-expression cells, HCC cells with higher active RhoA/ROCK expression were more likely to form VM channels, suggesting that the RhoA/ROCK signaling pathway was positively correlated with the potential of VM formation in HCC cells.

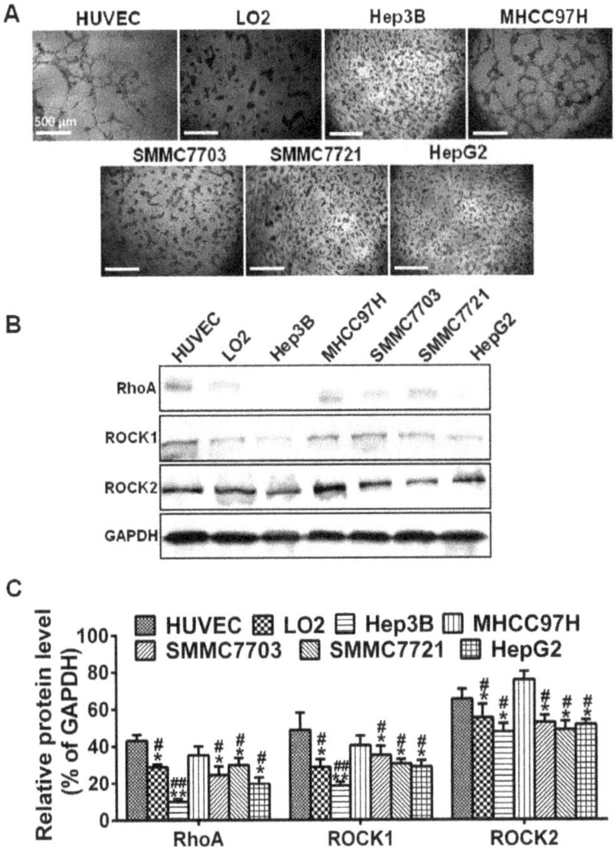

Figure 1. VM capacity and expression of RhoA, ROCK1 and ROCK2 in HCC cell lines. (**A**) Formation of tubular network structures on Matrigel by HUVEC and LO2 compared to HCC cell lines. Cells were seeded into Matrigel-coated 24-well plates and incubated at 37°C. Photographs were taken after 24 h, with original magnification of 40×, scale bars represent 500 μm. (**B**) Western blot was performed to confirm the protein expression of RhoA, ROCK1 and ROCK2 in HCC cell lines and LO2, using HUVEC as a positive control. (**C**) Relative densities (RD) are presented as mean ± S.E. (n = 3) of the fold change relative to the internal control. GAPDH was used as an internal control for protein loading. $^{*}P<0.05$ and $^{**}P<0.01$ *vs.* HUVEC and $^{\#}P<0.05$ and $^{\#\#}P<0.01$ *vs.* MHCC97H.

Effect of RhoA and ROCK inhibition on MHCC97H cell VM formation

Exoenzyme C3 and Y27632 were chosen as RhoA and ROCK inhibitors, respectively. To see whether blockage of RhoA/ROCK exerted an inhibitory effect on MHCC97H cell-mediated neovascularization *in vitro*, we observed the morphology of cell seizure activity in culture medium containing Y27632 or exoenzyme C3. MHCC97H cells were seeded onto Matrigel, and the formation of capillary-like structures was monitored and photographed after 8- and 24-h incubation (Figure. 2A and B). As shown in (Figure. 2B, left panel and C), Y27632 at concentrations of 10 μM and 50 μM dose-dependently reduced the formation of tubule-like structures ($^{**}P<0.01$ and $^{***}P<0.001$, *vs.* the control). Compared with the control, the formation of the tubular network was reduced almost by 80% at 50 μM of the compound, which provided the first evidence addressing the importance of this pathway in channel formation. Strikingly, there was no prominent dose-dependent destruction in the preformed VM structures with exoenzyme C3 treatment at the indicated concentrations in MHCC97H cells ($P>$ 0.05, Figure. 2B, right panel and D). These data suggest that

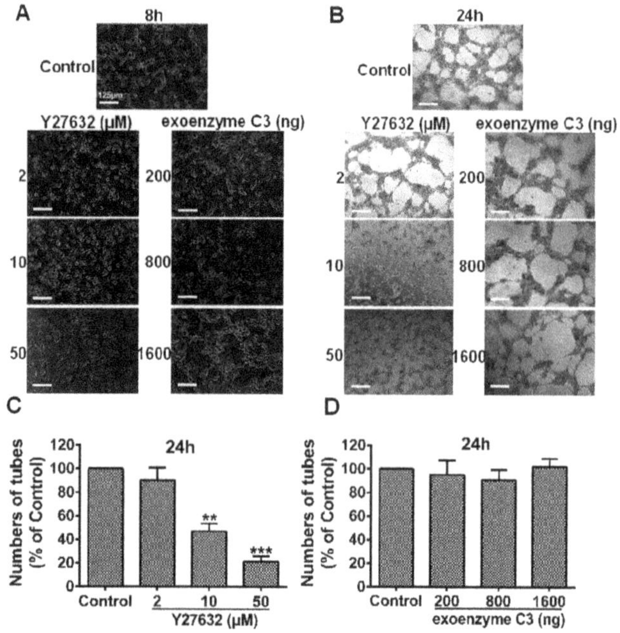

Figure 2. The impact of increased doses of Y27632 or exoenzyme C3 on VM formation. VM formation of MHCC97H cells cultured in Matrigel-coated 24-well plates, with culture medium containing Y27632 (2, 10 or 50 μM) or exoenzyme C3 (200, 800 or 1600 ng) for 8 h (**A**) or 24 h. (**B**). Photographs were taken at the indicated time points, and original magnification was 100×, scale bars represent 125 μm. (**C**), (**D**) Quantitative analysis of the mean number of tube-like structures formed from six randomly chosen areas in 3D cultures. Data are expressed as mean ± S.E. from three independent experiments, with significant differences from control designated as $^{**}P<0.01$ and $^{***}P<0.001$.

RhoA may not be essential for the VM process. Altogether, Y27632 treatment was sufficient to abolish tube structures through blocking ROCK activity, indicating the potential role of ROCK as a mediator of VM.

ROCK expression is consistent with the process of VM formation

It was found that MHCC97H cells began aggregating, adhering and gradually forming characteristic tubular structures within 8 h after plating on Matrigel, and this process was basically completed within 24 h (Figure. 3A). To see whether the up-regulation of RhoA/ROCK contributed to VM formation, western blot analysis of whole cell lysates from these experimental samples was conducted to assess the expression of ROCK and VM-associated marker (VE-cadherin). As shown in (Figure. 3B and C), the expression level of ROCK varied in a time-dependent manner similar to the case with VE-cadherin. In addition, the levels of both ROCK1 and ROCK2 began rising significantly at 8 h ($^{*}P<0.05$, *vs.* 0 h), and peaked at 24 h, which is consistent with the process of VM formation. These observations indicate that RhoA/ROCK signaling pathway was positively correlated with the potential of VM formation, which is consistent with the correlation that we observed between RhoA/ROCK signaling pathway and VM formation.

Blockage of ROCK inhibits VM formation by reducing EMT

Previous studies [15] suggested that EMT was involved in the VM formation in HCC. To determine the correlation between

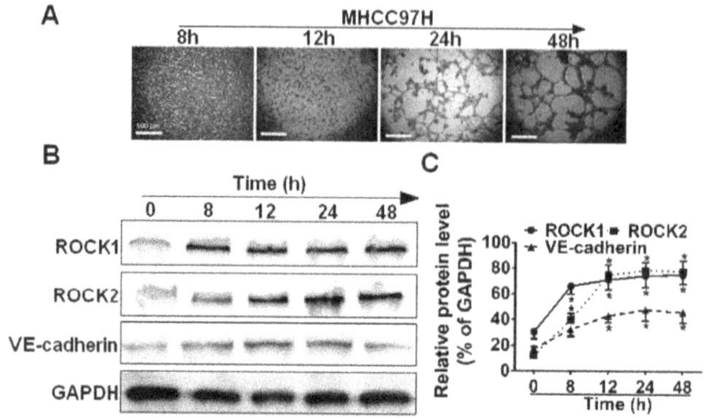

Figure 3. ROCK expression is consistent with the process of VM formation. (**A**) Formation of tubular network structures on Matrigel over 48 h. MHCC97H cells were subjected to Matrigel and photographed at 8, 12, 24 and 48 h, scale bars represent 500 μm. (**B**) Cell lysates from MHCC97H cells were seeded onto matrigel at the indicated time points and western blotted. (**C**) Relative protein level of each condition was quantitated using Image J and represented as line chart corresponding to pixels detected, (n = 3).

ROCK and EMT in VM formation, we decided to analyze the effect of Y27632 on EMT markers (Vimentin and E-cadherin). As shown in (Figure. 4A and B), MHCC97H significantly increased the expression of mesenchymal marker (Vimentin) and decreased the expression of epithelial marker (E-cadherin) in a time-dependent manner during VM formation, compared with 0 h ($^{*}P<0.05$). In contrast, the process was reversed upon Y27632 mediation at 10 and 50 μM (Figure. 4C and D). These data suggest that blockage of ROCK vanished VM formation in MHCC97H by reducing the occurrence of EMT.

Y27632 induces a robust alteration in protein and gene expression profiles related to VM

Signaling cascades involved in vasculogenic mimicry can be categorized into pathways associated with vascular, embryonic and/or stem cells, and hypoxia signaling [7], while vascular

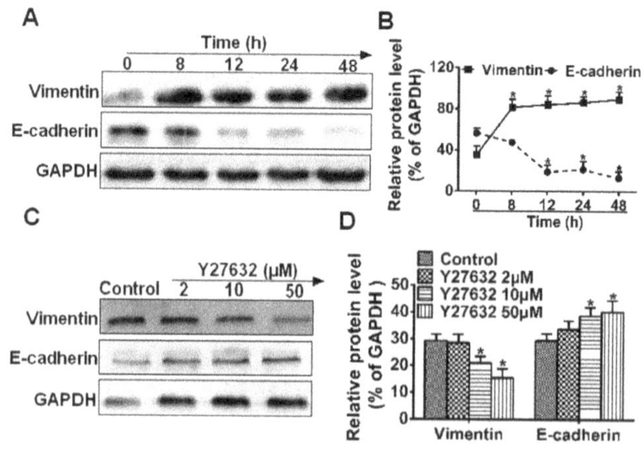

Figure 4. The effect of ROCK inhibition on the acquisition of an EMT phenotype. Western blot analysis showed that MHCC97H cells subjected to Matrigel with culture medium treated (**C**) or not treated (**A**) with Y27632 for 48 h regulated Vimentin and E-cadherin expression. GAPDH was used as a loading control. Quantification of EMT markers is shown in (**B**) and (**D**). The data are reported as mean ± S.E. ($^{*}P<0.05$ compared to 0 h or the control, n = 3).

signaling pathways are considered critical for vasculogenic events [17]. To further characterize the RhoA/ROCK signaling pathway mediating VM activation, western blot of whole cell lysates from these experimental samples was performed after addition of Y27632. As shown in (Figure. 5A and B), Y27632 suppressed the expression of protein in a dose-dependent manner. More specifically, VE-cadherin, MMP2 and MMP9 were down-regulated markedly after treatment with Y27632 (50 μM) as compared with the controls (*$P<0.05$), while the expressions of VE-cadherin and MMP9 were not affected significantly in the other two groups. The immunofluorescence analysis showed that no differences in VE-cadherin and MMP9 were observed between the control group and the Y27632 (2 and 10 μM) groups after 24 hours of incubation (Figure 5C), which is consistent with the results detected by western blot. To further deliberate the mechanism underlying the Y27632-mediated anti-vasculogenic effect, we evaluated six important tumor vasculogenic genes, using the primers shown in **Table 1**. Analyses of VE-cadherin, EphA2, PI3K, MMP14, MMP2 and MMP9 by real-time qPCR (Figure. 5D) showed that the Y27632 (50 μM) significantly inhibited mRNA levels, as compared with the controls (*$P<0.05$). Taken together, these results demonstrate that Y27632 had the potential to exogenously affect VM activity of MHCC97H cells in a consistent manner, strongly implying that the RhoA/ROCK pathway was involved in VM development.

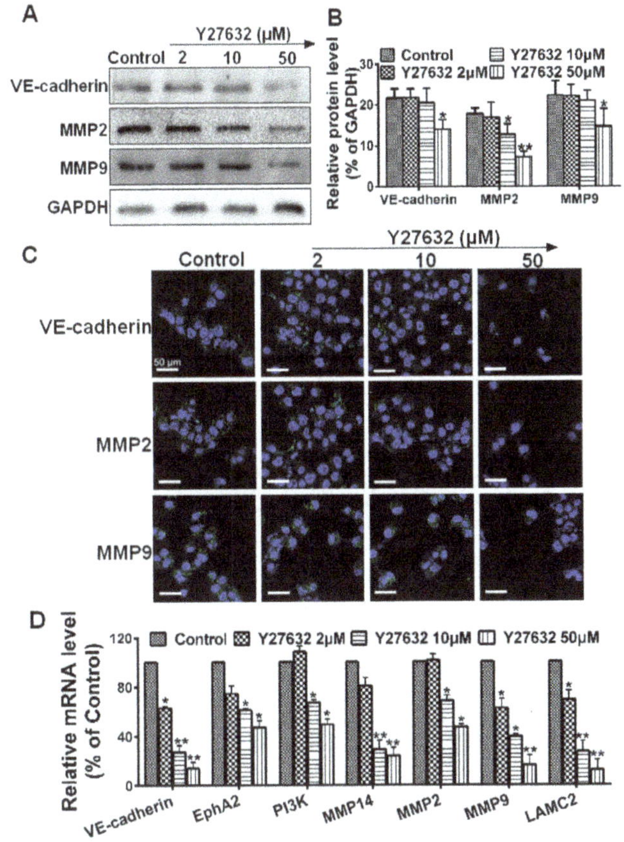

Figure 5. The effect of ROCK inhibition on the expression of VM-key factors. (**A**) Western blot assay was performed to evaluate the effect of ROCK inhibition on VM markers. (**B**) Relative protein level was quantitated using Image J (*$P<0.05$ and **$P<0.01$, ROCK inhibitor groups *vs.* the control, using GAPDH as an internal control for protein loading. (**C**) Representative confocal images (n = 3, five pictures per condition) of control and Y27632 (2, 10 or 50 μM) with 24 h incubation, after immunostaining for VE-cadherin, MMP2 or MMP9 (green) and the nuclear dye DAPI (blue), scale bars represent 50 μm. (**D**) Real-time qPCR analysis was used to determine changes in gene expression. Relative Y27632-induced change in gene expression compared with GAPDH is expressed as fold change calculated by $2^{-\Delta\Delta Cp}$ method. Data are expressed as mean ± S.E. from three independent experiments, with significant differences from control shown as *$P<0.05$ and **$P<0.01$.

ROCK inhibitors suppress HCC cell motility

VM is believed to be associated with cell migration and invasion. To further determine the active role of ROCK in the development of a vascular phenotype of MHCC97H, MHCC97H cells treated with Y27632 (2, 10 and 50 μM) were subjected to scratch wound assays and invasion assay. Cell migration toward the wounded area was observed (Figure. 6A). No treatment of MHCC97H led to nearly complete wound closure, while addition of Y27632 (50 μM) to cells led to a significant blockage of migration ($P>0.05$ *vs.* 0 h, Figure. 6B). These results indicate that Y27632 treated cultures exhibited a failure to migrate. In addition, cell invasion decreased by about 45% and 75% after blockage with in 10 μM and 50 μM Y27632 respectively, as compared with control cells (*$P<0.05$ and ***$P<0.001$, Figure. 6C and D). These findings indicate that the inhibition on cell motility by Y27632 was significant and concentration dependent.

Y27632 treatment did not affect cell apoptosis and viability

To eliminate any misinterpretation due to cell apoptosis or death caused by toxicity of the compound, we performed cell apoptosis and viability assessment on HCC cells. Flow cytometric analysis showed Y27632 up to 50 μM was found to be little cytotoxic to MHCC97H cells ($P>0.05$, *vs.* the control, Figure. 7A). Cell proliferation assay showed that Y27632 did not affect cell growth ($P>0.05$ *vs.* the control, Figure. 7B), confirming that inhibition of ROCK only affected HCC cell migration.

Discussion

Invasion of malignant tumor cells into neighboring tissues and formation of metastasis are crucially dependent on the migratory properties of the cancer cell. Most *in vitro* studies investigated Rho GTPase function in mesenchymal migration using a two-dimensional system: RhoA, B and C to stimulate the formation of stress fibers and focal adhesions, actomyosin-mediated cell contraction, and rear detachment [19]. In addition, Rho GTPases control the directionality of cell migration. In the present study, we examined the expression levels of RhoA, ROCK1 and ROCK2 in HCC cell lines and revealed a positive correlation between high RhoA/ROCK expression and high invasive potential. VM is defined as a fluid-conducting channel formed by highly invasive and genetically dysregulated melanoma cells [20] and has become a prognostic factor for poor clinical outcomes [8,21]. Our assay on the formation of tubular network structures demonstrated that higher levels of RhoA/ROCK were more prone to form VM networks, compared with RhoA/ROCK low-expressing cells, suggesting that the RhoA/ROCK signaling pathway is positively correlated with the potential of VM formation in HCC cells. In addition, the expression level of ROCK altered in a time-dependent manner as was the case with the formation of VM, confirming the contribution of RhoA/ROCK to VM formation.

Tumor cell invasion and metastasis require a complex cascade of events including changes in the cytoskeleton. Accumulating evidence indicates that the RhoA and downstream target ROCK

Table 1. Sequences of primers.

Gene	Forward Primer (5′-3′)	Reverse Primer (5′-3′)	Size
VE-cadherin	CATTTGTCGTGCCTGAAGAC	ATGGTGAAAGCGTCCTGGTA	133
EphA2	CCCGGAGGACGTTTACTTCT	GGATGGATGGATCTCGGTAG	124
PI3K	CGTTTCTGCTTTGGGACAAC	CCTGATGATGGTCGTGGAG	100
MMP14	GAGGGTCTTCGTTGCTCAGT	GGGTTTCTTCTGCCCACTT	120
LAMC2	ACATTCCTGCCTCAGACCAC	TCCCTTGTCAGTTGCTCCAT	121
MMP2	TATGGCTTCTGCCCTGAGAC	CACACCACATCTTTCCGTCA	142
MMP9	CAGTCCACCCTTGTGCTCTT	ACTCTCCACGCATCTCTGC	118

All the sequences were based on the published data on the National Center for Biotechnology Information followed by the accession number.

plays an important role in oncogenesis. The interaction of GTP-bound RhoA to Rho-binding domain (RBD) of ROCK increases ROCK activity through de-repression of the carboxyl-terminal RBD-pleckstrin homology (PH) domains on the amino-terminal kinase domain, leading to an active "open" kinase conformation [22]. It was reported that gastric cancer cell invasion could be induced via activation of the RhoA/ROCK pathway by IL-6 [23], and RhoA and RhoC siRNA gene therapy mediated by adenovirus has been suggested as useful for inhibiting the growth and invasion of human gastric carcinoma via the PI3K/Akt pathway [24]. However, our finding that exoenzyme C3 did not destruct VM structure formation suggests that RhoA is not essential for the VM formation process, probably because ROCK is an evolutionarily conserved downstream effector of RhoA, RhoB, RhoC and RhoE, all of which are potential activators [25]. Therefore, blockage of each GTPase above directly binds to ROCK and inhibits its kinase activity. Differently, RhoA activates ROCK1 through interaction with the carboxy-terminal site. RhoE and RhoA are unable to bind ROCK1 simultaneously [26], and RhoE phosphorylation events seem to antagonize RhoA-induced stress fiber assembly [27]. Interestingly, ROCK could also be activated independently of RhoA through amino-terminal trans-phosphorylation caused by protein oligomerization. Other small GTP-binding proteins such as Gem and Rad specifically regulate either ROCK1- and ROCK2-mediated cell rounding and neurite retraction [28]. In addition, ROCK can be auto-phosphorylated, suggesting that the function of ROCK may be, in part, dependent on auto-regulation [29]. However, which mechanism induces RhoA as not essential for the VM formation process needs to be determined by further investigation.

The ROCK family includes ROCK1 and ROCK2 that share 65% overall identity and 92% identity in the kinase domain. Both kinases contain a catalytic kinase domain at the N-terminus, followed by a central coiled-coil domain, including a RBD and a C-terminal PH domain, with an internal cysteine-rich domain. ROCK promotes actin filament stabilization and the generation of actin-myosin contractility by phosphorylating numerous downstream target proteins, including the myosin binding subunit of myosin light chain (MLC) phosphatase (MYPT1), MLC2, LIM kinases, ezrin/radixin/moesin and adducin. Y27632 or fasudil, inhibitors of ROCK, cause loss of actin stress fibers and focal adhesion complexes [30]. This is predominantly due to the phosphorylation and inhibition of MLCP by ROCK, which increases MLC phosphorylation and cellular contraction by facilitating interaction of myosin with F-actin [22]. Thus, ROCK regulates cell polarity and migration through cellular contractions, protrusions, and focal adhesions. It was found in the present study that Y27632 reduced the formation of tubule-like structures in a dose-dependent manner, indicating the potential role of ROCK as a mediator of VM. However, further studies are required to reveal which ROCK isoform dominates the VM activity.

Epithelial cells can convert into mesenchymal cells through a process known as EMT. EMT refers to a series of events in which epithelial cells lose many of their epithelial characteristics and take on properties typical of mesenchymal cells that require complex changes in cell architecture and behavior. The mechanism between the VM channels in highly aggressive human tumor cells and the EMT process may share the same process or similar relevance. These findings in (Figure. 4) suggest that VM formation is correlated with the EMT-marker and ROCK inhibition reverses the process of EMT, supporting the idea that VM formation may be part of EMT [31].

The key signaling pathway of VM formation is described as colocalization of VE-cadherin and activation of PI3K by EphA2, which subsequently induce the expression and activation of MMP14, which subsequently triggers MMP2 activation. Altogether, MMP14 and MMP2 promote the cleavage of LAMC2 to the pro-migratory $\gamma 2'$ and $\gamma 2\times$ fragments. It was suggested that up-regulation of any molecule in the above tumor microenvironment could increase migration and invasion, and may ultimately result in VM. However, what initially triggers this pathway to become activated remains unknown. In recent years, many more studies linking various angiogenesis-promoting factors to VM have been published. Vascular endothelial growth factor-A (VEGF-A) promoted the up-regulation of VM-associated genes for VE-cadherin, EphA2, MMP2 and MMP9 [32]. In contrast, our investigation showed that VM-associated genes was down-regulated, suggesting that ROCK inhibition could attenuate the characteristics associated with tumor cell plasticity essential for VM. Therefore, we conclude that VEGF-A and ROCK may have the same effect on VM formation. Similar findings in other studies [33] demonstrated that selective blockage of ROCK with Y27632 dose-dependently inhibited VEGF-induced venular hyperpermeability. We therefore hypothesize that VE-cadherin up-regulation through specific induction by ROCK activates the subsequent signaling cascade, similar to VEGF-A. Our future study will address the potential significance of this relationship. The recent progress in Rho/ROCK research continuously supports the therapeutic importance of the ROCK pathway in migration. MMPs have been implicated in a variety of mechanisms that promote tumor progression [34]. In particular, MMP2 and MMP9 are key mediators of invasion, metastasis and tumor angiogenesis [35]. Our western blot and real-time qPCR assays showed that both MMP2 and MMP9 were down-regulated. This finding could serve as an explanation why Y27632 not only suppressed cell migration but cell invasion that involves the

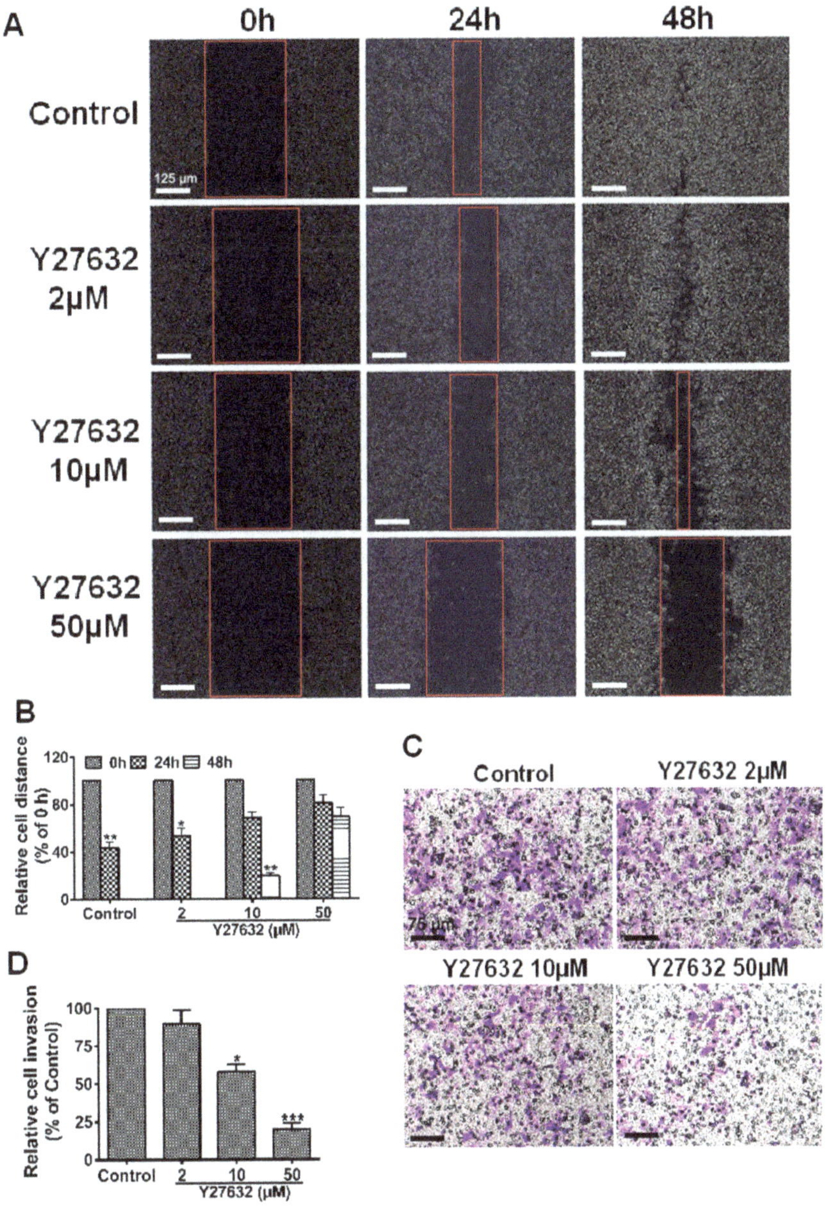

Figure 6. ROCK inhibition decreases the motility of MHCC97H cells. (**A**) Y27632 inhibition delayed wound healing. Representative images of scratch wounds formed at 0, 24 and 48 h after wounding. Original magnification was 100×, scale bars represent 125 μm. (**C**) Y27632 inhibition decreased invasiveness. Invaded cells attached at the lower surface of the filters were stained with crystal violet. Original magnification was 200×, scale bars represent 75 μm. (**B**) and (**D**) Data were normalized to untreated cells and the relative migration or invasion is expressed as mean ± S.E. of triplicate experiments. Fewer cells migrated or invaded 48 h after incubation with Y27632 (50 μM), compared with the control cells, *$P<0.05$, **$P<0.01$ and ***$P<0.001$.

extracellular matrix barrier (Figure. 6). In contrast, other studies reported contradictory findings. One study [2] reported that MMP9 but not MMP2 was correlated with VM formation in HCC, and another study [36] reported that Y27632 promoted human trabecular meshwork cells in adhesion, contraction and motility. However, there is also growing evidence to support the importance of Rho/ROCK in multiple aspects of migration activities [37–39]. Given the volume of the literature supporting a role for Rho/ROCK in controlling cell movement, it is not surprising to find that inhibition of ROCK blocks MHCC97H migration and invasion as demonstrated in our study.

In the current study, we demonstrated that the expression level of RhoA/ROCK was different in HCC cells, and that higher active RhoA/ROCK expression was prone to form VM channels. In addition, ROCK, but not RhoA, played a crucial role in the development and progression of cancer VM formation *in vitro* in MHCC97H cell line. Moreover, EMT was correlated with ROCK-induced VM formation. In brief, our results suggest that the RhoA/ROCK pathway is involved in numerous aspects of the VM process, and ROCK may prove to be a therapeutic target for VM in HCC.

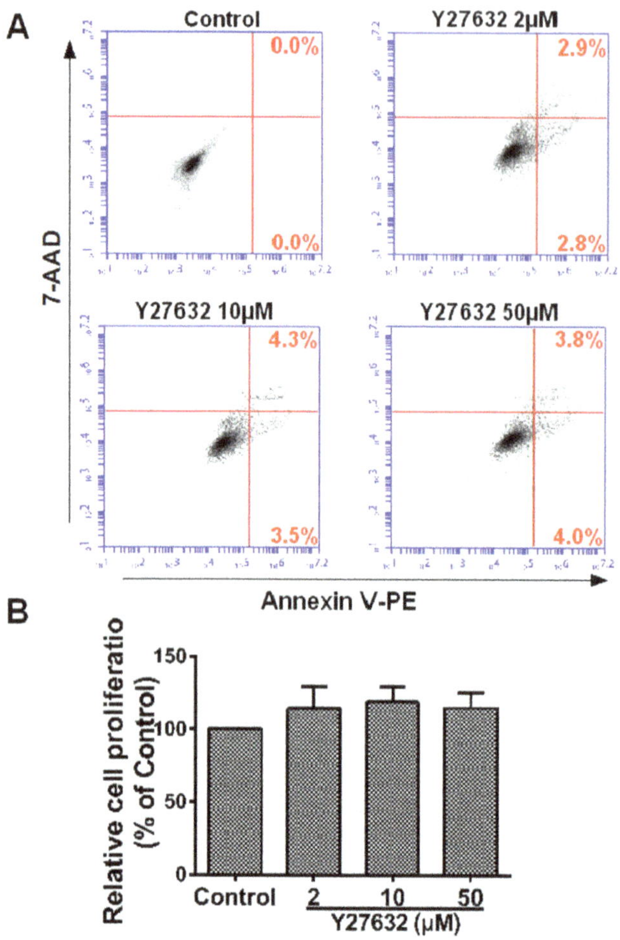

Figure 7. Y27632 treatment did not affect cell apoptosis and viability. (**A**) The concentrations of Y27632 (up to 50 μM) did not induce apoptosis of MHCC97H cells according to flow cytometric analysis. (**B**) Y27632 treatment did not affect cell viability. There was no statistically significant difference from three independent experiments ($P>0.05$, n = 5 in each group).

Materials and Methods

Chemical and antibodies

Chemical and antibodies used in this study included Matrigel (BD Biosciences); cell culture media (RPMI 1640, DMEM and MEM); fetal bovine serum and antibiotics (Gibco); exoenzyme C3, Y27632 and other chemicals (Sigma-Aldrich); anti-VE-cadherin antibody (Cell Signaling); PE Annexin V Apoptosis Detection Kit (BD Pharmingen). The rest were purchased from Abcam Inc. (Cambridge).

Cell culture

HUVEC, human hepatocyte cell line LO2 and MHCC97H cells were obtained from the Liver Cancer Institute, Zhongshan Hospital, Fudan University (Shanghai, China). SMMC7703, SMMC7721, HepG2 and Hep3B were from the cell bank of the Chinese Academy of Sciences. All the cell lines were cultured separately in RPMI 1640 (HUVEC, SMMC7703, SMMC7721 and LO2), MEM (HepG2 and Hep3B) and DMEM (MHCC97H), supplemented with 10% FBS and antibiotics. All cultures were maintained at 37°C in a humidified atmosphere of 5% CO_2.

Matrigel tube formation assay

The Matrigel tube formation assay is a technique used to determine *in vitro* VM capacity of cancer cells. Briefly, each well of a 24-well plate was coated with 100 μl Matrigel (10 mg/ml) and allowed to solidify at 37°C for 1 h. The cell suspension in culture medium (4×10^4/200 μl) was seeded into the Matrigel-coated 24-well plate and incubated at 37°C in a humidified atmosphere of 5% CO2. The effect of RhoA/ROCK inhibition on tube formation was studied by adding culture medium containing exoenzyme C3 or Y27632 into the wells immediately after cell seeding to a final concentration of 200, 800 or 1600 ng (exoenzyme C3) or 2, 10 or 50 μM (Y27632).

Western blot analysis

Total protein was extracted and electrophoresed using SDS-PAGE. Proteins on the gel were transferred onto PVDF membrane (Merck-Millipore), followed by blocking with 5% skimmed milk dissolved in TBS containing 1% Tween-20 (TBST) for 1 h at room temperature. The membrane was incubated with primary antibody at 4°C overnight, washed with 1% TBST three times, and incubated in alkaline phosphatase-conjugated secondary antibody for 1 h at room temperature. After washing, the chemiluminescence signal was imaged using a ChemiDoc XRS (Bio-Rad) and quantitated using Image J.

cDNA generation and real-time qPCR

Cells were treated with 2, 10 or 50 μM of Y27632 for 16 h. Total RNA was extracted from cells using Trizol (Invitrogen) and verified by electrophoresis. The mRNA was reverse-transcribed into cDNA with a reverse-transcription kit (Thermo Fisher Scientific). Human GAPDH Endogenous Reference Genes Primers (Order NO.: PHS04) and Primer sequences listed in **Table 1** used for PCR were from Sangon Biotech. SYBR Green I (Amersco) was added into the reaction mixture. Quantitative real-time PCR was performed on an MJ Opticon 2 thermal cycler (MJ Research Inc.) following the manufacturer's instruction.

Immunostaining

After fixation for 20 min in 4% paraformaldehyde at 37°C, cells were permeabilized for 15 min in 0.5% Triton-X and subsequently blocked in 5% goat serum for 1 h. After incubation with the appropriate primary (overnight incubation at 4°C) and secondary (2 h at 37°C) antibodies, the cells were imaged using a confocal laser scanning microscope (Leica TCS SP8).

Cell migration assay

Cell migration was evaluated using an *in vitro* wound healing assay. In brief, MHCC97H cells containing Y27632 at a final concentration of 2, 10 or 50 μM were seeded to a six-well plate and incubated for 8 h to allow the formation of a cell monolayer. Cells were scratched with the tip of a 200 μl pipette and then incubated at 37°C in a humidified atmosphere of 5% CO_2 for 48 h. To observe the scratch healing, each well was observed at 0, 24 and 48 h after scratching.

Matrigel invasion assay

Invasion was assayed in Transwell cell culture chambers (Corning Costar) attached with a membrane filter (8.0 μm pore size; Nucleopore) as previously described with some modifications [40]. Briefly, the inserts in the membrane filter were coated with Matrigel on the upper surface. MHCC97H cells were adjusted to a density of 1×10^6 cells/ml in serum-free DMEM high glucose culture medium. Cell suspension (200 μl) was seeded into the upper surface, while the lower chambers were filled with 500 µl DMEM medium with 20% FBS. After culture at 37°C in a humidified atmosphere of 5% CO_2 for 48 h, the cells on the upper surface of the filter were removed by wiping with a cotton swab and the number of cells that migrated through the Matrigel to the lower chamber was determined. Assays were performed in duplicate wells.

Cell apoptosis and viability assessment

Apoptosis assay of MHCC97H cells exposed to Y27632 (2, 10 and 50 µM) for 24 h were examined by flow cytometry (BD Accuri C6). MHCC97H cells were stained with PE Annexin V and 7-Amino-Actinomycin (7-AAD) following the manufacturer's instructions to detect early apoptotic cells (PE Annexin V^+/7-AAD^- events) and late apoptotic cells (PE Annexin V^+/7-AAD^+ events). Additionally, MHCC97H cells were trypsinized and seeded at 1×10^4 cells/well in 96 well plates. After 24 h, various concentrations of Y27632 were added, followed by incubation for another 48 h. Then, 10 µl Cell Counting Kit-8 (CCK8, Dojindo) solution was added to each well. Plates were incubated for additional 2 h. Absorbance readings at 490 nm were obtained using a spectrophotometer (Thermo Varioskan).

Statistical analysis

The data were expressed as mean ± standard errors (S.E.) and examined for their statistical significance of difference with ANOVA and the Student's *t*-test. *P*-values of less than 0.05 were considered statistically significant.

Author Contributions

Conceived and designed the experiments: XYL QL GLL. Performed the experiments: JGZ YZW QDZ. Analyzed the data: XYL SYG. Contributed reagents/materials/analysis tools: XW GHZ. Wrote the paper: JGZ QL XYL.

References

1. Maniotis AJ, Folberg R, Hess A, Seftor EA, Gardner LM, et al. (1999) Vascular Channel Formation by Human Melanoma Cells in Vivo and in Vitro: Vasculogenic Mimicry. Am J Pathol 155: 739–752.
2. Sun T, Zhao N, Zhao XL, Gu Q, Zhang SW, et al. (2010) Expression and functional significance of Twist1 in hepatocellular carcinoma: its role in vasculogenic mimicry. Hepatology 51: 545–556.
3. Wong CCL, Wong CM, Tung EKK, Man K, Ng IOL (2009) Rho-kinase 2 is frequently overexpressed in hepatocellular carcinoma and involved in tumor invasion. Hepatology 49: 1583–1594.
4. Jin LM, Su XH, Qing Z, Jing Z, Dan Z, et al. (2011) Role of Twist in vasculogenic mimicry formation in hypoxic hepatocellular carcinoma cells in vitro. Biochem Biophys Res Commun 408: 686–691.
5. El-Serag HB, Rudolph KL (2007) Hepatocellular Carcinoma: Epidemiology and Molecular Carcinogenesis. Gastroenterology 132: 2557–2576.
6. Karlsson R, Pedersen ED, Wang Z, Brakebusch C (2009) Rho GTPase function in tumorigenesis. Biochim Biophys Acta 1796: 91–98.
7. Kirschmann DA, Seftor EA, Hardy KM, Seftor RE, Hendrix MJ (2012) Molecular Pathways: Vasculogenic Mimicry in Tumor Cells: Diagnostic and Therapeutic Implications. Clin Cancer Res 18: 2726–2732.
8. Wang SY, Yu L, Ling GQ, Xiao S, Sun XL, et al. (2012) Vasculogenic mimicry and its clinical significance in medulloblastoma. Cancer Biol Ther 13: 341–348.
9. Quigley JP, Armstrong PB (1998) Tumor cell intravasation alu-cidated: the chick embryo opens the window. Cell 94: 281–284.
10. Grise F, Bidaud A (2009) Moreau V. Rho GTPases in hepatocellular carcinoma. Biochim Biophys Acta 1795: 137–151.
11. Shi J, Wu X, Surma M, Vemula S, Zhang L, et al. (2013) Distinct roles for ROCK1 and ROCK2 in the regulation of cell detachment. Cell Death Dis 4: 483
12. Thiery JP (2002) Epithelial-mesenchymal transitions in tumour progression. Nat Rev Cancer 2: 442–454.
13. Gulhati P, Bowen KA, Liu J, Stevens PD, Rychahou PG, et al. (2011) mTORC1 and mTORC2 Regulate EMT, Motility, and Metastasis of Colorectal Cancer via RhoA and Rac1 Signaling Pathways. Cancer Res 71: 3246–3256.
14. Lee J, Moon HJ, Lee JM, Joo CK (2010) Smad3 Regulates Rho Signaling via NET1 in the Transforming Growth Factor-β-induced Epithelial-Mesenchymal Transition of Human Retinal Pigment Epithelial Cells. J Biol Chem 285: 26618–26627.
15. Hendrix MJ, Seftor EA, Meltzer PS, Gardner LM, Hess AR, et al. (2001) Expression and functional significance of VE-cadherin in aggressive human melanoma cells: role in vasculogenic mimicry. Proc Nat Acad Sci USA 98: 8018–8023.
16. Seftor RE, Seftor EA, Koshikawa N, Meltzer PS, Gardner LM, et al. (2001) Cooperative Interactions of Laminin 5γ2 Chain, Matrix Metalloproteinase-2, and Membrane Type-1-Matrix/Metalloproteinase Are Required for Mimicry of Embryonic Vasculogenesis by Aggressive Melanoma. Cancer Res 61: 6322–6327.
17. Paulis YW, Soetekouw PM, Verheul HM, Tjan-Heijnen VC, Griffioen AW (2010) Signalling pathways in vasculogenic mimicry. Biochim Biophys Acta 1806: 18–28.
18. Vega FM, Ridley AJ (2008) Rho GTPases in cancer cell biology. FEBS Lett 582: 2093–2101
19. Wheeler AP, Ridley AJ (2004) Why three Rho proteins? RhoA, RhoB, RhoC, and cell motility. Exp Cell Res 301: 43–49
20. Hendrix MJ, Seftor EA, Hess AR, Seftor RE (2003) Vasculogenic mimicry and tumour-cell plasticity: lessons from melanoma. Nat Rev Cancer 3: 411–421.
21. Sun B, Qie S, Zhang S, Sun T, Zhao X, et al. (2008) Role and mechanism of vasculogenic mimicry in gastrointestinal stromal tumors. Hum Pathol 39: 444–451.
22. Noma K, Kihara Y, Higashi Y (2012) Striking crosstalk of ROCK signaling with endothelial function. J Cardiol 60: 1–6.
23. Lin MT, Lin BR, Chang CC, Chu CY, Su HJ, et al. (2007) IL-6 induces AGS gastric cancer cell invasion via activation of the c-Src/RhoA/ROCK signaling pathway. Int J Cancer 120: 2600–2608.
24. Sun HW, Tong SL, He J, Wang Q, Zou L, et al. (2007) RhoA and RhoC -siRNA inhibit the proliferation and invasiveness activity of human gastric carcinoma by Rho/PI3K/Akt pathway. World J Gastroenterol 13: 3517–3522.
25. Nunes KP, Rigsby CS, Webb RC (2010) RhoA/Rho-kinase and vascular diseases: what is the link? Cell Mol Life Sci 67: 3823–3836.
26. Riento K, Totty N, Villalonga P, Garg R, Guasch R, et al. (2005) RhoE function is regulated by ROCK I-mediated phosphorylation. EMBO J 24: 1170–1180.
27. Komander D, Garg R, Wan PT, Ridley AJ, Barford D (2008) Mechanism of multi-site phosphorylation from a ROCK-I: RhoE complex structure. EMBO J 27: 3175–3185.
28. Carton I, Trouet D, Hermans D, Barth H, Aktories K, et al. (2002) RhoA exerts a permissive effect on volume-regulated anion channels in vascular endothelial cells. Am J Physiol Cell Physiol 283: C115–125.
29. Leung T, Chen XQ, Manser E, Lim L (1996) The p160 RhoA-binding kinase ROK alpha is a member of a kinase family and is involved in the reorganization of the cytoskeleton. Mol Cell Biol 16: 5313–5327.
30. Shi J, Wei L (2013) Rho kinases in cardiovascular physiology and pathophysiology: the effect of fasudil. J Cardiovasc Pharmacol 62: 341–354.
31. Zhao Xl, Sun T, Che N, Sun D, Zhao N, et al. (2011) Promotion of hepatocellular carcinoma metastasis through matrix metalloproteinase activation by epithelial-mesenchymal transition regulator Twist1. J Cell Mol Med 15: 691–700.
32. Wang JY, Sun T, Zhao XL, Zhang SW, Zhang DF, et al. (2008) Functional significance of VEGF-a in human ovarian carcinoma: role in vasculogenic mimicry. Cancer Biol Ther 7: 758–766.
33. Sun H, Breslin JW, Zhu J, Yuan SY, Wu MH (2006) Rho and ROCK Signaling in VEGF-Induced Microvascular Endothelial Hyperpermeability. Microcirculation 13: 237–247.
34. Chang C, Werb Z (2001) The many faces of metalloproteases: cell growth, invasion, angiogenesis and metastasis. Trends Cell Biol 11: S37–43.
35. Xu B, Nakhla S, Makris A, Hennessy A (2011) TNF-α inhibits trophoblast integration into endothelial cellular networks. Placenta 32: 241–246.
36. Koga T, Koga T, Awai M, Tsutsui J, Yue BY, et al. (2006) Rho-associated protein kinase inhibitor, Y-27632, induces alterations in adhesion, contraction and motility in cultured human trabecular meshwork cells. Exp Eye Res 82: 362–370.
37. Bryan BA, Dennstedt E, Mitchell DC, Walshe TE, Noma K, et al. (2010) RhoA/ROCK signaling is essential for multiple aspects of VEGF-mediated angiogenesis. FASEB J 24: 3186–3195.
38. Vega FM, Fruhwirth G, Ng T, Ridley AJ (2011) RhoA and RhoC have distinct roles in migration and invasion by acting through different targets. J Cell Biol 193: 655–665.
39. Narumiya S, Tanji M, Ishizaki T (2009) Rho signaling, ROCK and mDia1, in transformation, metastasis and invasion. Cancer Metastasis Rev 28: 65–76.
40. Lirdprapamongkol K, Kramb JP, Suthiphongchai T, Surarit R, Srisomsap C, et al. (2009) Vanillin suppresses metastatic potential of human cancer cells through PI3K inhibition and decreases angiogenesis in vivo. J Agric Food Chem 57: 3055–3063.

14

Inhibition of IL-17A Suppresses Enhanced-Tumor Growth in Low Dose Pre-Irradiated Tumor Beds

Eun-Jung Lee[1], Hyo Jin Park[2], Ik-Jae Lee[1], Won Woo Kim[1], Sang-Jun Ha[2], Yang-Gun Suh[1], Jinsil Seong[1]*

1 Department of Radiation Oncology, Yonsei University College of Medicine, Seoul, Korea, **2** Department of Biochemistry, Yonsei University, Seoul, Korea

Abstract

Ionizing radiation induces modification of the tumor microenvironment such as tumor surrounding region, which is relevant to treatment outcome after radiotherapy. In this study, the effects of pre-irradiated tumor beds on the growth of subsequently implanted tumors were investigated as well as underlying mechanism. The experimental model was set up by irradiating the right thighs of C3H/HeN mice with 5 Gy, followed by the implantation of HCa-I and MIH-2. Both implanted tumors in the pre-irradiated bed showed accelerated-growth compared to the control. Tumor-infiltrated lymphocyte (TIL) levels were increased, as well as pro-tumor factors such as IL-6 and transforming growth factor-beta1 (TGF-β1) in the pre-irradiated group. In particular, the role of pro-tumor cytokine interleukin-17A (IL-17A) was investigated as a possible target mechanism because IL-6 and TGF-β are key factors in Th17 cells differentiation from naïve T cells. IL-17A expression was increased not only in tumors, but also in CD4+ T cells isolated from the tumor draining lymph nodes. The effect of IL-17A on tumor growth was confirmed by treating tumors with IL-17A antibody, which abolished the acceleration of tumor growth. These results indicate that the upregulation of IL-17A seems to be a key factor for enhancing tumor growth in pre-irradiated tumor beds.

Editor: David D. Roberts, Center for Cancer Research, National Cancer Institute, United States of America

Funding: This study was supported by the National Nuclear R&D Program through a National Research Foundation of Korea (NRF) grant (2010-001854) funded by the Ministry of Science, ICT and Future planning. This study was also supported by a grant of the Korean Health Technology R&D Project (A121982), Ministry of Health & Welfare, Republic of Korea. The funders had no role in study design, data collection and analysis, decision to publish, or preparation of the manuscript.

Competing Interests: The authors have declared that no competing interests exist.

* Email: jsseong@yuhs.ac

Introduction

In cancer radiotherapy (RT), high dose irradiated regions are always surrounded by areas of graded exposure doses ranging from medium- to low-doses [1]. Since tumor cells can be distributed at the microscopic level in a relatively wide area, circulating tumor cells might be present in surrounding areas that have received lower doses of irradiation. When tumor recurrence occurs in these low-dose irradiated areas, the recurrent tumor exhibits a more aggressive behavior than the primary counterpart [2]. However, this phenomenon has not been proved in a clinical setting yet, although the possibility that it could have a clinical implication has not been excluded. Therefore, surrounding areas receiving low-doses of irradiation, such as normal tissue in the vicinity of tumor or pre-irradiated areas, require special attention to achieve effective cancer control.

Many recent studies have shown radiation effects at lower-than-ablative doses in normal tissues. Irradiating normal tissue with low-doses could lead to the accumulation of DNA damage [3]. Chou *et al.* showed that irradiating endothelial cells with 4 Gy induced IL-6 expression, which acts through Mcl-1 expression to protect endothelial cells from irradiation-induced cell death [4]. It has been reported that irradiation-induced differential changes in the profiles of cytokines, including IL-6, IL-1α, keratinocyte-derived chemokine (KC), granulocyte colony-stimulating factor (G-CSF), and IL-17 in lung tissue irradiated with 12 Gy [5]. Several inflammatory cytokines are considered to be key factors that lead to tumor recurrence and metastasis in RT, and many recent studies have reported a role of IL-17 in tumor progression [6,7].

IL-17, a proinflammatory cytokine that plays a critical role in the inflammatory response, autoimmune diseases, and cancer immunity, acts as a potent regulator of tumor growth as well as an important mediator in inflammatory reactions through the recruitment of monocytes and neutrophils [8,9]. However, the role of IL-17 in tumor growth and metastasis is still unclear.

The role of pre-irradiated tumor beds on the growth of subsequently implanted tumors has been investigated extensively. Saeki *et al.* showed that pre-irradiated tumor beds that received injury induced by a single high-dose to the host vasculature and connective tissue showed impaired neovascularization in the implanted tumor [10]. However, high ablative-doses are seldom given to a substantial area of normal tissue. In current practice in stereotactic radiosurgery, where very high-dose irradiation is administered in one fraction, only a very small volume of normal tissue is included in the radiation field. Therefore, the effect of irradiating tumor beds with medium- to low-doses on the growth of subsequently implanted tumors require clinical attention and mechanism study. In the present study, we investigated the effect of medium- to low-dose pre-irradiation of tumor beds on the growth of subsequently implanted tumors. In particular, the role of the pro-inflammatory cytokine IL-17A was investigated *in vitro* and *in vivo* as a possible factor in the target mechanism.

Materials and Methods

Reagents

Anti-bodies of TGF-β and ROR-γ were purchased from Santa Cruz Biotechnology (CA). IL-6 and IL-17A anti-bodies were purchased from abcam (MA). p-stat-3 was purchased from Bio World (MN). IL-6 ELISA kit and CD4 anti-body were obtained from BD Bioscience (CA). TGF-β ELISA kit were purchased from BioLegend (CA). mIL-17A antibody was purchased to IL-17A neutralization from R&D system (MN). A reverse transcription system for cDNA synthesis and the primer sets of TGF-β and IL-6 were purchased from Qiagen (Hilden, Germany).

Animal experimental design and X-ray irradiation

Five male C3H/HeN mice, 6 to 7 weeks old (Central Lab, Japan), were used per each experimental group for this study. Mice were immobilized in specially designed mice jig and the right thighs of the mice were irradiated with 5 Gy in a single fraction using an X-Rad 320 irradiator (Precision X-ray, North Branford, CT). Mice were treated 69 cm from the radiation source (SSD) with a dose rate of 150 cGy/min with 300 kVp X-rays, using 12.5 mA and a X-ray beam filter consisting of 2.0 mm Al. On day 1 and 3 after irradiation, HCa-I [11,12] and MIH-2 [13,14] murine hepatocarcinoma cells (1×10^6 cells) in 100 µl phosphate-buffered saline (PBS) were injected intramuscularly into irradiated the site. Tumor volume was calculated as volume $=\pi/6$ X ab^2, where a is the long axis and b is the short axis of two orthogonal diameters. The maximum allowable size of tumors in mice is 20 mm in diameter according to the IACUC (Institutional Animal Care and Use Committee) guidelines of the Yonsei University Health System. After experiments, the experimental mice were sacrificed before reaching the maximum allowable size using carbon dioxide (CO_2).

Tumor infiltrating lymphocytes (TILs) isolation and Flow cytometry analysis

For the isolation of TILs, tumor were chopped by clipper then incubated in 1 mg/ml collagenase type IV (Worthington, Lake wood, NJ) solution containing 0.01 mg/ml DNase I (sigma, CA) at 37°C for 20 min. TILs were isolated by Percoll gradient (sigma, CA) after washing the dissociated tissues by chilled complete RPMI medium. Isolated TILs were resuspended in PBS and stained with the indicated reagents. Cells were then washed twice, fixed in 2% paraformaldehyde solution, and immediately analyzed using a FACS Canto flow cytometer (Becton Dickinson, CA).

Analysis of gene expression

Total RNA was isolated from tumor cells using TRIzol reagent (Invitrogen Corp., Carlsbad, CA). PCR was performed using the Step One Plus (Applied Biosystems, CA) and a QuantiTect SYBR Green PCR Kit (Applied Biosystems, Warrington, UK). The amplification program consisted of 1 cycle of 95°C with a 10 min hold (hot start), followed by 35 cycles of 95°C with a 20 sec hold, 60°C with a 20 sec hold, and 72°C with a 20 sec hold. After normalization with GAPDH, the median target level of implanted tumor only and non-irradiated bed were used as calibrators.

Immunohistochemical and immunofluorescence staining

Tumor samples were fixed in 10% formalin and were embedded in paraffin, which was cut into 5-µm-thick sections. For immunohistochemical staining, deparaffinized sections were blocked with 10% normal horse serum for 1 h and then incubated with primary antibodies against TGF-β, CD-31 and IL-17A (1:100). The samples were incubated with biotinylated secondary antibody (DAKO code K0675; DAKO Corp., Carpinteria, CA) and peroxidase-labeled streptavidin (DAKO code K0675). Staining was developed using the 3-3 diaminobenzidine (DAB) substrate chromogen system (DAKO Corp.).

To immunofluorescence staining, deparaffinized sections were blocked with 10% normal horse serum for 1 h and then incubated with primary antibodies against TGF-β and IL-6. And then, the samples were incubated with Alexa 594-conjugated donkey anti-rabbit IgG (Invitrogen).

Co-immunofluorescence staining was also performed to assess co-localization of CD4 and Ror-γ. The sections were incubated overnight with a mixture of anti-CD4 and anti-Ror-γ in 4°C followed by washes with PBS and incubation with a mixture of Alexa 488-conjugated donkey anti-goat IgG and Alexa 594-conjugated goat anti-rat IgG (Invitrogen). The reactions were examined using an immunofluorescence microscope.

Cytokine detection

IL-6 and IL-17A protein were measured in culture supernatants by enzyme immunometric assays (ELISA). ELISAs were performed using specific mAb pairs for the detection of both IL-6 and IL-17A. For sandwich ELISAs, purified antimouse IL-6 and IL-17A antibodies were adsorbed to capture cytokines on 96-well immunoassay plates. The culture supernatant at the appropriate dilution was incubated following the addition of biotinylated antimouse IL-6/IL-17A mAbs. Streptavidin-HRP (BD Pharmingen) was used for detection, followed by the addition of the TMB substrate reagent set (BD Pharmingen, San Diego, CA).

Th17 cell differentiation from naïve $CD4^+$ T cells

Naive $CD4^+$ T cells were isolated from spleen of C3H/HeN mice by negative selection using mouse $CD4^+$ T cell isolation kit (Miltenyi Biotec). Purified-naïve $CD4^+$ T cells were stimulated *in vitro* with anti-CD3 (1 µg/ml) anti-CD28 (1 µg/ml) antibodies in 5 Gy irradiated- or no irradiated media. For Th17 polarizing *in vitro*, Th17 polarizing factors except TGF-β (anti-IFNγ (2 µlg/ml), anti-IL-4 (2 µlg/ml), rmIL-6 (10 ng/ml) were added to culture media. These were cultured for 4 days.

IL-17 neutralization in vivo

Approximately 1×10^6 HCa-I and MIH-2 were injected intramuscularly in the pre-irradiated site day 3 after the implantation site had been irradiated with 5 Gy. 100 µg α-IL-17A antibody was treated with intraperitoneally (*i.p.*) at day 3 and day 10 after inoculation of tumor cells and with intratumoral (*i.t.*) twice a week for 2 weeks after tumor formation reached 8 mm. IgG2a antibody was administered to control mice using the same method.

Ethics statement

All procedure of animal research was provided in accordance with the Laboratory Animals Welfare Act, the Guide for the Care and Use of Laboratory Animals and the Guidelines and Policies for Rodent experiment provided by the IACUC in Yonsei University Health System (Permit Number: 2011-0114). All animal surgery was performed after euthanasia using CO^2, and all efforts were made to minimize suffering.

Statistical analysis

Data are expressed as means ± SEM. Comparisons among multiple groups were performed by factorial analysis of variance (ANOVA) followed by Scheffe's test or statistical comparisons

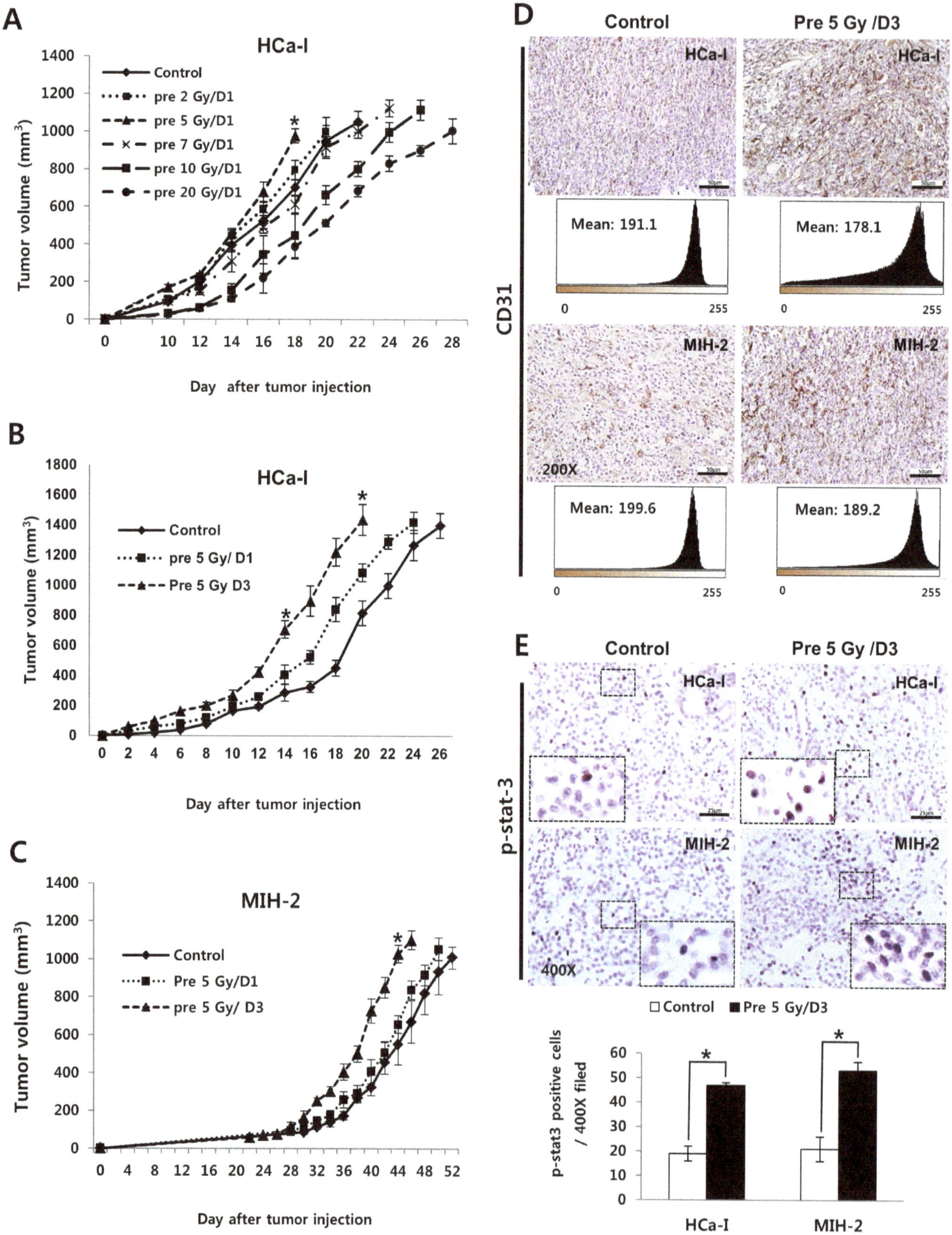

Figure 1. Tumor Growth and tumor related factors of implanted tumor in non-irradiated or pre-irradiated tumor beds with 5 Gy. (A) Growth rate of HCa-1 in various dose irradiated tumor beds. 1×10^6 murine hepatocarcinoma cells (HCa-1) were injected intramuscularly in the right thigh of the mice on day 1 after the implantation site had been irradiated. (n = 5 mice per group) *p<0.05, pre 5 Gy/D1 *vs* control (ANOVA) (B) Growth rate of HCa-I and (C) MIH-2 tumors (n = 5 mice per group), (D) expression of CD31 and (E) p-stat3 in implanted tumor. Approximately 1×10^6 murine

hepatocarcinoma cells (HCa-1 and MIH-2) were injected intramuscularly in the right thigh of the mice on day 1 and 3 after the implantation site had been irradiated. Error bars denote ± SEM. *p<0.05, pre 5Gy/D3 *vs* control (ANOVA). The tumors were resected for histologic examination when the tumor volume reached 800 to 1200 mm^3 and CD31 and p-stat3 were stained.

between groups were made by unpaired two-sided *t*-tests. Differences of $p<0.05$ (*) and $p<0.01$ (**) were considered significant.

Results

The growth of implanted tumors into low-dose pre-irradiated the tumor bed was accelerated compared with non-irradiated the tumor bed

When patients with HCC are treated in single fraction of 20 Gy, the surrounding regions of the tumor are exposure to graded doses (Sup Fig. 1). Tumor cells are distributed at the microscopic level in the surrounding area that has received lower doses of irradiation. The tumor growth can be affected by low-dose pre-irradiation. Therefore, to investigate the effect of pre-irradiation on the growth of subsequently implanted tumors after pre-irradiating the tumor bed, experimental models were developed by irradiating the right thighs of C3H/HeN mice with various doses followed by implantation of syngeneic tumor cells of murine hepatocarcinoma (HCa-I). As shown in Fig 1, tumor growth was accelerated in areas that received below 5 Gy, while the growth of the implanted tumor into the high-dose irradiated tumor bed (more than 7 Gy) was slow (Fig 1A). Therefore, we investigated the effect of the low-dose pre-irradiating tumor bed and the change of tumor microenvironment by pre-irradiation using 5 Gy and syngeneic murine hepatocarcinomas (HCa-I and MIH-2) in this study. HCa-I is a rapidly growing tumor that is resistant to radiation, while MIH-2 is a slow-growing tumor that is sensitive to radiation in relative comparison to HCa-I. The growth of both tumors was faster in the pre-irradiated bed than that in the non-irradiated bed (Figure 1, B and C). In addition, expression of pro-tumor factors, such as platelet endothelial cell adhesion molecule (PECAM-1, CD 31) and p-stat3, increased in both tumors in the pre-irradiated beds (Figure 1D and E).

Pre-irradiation on tumor bed increased TGF-β in implanted tumors and the tumor bed

TGF-β has multiple tumor-promoting effects and it can be induced by irradiation [15]; therefore, its expression was measured in the implanted tumors. TGF-β expression and its mRNA levels were higher at the tumor edges as well as in both the tumors implanted in the pre-irradiated beds than those in the control were (Figure 2A, B and Figure S2). TGF-β expression and mRNA level in the irradiated skin and muscles of the mice on day 3 of irradiating their thighs with 5 Gy was investigated because skin and muscles acted as tumor beds. It was highly expressed in vascular endothelial cells as well as in fibroblasts of dermis (Figures 2C and D). Thus, irradiation can induce TGF-β production in a tumor and its microenvironment, which includes the stroma and vascular endothelial cells.

Pre-irradiation on tumor bed increased TIL and IL-6 levels in implanted tumors

IL-6 is believed to have a pro-tumor effect as well as an inflammatory effect [16]. It is secreted by immune cells and some non-immune cells such as smooth muscle cells and fibroblasts [17]. Therefore, we investigated TIL and IL-6 production in this study. TIL increased in both tumors implanted into the pre-irradiated beds compared to the control (Figure 3A and B). Similarly, IL-6 expression also increased (Figure 3C). Immunofluorescence staining was performed to check IL-6 levels of pre-irradiated tumor beds (Figure D). A 5 Gy-irradiation led to increased IL-6 levels in the tumor bed and infiltration of immune cells (Figures 3D, E, F, and G).

Pre-irradiation on tumor bed increased IL-6 levels in the tumor-draining lymph node

We next set out to assess whether pre-irradiation of tumor beds can influence IL-6 levels in tumor-draining lymph nodes, as the lymph nodes, among lymphoid tissues, show the greatest involvement in mediating inflammatory responses. As shown in Figure 4, IL-6 levels were slightly increased in the tumor-draining lymph nodes of the pre-irradiated group, compared to control. These results potentially suggest that the enhancement of tumor growth in pre-irradiated tumor beds might be influenced by factors other than IL-6.

Pre-irradiation on tumor bed showed increased IL-17A in tumor-draining lymph node

Our results showed that IL-6 and TGF-β expressions increased in tumors implanted in pre-irradiated beds. TGF-β and IL-6 are required to induce Th17 differentiation from naive T cells [18]. IL-17A, in particular, plays an important role in cancer development and in inflammatory responses [6]; therefore, we investigated IL-17A and Th17 cell populations. To investigate IL-17A and Th17 cells in tumors, both tumor tissues were stained with IL-17A antibody and co-stained with CD4 and Ror-γt antibodies because Th17 cells are CD4- and Ror-γt-positive. We found an increase in IL-17A in both tumors implanted in the pre-irradiated beds, compared to controls (Figure 5A). Th17 cells also increased in number in both tumors implanted in the pre-irradiated beds, compared to controls (Figure 5B). To evaluate IL-17A levels in T cells, CD4$^+$ T cells were isolated from tumor-draining lymph nodes in mice and were cultured for 4 days in the presence of α-CD3 and α-CD28. IL-17A mRNA levels and secreted-IL-17A into the media from CD4$^+$ T cells increased in the pre-irradiated group, compared to the control group (Figure 5C and D). These data show that enhanced-tumor growth is closely correlated with IL-17A in pre-irradiated tumor beds.

Th17 cell differentiation was enhanced by irradiation in vitro

Next, to determine how irradiation to the tumor beds could induce Th17 cells, we examined Th17 cell differentiation by irradiation *in vitro*. First, we isolated dermal fibroblasts from mice and these were irradiated with 5 Gy. An irradiation of 5 Gy increased IL-6 and TGF-β levels in dermal fibroblasts (Figure S3). Isolated-naïve CD4$^+$ T cells from spleen were cultured for 4 days in conditioned medium derived from irradiated-dermal fibroblasts or no irradiated-dermal fibroblasts. For Th17 polarizing *in vitro*, Th17 polarizing factors except TGF-β were added to culture media (Anti-IFN-γ (2 μlg/ml), Anti-IL-4 (2 μlg/ml) and small amount rmIL-6 (10 ng/ml) than commonly used rmIL-6 for Th17 polarization *in vitro*. As shown Figure 5E, the differentiation of naïve T cells towards Th17 cells was enhanced in the conditioned medium derived from irradiated fibroblasts.

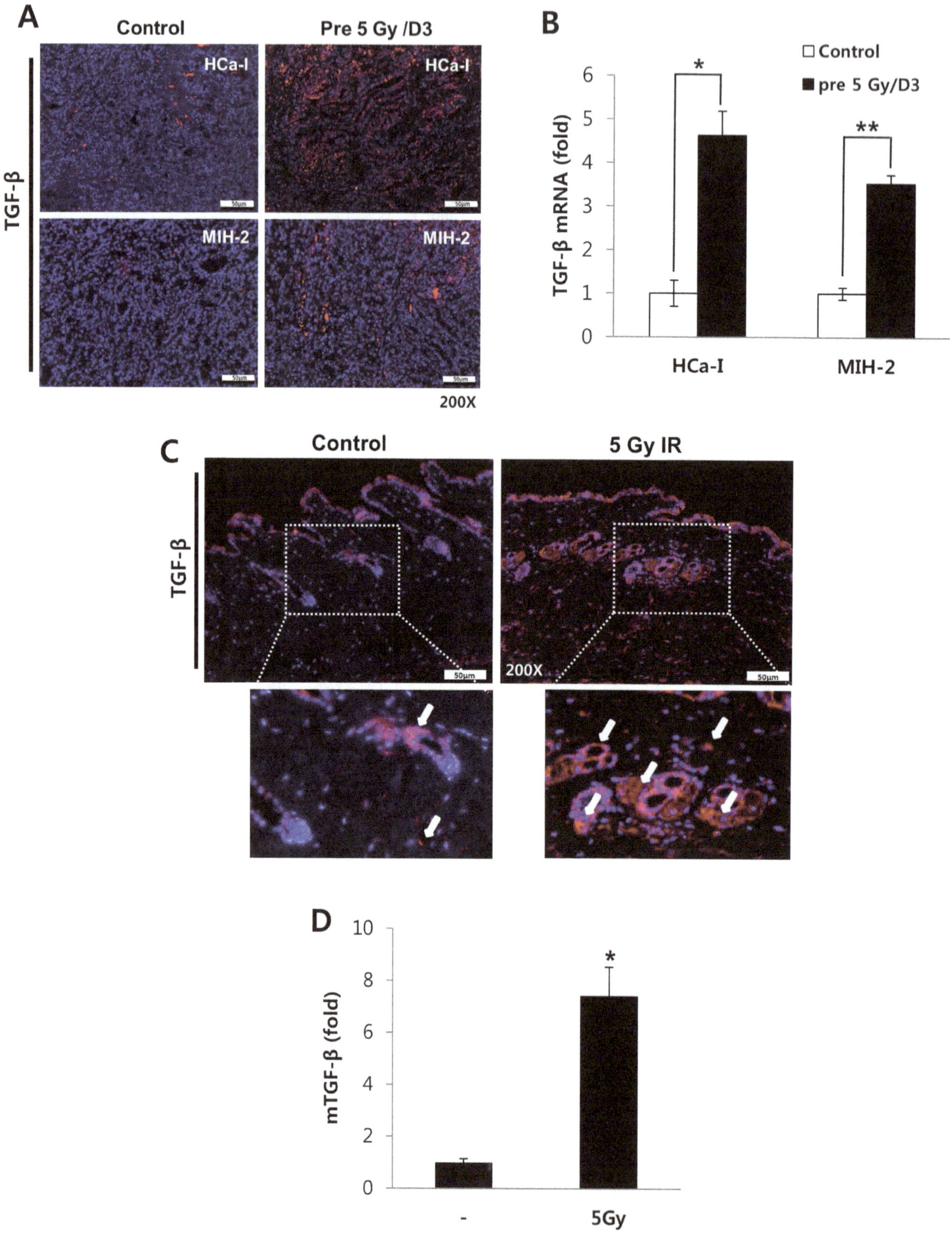

Figure 2. TGF-β expression. (A) TGF-β expression and (B) mRNA level in both tumors implanted into irradiated tumor beds or non-irradiated tumor beds at day 3 after irradiation. (C) TGF-β expression and (D) TGF-β mRNA level of tumor beds with or without 5 Gy-irradiation. $p<0.05$ (*) and $p<0.01$ (**) (*t*-test).

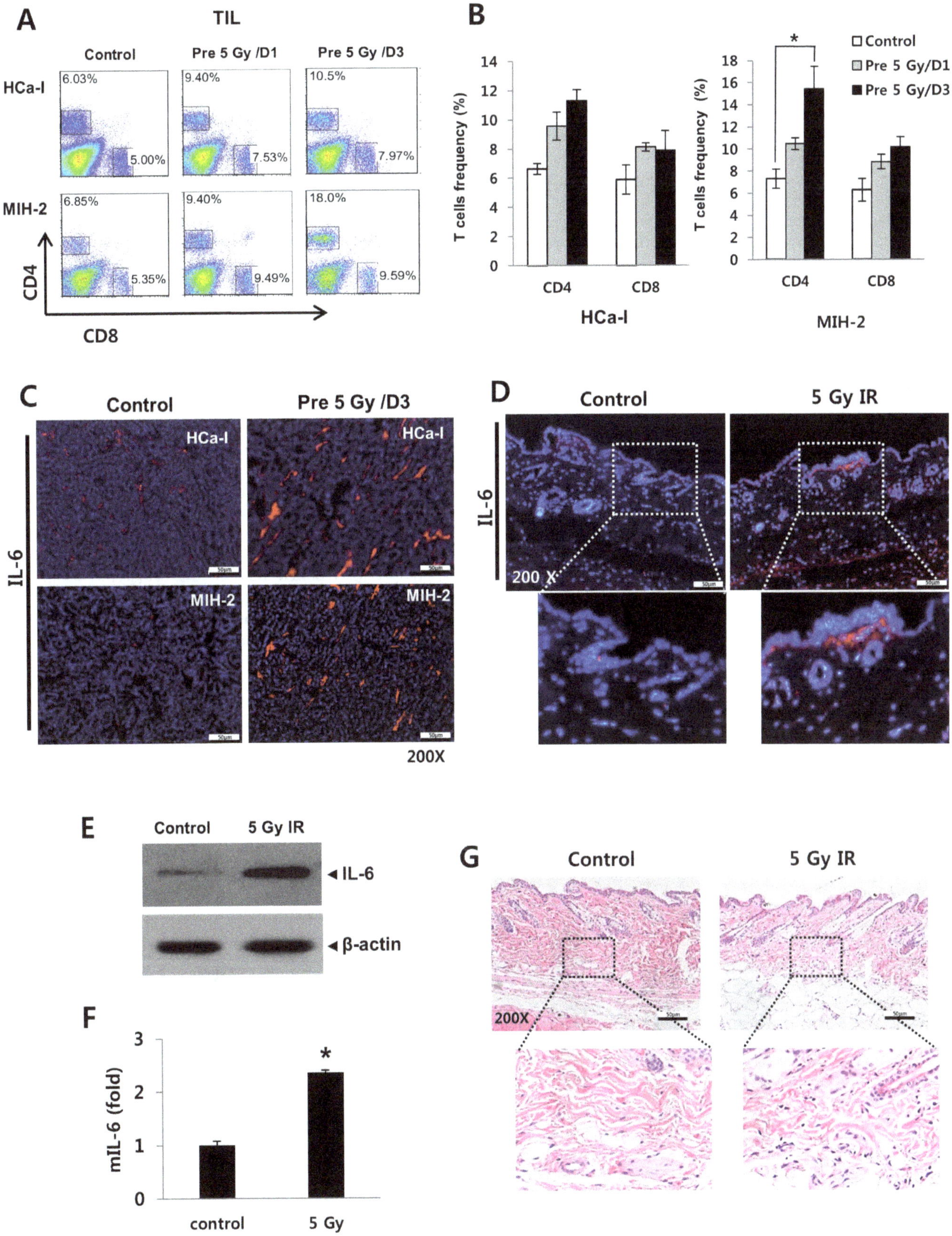

Figure 3. TIL frequency and IL-6 expression in implanted tumors and irradiated beds. TILs were isolated from the tumor and stained with $CD4^+$ and $CD8^+$ antibodies which was analyzed by FACS. (A) frequency of infiltrated $CD4^+$ and $CD8^+$ T cells and (B) Summary of TIL frequency in HCa-I and MIH-2 tumors. (C) IL-6 expression in both tumors. Irradiated beds were analyzed at day 3 after 5 Gy irradiation. (D) Representative

immunofluorescence staining for IL-6, (E) western blotting for IL-6, (F) IL-6 mRNA level and (G) histology in 5 Gy irradiated beds. $p<0.05$ (*) and $p<0.01$ (**) (*t*-test).

Tumor progression was inhibited by IL-17A neutralization in implanted tumors in pre-irradiated beds

When tumor cells were inoculated into irradiated tumor beds, the tumor growth rate and IL-17A expression drastically were increased relative to the controls. In addition, recombinant hIL-17A (rhIL-17A) treatment increased the proliferation of human hepatocellular carcinoma, HepG2 cells *in vitro* (Figure S4). Therefore, we further examined whether IL-17A neutralization can rescue accelerated tumor growth in pre-irradiated beds. As shown in figure 6A and C, neutralization of IL-17A suppressed the accelerated tumor growth in pre-irradiated tumor beds. Moreover, IL-17A decreased following IL-17A neutralization in both tumors implanted in the pre-irradiated beds (Figure 6B and D). Therefore, irradiating tumor beds might enhance the growth of subsequently implanted tumors via IL-17A.

Discussion

The effect of a high, ablative-radiation dose to the tumor bed on the growth of subsequently an implanted tumor has been extensively investigated, and is known as the tumor bed effect (TBE). The TBE was first described by Frankl and Kimball and was named the TBE by Senstrom [19]. A high-dose of irradiation to the tumor bed induced injury to the host vasculature and connective tissue, resulting in impaired neovascularization in the implanted tumor [10]. It has been reported that implanted tumor growth was inhibited in high-dose (20 Gy) pre-irradiated beds, while tumor metastasis increased through increased hypoxia-associated factors [20]. Although the nature of TBE has long been recognized, its mechanism is still uncertain.

In this study, we investigated the effect of low-dose pre-irradiation (5 Gy) on the tumor bed where tumor cells were subsequently implanted. In current practice hypofractionated RT, a low-dose region usually present around the region exposed to a high, lethal dose. Tumor of areas receiving low-doses of irradiation may be affected to tumor growth by pre-irradiation. Fig 1A showed that tumor growth was accelerated in areas that received below 5 Gy. More frequently, 5 Gy-fraction hypofractionated RT is used in a clinical setting [21,22], thus 5 Gy was used in this study.

The growth of implanted tumors in 5 Gy pre-irradiated beds was accelerated by IL-17A, compared to the controls. In HCa-I, tumor growth in the pre-irradiated beds was faster in the pre-5 Gy/D1 and D3 groups than in the control group, and was correlated with IL-17A production. However, MIH-2 showed faster growth only in the pre-5 Gy/D3 group, and there was only a slight difference in tumor growth between the control and pre-5 Gy/D1 groups. This might be attributable to a decrease in the potency of IL-17A in the pre-5 Gy/D1 group of MIH-2 than that in HCa-I.

In this study, tumor growth was suppressed by IL-17A neutralization; however, growth was still slightly faster than that in the non-irradiated control. This suggests that other factors in addition to IL-17A might promote tumor growth in pre-irradiated beds.

Several studies have shown that IL-6 inhibits radiation-induced apoptosis and enhances cell survival via stat3 activation [23,24]. Fujikawa *et al.* reported that the IL-6-induced inflammatory response can suppress immune-mediated anti-tumor effects [25]. In this study, IL-6 level in the tumor-draining lymph nodes of irradiated group was slightly induced compared to control. Our results also showed that a 5 Gy irradiation increased TGF-β. TGF-β suppresses tumor growth during tumor initiation, but it may in fact promote tumor progression and cancer cell invasiveness in later stages [26]. Accordingly, irradiation-induced IL-6 and TGF-β could act separately as a pro-tumor factor as well as accelerated tumor growth through the induction of IL-17A in this study. However, IL-17A was significantly increased in

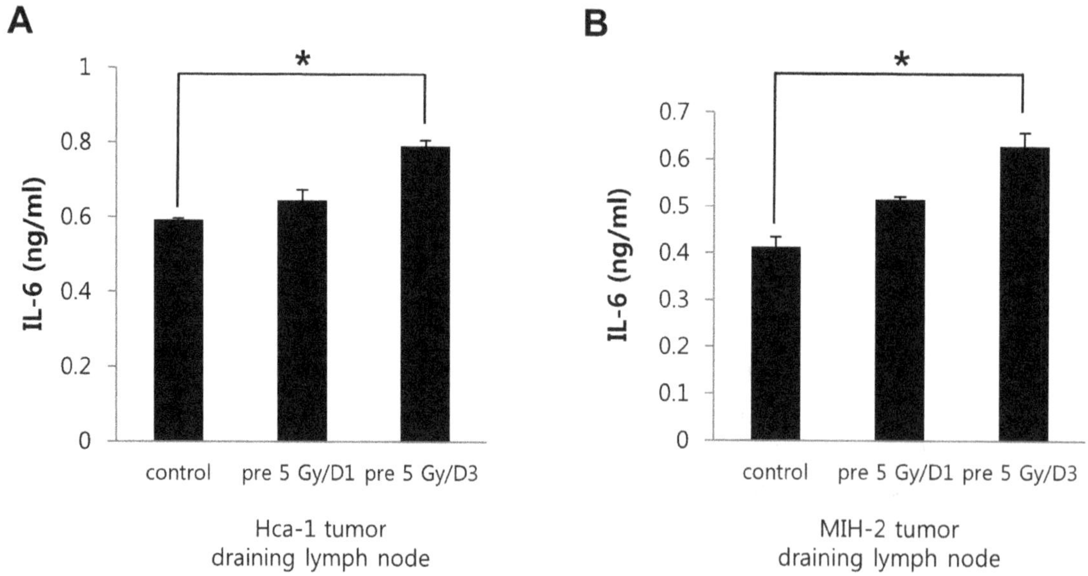

Figure 4. IL-6 expression in the tumor-draining lymph node of tumor bearing mice. (A and B) IL-6 expression in the tumor draining lymph node from HCa-I and MIH-2 bearing mice. $p<0.05$ (*) and $p<0.01$ (**) (*t*-test).

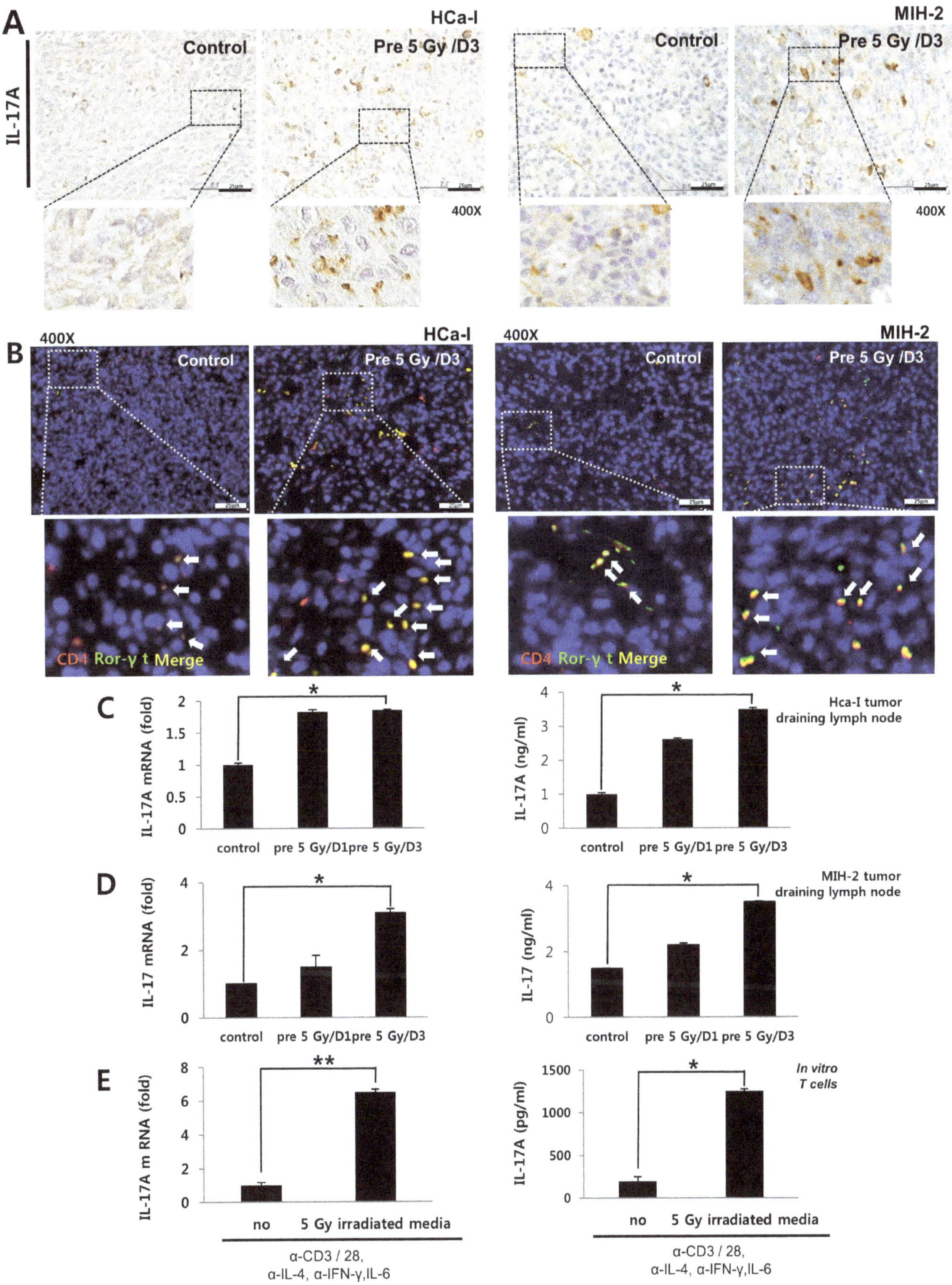
A
IL-17A
HCa-I
Control
Pre 5 Gy /D3
MIH-2
Control
Pre 5 Gy /D3
400X
B
400X
HCa-I
Control
Pre 5 Gy /D3
MIH-2
Control
Pre 5 Gy /D3
CD4 Ror-γ t Merge
C
IL-17A mRNA (fold)
control
pre 5 Gy/D1
pre 5 Gy/D3
IL-17A (ng/ml)
Hca-I tumor draining lymph node
D
IL-17 mRNA (fold)
IL-17 (ng/ml)
MIH-2 tumor draining lymph node
E
IL-17A m RNA (fold)
IL-17A (pg/ml)
In vitro T cells
no
5 Gy irradiated media
α-CD3 / 28,
α-IL-4, α-IFN-γ,IL-6

Figure 5. IL-17A expression in the tumor-draining lymph node of tumor bearing mice and Th17 differentiation by irradiation *in vitro*. (A) Expressions of IL-17A and (B) Th17 cells ($CD4^+$ and Ror-γt double positive cells) in both tumors. (C) IL-17A mRNA level and protein expression in the tumor draining lymph node of HCa-I bearing mice. (D) IL-17A mRNA level and protein expression in the tumor-draining lymph node of MIH-2 bearing mice. (E) Th17 differentiation by irradiation *in vitro*. Murine fibroblasts were cultured for 3 days after irradiating cells with 5 Gy. Naïve CD4+ T cells were isolated from the spleen, which were then cultured for 4 days in conditioned medium derived from irradiated fibroblasts or non-irradiated fibroblasts. Secreted IL-17A from Th17 cells was analyzed by ELISA. IL-17A mRNA level was evaluated using quantitative real time PCR. rmIL-6 (10 ng/ml), α-IFN-γ (2 μg/ml), and α-IL-4 (2 μg/ml) were added to the culture media. $p<0.05$ (*) and $p<0.01$ (**) (*t*-test).

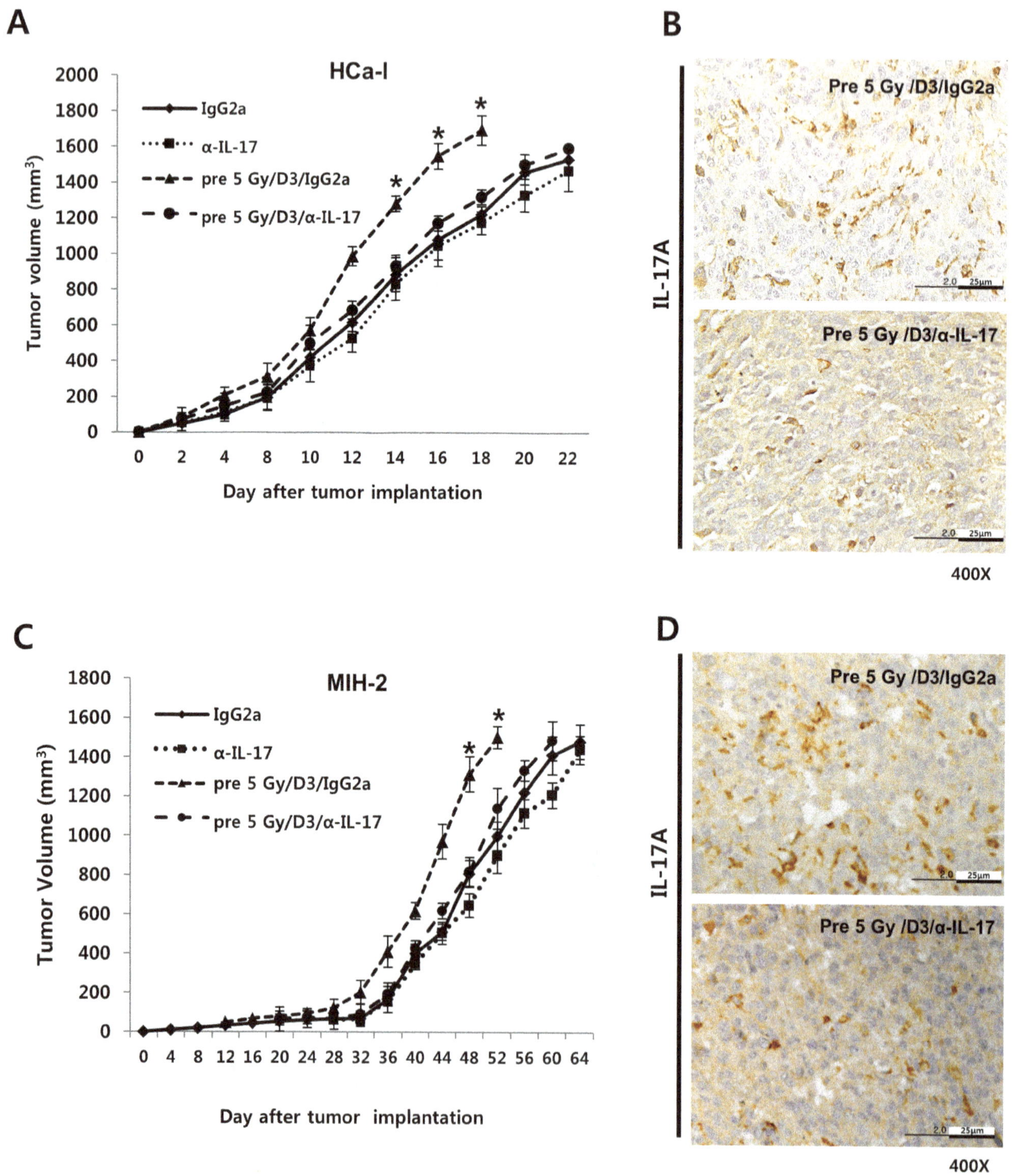

Figure 6. The effect of treatment with α-IL-17A neutralizing antibody on tumor growth. (A and C) Growth delay and (B and D) IL-17A expression of HCa-I and MIH-2 tumors implanted in 5 Gy irradiated beds or non-irradiated beds by α-IL-17A treatment, respectively (n = 5 mice per group). Error bars denote ± SEM. *p<0.05, pre 5 Gy/D3/α-IL-17 *vs* pre 5 Gy/D3/IgG2a (ANOVA).

draining lymph nodes of the irradiated group, compared to IL-6 and its expression exhibited a correlation with enhanced tumor growth. Therefore, IL-17A might be a major factor for enhancing tumor growth in low-dose pre-irradiated tumor beds.

IL-17A is mainly secreted by Th17 cells, which may influence cancer progression. IL-17B, IL-17C, IL-17D, IL-17E/IL-25, and IL-17F have all been identified in humans and cloned [27]. Among these, IL-17A has been detected in several human cancers. IL-17A promotes hepatocellular carcinoma (HCC) metastasis via matrix metalloproteinase (MMP) 2 and 9 [28]. In contrast, another study showed that endogenous IL-17 reduces tumor growth and metastasis [29]. Although, the role of IL-17 in cancer has not been fully studied, the clinical evidence of IL-17A and Th17 cells as pro-tumor factors in HCC have recently been reported. It has shown that increased IL-17 production in T cells from tumors or blood of HCC patients is correlated with both micro-vessel density and poor prognosis, suggesting the potential role of IL-17 as a pro-tumor factor [30,31]. It was also reported that the inhibition of monocytes/macrophage-derived inflammation in hepatoma-bearing mice suppresses tumor-infiltrating Th17 cell numbers, resulting in a reduction of tumor growth [32]. Thus, IL-17A seems to be a specific target in HCC. Indeed, this study demonstrated that low-dose pre-irradiation of tumor beds subsequently enhanced implanted-hepatoma growth *in vivo*, which was suppressed by IL-17A neutralization. Therefore, we suggest that IL-17A may be used as a novel therapeutic approach to improve the outcome of patients with HCC receiving RT through preventing recurrence in low-dose normal liver. However, further studies are needed to determine whether blocking IL-17A helps in preventing recurrence of both the primary irradiated tumor and recurrence in low-dose normal livers.

In conclusion, the results of our study suggest that low-dose irradiation of tumor beds can induce IL-17A production via IL-6 and TGF-β production, and promote the growth of subsequently implanted tumors. IL-17A seems to be a key factor for enhancing tumor growth in pre-irradiated tumor beds.

Supporting Information

Figure S1 Iso dose lines of the patient with Hepatocellular carcinoma receiving 20 Gy single fractionation RT.

Figure S2 Expression of TGF-β by pre-irradiation of tumor bed in tumor border and tumor. Approximately 1×10^6 HCa-1 cells were injected intramuscularly in the right thigh of the mice on day 3 after the implantation site had been irradiated with 5 Gy.

Figure S3 Murine fibroblasts were isolated from mice skin that were irradiated with 5 Gy. (A) TGF-β and (B) IL-6 expression was assessed by ELISA in irradiated-murine fibroblasts cultured media 3 day after irradiation, respectively. Data are representative of three independent experiments.

Figure S4 Proliferation of HepG2 cells by rhIL-17. HepG2 cells were treated with rhIL-17A of concentration from 0 to 100 ng/ml. Data are representative of three independent experiments.

Author Contributions

Conceived and designed the experiments: EJL JS. Performed the experiments: EJL HJP WWK. Analyzed the data: EJL JS IJL YGS SJH. Contributed reagents/materials/analysis tools: JS SJH. Wrote the paper: EJL JS.

References

1. Purdy JA (2008) Dose to normal tissues outside the radiation therapy patient's treated volume: a review of different radiation therapy techniques. Health physics 95: 666–676.
2. Kuonen F, Secondini C, Ruegg C (2012) Molecular pathways: emerging pathways mediating growth, invasion, and metastasis of tumors progressing in an irradiated microenvironment. Clinical cancer research 18: 5196–5202.
3. Pogribny I, Koturbash I, Tryndyak V, Hudson D, Stevenson SM, et al. (2005) Fractionated low-dose radiation exposure leads to accumulation of DNA damage and profound alterations in DNA and histone methylation in the murine thymus. Molecular cancer research 3: 553–561.
4. Chou C, Chen S, Cheng JC (2009) Radiation-induced interleukin-6 expression through MAPK/p38/NF-kappaB signaling pathway and the resultant anti-apoptotic effect on endothelial cells through Mcl-1 expression with sIL6-Ralpha. International journal of radiation oncology, biology, physics 75: 1553–1561.
5. Ao X, Zhao L, Davis M, Lubman D, Lawrence T, et al. (2009) Radiation produces differential changes in cytokine profiles in radiation lung fibrosis sensitive and resistant mice. J Hematol Oncol 2:6.
6. Numasaki M, Fukushi J, Ono M, Narula SK, Zavodny PJ, et al. (2003) Interleukin-17 promotes angiogenesis and tumor growth. Blood 101: 2620–2627.
7. Zou W, NP R (2010) Th17 cells in tumour immunity and immunotherapy. Nature Review 10: 248–256.
8. Park H, Li Z, Yang XO, Chang SH, Nurieva R, et al. (2005) A distinct lineage of CD4 T cells regulates tissue inflammation by producing interleukin 17. Nature Immunology 6: 1133–1141.
9. Van den Berg WB, Miossec P (2009) IL-17 as a future therapeutic target for rheumatoid arthritis. Nature Reviews Rheumatology 5: 549–553.
10. Saeki Y, Shimazaki S, Urano M (1971) Radiation effect on the vascularization of a C3H mouse mammary carcinoma. Microangiographic studies of the tumor in preirradiated tissue and of the recurrent tumor. Radiology 101: 175–180.
11. Milross CG, Mason KA, Hunter NR, Chung WK, Peters LJ, et al. (1996) Relationship of mitotic arrest and apoptosis to antitumor effect of paclitaxel. Journal of the National Cancer Institute 88: 1308–1314.
12. Kim W, Seong J, Oh HJ, Koom WS, Choi K, et al. (2011) A novel combination treatment of armed oncolytic adenovirus expressing IL-12 and GM-CSF with radiotherapy in murine hepatocarcinoma. journal of radiation research 52: 646–654.
13. Irie M, Homma S, Komita H, Zeniya M, Kufe D, et al. (2004) Inhibition of spontaneous development of liver tumors by inoculation with dendritic cells loaded with hepatocellular carcinoma cells in C3H/HeNCRJ mice. International journal of cancer 111: 238–245.
14. Park HJ, Kusnadi A, Lee EJ, Kim WW, Cho BC, et al. (2012) Tumor-infiltrating regulatory T cells delineated by upregulation of PD-1 and inhibitory receptors. Cellular immunology 278: 76–83.
15. Maehara Y, Kakeji Y, Kabashima A, Emi Y, Watanabe A, et al. (1999) Role of transforming growth factor-beta 1 in invasion and metastasis in gastric carcinoma. Journal of clinical oncology 17: 607–614.
16. Hodge DR, Hurt EM, Farrar WL (2005) The role of IL-6 and STAT3 in inflammation and cancer. European journal of cancer 41: 2502–2512.
17. Romano M, Sironi M, Toniatti C, Polentarutti N, Fruscella P, et al. (1997) Role of IL-6 and its soluble receptor in induction of chemokines and leukocyte recruitment. Immunity 6: 315–325.
18. Morishima N, Mizoguchi I, Takeda K, Mizuguchi J, Yoshimoto T (2009) TGF-beta is necessary for induction of IL-23R and Th17 differentiation by IL-6 and IL-23. Biochemical and biophysical research communications 386: 105–110.
19. Stenstrom KW, Vermund H, Mosser DG, Marvin JF (1955) Effects of roentgen irradiation on the tumor bed. I. The inhibiting action of local pretransplantation roentgen irradiation (1500 r alpha) on the growth of mouse mammary carcinoma. Radiation Research 2: 180–191.
20. Rofstad EK, Mathiesen B, Henriksen K, Kindem K, Galappathi K (2005) The tumor bed effect: increased metastatic dissemination from hypoxia-induced up-regulation of metastasis-promoting gene products. Cancer research 65: 2387–2396.
21. Hasselle MD, Haraf DJ, Rusthoven KE, Golden DW, Salgia R, et al. (2012) Hypofractionated image-guided radiation therapy for patients with limited volume metastatic non-small cell lung cancer. Journal of thoracic oncology 7: 376–381.
22. Bae SH, Park HC, Lim DH, Gwak GY, Choi MS, et al. (2012) Salvage treatment with hypofractionated radiotherapy in patients with recurrent small hepatocellular carcinoma. International journal of radiation oncology, biology, physics 82: e603–e607.
23. Horiguchi A, Oya M, Marumo K, Murai M (2002) STAT3, but not ERKs, mediates the IL-6-induced proliferation of renal cancer cells, ACHN and 769P. Kidney international 61: 926–938.

24. Miyamoto Y, Hosotani R, Doi R, Wada M, Ida J, et al. (2001) Interleukin-6 inhibits radiation induced apoptosis in pancreatic cancer cells. Anticancer research 21: 2449–2456.
25. Fujikawa K, Matsui Y, Miura K, Kobayashi T, Oka H, et al. (2000) Serum immunosuppressive acidic protein and natural killer cell activity in patients with metastatic renal cell carcinoma before and after nephrectomy. The Journal of urology 164: 673–675.
26. Basanta D, Strand DW, Lukner RB, Franco OE, Cliffel DE, et al. (2009) The role of transforming growth factor-beta-mediated tumor-stroma interactions in prostate cancer progression: an integrative approach. Cancer research 69: 7111–7120.
27. Moseley TA, Haudenschild DR, Rose L, Reddi AH (2003) Interleukin-17 family and IL-17 receptors. Cytokine & growth factor reviews 14: 155–174.
28. Li J, Lau GK, Chen L, Dong S, Lan H, et al. (2011) Interleukin 17A promotes hepatocellular carcinoma metastasis via NF-kB induced matrix metalloproteinases 2 and 9 expression. PLoS ONE 6: e21816–e21816.
29. Kryczek I, Wei S, Szeliga W, Vatan L, Zou W (2009) Endogenous IL-17 contributes to reduced tumor growth and metastasis. Blood 114: 357–359.
30. Zhang J, Yan J, Xu J, Pang X, Chen M, et al. (2009) Increased intratumoral IL-17-producing cells correlate with poor survival in hepatocellular carcinoma patients. Journal of hepatology 50: 980–989.
31. Wang W, Wang Z, Liu Y, Qin Y, Shen Q (2010) Increased level of Th17 cells in peripheral blood correlates with the development of hepatocellular carcinoma. J chinese Oncol 32: 757–761.
32. Kuang DM, Peng C, Zhao Q, Wu Y, Chen MS, et al. (2010) Activated Monocytes in Peritumoral Stroma of Hepatocellular Carcinoma Promote Expansion of Memory T Helper 17 Cells. Hepatology 51: 154–164.

15

Single Nucleotide Polymorphisms of One-Carbon Metabolism and Cancers of the Esophagus, Stomach, and Liver in a Chinese Population

Shen-Chih Chang[1], Po-Yin Chang[1], Brendan Butler[1], Binh Y. Goldstein[1], Lina Mu[2], Lin Cai[3], Nai-Chieh Y. You[1], Aileen Baecker[1], Shun-Zhang Yu[4], David Heber[5], Qing-Yi Lu[5], Liming Li[6], Sander Greenland[1,7], Zuo-Feng Zhang[1]*

1 Department of Epidemiology, University of California Los Angeles Fielding School of Public Health, Los Angeles, CA, United States of America, **2** Department of Social and Preventive Medicine, State University of New York at Buffalo, Buffalo, NY, United States of America, **3** Department of Epidemiology, Fujian Medical University, Fuzhou, Fujian, China, **4** Department of Epidemiology, Fudan University School of Public Health, Shanghai, China, **5** Center for Human Nutrition, University of California Los Angeles David Geffen School of Medicine, Los Angeles, CA, United States of America, **6** Department of Epidemiology, Peking University School of Public Health, Beijing, China, **7** Department of Statistics, University of California Los Angeles College of Letters and Science, Los Angeles, CA, United States of America

Abstract

One-carbon metabolism (folate metabolism) is considered important in carcinogenesis because of its involvement in DNA synthesis and biological methylation reactions. We investigated the associations of single nucleotide polymorphisms (SNPs) in folate metabolic pathway and the risk of three GI cancers in a population-based case-control study in Taixing City, China, with 218 esophageal cancer cases, 206 stomach cancer cases, 204 liver cancer cases, and 415 healthy population controls. Study participants were interviewed with a standardized questionnaire, and blood samples were collected after the interviews. We genotyped SNPs of the *MTHFR*, *MTR*, *MTRR*, *DNMT1*, and *ALDH2* genes, using PCR-RFLP, SNPlex, or TaqMan assays. To account for multiple comparisons and reduce the chances of false reports, we employed semi-Bayes (SB) shrinkage analysis. After shrinkage and adjusting for potential confounding factors, we found positive associations between *MTHFR* rs1801133 and stomach cancer (any T versus C/C, SB odds-ratio [SBOR]: 1.79, 95% posterior limits: 1.18, 2.71) and liver cancer (SBOR: 1.51, 95% posterior limits: 0.98, 2.32). There was an inverse association between *DNMT1* rs2228612 and esophageal cancer (any G versus A/A, SBOR: 0.60, 95% posterior limits: 0.39, 0.94). In addition, we detected potential heterogeneity across alcohol drinking status for ORs relating *MTRR* rs1801394 to esophageal (posterior homogeneity $P = 0.005$) and stomach cancer (posterior homogeneity $P = 0.004$), and ORs relating *MTR* rs1805087 to liver cancer (posterior homogeneity $P = 0.021$). Among non-alcohol drinkers, the variant allele (allele G) of these two SNPs was inversely associated with the risk of these cancers; while a positive association was observed among ever-alcohol drinkers. Our results suggest that genetic polymorphisms related to one-carbon metabolism may be associated with cancers of the esophagus, stomach, and liver. Heterogeneity across alcohol consumption status of the associations between *MTR/MTRR* polymorphisms and these cancers indicates potential interactions between alcohol drinking and one-carbon metabolic pathway.

Editor: Nathan A. Ellis, University of Arizona, United States of America

Funding: This work is supported in part by the International Union Against Cancer (UICC) Technology Transfer fellowship (ICRETT) awarded to Dr. Li-Na Mu and by the Foundation for the Author of National Excellent Doctoral Dissertation of P.R. China, No. 200157, awarded to Dr. Lin Cai. The study was also partially supported by the NIH National Institute of Environmental Health Sciences, National Cancer Institute, Department of Health and Human Services, grants ES06718, ES 011667, CA09142, as well as the Alper Research Program of Environmental Genomics of the UCLA Jonsson Comprehensive Cancer Center and the UCLA Clinical Nutrition Research Unit. The funders had no role in study design, data collection and analysis, decision to publish, or preparation of the manuscript.

Competing Interests: The authors have declared that no competing interests exist.

* Email: zfzhang@ucla.edu

Introduction

Upper gastrointestinal (GI) cancers are major causes of morbidity and mortality throughout the world. Based on GLOBOCAN 2012 estimates, stomach, liver, and esophageal cancers are the fifth, sixth, and eighth most common cancers, respectively, with a global incidence of approximately 2,189,829 new cancer cases (15.5% of the total), and 1,868,700 deaths (22.8% of the total) [1]. The majority of these cancer cases (1,694,874 cases, 77.4%) occur in less developed countries. China alone accounts for almost half of all incident GI cancers (1,023,072 cases, 46.7%) [1].

Continued research regarding the involvement of single nucleotide polymorphisms (SNPs) in the etiology of these three upper GI cancers has been fruitful. Of particular interest are the SNPs located within genes involved in folate metabolism [2–4]. Folate maintains DNA stability by regulating DNA biosynthesis, DNA repair and DNA methylation [5]. Neoplasms may develop when this pathway is disregulated by the depletion of micronutrients or through the incorporation of polymorphisms [5]. Several enzymes are involved in one-carbon metabolism, including the methylenetetrahydrofolate reductase (MTHFR), methionine synthase (MTR), methionine synthase reductase (MTRR), DNA methyltransferases (DNMTs), and mitochondrial aldehyde dehydrogenase 2 (ALDH2). MTHFR, MTR, and MTRR are involved in DNA synthesis, and the generation of S-adenosylmethionine (SAM)—a universal methyl-donor for methylation reactions. DNMTs catalyze DNA methylation and replicate methylation patterns. ALDH2 is responsible for metabolizing acetaldehyde generated during alcohol metabolism. Alcohol and acetaldehyde can inhibit folate absorption and impair DNA methylation [6].

The role of folate and one-carbon metabolism in upper GI cancers is not fully understood. Animal studies provided some evidence for an effect of low folate levels in oxidative stress, DNA methylation, and hepatocarcinogenesis [7,8]; while high folate intake can increase global DNA methylation and reduce gastric cancer risk [9,10]. Epidemiologic studies have suggested that genetic polymorphisms of genes in one-carbon metabolic pathway might modulate the risk of esophageal and gastric cancer [4]. However, published results are inconclusive and limited in terms of the number of genes/polymorphisms being investigated. Possible modification by related micronutrients and known risk factors has seldom been explored. Therefore, considering the importance of one-carbon metabolism in upper GI cancer development, we examined the associations between eight SNPs in genes in one-carbon metabolic pathway and cancers of the esophagus, stomach, and liver in a Chinese population. We also evaluated heterogeneity of the associations across different strata of plasma micronutrients (including folate, vitamin B12, and total homocysteine) and known risk factors for these cancers.

Materials and Methods

Ethics statement

This study was exempted by the institutional review board of University of California at Los Angeles (Certified Exempt 02-248).

Study Design and Population

A detailed description of the study design has been published previously [11,12]. Briefly, this was a population-based case-control study conducted in Taixing City, Jiangsu Province, China. Eligible cases were newly diagnosed patients with pathologically or clinically confirmed esophageal cancer (between June 1 and December 30, 2000), stomach cancer (between June 1 and December 30, 2000), and liver cancer (between January 1 and June 30, 2000) reported to the Taixing CDC Tumor Registry. Other inclusion criteria including being 20 years of age or older, in stable medical condition as determined by a physician, residency in Taixing for 10 years or more, and willingness to participate. A total of 218 esophageal cancer cases, 206 stomach cancer cases, and 204 liver cancer cases participated, representing 67, 65 and 57%, respectively, of all newly diagnosed cancer patients.

Controls were randomly selected among healthy residents of Taixing City with a 2:3 frequency matching ratio to the combined case group on 5-year age categories (20–24 to 80–84), sex, and residency (village in rural township or in an urban residential block in central Taixing City). There are 23 townships (rural areas) and one central town (urban area) in Taixing City. Each rural township consists of 10–12 villages, and the central urban area consists of 10–12 residential blocks. Other inclusion criteria were the same as the cases. A total of 464 potential controls were approached, and 415 (89.4%) consented to participate.

Epidemiologic data collection

All of the recruited cases and controls completed a standard questionnaire administered by trained interviewers. Interviews took place either at the participants' homes, in the hospitals (for cases), or in the county doctor's office (for controls). Cancer cases were usually interviewed within 6 months of diagnoses. The questionnaire collected detailed information on demographic factors, current height and weight, dietary history, tobacco smoking history, alcohol drinking history, tea drinking habits, occupational history, family history of cancers, and physical activities.

Laboratory assays

Each study participant provided a 5-ml peripheral blood sample after their interviews. DNA was isolated from blood clots, using the phenol-chloroform method. Hepatitis B virus surface antigen (HBsAg), IgG antibodies for hepatitis C virus (HCV), and IgG antibodies for CagA-*Helicobacter pylori* (H. *pylori*) were measured by enzyme-linked immunosorbant assay (ELISA) using kits from the Reagent Company of the Shanghai Hospital for Infectious Diseases (Shanghai, China), the Shanghai Huamei Biological Company (Shanghai, China), and the Reagent Company of the Shanghai Biotechnology Industry Park (Pudong, Shanghai, China), respectively. Plasma aflatoxin B1 (AFB1)-albumin adduct levels were determined by ELISA assay, as previously described [13], using free aflatoxin (Supelco) for the aflatoxin standards. A comparison between free and bound aflatoxin standards revealed a log-linear relationship, allowing us to estimate the absolute values of the samples. Plasma folate and vitamin B12 levels were measured using a competitive radioassay with iodine 125-labeled folate and cobalt 57-labeled vitamin B12 as tracers (Quantaphase II B12/folate radiobinding kit, Bio-Rad, CA). Plasma total homocysteine (tHcy) levels were measured using a commercially available chemiluminescent immunoassay system (IMMULITE 1000 Automated Analyzer, DPC, Los Angeles, CA).

We selected eight SNPs from *MTHFR*, *MTR*, *MTRR*, *DNMT1*, and *ALDH2* genes, based on the following criteria: 1) SNPs which are functional or potentially functional (SNPs located in the coding, 3′-, and 5′-untranslated regions); 2) SNPs previously reported to be associated with upper GI cancers; and 3) SNPs with minor allele frequency of at least 5% in the National Center for Biotechnology Information SNP database. Genotyping was performed using the TaqMan (*MTR* rs1805087, *MTRR* rs1532268/rs1801394, and *ALDH2* rs886205) or the SNPlex (*DNMT1* rs2228612 and *ALDH2* rs2238151) assay, as previously described (Applied Biosystems by Life Technologies, Foster City, CA) [14], or the PCR-RFLP analysis (*MTHFR* rs1801133 and *ALDH2* rs671) modified from previously published methods [15,16]. Genotyping call rates were over 97% for TaqMan and PCR-RFLP methods, and over 80% for the SNPlex assay. Reproducibility was 98% for the SNPlex assay (3% random duplicate samples) [17], and 100% for the TaqMan assay (10% random duplicate samples).

Statistical analysis

We used Pearson's chi-square test for Hardy-Weinberg equilibrium (HWE) for the distributions of genotype frequencies of the eight SNPs in the controls only. Testing for HWE among the controls is a commonly used preliminary quality-control method in genetic association studies to identify systematic genotyping errors in unrelated individuals. We analyzed each SNP-cancer association under co-dominant, log-linear, dominant, and recessive genetic models, using unconditional logistic regression models to calculate odds ratios (ORs) and 95% confidence intervals (CIs). Models included age-matched categories, sex, residency (urban/rural), education (illiteracy/primary school/higher than middle school), body mass index (BMI, continuous), smoking pack-years (continuous), alcohol consumption frequency (never/occasionally/often/everyday), *H. pylori* infection (stomach cancer; negative/

positive), HBsAg status (liver cancer; negative/positive) and plasma AFB1-albumin adduct levels in quintiles (liver cancer; estimated quintile: <222.7, 222.7–344.2, 344.2–442.6, 442.6–588.5, and >588.5 fmol/mg). To adjust for residual confounding effects from age, we also included the deviation of each person's age from the mean age in each age category [18]. We caution that a number of adjustment variables may be affected by genetic variations, as these variables occur afterward. At best, our estimates are for direct genotype effects, and otherwise may be over-adjusted or confounded by uncontrolled factors that affect both the adjustment variables and the outcomes [19]. Thus, we checked estimates for direct genotype effects against estimates adjusted only for age and sex.

We further conducted stratified analyses to check heterogeneity across strata of micronutrients or modifiable risk factors, including plasma micronutrients (folate, vitamin B12, and tHcy), smoking status, alcohol consumption, H. *pylori* infection (stomach cancer), HBsAg status (liver cancer), and plasma AFB1 levels (liver cancer). We used estimated median levels in controls to dichotomize plasma levels of folate (12.76 nmol/l), vitamin B12 (228.88 pmol/l), tHcy (9.5 μmol/l), and AFB1 (388.95 fmol/mg). We used the dominant genetic model, which assumed that the effect of the variant allele is dominant if the ratio of the ORs comparing variant allele homozygotes to heterozygotes was smaller than that comparing heterozygotes to common allele homozygotes; otherwise we used the recessive genetic model. We assessed heterogeneity across strata using likelihood ratio tests by comparing models with and without product terms.

To reduce the risks of multiple-comparison artefacts and sparse-data bias, we used a semi-Bayes (SB) shrinkage (penalized-likelihood) method to estimate genotype coefficients [20]; the odds-ratio estimates we report are the antilogs of these coefficients. Shrinkage estimation has been recommended extensively as an alternative superior to Bonferroni in the statistical literature for eliminating multiple-testing artefacts in comparative studies [21–24]. In shrinkage estimation, instead of changing the alpha level, we regress ('shrink') the estimates toward zero to a degree proportional to their estimated variances and inversely proportional to the prior variances v. The prior variance plays a role analogous to the adjusted α-level, in that smaller values correspond to more stringent rejection/detection criteria, with $\alpha = 0$ and $v = 0$ being the lower limits of adjustment at which rejection of the null becomes impossible. At the other extreme, no adjustment occurs when using the original value of α or a huge (effectively infinite) value for v.

In our study, we assigned a prior variance of 0.50, and a prior median OR = 1 (no association) which results in a 95% prior probability of falling within the interval 0.25, 4. This pulls the observed associations toward the null to the degree that would result if there had been a previous null experiment observing 4/v = 8 cases total and it had been merged with the current data [20,25]. When differing stratum-specific SNP effects were allowed, such as in stratified analyses, the prior variance was reduced to 0.25, which corresponds to a variance of 0.50 for the coefficient of the stratum-SNP product (interaction). For each SB posterior estimate, we further provide the directional (one-sided) SB P-values, which equal the posterior probability that the point estimate is on the wrong side of the null under the fitted model and the shrinkage priors [26,27].

To summarize the associations of the 8 SNPs for each of the three upper GI cancers, we constructed a polygenetic risk score (PRS) [28]. The PRS was calculated as the weighted sum of the risk genotype (under either dominant or recessive model as in the stratified analyses) counts, where the weight for each SNP was determined by the semi-Bayes log OR of its association with each cancer in the fully adjusted model. PRS was only estimated among those with complete genotype data on all of the 8 SNPs, which include 126 esophageal cancer cases, 125 stomach cancer cases, 142 liver cancer cases, and 287 controls. The range (maximum minus minimum) of PRS for each cancer was divided into three equally spaced categories; these ranges were 0.11 to 2.05 for esophageal cancer, 0 to 1.91 for stomach cancer, and 0 to 1.40 for liver cancer. Data analyses were performed using SAS 9.1.3 (SAS Institute, Cary, NC).

Results

Compared to population controls, cancer cases tended to be smokers, had lower BMI, and lower education levels (Table 1). Esophageal and stomach cancer cases were older than the controls, while liver cancer cases were the youngest. Liver cancer patients had the highest male-to-female ratio of 3.53, and were most likely to consume alcohol; esophageal cancer patients drank more frequently than the other cancer cases and controls in this study. For risk factors specific to each cancer site, we did not observe differing frequency of *H. pylori* infection between stomach cancer patients and controls. Compared with controls, liver cancer patients showed a higher percentage of HBsAg positive (65 vs. 25%), anti-HCV positive (9 vs. 3%), and had higher plasma AFB1-albumin adduct levels (30 vs. 20% in the 5th quintile).

Table 2 presents the SB odds-ratio estimates (SBOR) for each SNP-cancer association of the eight SNPs; Table S1, S2, S3, S4, S5, S6 shows stratified associations and Figure 1 summarizes selected results. Genotype distributions among controls appeared compatible with Hardy-Weinberg equilibrium, except possibly for *DNMT1* rs2228612, which had $P = 0.010$, below the traditional alpha level of 0.05, but larger than the Bonferroni-adjusted alpha level of 0.05/8 = 0.006 (testing all eight SNPs). However, we note that matching may bias controls away from equilibrium if the matching factors are associated with both the SNPs and cancer.

We have previously reported positive associations of the T allele of *MTHFR* rs1801133 with stomach and liver cancer [11,12]. In the present analysis, these associations remained apparent after confounder adjustment and SB shrinkage (any T versus C/C, fully adjusted SBOR: 1.79, 95% posterior limits: 1.18, 2.71 for stomach cancer; SBOR: 1.51, 95% posterior limits: 0.98, 2.32 for liver cancer). In stratified SB analyses, the association between *MTHFR* rs1801133 and stomach cancer appeared stronger among individuals who had lower plasma folate levels, higher plasma vitamin B12 or tHcy levels, and among smokers (Figure 1). There was no clear association of *MTHFR* rs1801133 with esophageal cancer (Table 2 and Tables S1, S2, S3, S4, S5).

While there was no clear overall association between SNPs in *MTR* and *MTRR* and any cancer in main effect analyses (Table 2), heterogeneity of association was suggested in stratified analyses on alcohol consumption, including associations of *MTR* rs1805087 with liver cancer (homogeneity $P = 0.021$), and *MTRR* rs1801394 with both esophageal (homogeneity $P = 0.005$) and stomach cancer (homogeneity $P = 0.004$). While G allele carriers of *MTR* rs1805087 were inversely associated with liver cancer among non-drinkers (SBOR: 0.57, 95% posterior limits: 0.31, 1.04), they were positively associated with liver cancer among drinkers (SBOR: 1.48, 95% posterior limits: 0.85, 2.57) (Figure 1). Similarly, G allele carriers of *MTRR* rs1801394 were inversely associated with esophageal and stomach cancer among non-drinkers (SBOR: 0.59, 95% posterior limits: 0.37, 0.94 for esophageal cancer; SBOR: 0.49, 95% posterior limits: 0.30, 0.79 for stomach cancer) but positively associated with cancer among

Table 1. Distribution for selected demographic and health characteristics comparing esophageal, stomach, and liver cancer cases with controls.

	Controls	Cancer Cases					
		Esophageal Cancer		Stomach Cancer		Liver Cancer	
	(N, %)	(N, %)	One-Sided	(N, %)	One-Sided	(N, %)	One-Sided
	(N=415)	(N=218)	*P*-value†	(N=206)	*P*-value†	(N=204)	*P*-value†
Age*, mean ± SD	57.7±11.8	60.6±9.6	0.001	62.8±9.8	<0.001	53.9±13.0	<0.001
Sex*							
Female	128 (30.8)	77 (35.3)	0.25	68 (33.0)	0.58	45 (22.1)	0.022
Male	287 (69.2)	141 (64.7)		138 (67.0)		159 (77.9)	
BMI, mean ± SD	22.4±2.6	21.9±2.8	0.035	21.4±2.7	<0.001	21.5±2.7	<0.001
Education							
Illiterate	73 (17.6)	83 (38.6)	<0.001	66 (32.0)	<0.001	44 (21.6)	0.19
Primary school	142 (34.2)	101 (47.0)		107 (51.9)		77 (37.8)	
Middle school or higher	200 (48.2)	31 (14.4)		33 (16.0)		83 (40.7)	
Smoking							
Never	217 (52.4)	94 (44.6)	0.063	92 (45.8)	0.12	85 (44.3)	0.062
Ever	197 (47.6)	117 (55.5)		109 (54.2)		107 (55.7)	
pack-years, mean ± SD	23.7±15.6	28.9±21.9	0.030	27.7±19.2	0.068	21.2±14.0	0.20
Alcohol drinking							
Never	207(50.2)	116 (55.0)	0.015	111 (55.2)	0.70	87 (45.3)	0.13
Occasionally	72(17.5)	18 (8.5)		31 (15.4)		29(15.1)	
Often	75(18.2)	37 (17.5)		32 (15.9)		51(26.6)	
Everyday	58(14.1)	40 (19.0)		27 (13.4)		25(13.0)	
H. *pylori* CagA status							
+	251 (68.8)			130 (64.7)	0.32		
−	114 (31.2)			71 (35.3)			
HBsAg status							
+	102 (24.6)					132 (64.7)	<0.001
−	312 (75.4)					72 (35.3)	
Anti-HCV status							
+	12 (2.9)					18 (9.0)	0.001
−	403 (97.1)					183 (91.0)	
Plasma AFB1-albumin adduct levels (qunitile)							
1	75 (19.9)					26 (14.4)	0.054
2	76 (20.2)					36 (19.9)	
3	75 (19.9)					36 (19.9)	

Table 1. Cont.

	Controls	Cancer Cases					
		Esophageal Cancer		Stomach Cancer		Liver Cancer	
	(N, %)	(N, %)	One-Sided	(N, %)	One-Sided	(N, %)	One-Sided
	(N = 415)	(N = 218)	*P*-value†	(N = 206)	*P*-value†	(N = 204)	*P*-value†
4	76 (20.2)					28 (15.5)	
5	75 (19.9)					55 (30.4)	

*: Matching factors.
†: Two-sided *P*-values derived from t-tests for continuous variables and $\chi 2$ tests for categorical variables comparing cancer cases to controls.

drinkers (SBOR: 1.56, 95% posterior limits: 0.95, 2.56 for esophageal cancer; SBOR: 1.39, 95% posterior limits: 0.83, 2.32 for stomach cancer) (Figure 1).

For *DNMT1* polymorphism, rs2228612 was inversely associated with esophageal cancer in the dominant genetic model (any G versus A/A, SBOR: 0.60, 95% posterior limits: 0.39, 0.94) (Table 2). Among three *ALDH2* SNPs, rs671 was associated with esophageal cancer in the recessive genetic model (A/A versus any G, SBOR: 1.76, 95% posterior limits: 0.96, 3.24). In stratified adjusted analyses, *ALDH2* rs671 appeared associated with esophageal cancer among individuals with lower plasma folate levels (A/A versus any G, SBOR: 2.12, 95% posterior limits: 1.01, 4.44) (Figure 1). The *ALDH2* rs2238151 appeared inversely associated with liver cancer when comparing T allele carriers to those with the C/C genotype (age and sex-adjusted SBOR: 0.47, 95% posterior limits: 0.24, 0.92). While we did not find associations between *ALDH2* rs886205 and cancer susceptibility in main effect analyses, stratum-specific SBOR suggested that *ALDH2* rs886205 was positively associated with stomach cancer among participants with higher plasma vitamin B12 levels (SBOR: 1.87, 95% posterior limits: 1.09, 3.20) (Figure 1).

Except for analysis on single SNP models, we also did joint SNPs analysis by including all of the 8 SNPs in a model (Table 3). The results from joint SNPs analysis suggested similar associations as in the single SNP models, but the 95% posterior intervals were wider.

The analysis on PRS suggested roughly a doubling of odds for esophageal and liver cancers among individuals in the highest PRS category compared to those in the lowest category (SBOR: 2.06; 95% posterior limits: 1.13, 3.77 for esophageal cancer and SBOR: 2.09, 95% posterior limits: 1.05, 4.17 for liver cancer), with somewhat less consistency across categories for stomach cancer. In the continuous PRS analysis, the results suggested a doubling of odds for these three upper GI cancers with one unit (in log OR) increase of PRS (Table 4). We caution however that PRS analyses do not account for the score construction from the data, and thus may overestimate effects and underestimate variability in the resulting estimates.

Discussion

We examined the associations between eight SNPs in genes involved in the one-carbon metabolic pathway and susceptibility of esophageal, stomach, and liver cancers in a Chinese population. After applying SB shrinkage methods and controlling for potential confounders, we observed that any T genotype of *MTHFR* rs1801133 was positively associated with both stomach and liver cancer. We also found an inverse association between the variant G allele of *DNMT1* rs2228612 and esophageal cancer. In addition, our study suggested potential OR variations across strata of alcohol consumption, including associations of *MTRR* rs1801394 with esophageal and stomach cancer, and *MTR* rs1805087 with liver cancer. The odds for upper GI cancers were roughly doubled for Chinese participants with one unit (in log OR) increase of PRS.

In one-carbon metabolism, MTHFR irreversibly catalyzes the conversion of 5,10-methylenetetrahydrofolate (5,10-methyleneTHF) to 5-methyltetrahydrofolate (5-methylTHF). The 5,10-methyleneTHF is essential in purine and thymidilate synthesis, and 5-methylTHF is a co-substrate for remethylation of homocysteine to methionine, which is further converted to SAM for methylation reactions [5]. The *MTHFR* C677T (rs1801133) polymorphism, which results in an alanine to valine substitution, leads to reduced MTHFR enzyme activity [29], decreased 5-

Table 2. Associations between SNPs of MTHFR, MTR, MTRR, DNMT1, and ALDH2 genes and cancers of the esophagus, stomach, and liver.

	Esophageal Cancer					Stomach Cancer					Liver Cancer				
	Ca/Co	SBOR[1] (95% posterior limit)	One-sided P^*	SBOR[2] (95% posterior limit)	One-sided P^*	Ca/Co	SBOR[1] (95% posterior limit)	One-sided P^*	SBOR[2] (95% posterior limit)	One-sided P^*	Ca/Co	SBOR[1] (95% posterior limit)	One-sided P^*	SBOR[2] (95% posterior limit)	One-sided P^*
MTHFR															
rs1801133															
CC	65/135	1.00		1.00		50/135	1.00		1.00		50/135	1.00		1.00	
CT	105/199	1.15 (0.79, 1.65)	0.24	1.19 (0.80, 1.77)	0.20	106/199	1.38 (0.94, 2.02)	0.050	1.53 (1.00, 2.33)	0.024	114/199	1.46 (1.00, 2.13)	0.026	1.57 (1.02, 2.42)	0.021
TT	32/57	1.13 (0.69, 1.86)	0.32	1.35 (0.78, 2.32)	0.14	38/57	1.66 (1.02, 2.71)	0.021	2.26 (1.30, 3.91)	0.002	30/57	1.31(0.78, 2.19)	0.15	1.17 (0.64, 2.12)	0.31
P_{trend}[†]		0.50		0.21			0.021		0.001			0.12		0.24	
Dominant		1.15 (0.81, 1.64)	0.22	1.25 (0.85, 1.84)	0.13		1.49 (1.03, 2.16)	0.018	1.79 (1.18, 2.71)	0.003		1.46 (1.00, 2.12)	0.024	1.51 (0.98, 2.32)	0.029
Recessive		1.05 (0.67, 1.66)	0.41	1.23 (0.74, 2.03)	0.21		1.38 (0.90, 2.14)	0.072	1.78 (1.09, 2.91)	0.011		1.05 (0.66, 1.67)	0.41	0.91 (0.53, 1.56)	0.37
MTR															
rs1805087															
A/A	161/310	1.00		1.00		142/310	1.00		1.00		149/310	1.00		1.00	
A/G	35/76	0.90 (0.58, 1.37)	0.31	0.79 (0.50, 1.27)	0.17	46/76	1.31 (0.87, 1.96)	0.096	1.16 (0.74, 1.83)	0.26	40/76	1.03 (0.68, 1.56)	0.45	0.92 (0.57, 1.47)	0.36
G/G	4/0	–		–		1/0	–		–		1/0	–		–	
Dominant		1.01 (0.66, 1.52)	0.49	0.90 (0.57, 1.42)	0.32		1.34 (0.90, 2.00)	0.078	1.19 (0.76, 1.87)	0.22		1.05 (0.69, 1.59)	0.41	0.93 (0.58, 1.49)	0.38
MTRR															
rs1532268															
C/C	145/283	1.00		1.00		144/283	1.00		1.00		149/283	1.00		1.00	
C/T	47/94	0.99 (0.67, 1.46)	0.47	1.16 (0.76, 1.78)	0.25	44/94	0.96 (0.65, 1.43)	0.42	0.98 (0.63, 1.53)	0.47	39/94	0.77 (0.51, 1.15)	0.10	0.83 (0.52, 1.32)	0.21
T/T	11/11	1.80 (0.86, 3.80)	0.060	1.96 (0.89, 4.31)	0.047	5/11	1.08 (0.45, 2.56)	0.43	1.05 (0.43, 2.57)	0.46	4/11	0.75 (0.31, 1.82)	0.27	1.09 (0.42, 2.82)	0.43
P_{trend}[†]		0.27		0.070			0.98		0.97			0.14		0.61	
Dominant		1.11 (0.77, 1.61)	0.29	1.32 (0.88, 1.98)	0.089		0.98 (0.67, 1.44)	0.45	1.00 (0.65, 1.52)	0.49		0.75 (0.50, 1.11)	0.075	0.85 (0.54, 1.34)	0.25
Recessive		1.81 (0.86, 3.80)	0.059	1.91 (0.87, 4.19)	0.052		1.09 (0.46, 2.58)	0.43	1.06 (0.43, 2.57)	0.45		0.78 (0.33, 1.89)	0.30	1.12 (0.43, 2.90)	0.41
rs1801394															
A/A	117/204	1.00		1.00		119/204	1.00		1.00		114/204	1.00		1.00	
A/G	74/149	0.88 (0.62, 1.25)	0.24	0.92 (0.63, 1.35)	0.34	63/149	0.75 (0.53, 1.08)	0.063	0.74 (0.49, 1.11)	0.070	64/149	0.78 (0.54, 1.12)	0.092	0.74 (0.49, 1.12)	0.078

Table 2. Cont.

	Esophageal Cancer					Stomach Cancer					Liver Cancer				
	Ca/Co	SBOR[1] (95% posterior limit)	One-sided*P**	SBOR[2] (95% posterior limit)	One-sided*P**	Ca/Co	SBOR[1] (95% posterior limit)	One-sided *P**	SBOR[2] (95% posterior limit)	One-sided *P**	Ca/Co	SBOR[1] (95% posterior limit)	One-sided *P**	SBOR[2] (95% posterior limit)	One-sided *P**
G/G	10/25	0.81 (0.42, 1.59)	0.27	0.95 (0.47, 1.93)	0.44	9/25	0.76 (0.38, 1.50)	0.21	0.77 (0.37, 1.60)	0.24	13/25	0.93 (0.49, 1.75)	0.41	1.39 (0.70, 2.78)	0.17
P_{trend}†		0.36		0.70			0.10		0.13			0.30		0.87	
Dominant		0.86 (0.61, 1.21)	0.20	0.92 (0.64, 1.34)	0.33		0.74 (0.52, 1.05)	0.046	0.73 (0.49, 1.07)	0.055		0.80 (0.56, 1.13)	0.10	0.83 (0.56, 1.24)	0.19
Recessive		0.85 (0.44, 1.64)	0.31	0.97 (0.48, 1.96)	0.47		0.82 (0.41, 1.62)	0.29	0.84 (0.41, 1.74)	0.32		1.00 (0.54, 1.88)	0.50	1.53 (0.78, 3.03)	0.11
DNMT1															
rs2228612															
A/A	52/100	1.00		1.00		43/100	1.00		1.00		48/100	1.00		1.00	
A/G	56/200	0.58 (0.38, 0.88)	0.006	0.52 (0.33, 0.82)	0.003	72/200	0.84 (0.55, 1.28)	0.21	0.82 (0.51, 1.31)	0.20	74/200	0.79 (0.52, 1.19)	0.13	0.79 (0.49, 1.28)	0.17
G/G	29/57	1.03 (0.61, 1.73)	0.46	0.96 (0.55, 1.68)	0.44	28/57	1.11 (0.65, 1.89)	0.36	1.12 (0.62, 2.04)	0.35	36/57	1.33 (0.80, 2.22)	0.13	1.35 (0.76, 2.42)	0.15
P_{trend}†		0.57		0.37			0.88		0.88			0.42		0.42	
Dominant		0.67 (0.45, 1.00)	0.026	0.60 (0.39, 0.94)	0.012		0.90 (0.59, 1.36)	0.31	0.89 (0.56, 1.41)	0.31		0.92 (0.62, 1.37)	0.34	0.93 (0.58, 1.50)	0.39
Recessive		1.38 (0.86, 2.21)	0.092	1.35 (0.81, 2.25)	0.13		1.22 (0.76, 1.97)	0.20	1.26 (0.74, 2.15)	0.20		1.53 (0.97, 2.40)	0.033	1.54 (0.92, 2.59)	0.051
ALDH2															
rs671															
G/G	118/213	1.00		1.00		108/213	1.00		1.00		109/213	1.00		1.00	
A/G	60/160	0.70 (0.49, 1.01)	0.029	0.76 (0.51, 1.13)	0.088	76/160	0.97 (0.68, 1.38)	0.44	1.06 (0.71, 1.57)	0.39	74/160	0.91 (0.64, 1.30)	0.31	1.05 (0.70, 1.58)	0.41
A/A	25/20	1.97 (1.11, 3.49)	0.010	1.61 (0.86, 3.00)	0.066	12/20	1.13 (0.58, 2.21)	0.36	0.99 (0.48, 2.03)	0.49	10/20	1.03 (0.51, 2.06)	0.47	0.96 (0.45, 2.06)	0.46
P_{trend}†		0.49		0.67			0.88		0.88			0.77		0.94	
Dominant		0.88 (0.63, 1.24)	0.24	0.90 (0.62, 1.31)	0.29		1.00 (0.71, 1.40)	0.49	1.05 (0.71, 1.54)	0.41		0.93 (0.66, 1.31)	0.33	1.04 (0.70, 1.54)	0.43
Recessive		2.20 (1.25, 3.86)	0.003	1.76 (0.96, 3.24)	0.035		1.14 (0.59, 2.21)	0.35	0.97 (0.48, 1.97)	0.47		1.06 (0.53, 2.10)	0.44	0.95 (0.45, 2.01)	0.44
rs2238151															
C/C	173/293	1.00		1.00		151/293	1.00		1.00		166/293	1.00		1.00	
C/T	11/34	0.66 (0.35, 1.22)	0.093	0.66 (0.34, 1.29)	0.11	18/34	1.08 (0.61, 1.89)	0.40	1.21 (0.65, 2.23)	0.28	7/34	0.44 (0.22, 0.87)	0.009	0.51 (0.23, 1.11)	0.045

Table 2. Cont.

	Esophageal Cancer					Stomach Cancer					Liver Cancer				
	Ca/Co	**SBOR[1] (95% posterior limit)**	**One-sided P^***	**SBOR[2] (95% posterior limit)**	**One-sided P^***	**Ca/Co**	**SBOR[1] (95% posterior limit)**	**One-sided P^***	**SBOR[2] (95% posterior limit)**	**One-sided P^***	**Ca/Co**	**SBOR[1] (95% posterior limit)**	**One-sided P^***	**SBOR[2] (95% posterior limit)**	**One-sided P^***
T/T	0/1	–		–		0/1	–		–		1/1	1.15 (0.33, 4.03)	0.41	1.43 (0.39, 5.33)	0.30
P_{trend}[†]		–		–			–		–			0.045		0.29	
Dominant		0.64 (0.35, 1.19)	0.079	0.65 (0.33, 1.28)	0.11		1.05 (0.60, 1.83)	0.43	1.20 (0.65, 2.21)	0.29		0.47 (0.24, 0.92)	0.013	0.58 (0.27, 1.25)	0.082
Recessive		–		–			–		–			1.16 (0.33, 4.07)	0.41	1.44 (0.39, 5.37)	0.29
rs886205															
G/G	173/315	1.00		1.00		150/315	1.00		1.00		149/315	1.00		1.00	
A/G	29/69	0.81 (0.51, 1.26)	0.17	0.78 (0.48, 1.28)	0.17	41/69	1.23 (0.81, 1.87)	0.17	1.47 (0.92, 2.34)	0.054	40/69	1.19 (0.78, 1.81)	0.21	1.38 (0.85, 2.24)	0.096
A/A	2/4	1.07 (0.36, 3.18)	0.45	1.00 (0.33, 3.08)	0.50	2/4	1.10 (0.37, 3.30)	0.43	1.18 (0.39, 3.65)	0.38	2/4	1.00 (0.34, 2.96)	0.50	1.27 (0.40, 4.10)	0.34
P_{trend}[†]		0.45		0.39			0.32		0.098			0.47		0.14	
Dominant		0.82 (0.53, 1.28)	0.19	0.79 (0.49, 1.29)	0.17		1.23 (0.82, 1.86)	0.16	1.48 (0.93, 2.34)	0.047		1.18 (0.78, 1.79)	0.22	1.41 (0.88, 2.28)	0.076
Recessive		1.08 (0.36, 3.23)	0.44	1.02 (0.33, 3.13)	0.49		1.08 (0.36, 3.24)	0.44	1.16 (0.38, 3.55)	0.40		0.98 (0.33, 2.92)	0.49	1.25 (0.39, 4.03)	0.35

[1]: Semi-Bayes odds ratio (SBOR) adjusted for age (5-year categories and deviation from stratum mean) and sex.

[2]: SBOR further adjusted for residency (city, rural), alcohol drinking frequency, smoking pack-years, BMI, education, H. *pylori* infection (in stomach cancer analyses), HBsAg (in liver cancer analyses), and plasma AFB1 levels (in liver cancer analyses), based on the assumption that genotype did not affect any of these variables.

*: One-sided semi-Bayes *P*-values; the posterior probability that the point estimate is on the wrong side of the null [26,27].

[†]: *P*-value from Chi-Square test for trend.

Cancer	SNP	Stratum	P*	SBOR	95% Posterior Limits
Esophagus	ALDH2 rs671	Lower plasma folate	0.094	2.12	1.01-4.44
		Higher plasma folate		0.97	0.49-1.91
	MTRR rs1801394	Non-alcohol drinkers	0.005	0.59	0.37-0.94
		Alcohol drinkers		1.56	0.95-2.56
Stomach	MTHFR rs1801133	Lower plasma folate	0.43	1.82	1.06-3.13
		Higher plasma folate		1.40	0.85-2.30
		Lower plasma vit B12	0.69	1.39	0.80-2.42
		Higher plasma vit B12		1.69	1.03-2.77
		Lower plasma tHcy	0.38	1.33	0.80-2.22
		Higher plasma tHcy		1.84	1.08-3.12
		Non-smokers	0.56	1.37	0.81-2.32
		Smokers		1.75	1.06-2.88
	MTRR rs1801394	Non-alcohol drinkers	0.004	0.49	0.30-0.79
		Alcohol drinkers		1.39	0.83-2.32
	ALDH2 rs886206	Lower plasma vit B12	0.097	0.90	0.48-1.68
		Higher plasma vit B12		1.87	1.09-3.20
Liver	MTR rs1805087	Non-alcohol drinkers	0.021	0.57	0.31-1.04
		Alcohol drinkers		1.48	0.85-2.57

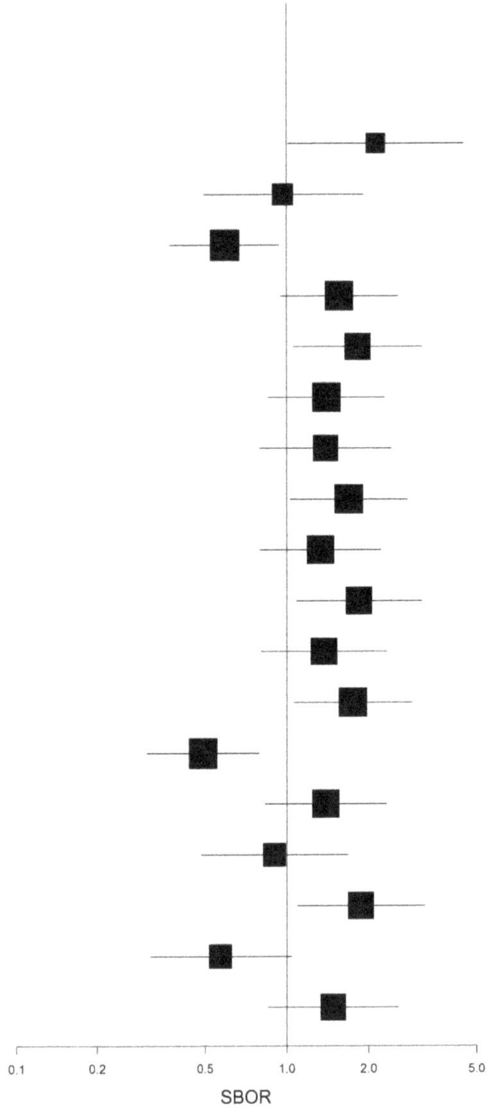

Figure 1. Selected semi-Bayes stratum-specific associations. Selected semi-Bayes stratum-specific associations between SNPs in *MTHFR, MTR, MTRR, DNMT1, ALDH2,* and upper GI cancer susceptibility, by plasma levels of micronutrients (folate, vitamin B12, and homocysteine) and environmental factors (smoking, alcohol drinking, H. *pylori* CagA status, HBsAg status, and plasma AFB1-albumin adduct levels). Semi-Bayes adjusted ORs (SBOR) and 95% posterior limits were under dominant genetic models, except for the SBOR relating *ALDH2* rs671to esophageal cancer, where recessive genetic model was used. *P** denotes *P*-value for homogeneity test.

methylTHF and an accumulation of 5,10-methyleneTHF in red blood cells [30].

Low MTHFR activity is associated with increase cancer risk due to low blood 5-methylTHF and impaired DNA methylation. Conversely, it could reduce cancer risk by increasing the availability of 5,10-methyleneTHF for normal DNA synthesis and preventing uracil misincorporation and chromosomal breakage [5]. Although evidence in support of these hypotheses is weak and inconsistent [5], an *in vitro* study suggested that the effect of *MTHFR* rs1801133 on DNA stability and methylation is site-specific and may depend on folate availability [31]. When folate supply is adequate or high, the T allele of *MTHFR* is associated with increased genomic DNA methylation in colon cancer cells, but decreased DNA methylation in breast cancer cells. When folate supply is limited, this variant is associated with decreased and unchanged DNA methylation in colon and breast cancer cells, respectively [31]. Uracil misincorporation is decreased in colon cancer cells expressing the *MTHFR* T allele, and increased in breast cancer cells expressing the same variant [31]. This site-specific difference may partly explain the difference in cancer risk associated with the *MTHFR* rs1801133 polymorphism [4]. In epidemiologic studies, the T allele appears to decrease the risk of colorectal and breast cancers [32,33], but increase the risk of cancers of the esophagus, stomach, liver, bladder, cervix uteri, and lung [2–4,34–36].

In the present analysis using SB shrinkage, we confirmed our previous findings of positive associations between the T allele of *MTHFR* rs1801133 and cancers of the stomach and liver in this Taixing population [11,12], implying that the disturbance of DNA methylation resulting from this variant plays a major role in stomach and liver carcinogenesis. Recent meta-analyses reported similar associations (T/T versus C/C, OR: 1.40, 95% CI: 1.19–1.66 for stomach cancer; OR: 1.21, 95% CI: 0.95–1.56 for liver cancer) [3,4]. In addition, Zacho et al. [4] reported a larger

Table 3. Associations between SNPs of MTHFR, MTR, MTRR, DNMT1, and ALDH2 genes and cancers of the esophagus, stomach, and liver –the comparison between results from single SNP model[1] and joint SNPs model[2].

	Esophageal Cancer					Stomach Cancer					Liver Cancer				
	Ca/Co	SBOR[1] (95% posterior limit)	One-sided P^*	SBOR[2] (95% posterior limit)	One-sided P^*	Ca/Co	SBOR[1] (95% posterior limit)	One-sided P^*	SBOR[2] (95% posterior limit)	One- sided P^*	Ca/Co	SBOR[1] (95% posterior limit)	One- sided P^*	SBOR[2] (95% posterior limit)	One- sided P^*
MTHFR															
rs1801133															
CC	65/135	1.00		1.00		50/135	1.00		1.00		50/135	1.00		1.00	
CT	105/199	1.19 (0.80, 1.77)	0.20	1.20 (0.73, 1.96)	0.24	106/199	1.53 (1.00, 2.33)	0.024	1.33 (0.79, 2.21)	0.14	114/199	1.57 (1.02, 2.42)	0.021	1.34 (0.80, 2.25)	0.14
TT	32/57	1.35 (0.78, 2.32)	0.14	1.72 (0.91, 3.27)	0.048	38/57	2.26 (1.30, 3.91)	0.002	2.15 (1.13, 4.08)	0.010	30/57	1.17 (0.64, 2.12)	0.31	1.07 (0.52, 2.20)	0.42
P_{trend}†		0.21		0.033			0.001		0.003			0.24		0.18	
Dominant		1.25 (0.85, 1.84)	0.13	1.37 (0.85, 2.21)	0.10		1.79 (1.18, 2.71)	0.003	1.64 (1.01, 2.66)	0.022		1.51 (0.98, 2.32)	0.029	1.40 (0.88, 2.24)	0.078
Recessive		1.23 (0.74, 2.03)	0.21	1.55 (0.87, 2.75)	0.069		1.78 (1.09, 2.91)	0.011	1.93 (1.11, 3.35)	0.009		0.91 (0.53, 1.56)	0.37	1.00 (0.54, 1.83)	0.49
MTR															
rs1805087															
A/A	161/310	1.00		1.00		142/310	1.00		1.00		149/310	1.00		1.00	
A/G	35/76	0.79 (0.50, 1.27)	0.17	0.83 (0.48, 1.45)	0.26	46/76	1.16 (0.74, 1.83)	0.26	1.23 (0.73, 2.09)	0.22	40/76	0.92 (0.57, 1.47)	0.36	0.94 (0.54, 1.63)	0.41
G/G	4/0	–		–		1/0	–		–		1/0	–		–	
Dominant		0.90 (0.57, 1.42)	0.32	0.94 (0.55, 1.62)	0.42		1.19 (0.76, 1.87)	0.22	1.30 (0.78, 2.15)	0.16		0.93 (0.58, 1.49)	0.38	1.20 (0.73, 1.98)	0.23
MTRR															
rs1532268															
C/C	145/283	1.00		1.00		144/283	1.00		1.00		149/283	1.00		1.00	
C/T	47/94	1.16 (0.76, 1.78)	0.25	0.99 (0.57, 1.70)	0.48	44/94	0.98 (0.63, 1.53)	0.47	1.01 (0.58, 1.77)	0.48	39/94	0.83 (0.52, 1.32)	0.21	1.03 (0.59, 1.81)	0.46
T/T	11/11	1.96 (0.89, 4.31)	0.047	1.61 (0.61, 4.25)	0.17	5/11	1.05 (0.43, 2.57)	0.46	0.83 (0.25, 2.70)	0.38	4/11	1.09 (0.42, 2.82)	0.43	1.58 (0.54, 4.63)	0.20
P_{trend}†		0.070		0.21			0.97		0.49			0.61		0.50	
Dominant		1.32 (0.88, 1.98)	0.089	1.12 (0.67, 1.87)	0.34		1.00 (0.65, 1.52)	0.49	1.06 (0.63, 1.80)	0.41		0.85 (0.54, 1.34)	0.25	0.97 (0.59, 1.60)	0.46
Recessive		1.91 (0.87, 4.19)	0.052	1.70 (0.66, 4.40)	0.14		1.06 (0.43, 2.57)	0.45	0.87 (0.27, 2.81)	0.41		1.12 (0.43, 2.90)	0.41	1.41 (0.51, 3.86)	0.25
rs1801394															
A/A	117/204	1.00		1.00		119/204	1.00		1.00		114/204	1.00		1.00	

Table 3. Cont.

	Esophageal Cancer					Stomach Cancer					Liver Cancer				
	Ca/Co	SBOR[1] (95% posterior limit)	One-sided P^{*}	SBOR[2] (95% posterior limit)	One-sided P^{*}	Ca/Co	SBOR[1] (95% posterior limit)	One-sided P^{*}	SBOR[2] (95% posterior limit)	One-sided P^{*}	Ca/Co	SBOR[1] (95% posterior limit)	One-sided P^{*}	SBOR[2] (95% posterior limit)	One-sided P^{*}
A/G	74/149	0.92 (0.63, 1.35)	0.34	0.84 (0.51, 1.36)	0.24	63/149	0.74 (0.49, 1.11)	0.070	0.66 (0.40, 1.08)	0.049	64/149	0.74 (0.49, 1.12)	0.078	0.79 (0.47, 1.31)	0.18
G/G	10/25	0.95 (0.47, 1.93)	0.44	1.16 (0.52, 2.59)	0.36	9/25	0.77 (0.37, 1.60)	0.24	0.98 (0.41, 2.34)	0.49	13/25	1.39 (0.70, 2.78)	0.17	1.60 (0.72, 3.55)	0.12
P_{trend}†		0.70		0.50			0.13		0.075			0.87		0.33	
Dominant		0.92 (0.64, 1.34)	0.33	0.89 (0.56, 1.43)	0.32		0.73 (0.49, 1.07)	0.055	0.65 (0.41, 1.03)	0.034		0.83 (0.56, 1.24)	0.19	0.95 (0.61, 1.49)	0.42
Recessive		0.97 (0.48, 1.96)	0.47	1.35 (0.62, 2.92)	0.23		0.84 (0.41, 1.74)	0.32	1.09 (0.48, 2.47)	0.42		1.53 (0.78, 3.03)	0.11	1.49 (0.71, 3.13)	0.14
DNMT1															
rs2228612															
A/A	52/100	1.00		1.00		43/100	1.00		1.00		48/100	1.00		1.00	
A/G	56/200	0.52 (0.33, 0.82)	0.003	0.52 (0.31, 0.85)	0.005	72/200	0.82 (0.51, 1.31)	0.20	0.81 (0.48, 1.36)	0.21	74/200	0.79 (0.49, 1.28)	0.17	0.69 (0.40, 1.18)	0.088
G/G	29/57	0.96 (0.55, 1.68)	0.44	0.87 (0.47, 1.58)	0.32	28/57	1.12 (0.62, 2.04)	0.35	1.06 (0.55, 2.04)	0.43	36/57	1.35 (0.76, 2.42)	0.15	1.25 (0.66, 2.35)	0.25
P_{trend}†		0.37		0.12			0.88		0.48			0.42		0.32	
Dominant		0.60 (0.39, 0.94)	0.012	0.58 (0.36, 0.94)	0.013		0.89 (0.56, 1.41)	0.31	0.90 (0.55, 1.48)	0.34		0.93 (0.58, 1.50)	0.39	0.82 (0.51, 1.32)	0.21
Recessive		1.35 (0.81, 2.25)	0.13	1.20 (0.69, 2.09)	0.25		1.26 (0.74, 2.15)	0.20	1.19 (0.69, 2.07)	0.26		1.54 (0.92, 2.59)	0.051	1.62 (0.97, 2.71)	0.033
ALDH2															
rs671															
G/G	118/213	1.00		1.00		108/213	1.00		1.00		109/213	1.00		1.00	
A/G	60/160	0.76 (0.51, 1.13)	0.088	0.78 (0.48, 1.27)	0.16	76/160	1.06 (0.71, 1.57)	0.39	0.99 (0.61, 1.62)	0.49	74/160	1.05 (0.70, 1.58)	0.41	1.04 (0.63, 1.70)	0.44
A/A	25/20	1.61 (0.86, 3.00)	0.066	1.10 (0.52, 2.31)	0.40	12/20	0.99 (0.48, 2.03)	0.49	1.12 (0.51, 2.47)	0.39	10/20	0.96 (0.45, 2.06)	0.46	0.80 (0.34, 1.92)	0.31
P_{trend}†		0.67		0.31			0.88		0.49			0.94		0.33	
Dominant		0.90 (0.62, 1.31)	0.29	0.80 (0.51, 1.26)	0.17		1.05 (0.71, 1.54)	0.41	1.00 (0.63, 1.58)	0.50		1.04 (0.70, 1.54)	0.43	0.94 (0.61, 1.47)	0.40
Recessive		1.76 (0.96, 3.24)	0.035	1.16 (0.56, 2.37)	0.35		0.97 (0.48, 1.97)	0.47	1.01 (0.48, 2.14)	0.49		0.95 (0.45, 2.01)	0.44	0.84 (0.37, 1.87)	0.33
rs2238151															
C/C	173/293	1.00		1.00		151/293	1.00		1.00		166/293	1.00		1.00	

Table 3. Cont.

	Esophageal Cancer					Stomach Cancer					Liver Cancer				
	Ca/Co	SBOR[1] (95% posterior limit)	One-sided P*	SBOR[2] (95% posterior limit)	One-sided P*	Ca/Co	SBOR[1] (95% posterior limit)	One-sided P*	SBOR[2] (95% posterior limit)	One- sided P*	Ca/Co	SBOR[1] (95% posterior limit)	One- sided P*	SBOR[2] (95% posterior limit)	One- sided P*
C/T	11/34	0.66 (0.34, 1.29)	0.11	0.81 (0.35, 1.86)	0.31	18/34	1.21 (0.65, 2.23)	0.28	1.00 (0.45, 2.22)	0.50	7/34	0.51 (0.23, 1.11)	0.045	0.36 (0.14, 0.92)	0.016
T/T	0/1	–		–		0/1	–				1/1	1.43 (0.39, 5.33)	0.30	1.00 (0.25, 4.00)	0.50
P_{trend} †		–		–			–					0.29		0.006	
Dominant		0.65 (0.33, 1.28)	0.11	0.80 (0.35, 1.84)	0.30		1.20 (0.65, 2.21)	0.29	1.08 (0.49, 2.35)	0.43		0.58 (0.27, 1.25)	0.082	0.31 (0.13, 0.75)	0.005
Recessive		–		–			–					1.44 (0.39, 5.37)	0.29	1.00 (0.25, 4.00)	0.50
rs886205															
G/G	173/315	1.00		1.00		150/315	1.00		1.00		149/315	1.00		1.00	
A/G	29/69	0.78 (0.48, 1.28)	0.17	1.05 (0.55, 2.00)	0.44	41/69	1.47 (0.92, 2.34)	0.054	1.76 (0.93, 3.33)	0.041	40/69	1.38 (0.85, 2.24)	0.096	1.41 (0.75, 2.66)	0.14
A/A	2/4	1.00 (0.33, 3.08)	0.50	0.82 (0.25, 2.69)	0.37	2/4	1.18 (0.39, 3.65)	0.38	0.65 (0.19, 2.23)	0.25	2/4	1.27 (0.40, 4.10)	0.34	1.07 (0.31, 3.76)	0.46
P_{trend} †		0.39		0.37			0.098		0.31			0.14		0.17	
Dominant		0.79 (0.49, 1.29)	0.17	0.99 (0.52, 1.86)	0.48		1.48 (0.93, 2.34)	0.047	1.38 (0.76, 2.51)	0.15		1.41 (0.88, 2.28)	0.076	1.34 (0.76, 2.37)	0.16
Recessive		1.02 (0.33, 3.13)	0.49	0.85 (0.26, 2.75)	0.39		1.16 (0.38, 3.55)	0.40	0.70 (0.20, 2.40)	0.28		1.25 (0.39, 4.03)	0.35	0.93 (0.28, 3.04)	0.45

[1]: Single SNP model: models included one SNP only; Semi-Bayes odds ratio (SBOR) adjusted for age (5-year categories and deviation from stratum mean), sex, residency (city, rural), alcohol drinking frequency, smoking pack-years, BMI, education, H. *pylori* infection (in stomach cancer analyses), HBsAg (in liver cancer analyses), and plasma AFB1 levels (in liver cancer analyses), based on the assumption that genotype did not affect any of these variables.
[2]: Joint SNPs model: models included all of the 8 SNPs; SBOR adjusted for the same set of covariates. All of the SNPs combined together were under the same genetic models (genotype-specific, log-additive, dominant, or recessive).
*: One-sided semi-Bayes *P*-values; the posterior probability that the point estimate is on the wrong side of the null [26,27].
†: *P*-value from Chi-Square test for trend.

Table 4. Association between polygenetic risk score and cancers of the esophagus, stomach, and liver[¶].

Polygenetic risk score (8 SNPs)	Esophageal cancer			Stomach cancer			Liver cancer		
	Ca/Co	SBOR[†]	One-sided P[*]	Ca/Co	SBOR[†]	One-sided P[*]	Ca/Co	SBOR[†]	One-sided P[*]
Equal-spaced categories									
Lowest	20/65	1.00		37/131	1.00		27/64	1.00	
Middle	65/165	1.21 (0.70, 2.08)	0.25	74/123	2.07 (1.28, 3.35)	0.001	88/194	0.95 (0.55, 1.64)	0.43
Highest	41/57	2.06 (1.13, 3.77)	0.010	14/33	1.55 (0.77, 3.11)	0.11	27/29	2.09 (1.05, 4.17)	0.019
Continuous (1 unit increase in PRS)		2.13 (1.23, 3.69)	0.004		2.37 (1.34, 4.19)	0.002		2.17 (1.11, 4.25)	0.012

†: Semi-Bayes odds ratio (SBOR) adjusted for age (5-year categories and deviation from stratum mean), sex, residency (city, rural), alcohol drinking frequency, smoking pack-years, BMI, education, H. *pylori* infection (in stomach cancer analyses), HBsAg (in liver cancer analyses), and plasma AFB1 levels (in liver cancer analyses), based on the assumption that genotype did not affect any of these variables.
*: One-sided semi-Bayes *P*-values; the posterior probability that the point estimate is on the wrong side of the null [26,27].
¶: Polygenetic risk score (PRS) was calculated only among subjects with complete data on all 8 SNPs.

association between *MTHFR* rs1801133 and stomach cancer among study populations without folic acid fortification (OR: 1.60, 95% CI: 1.36–1.88), as compared to those with fortification (OR: 1.15, 95% CI: 0.81–1.63), which is similar to our finding of a stronger association among individuals with lower plasma folate levels. For esophageal cancer, our data suggested an increased risk among *MTHFR* rs1801133 T allele carriers (any T vs. C/C, SBOR: 1.25, 95% posterior limits: 0.85, 1.84), which is consistent with findings from a meta-analysis of 19 studies (C/T versus C/C, OR: 1.47, 95% CI: 1.32–1.63; T/T versus C/C, OR: 1.69, 95% CI: 1.49–1.91) [2].

MTR and MTRR are two other important enzymes involved in one-carbon metabolism. MTR catalyzes the methylation of homocysteine to methionine. *MTR* A2756G (rs1805087), a common SNP leading to the substitution of aspartic acid with glycine, has been largely studied. However, no apparent associations have been observed with cancer at the following sites: lung, prostate, head and neck, bladder, esophagus, stomach, breast, or colon and rectal [37–46]. MTRR regenerates a functional MTR via reductive methylation. Two common polymorphisms, *MTRR* A66G (rs1801394, converts isoleucine to methionine) and C524T (rs1532268, changes serine to leucine), have been indicated to regenerate MTR less efficiently [47]. G allele carriers of *MTRR* rs1801394 have been associated with increased risk for hepatocellular carcinoma (HCC) [48]. Conversely, associations are inconsistent with other malignancies, including esophageal squamous cell carcinoma (ESCC), stomach cancer, and colorectal cancer [37,44,49–53]. Most studies that have investigated *MTRR* rs1532268 reported no associations with colorectal, gastric, breast, and lung cancer [44,51,53–56]. One should bear in mind however that apparent inconsistencies and reports of no association may only reflect expected variation in *P*-values ("statistical significance") rather than any real conflicts.

Our study observed odds-ratio variation of the associations between these *MTR/MTRR* polymorphisms and upper GI cancers across alcohol consumption, even after conservative SB shrinkage. Alcohol consumption appeared to have modified odds-ratios relating *MTR* rs1805087 to liver cancer, and *MTRR* rs1801394 to esophageal and stomach cancer. G allele carriers of these two SNPs were positively associated with cancer among drinkers, and inversely associated with cancer among non-drinkers. Matsuo et al., observed a similar OR variation [57]: G/G genotype carriers of *MTR* rs1805087 showed higher colorectal cancer risk among alcohol drinkers and lower risk among non-drinkers. Although the functional effect of *MTR/MTRR* polymorphisms has not been established, our results are biologically plausible as alcohol can disrupt one-carbon metabolism by inhibiting folate absorption, suppressing SAM synthesis, and impairing DNA methylation [6]. Alcohol can also cause inhibition of methionine synthase activity [6]. Therefore, it is possible that the variant allele of these two *MTR/MTRR* polymorphisms is protective for the upper GI cancers under the environment without alcohol exposures. However, it becomes deleterious when one-carbon metabolism is disrupted by alcohol and its metabolites.

ALDH2 is involved in alcohol metabolism by oxidizing acetaldehyde, a group 2B human carcinogen, to acetic acid. The *ALDH2* rs671 polymorphism—a well-known variant that occurs exclusively in Asian populations—causes a lower catalytic efficiency of ALDH2, and hence renders lower ability to eliminate acetaldehyde [58]. The *ALDH2* rs671 A allele (slow type) has been associated with increased risk of head and neck cancer, as well as esophageal cancer [59,60]. Consistent with previous findings, we observed a positive association between the A/A genotype and esophageal cancer in this study, and further reported a stronger association among individuals with lower plasma folate levels. Acetaldehyde also interferes with folate metabolism [6]. It is possible that the deleterious effect associated with rs671 polymorphism is more prominent under the condition of lower folate supply. Another common variation in the *ALDH2* gene—rs886205 with a G to A substitution in the promoter region—has been suggested to be functional. Chou et al., reported that the promoter constructs encoded by the G allele were more active than the A allele in hepatoma cells [61]. The G allele of rs886205 was reported to be associated with increased risk of ESCC [62,63] but not with stomach [64,65] and colorectal cancer [66]. It also showed inconsistent results with head and neck cancer [67–69]. We observed a positive association between the A allele of rs886205 and stomach cancer among those with higher plasma vitamin B12 levels. Although *ALDH2* rs886205 is suggested to be a functional polymorphism in hepatoma cells [61], further functionality studies are warranted.

There are several limitations due to the case-control design and the multiple comparisons in this study. Because we were not able to recruit all of the identified cases and controls, selection bias may occur if participation is affected by an un-identified factor which is associated with both the SNPs and cancer. On the other hand, cancers of the esophagus, stomach, and liver are fatal, and some patients with late clinical stages at diagnosis were either too ill to participate or passed away. This selection of patients may have resulted in biased estimates if the SNPs under study are associated with disease progression. Also, we collected plasma samples after cancer diagnoses. By stratification on plasma micronutrients, we may have introduced a "collider-stratification bias" if disease states, as well as treatments and/or diet and behavior changes among cancer patients would affect the levels of these biomarkers [70]. However, given that there may be only a weak association between SNPs and plasma micronutrients in one-carbon metabolic pathway [71], we believe that the size of the bias would be small. In addition, we conducted many comparisons and subgroup analyses, which led us to employ semi-Bayes shrinkage estimation to reduce the risk of misleading results. Using these methods, in this Chinese population, several polymorphisms in the one-carbon metabolic pathway appear to be associated with esophageal, stomach, and liver cancer, with heterogeneity across strata of alcohol consumption for the odds ratios relating *MTR/MTRR* polymorphisms to these cancers, suggesting potential interactions between alcohol drinking and genes of the one-carbon metabolic pathway. Confirmation of these results and research on the underlying mechanisms are needed.

Supporting Information

Table S1 Results of the associations between SNPs of MTHFR, MTR, MTRR, DNMT1, and ALDH2 genes and cancers of esophagus, stomach, and liver, stratified on plasma folate levels.

Table S2 Results of the associations between SNPs of MTHFR, MTR, MTRR, DNMT1, and ALDH2 genes and cancers of esophagus, stomach, and liver, stratified on plasma vitamin B12 levels.

Table S3 Results of the associations between SNPs of MTHFR, MTR, MTRR, DNMT1, and ALDH2 genes and cancers of esophagus, stomach, and liver, stratified on plasma homocysteine levels.

Table S4 Results of the associations between SNPs of MTHFR, MTR, MTRR, DNMT1, and ALDH2 genes and cancers of esophagus, stomach, and liver, stratified on tobacco smoking status.

Table S5 Results of the associations between SNPs of MTHFR, MTR, MTRR, DNMT1, and ALDH2 genes and cancers of esophagus, stomach, and liver, stratified on alcohol drinking status.

Table S6 Results of the associations between SNPs of MTHFR, MTR, MTRR, DNMT1, and ALDH2 genes and stomach cancer, stratified on H. Pylori infection status, and on liver cancer, stratified on HBsAg status and plasma aflatoxin B1 albumin adduct levels.

Acknowledgments

The authors would like to acknowledge Dr. Regina Santella (Columbia University) for her help with the measurement of plasma AFB1-albumin adducts, and all of the study participants.

Author Contributions

Conceived and designed the experiments: SCC LM LC SZY QYL ZFZ. Performed the experiments: SCC BYG LM NCYY AB. Analyzed the data: SCC PYC SG ZFZ. Contributed reagents/materials/analysis tools: DH. Wrote the paper: SCC. Interpreted the results: SCC PYC LL SG ZFZ. Participated in manuscript writing process: BB LM SZY QYL LL SG ZFZ.

References

1. Ferlay J, Soerjomataram I, Ervik M, Dikshit R, Eser S, et al. (2013) GLOBOCAN 2012 v1.0, Cancer Incidence and Mortality Worldwide. IARC CancerBase no 11. Lyon, France: International Agency for Research on Cancer.
2. Fang Y, Xiao F, An Z, Hao L (2011) Systematic review on the relationship between genetic polymorphisms of methylenetetrahydrofolate reductase and esophageal squamous cell carcinoma. Asian Pac J Cancer Prev 12: 1861–1866.
3. Qin X, Peng Q, Chen Z, Deng Y, Huang S, et al. (2013) The association between MTHFR gene polymorphisms and hepatocellular carcinoma risk: a meta-analysis. PLoS One 8: e56070.
4. Zacho J, Yazdanyar S, Bojesen SE, Tybjaerg-Hansen A, Nordestgaard BG (2011) Hyperhomocysteinemia, methylenetetrahydrofolate reductase c.677C>T polymorphism and risk of cancer: cross-sectional and prospective studies and meta-analyses of 75,000 cases and 93,000 controls. Int J Cancer 128: 644–652.
5. Duthie SJ (2011) Folate and cancer: how DNA damage, repair and methylation impact on colon carcinogenesis. J Inherit Metab Dis 34: 101–109.
6. Seitz HK, Stickel F (2007) Molecular mechanisms of alcohol-mediated carcinogenesis. Nat Rev Cancer 7: 599–612.
7. Ghoshal K, Li X, Datta J, Bai S, Pogribny I, et al. (2006) A folate- and methyl-deficient diet alters the expression of DNA methyltransferases and methyl CpG binding proteins involved in epigenetic gene silencing in livers of F344 rats. J Nutr 136: 1522–1527.
8. Huang RF, Hsu YC, Lin HL, Yang FL (2001) Folate depletion and elevated plasma homocysteine promote oxidative stress in rat livers. J Nutr 131: 33–38.
9. Gonda TA, Kim YI, Salas MC, Gamble MV, Shibata W, et al. (2012) Folic acid increases global DNA methylation and reduces inflammation to prevent Helicobacter-associated gastric cancer in mice. Gastroenterology 142: 824–833 e827.
10. Xiao SD, Meng XJ, Shi Y, Hu YB, Zhu SS, et al. (2002) Interventional study of high dose folic acid in gastric carcinogenesis in beagles. Gut 50: 61–64.
11. Mu LN, Cao W, Zhang ZF, Cai L, Jiang QW, et al. (2007) Methylenetetrahydrofolate reductase (MTHFR) C677T and A1298C polymorphisms and the risk of primary hepatocellular carcinoma (HCC) in a Chinese population. Cancer Causes Control 18: 665–675.
12. Mu LN, Cao W, Zhang ZF, Yu SZ, Jiang QW, et al. (2007) Polymorphisms of 5,10-methylenetetralydrofolate reductase (MTHFR), fruit and vegetable intake, and the risk of stomach cancer. Biomarkers 12: 61–75.
13. Chen SY, Chen CJ, Tsai WY, Ahsan H, Liu TY, et al. (2000) Associations of plasma aflatoxin B1-albumin adduct level with plasma selenium level and

genetic polymorphisms of glutathione S-transferase M1 and T1. Nutr Cancer 38: 179–185.
14. Oh SS, Chang SC, Cai L, Cordon-Cardo C, Ding BG, et al. (2010) Single nucleotide polymorphisms of 8 inflammation-related genes and their associations with smoking-related cancers. Int J Cancer 127: 2169–2182.
15. Harada S, Zhang S (1993) New strategy for detection of ALDH2 mutant. Alcohol Alcohol Suppl 1A: 11–13.
16. Stern LL, Mason JB, Selhub J, Choi SW (2000) Genomic DNA hypomethylation, a characteristic of most cancers, is present in peripheral leukocytes of individuals who are homozygous for the C677T polymorphism in the methylenetetrahydrofolate reductase gene. Cancer Epidemiol Biomarkers Prev 9: 849–853.
17. Oh SS, Chang SC, Cai L, Cordon-Cardo C, Ding BG, et al. (2010) Single nucleotide polymorphisms of 8 inflammation-related genes and their associations with smoking-related cancers. Int J Cancer 127: 2169–2182.
18. Greenland S (1997) Re: "Estimating relative risk functions in case-control studies using a nonparametric logistic regression". Am J Epidemiol 146: 883–885.
19. Robins JM, Greenland S (1992) Identifiability and exchangeability for direct and indirect effects. Epidemiology 3: 143–155.
20. Greenland S (2007) Bayesian perspectives for epidemiological research. II. Regression analysis. Int J Epidemiol 36: 195–202.
21. Efron B, Morris C (1973) Stein's estimation rule and its competitors - an empirical Bayes approach. J Am Stat Assoc 68: 117–130.
22. Thomas DC, Siemiatycki J, Dewar R, Robins J, Goldberg M, et al. (1985) The problem of multiple inference in studies designed to generate hypotheses. Am J Epidemiol 122: 1080–1095.
23. Greenland S, Robins JM (1991) Empirical-Bayes adjustments for multiple comparisons are sometimes useful. Epidemiology 2: 244–251.
24. Carlin B, Louis TA (2000) Bayes and Empirical-Bayes methods of data analysis. New York: Chapman and Hall.
25. Sullivan SG, Greenland S (2013) Bayesian regression in SAS software. Int J Epidemiol 42: 308–317.
26. Greenland S, Poole C (2013) Living with p values: resurrecting a Bayesian perspective on frequentist statistics. Epidemiology 24: 62–68.
27. Greenland S, Poole C (2013) Living with statistics in observational research. Epidemiology 24: 73–78.
28. Garcia-Closas M, Rothman N, Figueroa JD, Prokunina-Olsson L, Han SS, et al. (2013) Common genetic polymorphisms modify the effect of smoking on absolute risk of bladder cancer. Cancer Res 73: 2211–2220.
29. Rozen R (1997) Genetic predisposition to hyperhomocysteinemia: deficiency of methylenetetrahydrofolate reductase (MTHFR). Thromb Haemost 78: 523–526.
30. Bagley PJ, Selhub J (1998) A common mutation in the methylenetetrahydrofolate reductase gene is associated with an accumulation of formylated tetrahydrofolates in red blood cells. Proc Natl Acad Sci U S A 95: 13217–13220.
31. Sohn KJ1, Jang H, Campan M, Weisenberger DJ, Dickhout J, et al. (2009) The methylenetetrahydrofolate reductase C677T mutation induces cell-specific changes in genomic DNA methylation and uracil misincorporation: a possible molecular basis for the site-specific cancer risk modification. Int J Cancer 124: 1999–2005.
32. Teng Z, Wang L, Cai S, Yu P, Wang J, et al. (2013) The 677C>T (rs1801133) polymorphism in the MTHFR gene contributes to colorectal cancer risk: a meta-analysis based on 71 research studies. PloS one 8: e55332.
33. Yu L, Chen J (2012) Association of MTHFR Ala222Val (rs1801133) polymorphism and breast cancer susceptibility: An update meta-analysis based on 51 research studies. Diagnostic pathology 7: 171.
34. You W, Li Z, Jing C, Qian-Wei X, Yu-Ping Z, et al. (2013) MTHFR C677T and A1298C polymorphisms were associated with bladder cancer risk and disease progression: a meta-analysis. DNA Cell Biol 32: 260–267.
35. Yu L, Chang K, Han J, Deng S, Chen M (2013) Association between Methylenetetrahydrofolate reductase C677T polymorphism and susceptibility to cervical cancer: a meta-analysis. PloS one 8: e55835.
36. Liu ZB, Wang LP, Shu J, Jin C, Lou ZX (2013) Methylenetetrahydrofolate reductase 677TT genotype might be associated with an increased lung cancer risk in Asians. Gene 515: 214–219.
37. Ibiebele TI, Hughes MC, Pandeya N, Zhao Z, Montgomery G, et al. (2011) High intake of folate from food sources is associated with reduced risk of esophageal cancer in an Australian population. J Nutr 141: 274–283.
38. Marchal C, Redondo M, Reyes-Engel A, Perea-Milla E, Gaitan MJ, et al. (2008) Association between polymorphisms of folate-metabolizing enzymes and risk of prostate cancer. Eur J Surg Oncol 34: 805–810.
39. Moore LE, Hung R, Karami S, Boffetta P, Berndt S, et al. (2008) Folate metabolism genes, vegetable intake and renal cancer risk in central Europe. Int J Cancer 122: 1710–1715.
40. Moore LE, Malats N, Rothman N, Real FX, Kogevinas M, et al. (2007) Polymorphisms in one-carbon metabolism and trans-sulfuration pathway genes and susceptibility to bladder cancer. Int J Cancer 120: 2452–2458.
41. Ott N, Geddert H, Sarbia M (2008) Polymorphisms in methionine synthase (A2756G) and cystathionine beta-synthase (844ins68) and susceptibility to carcinomas of the upper gastrointestinal tract. J Cancer Res Clin Oncol 134: 405–410.
42. Suzuki T, Matsuo K, Hasegawa Y, Hiraki A, Wakai K, et al. (2007) One-carbon metabolism-related gene polymorphisms and risk of head and neck squamous cell carcinoma: case-control study. Cancer Sci 98: 1439–1446.
43. Suzuki T, Matsuo K, Hiraki A, Saito T, Sato S, et al. (2007) Impact of one-carbon metabolism-related gene polymorphisms on risk of lung cancer in Japan: a case control study. Carcinogenesis 28: 1718–1725.
44. Zhang FF, Terry MB, Hou L, Chen J, Lissowska J, et al. (2007) Genetic polymorphisms in folate metabolism and the risk of stomach cancer. Cancer Epidemiol Biomarkers Prev 16: 115–121.
45. Zhong S, Xu J, Li W, Chen Z, Ma T, et al. (2013) Methionine synthase A2756G polymorphism and breast cancer risk: an up-to-date meta-analysis. Gene 527: 510–515.
46. Ding W, Zhou DL, Jiang X, Lu LS (2013) Methionine synthase A2756G polymorphism and risk of colorectal adenoma and cancer: evidence based on 27 studies. PloS one 8: e60508.
47. Olteanu H, Munson T, Banerjee R (2002) Differences in the efficiency of reductive activation of methionine synthase and exogenous electron acceptors between the common polymorphic variants of human methionine synthase reductase. Biochemistry 41: 13378–13385.
48. Kwak SY, Kim UK, Cho HJ, Lee HK, Kim HJ, et al. (2008) Methylenetetrahydrofolate reductase (MTHFR) and methionine synthase reductase (MTRR) gene polymorphisms as risk factors for hepatocellular carcinoma in a Korean population. Anticancer Res 28: 2807–2811.
49. Han D, Shen C, Meng X, Bai J, Chen F, et al. (2012) Methionine synthase reductase A66G polymorphism contributes to tumor susceptibility: evidence from 35 case-control studies. Mol Biol Rep 39: 805–816.
50. Jokic M, Brcic-Kostic K, Stefulj J, Catela Ivkovic T, Bozo L, et al. (2011) Association of MTHFR, MTR, MTRR, RFC1, and DHFR gene polymorphisms with susceptibility to sporadic colon cancer. DNA Cell Biol 30: 771–776.
51. Pardini B, Kumar R, Naccarati A, Prasad RB, Forsti A, et al. (2011) MTHFR and MTRR genotype and haplotype analysis and colorectal cancer susceptibility in a case-control study from the Czech Republic. Mutation research 721: 74–80.
52. Stolzenberg-Solomon RZ, Qiao YL, Abnet CC, Ratnasinghe DL, Dawsey SM, et al. (2003) Esophageal and gastric cardia cancer risk and folate- and vitamin B(12)-related polymorphisms in Linxian, China. Cancer Epidemiol Biomarkers Prev 12: 1222–1226.
53. Yoo JY, Kim SY, Hwang JA, Hong SH, Shin A, et al. (2012) Association Study between Folate Pathway Gene Single Nucleotide Polymorphisms and Gastric Cancer in Koreans. Genomics Inform 10: 184–193.
54. Hazra A, Fuchs CS, Kawasaki T, Kirkner GJ, Hunter DJ, et al. (2010) Germline polymorphisms in the one-carbon metabolism pathway and DNA methylation in colorectal cancer. Cancer Causes Control 21: 331–345.
55. Lissowska J, Gaudet MM, Brinton LA, Chanock SJ, Peplonska B, et al. (2007) Genetic polymorphisms in the one-carbon metabolism pathway and breast cancer risk: a population-based case-control study and meta-analyses. Int J Cancer 120: 2696–2703.
56. Shen M, Rothman N, Berndt SI, He X, Yeager M, et al. (2005) Polymorphisms in folate metabolic genes and lung cancer risk in Xuan Wei, China. Lung Cancer 49: 299–309.
57. Matsuo K, Ito H, Wakai K, Hirose K, Saito T, et al. (2005) One-carbon metabolism related gene polymorphisms interact with alcohol drinking to influence the risk of colorectal cancer in Japan. Carcinogenesis 26: 2164–2171.
58. Crabb DW, Edenberg HJ, Bosron WF, Li TK (1989) Genotypes for aldehyde dehydrogenase deficiency and alcohol sensitivity. The inactive ALDH2(2) allele is dominant. J Clin Invest 83: 314–316.
59. Cadoni G, Boccia S, Petrelli L, Di Giannantonio P, Arzani D, et al. (2012) A review of genetic epidemiology of head and neck cancer related to polymorphisms in metabolic genes, cell cycle control and alcohol metabolism. Acta Otorhinolaryngol Ital 32: 1–11.
60. Yang SJ, Yokoyama A, Yokoyama T, Huang YC, Wu SY, et al. (2010) Relationship between genetic polymorphisms of ALDH2 and ADH1B and esophageal cancer risk: a meta-analysis. World J Gastroenterol 16: 4210–4220.
61. Chou WY, Stewart MJ, Carr LG, Zheng D, Stewart TR, et al. (1999) An A/G polymorphism in the promoter of mitochondrial aldehyde dehydrogenase (ALDH2): effects of the sequence variant on transcription factor binding and promoter strength. Alcohol Clin Exp Res 23: 963–968.
62. Bye H, Prescott NJ, Matejcic M, Rose E, Lewis CM, et al. (2011) Population-specific genetic associations with oesophageal squamous cell carcinoma in South Africa. Carcinogenesis 32: 1855–1861.
63. Ma WJ, Lv GD, Zheng ST, Huang CG, Liu Q, et al. (2010) DNA polymorphism and risk of esophageal squamous cell carcinoma in a population of North Xinjiang, China. World J Gastroenterol 16: 641–647.
64. Duell EJ, Sala N, Travier N, Munoz X, Boutron-Ruault MC, et al. (2012) Genetic variation in alcohol dehydrogenase (ADH1A, ADH1B, ADH1C, ADH7) and aldehyde dehydrogenase (ALDH2), alcohol consumption and gastric cancer risk in the European Prospective Investigation into Cancer and Nutrition (EPIC) cohort. Carcinogenesis 33: 361–367.
65. Zhang FF, Hou L, Terry MB, Lissowska J, Morabia A, et al. (2007) Genetic polymorphisms in alcohol metabolism, alcohol intake and the risk of stomach cancer in Warsaw, Poland. Int J Cancer 121: 2060–2064.
66. Yang H, Zhou Y, Zhou Z, Liu J, Yuan X, et al. (2009) A novel polymorphism rs1329149 of CYP2E1 and a known polymorphism rs671 of ALDH2 of alcohol metabolizing enzymes are associated with colorectal cancer in a southwestern Chinese population. Cancer Epidemiol Biomarkers Prev 18: 2522–2527.

67. Canova C, Richiardi L, Merletti F, Pentenero M, Gervasio C, et al. (2010) Alcohol, tobacco and genetic susceptibility in relation to cancers of the upper aerodigestive tract in northern Italy. Tumori 96: 1–10.
68. Chung CS, Lee YC, Liou JM, Wang CP, Ko JY, et al. (2012) Tag single nucleotide polymorphisms of alcohol-metabolizing enzymes modify the risk of upper aerodigestive tract cancers: HapMap database analysis. Dis Esophagus 27: 493–503.
69. Hashibe M, Boffetta P, Zaridze D, Shangina O, Szeszenia-Dabrowska N, et al. (2006) Evidence for an important role of alcohol- and aldehyde-metabolizing genes in cancers of the upper aerodigestive tract. Cancer Epidemiol Biomarkers Prev 15: 696–703.
70. Greenland S (2003) Quantifying biases in causal models: classical confounding vs collider-stratification bias. Epidemiology 14: 300–306.
71. Fredriksen A, Meyer K, Ueland PM, Vollset SE, Grotmol T, et al. (2007) Large-scale population-based metabolic phenotyping of thirteen genetic polymorphisms related to one-carbon metabolism. Human mutation 28: 856–865.

16

Design and Development of a Robotized System Coupled to μCT Imaging for Intratumoral Drug Evaluation in a HCC Mouse Model

Gaétan Bour[1]*, Fernand Martel[2], Laurent Goffin[3], Bernard Bayle[3], Jacques Gangloff[3], Marc Aprahamian[1], Jacques Marescaux[1], Jean-Marc Egly[1,2]*

1 Institut de Recherche contre les Cancers de l'Appareil Digestif (IRCAD), Strasbourg, France, **2** IGBMC, Department of Functional Genomics and Cancer, CNRS/INSERM/ Université de Strasbourg, BP 163, Illkirch, C. U. Strasbourg, Strasbourg, France, **3** ICube laboratory UMR, CNRS 7357, University of Strasbourg, Strasbourg, France

Abstract

Hepatocellular carcinoma (HCC) is one of the most common cancer related deaths worldwide. One of the main challenges in cancer treatment is drug delivery to target cancer cells specifically. Preclinical evaluation of intratumoral drugs in orthotopic liver cancer mouse models is difficult, as percutaneous injection hardly can be precisely performed manually. In the present study we have characterized a hepatoma model developing a single tumor nodule by implantation of Hep55.1C cells in the liver of syngeneic C57BL/6J mice. Tumor evolution was followed up by μCT imaging, and at the histological and molecular levels. This orthotopic, poorly differentiated mouse HCC model expressing fibrosis, inflammation and cancer markers was used to assess the efficacy of drugs. We took advantage of the high precision of a previously developed robotized system for automated, image-guided intratumoral needle insertion, to administer every week in the tumor of the Hep55.1C mouse model. A significant tumor growth inhibition was observed using our robotized system, whereas manual intraperitoneal administration had no effect, by comparison to untreated control mice.

Editor: Kalpana Ghoshal, The Ohio State University, United States of America

Funding: The work was supported by the following: European Research Council Advanced Scientists grants (JME, http://erc.europa.eu/advanced-grants); Institut National du Cancer (INCA-2008-041, http://www.e-cancer.fr/); and Association de la Recherche contre le Cancer (ARC-N°3153, http://www.recherche-cancer.net/) (MA JME). The funders had no role in study design, data collection and analysis, decision to publish, or preparation of the manuscript.

Competing Interests: The authors have declared that no competing interests exist.

* Email: bour.gaetan@gmail.com (GB); egly@igbmc.fr (JME)

Introduction

Hepatocellular carcinoma (HCC) represents 80–85% of the primary malignant liver tumors and is the 3rd most common cancer related death worldwide, with a high increase in developed countries [1]. One of the main challenges in cancer treatment is the targeting of the drug to the tumor to increase the local concentration of the therapeutic agent and avoid major side effects on healthy tissues [2]. This is addressed by using either specifically formulated drug vehicles [2] or targeted therapies delivered by intravenous administration. Some cancers like early HCC can also be treated by radiofrequency, thermal ablation or percutaneous ethanol or acetic acid injection in the tumor [3]. Moreover, among the recent developments in cancer treatment, viral based gene therapy often requires an intratumoral administration [4–7]. Intratumoral injection is also frequently performed in the preclinical steps on animal models to develop and assess the efficacy of new therapies [8–13].

For many decades, carcinogenesis studies as well as assays in drug therapy utilized tumor rodent models. The recent development of medical imaging especially micro CT scanner (μCT), allows to follow the evolution of the disease and/or the therapy at high resolution, on the same model animal; it also make it possible to perform preclinical drug evaluation in a non-invasive manner on orthotopic rodent cancer models [14,15]. Additionally such experimental procedures might avoid the intense use of animal models.

Several types of cancer animal models are reported to study hepatocellular carcinoma [16]: (i) genetically engineered mice developing spontaneous tumors; (ii) chemical induction using carcinogens; (iii) xenograft models, in which HCC cells or tumors from human origin are injected subcutaneously or orthotopically into the liver of immunocompromised mice; (iv) syngeneic graft of rodent HCC cells or tumors; (iv) viral hepatocarcinogenesis. Graft of HCC cell lines is the fastest model as it allows tumor growth within days after implantation [14,15].

In the present study, we characterized a hepatoma model in immunocompetent mice, obtained by implantation of Hep55.1C cells [17] in the liver of syngeneic C57BL/6J mice. We demonstrated that this mouse model can be used to assess the efficacy of drugs taking advantage of a robotized system developed for automated, image-guided intratumoral administration [18].

Results

Development of a restrainer bed system for *in vivo* imaging

Since most µCT scanners do not allow to perform robotized procedures under CT guidance in real-time, we designed a robotized-cell and a process to use pre-operative scan data to precisely target the affected organ. However, the use of µCT scanner analysis for further robotized investigations has to be performed in well-defined conditions. First of all, the animal has to be maintained anesthetized during the whole procedure. We then modeled a dedicated bed for 4–8 week-old mice by Computer Assisted Design (Figure 1A). This bed is composed of three different parts: (i) the support frame of the bed that can be placed inside the µCT scanner, lipped on the existing carbon bed for imaging, as well as in the robotized cell for the image-guided robotized intratumoral administration of the drug. The mouse is maintained under gaseous anesthesia during the entire procedure; (ii) the hemi-cylindrical mouse restrainer that is plugged and screwed in the support frame, firmly restraining the animal in a comfortable position on its back (Figure 1B) to expose the abdomen of the mouse. A sterile operative field stuck on the shaved abdomen ensures that the mouse does not slide during the transfer from the scanner to the robotized cell. In addition, tensing the skin and compressing the abdomen facilitates the penetration of the needle during the robotized insertion step; (iii) the removable registration cover [18,19] screwed on the support frame, overlaps the mouse on the restrainer part (Figure 1C) during the imaging recording after which it will be removed prior to the needle insertion. A needle insertion system was developed [18], keeping into account the size of the animal, the skin elasticity and the internal organ displacement. A particular attention was paid to the choice of the needle, which length, diameter, and bevel must be compatible with either drug injection or biopsy. Except for the final injection, all the steps are automated, from the positioning outside the animal, to the insertion in the animal.

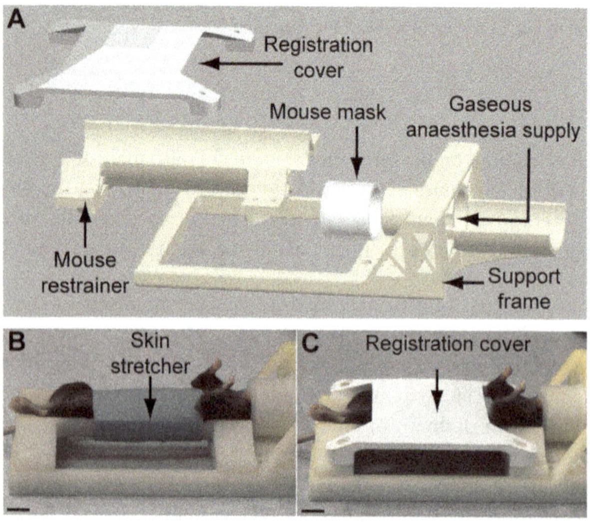

Figure 1. Mouse restrainer and robotized needle injector for intratumoral drug administration. (**A**) Description of the mouse restrainer bed. (**B**) View of a mouse restrained under gaseous anesthesia. The animal is tightly fixed on a hemicylindrical shell by a sterile operative field stuck on the abdomen. A sensor placed on the back of the mouse monitors respiration. (**C**) A dedicated registration cover is screwed on the bed frame during µCT scan imaging and registration by structured light projection.

Hepp55.1C cells induce fast growing orthotopic HCC

In parallel, to develop a HCC tumor model that would be accepted by immune competent mice, Hep55.1C and Hepa1.6 rodent HCC cell lines [17,20] were screened for their sensitivity to human standard therapeutic drugs for HCC and their tumorigenicity. We observed that Hep55.1C cells were more sensitive to Doxorubicin and Sorafenib than Hepa1.6 cells: IC50 values for Doxorubicin being around 0.10 µg/ml for Hep55.1C and 0.20 µg/ml for Hepa1.6, and in the range 6.6–10 µg/ml and 10–12.5 µg/ml respectively for Sorafenib (Figure 2A and 2B). Interestingly, Hep55.1C cells were found to be much more tumorigenic than Hepa1.6 cells, as all mice injected subcutaneously with Hep55.1C cells developed tumors, whereas Hepa1.6 tumors were observed in only 15% of the mice (Figure 2C).

We next followed HCC evolution in the Hep55.1C syngeneic orthotopic graft mouse model by recurrent µCT imaging and histological evaluation (Figure 3). An intrahepatic HCC was initiated by injection of 2×10^6 Hep55.1C cells either directly into the liver left lateral lobe or indirectly via the spleen. Macroscopically, Hep55.1C tumors appeared either as a white large nodule or as multiple small white nodules under liver capsule (Figure S1A and S1B). By micro CT imaging, contrast enhancement of the liver allowed a clear identification of the tumor nodules (TN) that remained hypo dense by comparison to normal contrast-enhanced liver (Figure S1C and S1D).

We focused on the intrahepatic graft model that developed single, well localized tumor nodules identified by µCT imaging, and more adapted to evaluate drug. The small nodule (initiated by the Hep55.1C cells) visualized at 2 weeks (in green on Figure 3A), expended progressively in the lobe (Figure 3B). The 3D reconstructions highlight the rapid increase in tumor volume from 5 to 9 weeks, rising from 2% to 40% (Figure 3B–C). Indeed, at 9 weeks, a large nodule invaded the left lateral liver lobe as well as the peritoneal cavity. We observed that the median survival was around 8 weeks, concurrently with the strong increase of tumor size (Figure S2). Similar results were also obtained by grafting Hep55.1C cells in male mice [21].

The progression of the tumor was also followed by histological examination. At 2 weeks after graft, Hep55.1C tumors presented small sized cells with an increasing nuclear/cytoplasm ratio and empty vesicles (right panel black arrows in Figure 3D) that could correspond to vesicular steatosis, in line with positive oil red O staining of tumor frozen section (Figure S3A). At that stage, Hep55.1C tumor cells were highly proliferative, as depicted by a Ki67 index of 40 (fraction of green positive nuclei in figure S3B), comparable to the Ki67 score observed in human HCC [22]. At 5 weeks the tumor exhibited a pseudo glandular aspect similar to a cholangiocarcinoma (Figure 3E, closed white arrows) and presented some features of non-alcoholic steatohepatitis (NASH) with vesicular steatosis (black arrow). At 9 weeks after graft, Hep55.1C tumors corresponded to a poorly differentiated human HCC (Grade III/IV) with a very dense fibrotic structure, and tumor cells with an almost invisible cytoplasm. Some glandular structures and vessels (indicated respectively by open and closed white arrows, Figure 3F) were observed at the periphery of the tumors. The presence of tumor neo-angiogenesis was assessed by immunofluorescence microscopy; we observed a labeling of vessels by the specific endothelial cell marker PECAM-1/CD31 (green staining in figure S3C). In addition, a very strong fibrosis appeared in early and advanced Hep55-1C tumors (Figure 3E–F) as visualized by silver and Sirius red staining for reticulin and collagen respectively

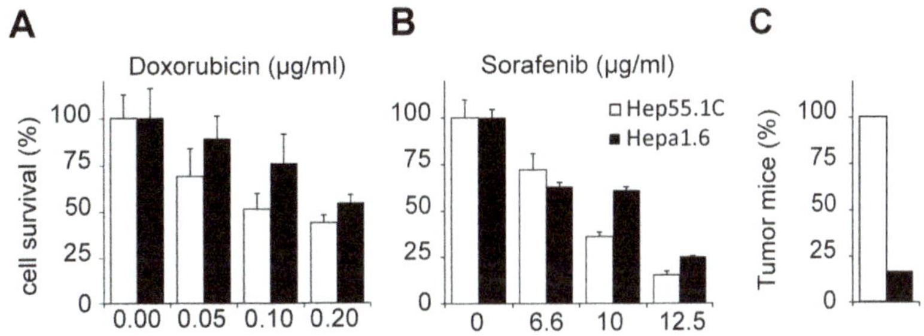

Figure 2. Screening of mouse hepatoma cell lines for chemical sensitivity and tumorigenicity. Hepa1.6 and Hep55.1C cells were exposed to Doxorubicin (**A**) and Sorafenib (**B**) for 3 days and assessed for toxicity using a cell proliferation assay. Results are shown as the mean +/− SD of triplicates. (**C**) Percentage of C57BL6J mice (n = 6) with palpable tumor two weeks after subcutaneous injection of either 10^6 Hepa1.6 or Hep55.1C in the back mice.

(Figure S3D and data not shown). Fibers of collagen and reticulin were scattered throughout the tumor, invading the anarchic Tumor cells and surrounding the pseudo glandular structures (white arrow in figure S3D. The presence of reticulin and collagen fibers inside the tumor is independent of animal sex, fibrosis deposition being observed following orthotopic graft of Hep55.1C cells in both male and female mice (data not shown).

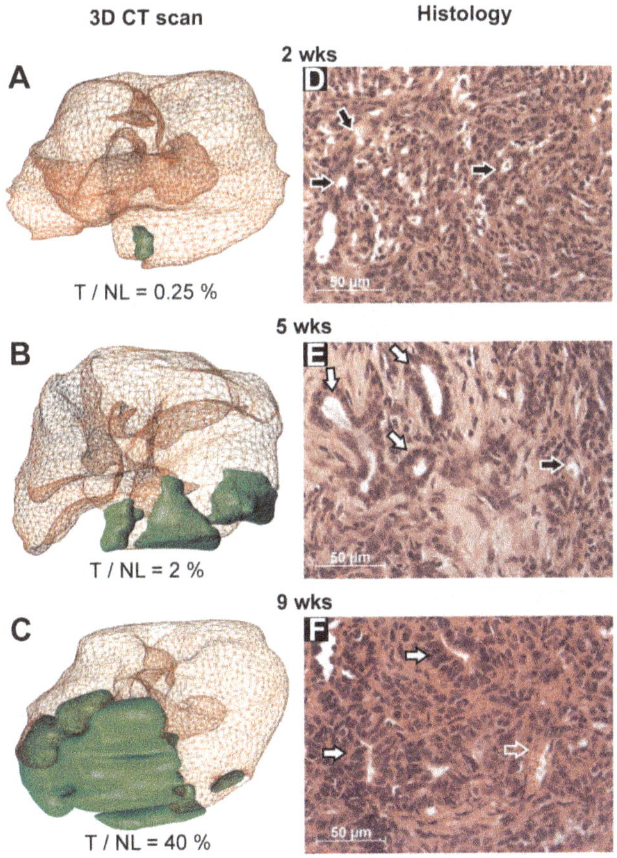

Figure 3. Evolution of tumor after intra liver injection of Hep55.1C cells. Evolution of liver tumor was followed by μCT scan imaging and histology two (**A, D**), five (**B, E**) and nine (**C, F**) weeks after Hep55.1C cells grafted in the liver of C57BL6/J mice. (**A–C**) 3D reconstructions from representative μCT scan showing the normal liver (red) and the tumor (green). Tumor/normal liver volume ratio (T/NL) computed from 3D reconstruction is indicated. (**D–F**) H&E staining of formalin fixed paraffin embedded tumors (black arrow: vesicle, closed white arrow: glandular structure; open white arrow: red blood cells).

We further investigated for the presence of fibrotic genes by RT-qPCR on Hep55.1C tumor extract (Figure 4). We observed a strong expression of type 1 collagen (COLA1), a major extracellular matrix component by comparison to surrounding normal liver cell extract. As collagen is mainly deposited by during fibrosis, the overexpression of both alpha smooth muscle actin (ASMA), and matrix metalloproteinase 3 (MMP3) genes, two activated stellate cells (HSC) markers was noted in tumor cells extract compared to wild type cells. Moreover, an increase in the mRNA level of signaling molecules associated with inflammation and hepatic stellate cell activation like interleukin-6 (IL-6), platelet derived growth factor beta (PDGFB); transforming growth factor beta (TGFB) was also marked by comparison to the surrounding liver cells (Figure 4). However, no expression of fibronectin 1 (FN-1), another extracellular matrix protein and fibrosis marker, was observed. Interestingly, we found that Hep55.1C tumor do not express albumin, a liver specific gene, in line with its poorly differentiated state. On the contrary, cyclin D1 (CCND1), implicated in cell cycle regulation and often dysregulated in cancers, and osteopontin (SPP1) a HCC marker [23–25], were highly expressed. The HCC specific marker alpha fetoprotein (AFP) was also overexpressed in the tumor extract (Figure 4), but also in the adjacent liver presumably as a consequence of liver

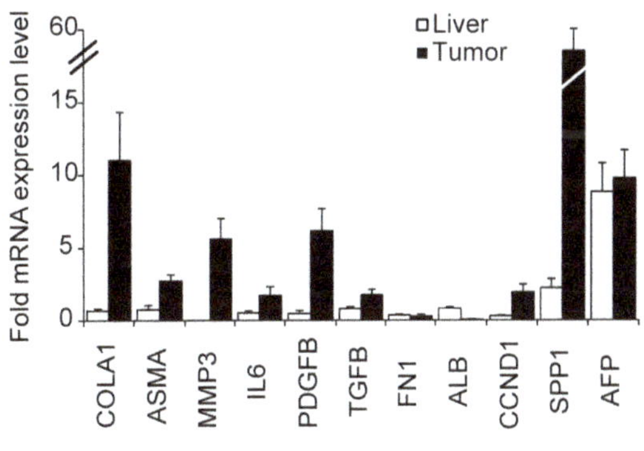

Figure 4. Hep55.1C tumors markers. Expression of COLA1, ASMA, MMP3, FN1 fibrosis markers, IL6, PDGFB, TGFB inflammation markers and ALB, CCND1, SPP1, AFP cancer markers was assessed by RTqPCR from Hep55.1C tumor and corresponding surrounding normal liver. Relative mRNA level of each gene was normalized to the level of the housekeeping gene 36B4. Results are expressed as the mean +/− SEM for at least 3 animals.

injury and regeneration consecutive to the graft and tumor growth [26].

The graft of Hep55.1C cells in the syngeneic mice liver allows the fast growth of a highly differentiated tumor, expressing fibrotic and cancer marker genes. Pretreatment of the mice with diethylnitrosamine for 4 weeks to induce liver fibrosis prior to Hep55.1C cell graft did not modify tumor growth and marker gene expression (Figure S4 and data not shown).

Robotized intratumoral injection inhibits Hep55.1C tumor growth

Having set up and followed the evolution of HCC tumor in mice, we evaluated the potency of intratumoral drug administration, using our system for image-guided robotized needle positioning [18]. μCT scan imaging helps to precisely position the needle of a disposable syringe filed with a test drug at the center of the tumor; the needle is positioned by a robot with a deviation lower than 0.3 mm (Figure S5 and [18]). We compared the growth of hepatic tumors in untreated mice to mice either treated intratumorally (IT) with Doxorubicin using our automated positioning system, or injected intraperitoneally (IP). For intratumoral injection, a 29G needle was used to facilitate the insertion while limiting damaging effects on tumors. In addition, it has been demonstrated in previous studies that the sole intratumoral injection of inactive compounds in rodent models of human cancers did not inhibit tumor growth [27,28]. Thus we postulated that a reduced tumor growth in the IT group could be attributed to the antineoplastic effect of Doxorubicin on tumor cells.

Treatment started two weeks after Hep55.1C cell inoculation in a liver lobe, once tumor was detected by μCT scan. In the IT group, each of the 3 mice was subjected to robotized administration of 10 μl of Doxorubicin, at the center of the tumor. In the IP group, the same amount of drug was injected manually in the peritoneum at the vicinity of the tumor. Tumor volume was determined for each mouse at each time point by 3D reconstruction from the μCT scan data (Figure 5A). Tumors resected at the end of the experiment after 3 weeks of treatment were smaller in the IT group than in the IP and control group. μCT scan follow up demonstrated that IT injection of Doxorubicin decreased tumor growing rate by comparison to untreated mice, as tumor volume in the IT group was significantly smaller than in the control group after 2 weeks (Figure 5B). However, no statistical difference was observed after manual IP injection of Doxorubicin, tumor growth being only slightly affected by drug administration (Figure 5B). In addition, a statistical increase in apoptosis was evidenced by TUNEL assay in the tumor injected intratumorally with Doxorubicin by comparison to the non-treated control group (Figure S6).

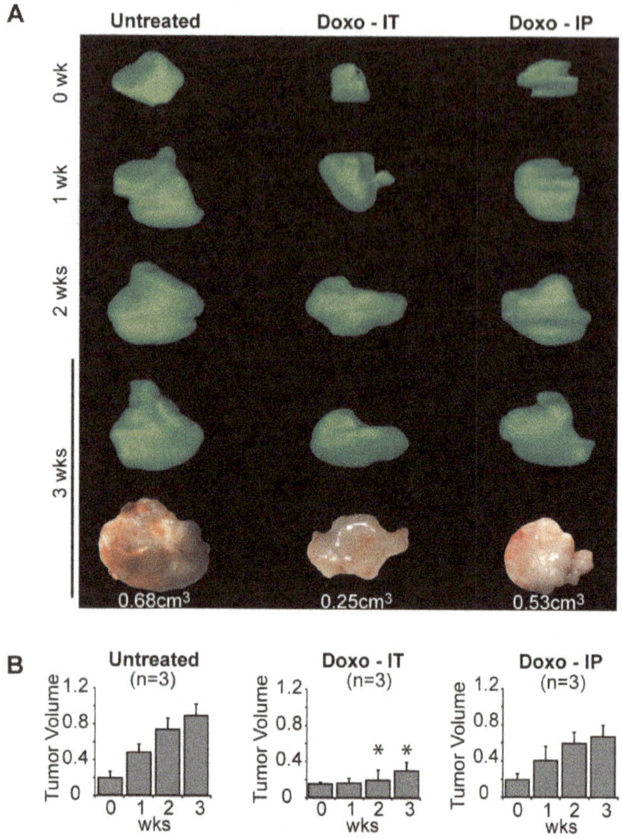

Figure 5. Treatment of Hep55.1C mouse HCC model by Doxorubicin. Mice bearing orthotopic HCC tumors were treated by recurrent automated robotized intratumoral injection (IT, n = 3) or manual intraperitoneal (IP, n = 3) of Doxorubicin; untreated mice (n = 3) were used as control of tumor growth. (**A**) Representative 3-weeks follow-up by μCT scan imaging and 3D reconstruction of tumor development. Volumes of the tumors resected at the end of the experiment were measured. (**B**) Tumor volume was computed at each time point from the 3D reconstructions of the tumors in untreated (left), IT (middle) or IP (right) injected mice (mean +/− SEM, star (*) indicates a difference with untreated control at the same time point with $p<0.05$).

Discussion

Here we have developed a HCC tumor mouse model and an automated image-guided system to follow the tumor evolution overtime and evaluate the potency of anti-cancer drugs. Among all HCC animal models, tumor cell graft is most appropriate for rapid development of a single tumor nodule. One of the main limitations of the tumor graft model in immune-competent animals is tumor rejection. The Hepa1.6 cells [20] are rejected in the majority of C57BL/6J mice [29–36], probably due to differences between cell line and host haplotypes. On the contrary, we observed that the Hep55.1C cell line, deriving from a C57BL/6J tumor [17], is tumorigenic after subcutaneous, intra hepatic or intra splenic injection, in 100% of both male and female mice. This model, based on the Hep55.1C cells harboring a mutation in the β-catenin pathway [17,37] represents a reproducible HCC model in the C57BL/6J mouse strain, which has a low susceptibility to spontaneous cancers.

At the histological level, these tumor cells resemble a poorly differentiated human HCC, with small sized cell, a high proliferation index, and duct like structures. A high level of fibrosis was also evidenced in the tumor as reported for other syngeneic or xenogeneic liver tumor models in mouse [38,39]. At the molecular level, an increased expression of inflammatory and pro-fibrotic genes has been observed, in line with hepatic stellate cell activation. Recent studies demonstrated that hepatic stellate cells not only play a major role in fibrosis, but also in liver development, regeneration, and cancer, notably by promoting HCC cell growth [40–42]. The Hep55.1C tumors being vascularized, expressing some human cancer and HCC markers like osteopontin, cyclin D1 and AFP, the model seemed suitable to analyze the effect of anti-cancer or anti-fibrotic drugs.

Several therapies in preclinical development or evaluated in clinical trials require intratumoral administration [4–6,43–45] that helps to reduce toxicity on normal tissue and improve treatment efficacy as concentration is locally increased. In rodents, one of the main constraints is the small size of the tumor necessitating to perform a laparotomy [35] for direct injection in orthotopic tumors. We here have designed a dedicated animal restrainer bed allowing both reproducible positioning of the animal in the µCT scan for longitudinal follow-up, and firm animal restrainment for accurate percutaneous needle insertion. Our image guided system for percutaneous drug administration did not damage surrounding tissues (see also [18,19]).

By combining µCT imaging and 3D reconstructions [15,21], we localized and computed the volume of liver tumors after intrahepatic or intrasplenic graft of Hep55.1C cells. As an example, we demonstrated that the robotized intratumoral injection of low amount of Doxorubicin, a drug used notably for transarterial chemoembolization of HCC [46], significantly reduced tumor growth by around 60% after 3 weeks, whereas manual intraperitoneal administration of the same amount of drug has no significant effect on tumor evolution.

The high accuracy of the system would also allow to perform recurrent tumor micro biopsy to analyze on the same animal at the molecular level, the evolution of specific markers, notably in response to drug administration. Due to the high level of fibrosis in the tumor, this model could also be used to test anti fibrotic drugs. Further developments will include the reduction of the duration of the robotized procedure for routine use on larger groups of animal, and also the development of a microbiopsy needle to retrieve biological samples from recurrent robotized biopsies.

Materials and Methods

Ethics statement

The project was approved by the local ethics committee (ICOMETH), under the permit number 38.2011.01.011. All experiments were performed under gaseous anesthesia, and animals were euthanized by overdosage of anesthesia followed by cervical dislocation.

Cell lines

Hep-55.1C derived from DENA induced HCC in C57BL/6J mouse [17] was obtained from Cell Lines Service (Eppelheim, Germany) and maintained in Dulbecco's modified Eagle's medium supplemented with 4.5 g/L glucose and 10% fetal bovine serum in a 5% CO2 humidified chamber. The Hepa1.6 cell line derived from an HCC tumor in a C57L/J mouse [20] was obtained from ATCC and maintained in Dulbecco's modified Eagle's medium supplemented with 1 g/L glucose and 10% fetal bovine serum in a 5% CO2 humidified chamber.

Cytotoxicity assay

24 h before treatment, 1.5 10^3 Hep55.1C or Hepa1.6 cells were seeded in 96 well plates. 50–70% confluent cells were treated with Sorafenib (Nexavar, Bayer), Doxorubicin (Adriamycin, Pfizer) or DMSO for 72 h and MTT (Sigma-Aldrich) dissolved in DMEM was added to the cells for 4 h. MTT formazan crystals were then dissolved in isopropanol: HCl (10:1) containing 0.01% NP-40. Background absorbance at 690 nm was subtracted from the measurement at 570 nm.

Mouse Hepatoma tumor model

C57BL/6J mice (Janvier Labs, France) experiments were realized under anesthesia, following FELASA recommendations and local ethics committee approval. For subcutaneous tumor, 10^6 cells resuspended in PBS (Sigma-Aldrich) where injected subcutaneously in the back of anaesthetized mice. For orthotopic tumor graft, 2×10^6 Hep55.1C cells were injected in the left liver lateral lobe of anaesthetized 8 week-old mice after midline laparotomy as described in [21]. Diffuse HCC was induced after injection of 2×10^6 Hep55.1C cells in PBS into the spleen of C57BL/6J mice following subcostal incision under gaseous anesthesia.

Mouse Scanning procedure

MicroCT images were obtained on a micro CAT II scanner (Imtek Inc, Siemens) at 80 kVp X-ray voltage and 500 µA anode current under general gaseous anesthesia with isoflurane (Abbott). Respiratory-gated images were acquired with a voxel size of 119×119×119 µm, corresponding to a scanned volume of 6.1×6.1×6.1 cm to encompass the whole registration cover.

Four hours before imaging, animals were injected intraperitoneally with 6 µl/g Fenestra LC (ART, Canada) liver contrast agent. This polyiodinated contrast agent is taken-up specifically by normal hepatocytes via the ApoE cell surface receptors [47,48]. Five min before µCT scan the mouse was anaesthetized, the abdomen was shaved and disinfected. The mouse was then positioned on the restrainer bed and fastened with a sterile sticky operative field. A pressure pad placed on the back of the mouse and connected to a pressure transducer served to gate µCT imaging and needle insertion on animal respiration.

µCT images exported by the AMIRA software were processed with VR-Render (available at http://www.ircad.fr/softwares) for visualization and planning or with 3DVPM for tumor segmentation, 3D reconstruction and to compute tumor volume [49,50].

Histology

Excised tumors and normal liver were fixed in 10% formalin and embedded in paraffin after dehydration in ethanol and xylene substitute. 5 µm thick sections were stained with Eosin and Haematoxylin for morphometric analyses. Reticulin was stained with silver according to Gordon and Sweet [51], collagen was stained with Sirius Red (Euromedex, France). For immunofluorescence, tissue was frozen in OCT embedding medium above liquid nitrogen. After permeabilization/fixation in 4% PFA, 0.1% Triton X-100 in PBS, 5 µm thick cryosection were saturated with PBS-5% BSA, and incubated with primary anti-PECAM-1 or anti-Ki-67 (Santa Cruz Biotech) and secondary AlexaFluor 488 anti-Rabbit antibodies. Lipid vesicles were stained using Oil Red O (Sigma-Aldrich, France) on frozen section. For apoptosis detection, TUNEL assay was performed on paraffin sections using the Apoptag Red in situ detection kit (Merck Millipore, France), according to the manufacturer recommendations. Images were acquired with an Axiophot microscope equipped with a CDD camera (Axiocam, Carl Zeiss) and processed with Photoshop CS4.

RT-PCR

Tumor and normal liver samples were homogenized in a Fastprep apparatus (MP Biomedical) in Lysis Matrix B tubes (MP Biomedical) containing lysis buffer (Sigma). RNAs were purified with the mammalian Genelute kit from Sigma, according to the manufacturer recommendations. 3 µg of RNA were used as template for reverse transcription with random hexamer in the presence of 200 units of Superscript II reverse transcriptase (Invitrogen). cDNA were analyzed by real time quantitative PCR on a Chromo4 (Biorad), using Quantitect mastermix (Qiagen). Primer sequences for the PCR were as follows: 36B4: 5′-GAGGTCACTGTGCCAGCTCA-3′ and 5′-GAAGGTGTACTCAGTCTCCA-3′; AFP: 5′-GGCAAAGCCC-TACAGACCA-3′ and 5′-TAAACGCCCAAAGCATCAC-3′; ALB: 5′-CCCTGTTGCTGAGACTTGCT-3′ and 5′-CTGAGGTGC-TTTCTGGGTGT-3′; ASMA: 5′-GGCTGTGCTGTCCCTCT-ATG-3′ and 5′-TCTCACGCTCGGCAGTAGTC-3′; CCND1:

5′-AACTACCTGGACCGCTTCCT-3′ and 5′-GCTTGTTCT-CATCCGCCTCT-3′; COLA1: 5′-TTTGGAGAGAGCATGAC-CGA-3′ and 5′-AAGTTCCGGTGTGACTCGTG-3′; IL-6: 5′-AGGATACCACTCCCAACAGAC-3′ and 5′-AGTGCATCATC-GTTGTTCATAC-3′; FN1: 5′-CCACCTCGAGCCCGTTATAG-3′ and 5′-GCAGAGGCTGCAGGGTAGTA-3′; MMP3: 5′-CAC-GAGGAGCTAGCAGGTTA-3′ and 5′-TCCAACTGCGAAGA-TCCACT-3′; PDGFB: 5′-CCGGTCCAGGTGAGAAAGAT-3′ and 5′-AATAACCCTGCCCACACTCT-3′; SPP1: 5′-GCTTG-GCTTATGGACTGAGG-3′ and 5′-CTCTCCTGGCTCTCT-TTGGA-3′; TGFB: 5′-ATTCAGCGCTCACTGCTCTT-3′ and 5′-ACTTCCAACCCAGGTCCTTC-3′.

Robotic System Design

The robotized procedure for image-guided percutaneous injection has been described [18]. Briefly, a specific mouse restrainer bed (Figure 1A–C) was developed and prototyped by stereolithography (Initial, France) in ABS-like epoxy resin (Protogen 18420) to maintain the animal during the different steps of the procedure. Animal respiration is monitored via a custom developed software using a pressure pad placed on the back of the animal and connected to a Unik5000 pressure transducer (GE, France) linked to a USB multifunction I/O NI 6800 (National Instruments, France). Following mouse imaging in the µCT scan, the needle insertion is performed in a robotized cell according to the trajectory defined in the µCT scan images, from the skin entry point to the center of the tumor. The robotized system is composed of a 6-degree of freedom (DOF) robotic arm RV-1A (Mitsubishi), holding a needle injector and able to reproduce the motion of a human arm with high accuracy and excellent repeatability (+/−0.02 mm). Two stereoscopic cameras (AVT Marlin, Stemmer Imaging, France) are fixed on a tripod to observe the mouse bed with an angle of about 55°. A grid projector fixed on the top of the robotized cell projects structured light on the bed as detailed in [18]. The needle injector is composed of a high speed linear motorized stage M-663 (PI France S.A.S) driven by a C-867 controller (PI France S.A.S). A disposable 29G Myjector syringe (Terumo/Thermo Fisher, France) filed with the drug is fixed on the needle injector prior to the calibration of the system.

Non-invasive follow-up of HCC evolution and intratumoral robotized drug administration

Nine mice bearing an orthotopic Hep55.1C hepatoma tumor were randomly assigned to 3 groups. IP mice received every week 10 µl of a solution of Doxorubicin at 2 mg/ml intraperitoneally under anesthesia; robotized intratumoral injection of Doxorubicin was applied to IT mice, and untreated mice were used as control. Tumor volume was determined every week by µCT imaging and 3D reconstruction of the tumors using 3DVPM [49]. Mean tumor volumes and standard deviations were determined for each group at each time point. When tumor volume reached 5% of total body weight, as determined by µCT imaging, (assuming 1 cm^3 of tumor weights 1 g) in one mouse, the experiments was stopped, all mice were sacrificed, and the tumors dissected.

Supporting Information

Figure S1 Orthotopic HCC development after inoculation of hepatoma cells in the liver or in the spleen. Hep55.1C cells were surgically injected either in the liver left lateral lobe (**A, C**) or in the spleen (**B, D**) of C57BL/6J mice. (**A**) Macroscopic appearance of a unique tumor nodule (TN) 6 weeks after Hep55.1C cell inoculation in the liver (L). (**B**) Macroscopic appearance of multiple sub capsular tumor nodules (TN) 6 weeks after Hep55.1C cells injection in the spleen. (**C, D**) Contrast enhanced µCT imaging was performed 6 weeks after Hep55.1C cell inoculation. Hypodense tumor nodules (TN) in normal liver lobes (L) and in the spleen (S) are delineated by dotted lines (scale bar: 3 mm).

Figure S2 Mice survival after intrahepatic Hep55.1C cell injection correlates with increased tumor volume determined by µCT-scan. The evolution Hep55.1C orthotopically grafted mice (n = 20) was followed over 18 weeks (black line). Tumor volume (dashed line) was measured on a subset of animals (n = 6) by contrast enhanced µCT scan. For ethical reasons, animal were sacrificed when tumor size exceeded the maximal ethical volume or when humane endpoints were reached.

Figure S3 Histological characterization of Hep55.1C tumors. (**A**) Oil red O staining of lipid vesicles in Hep55.1c tumor 2 weeks after graft. (**B**) Proliferative tumor cells evidenced by immunofluorescent staining of the nuclear Ki-67 cell proliferation marker (green). Nuclei were counterstained with DAPI (blue). (**C**) Tumor vascularization evidenced by PECAM-1 endothelial cell marker immunofluorescent staining (green) 5 weeks after graft. (**D**) Silver staining of reticulin fibers in Hep55.1C tumors demonstrating the presence of fibrosis (black arrow) surrounding duct like structures (white arrow) 9 weeks after graft.

Figure S4 Fibrosis induction by diethylnitrosamine. Fibrosis was induced in the liver of C57BL6/J mice prior to Hep55.1C cell graft by weekly DENA injection. (**A**) Liver fibrosis evidenced by increased Sirius red staining of the collagen fibers (black arrow). (**B**) Western Blot demonstrates the increased expression of ASMA following activation of Hepatic Stellate Cells by DENA.

Figure S5 In vitro evaluation of image guided robotized needle positioning. (**A**) Volume Rendering view from µCT scan of the mouse restrainer bed filed with an 80%parafin: 20%solvent phantom. 22 virtual targets were defined in this phantom (yellow sphere, only 7 targets (T1 to T7) are represented). (**B**) Axial view of the needle track observed on a post-operative µCT scan of the phantom after robotized positioning. The distance between the targeted position (T1) and the needle tip stop was measured to calculate the precision of the procedure. (**C**) Box plot representing the positioning precision in the three dimensions for from 3 independent experiments on 22 targets (mean: white dash; 1st and 3rd percentile: white rectangle; min/max values: black dashes).

Figure S6 Intratumoral injection of Doxorubicin increases apoptosis. Apoptosis was evidenced in tumors from the non-treated control group (**A, B**) and from the intratumorally injected group (**C, D**) by indirect TUNEL assay. Nuclei were counterstained with DAPI. (**E**) Mean positive nuclei observed per microscope field of view at magnification 40x.

Acknowledgments

We thank Francine Gosse for excellent technical expertise. Thanks are also due to Emmanuel Compe and Luc Soler for fruitful discussion.

Author Contributions

Conceived and designed the experiments: GB FM LG BB JG MA JM JME. Performed the experiments: GB FM LG. Analyzed the data: GB FM LG BB JG MA JM JME. Contributed reagents/materials/analysis tools: GBM FM LG. Contributed to the writing of the manuscript: GB FM LG BB JG MA JM JME.

References

1. Llovet JM, Burroughs A and Bruix J (2003) Hepatocellular carcinoma. Lancet 362: 1907–1917.
2. Arias JL (2011) Drug delivery strategies in targeting cancer: current concepts and future developments. Curr Drug Targets 12: 1094–1095.
3. Shiina S, Teratani T, Obi S, Sato S, Tateishi R, et al. (2005) A Randomized Controlled Trial of Radiofrequency Ablation With Ethanol Injection for Small Hepatocellular Carcinoma. Gastroenterology 129: 122–130.
4. Harrington KJ, Hingorani M, Tanay MA, Hickey J, Bhide SA, et al. (2010) Phase I/II study of oncolytic HSV GM-CSF in combination with radiotherapy and cisplatin in untreated stage III/IV squamous cell cancer of the head and neck. Clin Cancer Res 16: 4005–4015.
5. Harrington KJ, Karapanagiotou EM, Roulstone V, Twigger KR, White CL, et al. (2010) Two-stage phase I dose-escalation study of intratumoral reovirus type 3 dearing and palliative radiotherapy in patients with advanced cancers. Clin Cancer Res 16: 3067–3077.
6. Park BH, Hwang T, Liu TC, Sze DY, Kim JS, et al. (2008) Use of a targeted oncolytic poxvirus, JX-594, in patients with refractory primary or metastatic liver cancer: a phase I trial. Lancet Oncol 9: 533–542.
7. Sung MW, Yeh HC, Thung SN, Schwartz ME, Mandeli JP, et al. (2001) Intratumoral adenovirus-mediated suicide gene transfer for hepatic metastases from colorectal adenocarcinoma: results of a phase I clinical trial. Mol Ther 4: 182–191.
8. Borovjagin AV, McNally LR, Wang M, Curiel DT, MacDougall MJ, et al. (2010) Noninvasive monitoring of mRFP1- and mCherry-labeled oncolytic adenoviruses in an orthotopic breast cancer model by spectral imaging. Mol Imaging 9: 59–75.
9. Fernandes MS, Gomes EM, Butcher LD, Hernandez-Alcoceba R, Chang D, et al. (2009) Growth inhibition of human multiple myeloma cells by an oncolytic adenovirus carrying the CD40 ligand transgene. Clin Cancer Res 15: 4847–4856.
10. Kolodkin-Gal D, Zamir G, Edden Y, Pikarsky E, Pikarsky A, et al. (2008) Herpes simplex virus type 1 preferentially targets human colon carcinoma: role of extracellular matrix. J Virol 82: 999–1010.
11. Lun X, Chan J, Zhou H, Sun B, Kelly JJ, et al. (2010) Efficacy and safety/toxicity study of recombinant vaccinia virus JX-594 in two immunocompetent animal models of glioma. Mol Ther 18: 1927–1936.
12. Penheiter AR, Wegman TR, Classic KL, Dingli D, Bender CE, et al. (2010) Sodium iodide symporter (NIS)-mediated radiovirotherapy for pancreatic cancer. AJR Am J Roentgenol 195: 341–349.
13. Suggitt M and Bibby MC (2005) 50 years of preclinical anticancer drug screening: empirical to target-driven approaches. Clin Cancer Res 11: 971–981.
14. Akladios CY, Bour G, Balboni G, Mutter D, Marescaux J, et al. (2011) [Contribution of microCT structural imaging to preclinical evaluation of hepatocellular carcinoma chemotherapeutics on orthotopic graft in ACI rats]. Bull Cancer 98: 120–132.
15. Aprahamian M, Bour G, Akladios CY, Fylaktakidou K, Greferath R, et al. (2011) Myo-InositolTrisPyroPhosphate treatment leads to HIF-1alpha suppression and eradication of early hepatoma tumors in rats. Chembiochem 12: 777–783.
16. Leenders MW, Nijkamp MW and Borel Rinkes IH (2008) Mouse models in liver cancer research: a review of current literature. World J Gastroenterol 14: 6915–6923.
17. Kress S, Konig J, Schweizer J, Lohrke H, Bauer-Hofmann R, et al. (1992) p53 mutations are absent from carcinogen-induced mouse liver tumors but occur in cell lines established from these tumors. Mol Carcinog 6: 148–158.
18. Goffin L, Bour G, Martel F, Nicolau S, Gangloff J, et al. (2013) Design and In Vivo Evaluation of a Robotized Needle Insertion System for Small Animals. Biomedical Engineering, IEEE Transactions on 60: 2193–2204.
19. Ayadi A, Bour G, Aprahamian M, Bayle B, Graebling P, et al. (2007) Fully automated image-guided needle insertion: application to small animal biopsies. Conf Proc IEEE Eng Med Biol Soc 2007: 194–197.
20. Darlington GJ, Bernhard HP, Miller RA and Ruddle FH (1980) Expression of liver phenotypes in cultured mouse hepatoma cells. J Natl Cancer Inst 64: 809–819.
21. Bousserouel S, Bour G, Kauntz H, Gosse F, Marescaux J, et al. (2012) Silibinin inhibits tumor growth in a murine orthotopic hepatocarcinoma model and activates the TRAIL apoptotic signaling pathway. Anticancer Res 32: 2455–2462.
22. Grigioni WF, D'Errico A, Bacci F, Gaudio M, Mazziotti A, et al. (1989) Primary liver neoplasms: evaluation of proliferative index using MoAb Ki67. J Pathol 158: 23–29.
23. Luo JH, Ren B, Keryanov S, Tseng GC, Rao UN, et al. (2006) Transcriptomic and genomic analysis of human hepatocellular carcinomas and hepatoblastomas. Hepatology 44: 1012–1024.
24. Gotoh M, Sakamoto M, Kanetaka K, Chuuma M and Hirohashi S (2002) Overexpression of osteopontin in hepatocellular carcinoma. Pathol Int 52: 19–24.
25. Wu JC, Sun BS, Ren N, Ye QH and Qin LX (2010) Genomic aberrations in hepatocellular carcinoma related to osteopontin expression detected by array-CGH. J Cancer Res Clin Oncol 136: 595–601.
26. Bisgaard HC, Nagy Ton PPT, Hu Z and Thorgeirsson SS (1994) Modulation of keratin 14 and α-fetoprotein expression during hepatic oval cell proliferation and liver regeneration. Journal of Cellular Physiology 159: 475–484.
27. Angelova AL, Aprahamian M, Balboni G, Delecluse HJ, Feederle R, et al. (2009) Oncolytic rat parvovirus H-1PV, a candidate for the treatment of human lymphoma: In vitro and in vivo studies. Mol Ther 17: 1164–1172.
28. Li J, Bonifati S, Hristov G, Marttila T, Valmary-Degano S, et al. (2013) Synergistic combination of valproic acid and oncolytic parvovirus H-1PV as a potential therapy against cervical and pancreatic carcinomas. EMBO molecular medicine 5: 1537–1555.
29. Nakatsuka K, Sugiyama H, Nakagawa Y and Takahashi H (1999) Purification of antigenic peptide from murine hepatoma cells recognized by Class-I major histocompatibility complex molecule-restricted cytotoxic T-lymphocytes induced with B7-1-gene-transfected hepatoma cells. J Hepatol 30: 1119–1129.
30. Zhang BN, Watanabe S, Kohyama M, Saijo K, Kusakabe M, et al. (2000) Tumor formation suppressed in gammadeltaT knock-out mice. Cancer Lett 153: 63–66.
31. Dan Q, Sanchez R, Delgado C, Wepsic HT, Morgan K, et al. (2001) Non-immunogenic murine hepatocellular carcinoma Hepa1-6 cells expressing the membrane form of macrophage colony stimulating factor are rejected in vivo and lead to CD8+ T-cell immunity against the parental tumor. Mol Ther 4: 427–437.
32. Ohira M, Ohdan H, Mitsuta H, Ishiyama K, Tanaka Y, et al. (2006) Adoptive transfer of TRAIL-expressing natural killer cells prevents recurrence of hepatocellular carcinoma after partial hepatectomy. Transplantation 82: 1712–1719.
33. Si S, Sun Y, Li Z, Ge W, Zhang X, et al. (2006) Gene therapy by membrane-expressed superantigen for alpha-fetoprotein-producing hepatocellular carcinoma. Gene Ther 13: 1603–1610.
34. Nie F, Xu HX, Lu MD, Wang Y and Tang Q (2008) Anti-angiogenic gene therapy for hepatocellular carcinoma mediated by microbubble-enhanced ultrasound exposure: an in vivo experimental study. J Drug Target 16: 389–395.
35. Wang G, Dong X, Tian W, Lu Y, Hu J, et al. (2013) Evaluation of miR-122-regulated suicide gene therapy for hepatocellular carcinoma in an orthotopic mouse model. Chin J Cancer Res 25: 646–655.
36. Tamaki S, Homma S, Enomoto Y, Komita H, Zeniya M, et al. (2005) Autoimmune hepatic inflammation by vaccination of mice with dendritic cells loaded with well-differentiated hepatocellular carcinoma cells and administration of interleukin-12. Clin Immunol 117: 280–293.
37. Schwarz M, Wanke I, Wulbrand U, Moennikes O and Buchmann A (2003) Role of connexin32 and beta-catenin in tumor promotion in mouse liver. Toxicol Pathol 31: 99–102.
38. Shouval D, Schuger L, Levij IS, Reid LM, Neeman Z, et al. (1988) Comparative morphology and tumourigenicity of human hepatocellular carcinoma cell lines in athymic rats and mice. Virchows Arch A Pathol Anat Histopathol 412: 595–606.
39. Higashi N, Ishii H, Fujiwara T, Morimoto-Tomita M and Irimura T (2002) Redistribution of fibroblasts and macrophages as micrometastases develop into established liver metastases. Clin Exp Metastasis 19: 631–638.
40. Amann T, Bataille F, Spruss T, Muhlbauer M, Gabele E, et al. (2009) Activated hepatic stellate cells promote tumorigenicity of hepatocellular carcinoma. Cancer Sci 100: 646–653.
41. Yin C, Evason KJ, Asahina K and Stainier DYR (2013) Hepatic stellate cells in liver development, regeneration, and cancer. The Journal of Clinical Investigation 123: 1902–1910.
42. Coulouarn C, Corlu A, Glaise D, Guenon I, Thorgeirsson SS, et al. (2012) Hepatocyte-stellate cell cross-talk in the liver engenders a permissive inflammatory microenvironment that drives progression in hepatocellular carcinoma. Cancer Res 72: 2533–2542.
43. Carpentier A, Metellus P, Ursu R, Zohar S, Lafitte F, et al. (2010) Intracerebral administration of CpG oligonucleotide for patients with recurrent glioblastoma: a phase II study. Neuro Oncol 12: 401–408.
44. Kang YM, Kim GH, Kim JI, Kim DY, Lee BN, et al. (2011) In vivo efficacy of an intratumorally injected in situ-forming doxorubicin/poly(ethylene glycol)-b-polycaprolactone diblock copolymer. Biomaterials 32: 4556–4564.
45. Santamaria E, Mora MI, Carro-Roldan E, Molina M, Fernandez-Irigoyen J, et al. (2009) Identification of replication-competent HSV-1 Cgal+ strain targets in a mouse model of human hepatocarcinoma xenograft. J Proteomics 73: 153–160.

46. Huang K, Zhou Q, Wang R, Cheng D and Ma Y (2013) Doxorubicin-eluting Bead versus Conventional Transarterial Chemoembolization for the Treatment of HCC: a Meta-Analysis. J Gastroenterol Hepatol.
47. Weber SM, Peterson KA, Durkee B, Qi C, Longino M, et al. (2004) Imaging of murine liver tumor using microCT with a hepatocyte-selective contrast agent: accuracy is dependent on adequate contrast enhancement. J Surg Res 119: 41–45.
48. Weichert JP, Lee FT, Jr., Chosy SG, Longino MA, Kuhlman JE, et al. (2000) Combined hepatocyte-selective and blood-pool contrast agents for the CT detection of experimental liver tumors in rabbits. Radiology 216: 865–871.
49. Fasquel JB, Agnus V, Moreau J, Soler L and Marescaux J (2006) An interactive medical image segmentation system based on the optimal management of regions of interest using topological medical knowledge. Comput Methods Programs Biomed 82: 216–230.
50. Soler L, Nicolau S, Pessaux P, Mutter D and Marescaux J (2014) Real-time 3D image reconstruction guidance in liver resection surgery. Hepatobiliary surgery and nutrition 3: 73–81.
51. Gordon H and Sweet HH (1936) A simple method for the silver impregnation of reticulin. American Journal of Pathology 12: 545.

17

Nuclear Expression of the Deubiquitinase CYLD is Associated with Improved Survival in Human Hepatocellular Carcinoma

Stefan Welte[1]*, Toni Urbanik[1], Christin Elßner[1], Nicole Kautz[1], Bruno Christian Koehler[1], Nina Waldburger[2], Justo Lorenzo Bermejo[3], Federico Pinna[2], Karl-Heinz Weiss[4], Peter Schemmer[5], Dirk Jaeger[1], Thomas Longerich[2], Kai Breuhahn[2], Henning Schulze-Bergkamen[1,6]

1 National Center for Tumor Diseases, Department of Medical Oncology, Internal Medicine VI, Heidelberg University Hospital, Heidelberg, Germany, **2** Institute of Pathology, Heidelberg University Hospital, Heidelberg, Germany, **3** Institute of Medical Biometry and Informatics, Heidelberg University Hospital, Heidelberg, Germany, **4** Department of Gastroenterology, Toxicology, and Infectious Diseases, Heidelberg University Hospital, Internal Medicine IV, Heidelberg, Germany, **5** Department of General and Transplant Surgery, Heidelberg University Hospital, Heidelberg, Germany, **6** Department of Gastroenterology, Diabetology and Rheumatology, Internal Medicine II, Marien-Hospital, Wesel, Germany

Abstract

Background & Aims: The deubiquitinase CYLD removes (K-63)-linked polyubiquitin chains from proteins involved in NF-κB, Wnt/ß-catenin and Bcl-3 signaling. Reduced CYLD expression has been reported in different tumor entities, including hepatocellular carcinoma (HCC). Furthermore, loss of CYLD has been shown to contribute to HCC development in *knockout* animal models. This study aimed to assess subcellular CYLD expression in tumor tissues and its prognostic significance in HCC patients undergoing liver resection or liver transplantation.

Methods: Subcellular localization of CYLD was assessed by immunohistochemistry in tumor tissues of 95 HCC patients undergoing liver resection or transplantation. Positive nuclear CYLD staining was defined as an immunhistochemical (IHC) score ≥3. Positive cytoplasmic CYLD staining was defined as an IHC score ≥6. The relationship with clinicopathological parameters was investigated. Cell culture experiments were performed to analyze subcellular CYLD expression *in vitro*.

Results: Cytoplasmic CYLD expression was observed in 57 out of 95 (60%) HCC specimens (^{cyto}CYLD$^+$). Nuclear CYLD staining was positive in 52 out of 95 specimens (55%, ^{nuc}CYLD$^+$). 13 out of 52 ^{nuc}CYLD$^+$ patients (25%) showed a lack of cytoplasmic CYLD expression. ^{nuc}CYLD$^+$ was associated with prolonged overall survival in patients after resection or liver transplantation ($P = 0.007$). 5-year overall survival rates were 63% in ^{nuc}CYLD$^+$ *vs.* 26% in ^{nuc}CYLD$^-$ patients. Nuclear CYLD staining strongly correlated with tumor grading ($P<0.001$) and Ki67 positivity ($P = 0.005$). ^{nuc}CYLD$^+$ did not prove to be an independent prognostic parameter. *In vitro*, Huh7, Hep3B and HepG2 showed reduced CYLD levels compared to the non-malignant liver cell line THLE-2. Induction of CYLD expression by doxorubicin treatment led to increased cytoplasmic and nuclear expression of CYLD.

Conclusions: Expression of nuclear CYLD is a novel prognostic factor for improved survival in patients with HCC undergoing liver resection or transplantation.

Editor: Guy Brock, University of Louisville, United States of America

Funding: This study was supported by research grants from the Deutsche Forschungsgemeinschaft, http:/www.dfg.de/, DFG SCHU 1443/4-1 (SFB/TRR 77; associated project to HSB, BJL, TL, and KB) and the Virtual Liver Network of the BMBF (FKZ 0315761). The funders had no role in study design, data collection and analysis, decision to publish, or preparation of the manuscript.

Competing Interests: The authors have declared that no competing interests exist.

* Email: stefan.welte@med.uni-heidelberg.de

Introduction

Hepatocellular carcinoma (HCC) is the third most common cancer-related cause of death in both sexes worldwide [1,2]. In unresectable HCC, prognosis of patients is poor, with only limited treatment options. Thus, there is a need to identify new targets for diagnosis and treatment of the disease [3].

Ubiquitination controls the half-life of proteins, but also acts as modulator of the enzymatic activity or interaction of proteins. Ubiquitination is a dynamic process that can be counterbalanced by deubiquitinating enzymes such as Cylindromatosis (CYLD). CYLD has initially been identified as a tumor suppressor gene mutated in familial cylindromatosis, an autosomal-dominant predisposition to multiple tumors of skin appendages [4]. In

Table 1. Baseline characteristics of HCC patients corresponding to CYLD expression in the cytoplasma ($^{cyto}CYLD^{+/-}$) or nucleus ($^{nuc}CYLD^{+/-}$).

Variables	N		$^{nuc}CYLD^{-}$		$^{nuc}CYLD^{+}$		*P* value	$^{cyto}CYLD^{-}$		$^{cyto}CYLD^{+}$		*P* value
sex	95		43		52		0.46	38		57		0.84
men	74	(78%)	35	(81%)	39	(75%)		30	(78%)	44	(77%)	
women	21	(22%)	8	(19%)	13	(25%)		8	(21%)	13	(23%)	
grading	95		43		52		0.038	38		57		0.55
G1	13	(14%)	3	(7%)	10	(19%)		5	(13%)	8	(14%)	
G2	54	(57%)	22	(51%)	32	(62%)		19	(50%)	35	(61%)	
G3	25	(26%)	17	(40%)	8	(15%)		13	(34%)	12	(21%)	
G4	3	(3%)	1	(2%)	2	(4%)		1	(3%)	2	(4%)	
age	95		43		52		0.11	38		57		0.93
<60 y	37	(39%)	13	(30%)	24	(46%)		15	(40%)	22	(39%)	
>60 y	58	(61%)	30	(70%)	28	(54%)		23	(60%)	35	(61%)	
tumor size	83		38		45		0.68	33		50		0.9
<5 cm	37	(45%)	16	(42%)	21	(47%)		15	(46%)	22	(44%)	
>5 cm	46	(55%)	22	(58%)	24	(53%)		18	(54%)	28	(56%)	
vascular invasion	83		37		46		0.83	33		50		0.01
negative	37	(45%)	16	(43%)	21	(46%)		9	(27%)	28	(56%)	
positive	46	(55%)	21	(57%)	25	(54%)		24	(73%)	22	(44%)	
AFP	81		36		45		0.065	32		49		0.02
<8 IU/ml	43	(53%)	15	(83%)	28	(62%)		12	(37,5%)	31	(63%)	
>8 IU/ml	38	(47%)	21	(17%)	17	(38%)		20	(62,5%)	18	(37%)	
CHILD	89		41		48		0.55	34		55		0.85
A	68	(77%)	33	(81%)	35	(73%)		25	(73%)	43	(78%)	
B	11	(12%)	5	(12%)	6	(12%)		5	(15%)	6	(11%)	
C	10	(11%)	3	(7%)	7	(15%)		4	(12%)	6	(11%)	
alcohol consumption	91		41		50		0.76	36		55		0.66
negative	68	(75%)	30	(73%)	38	(76%)		26	(72%)	42	(76%)	
positive	23	(25%)	11	(27%)	12	(24%)		10	(28%)	13	(24%)	
viral hepatitis	87		40		47		0.89	34		53		0.33
B	16	(18%)	7	(17,5%)	9	(20%)		8	(23,5%)	8	(15%)	
C	19	(22%)	8	(20%)	11	(23%)		9	(26,5%)	10	(19%)	
bilirubin	87		40		47		0.54	32		55		0.53
normal	58	(67%)	28	(70%)	30	(33%)		20	(63%)	38	(70%)	
increased	29	(33%)	12	(30%)	17	(67%)		12	(38%)	17	(30%)	

Bilirubin levels >1 mg/dl were depicted as "increased". AFP serum levels: normal range <8 IU/ml).

addition, dysregulation of CYLD has been demonstrated in various other cancer entities [5]. CYLD removes lysine (K-63)-linked polyubiquitin chains from proteins regulating signaling pathways involved in cancer development and progression. Various deubiqitinating enzymes are predominantly localized in the nucleus and have been identified to target histones, influencing chromatin structure and downstream DNA-based processes [6]. CYLD was shown to be located in the cytoplasma and, upon stimulation, translocates to the perinuclear region where it binds to the IκB family member Bcl-3 and removes K63-linked polyubiquitin chains, thus preventing nuclear translocation of Bcl-3-p50 and Bcl-3-p52 complexes [7]. Recently, a small zinc-binding B box domain within the core of USP domain, contributing to nuclear localization of CYLD, was identified [8]. However, the precise function of nuclear CYLD still remains elusive. Cytoplasmic CYLD acts as a negative regulator of NF-κB activation by deubiquitination of TNF receptor-associated factor (TRAF)-2/-6 and NF-κB essential modulator (NEMO) [9]. Little is known about the relevance of deubiquitinating enzymes for HCC development. We and others observed decreased levels of CYLD mRNA and protein in human HCC tissues [10,11]. In addition, a negative correlation between CYLD and oncogenic c-MYC expression has been described [12]. In CYLD *knockout* mouse models, a central role of CYLD for liver injury and hepatocarcinogenesis was demonstrated. Liver-specific deletion of "full-length" CYLD, accompanied by expression of an ablated CYLD splice variant, resulted in chronic liver injury and profoundly increased sensitivity towards carcinogen-induced liver cancer [13]. Deletion of full-length CYLD resulted in spontaneous HCC development in another murine model [14]. Moreover, downregulation of CYLD was shown to contribute to apoptosis resistance of human HCC cells [11]. However, the exact role of CYLD in human HCC development and progression remains unclear.

In early stages HCC is curable by liver transplantation, surgical resection or local ablation [15], but most patients present with locally advanced and/or metastasized HCC at first diagnosis. Even after curative surgery or local ablation, long-term survival remains limited due to high incidence of intrahepatic recurrence. Identification of prognostic biomarkers would help to identify patients at high risk for recurrence. Here we show for the first time that lacking nuclear expression of the deubiquitinase CYLD in HCC tumor tissues strongly correlates with poor outcome of patients.

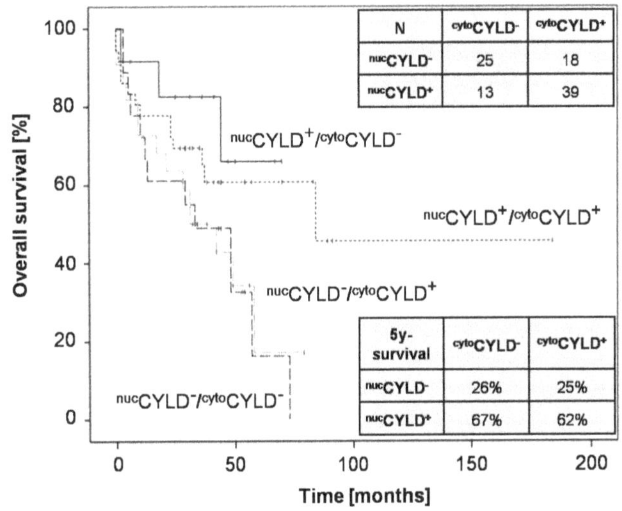

Figure 1. Survival of HCC patients after liver surgery according to subcellular CYLD expression. Kaplan-Meier analysis (N = 95) for overall survival (OS) of patients receiving liver resection, for the following subgroups: (^{nuc}CYLD$^+$/^{cyto}CYLD$^-$, ^{nuc}CYLD$^+$/^{cyto}CYLD$^+$, ^{nuc}CYLD$^-$/^{cyto}CYLD$^+$ and ^{nuc}CYLD$^-$/^{cyto}CYLD$^-$ ($P = 0.06$). Positive nuclear (^{nuc}CYLD$^+$) and cytoplasmic (^{cyto}CYLD$^+$) CYLD staining was defined as an immunohistochemical score (IHS) $\geq$3 for ^{nuc}CYLD$^+$ and $\geq$6 for ^{cyto}CYLD$^+$ (IHS ranging from 0 to 12, obtained by multiplication of the intensity and the quantity score).

Patients and Methods

Patients' cohort and immunohistochemistry

All experiments were done in accordance with the governmental and institutional guidelines of the ICH-GCP (according to the principles expressed in the Declaration of Helsinki) and were performed under the written approval by the local ethics committee of the Medical Faculty of Heidelberg University (206/2005). For the evaluation of CYLD expression, a tissue microarray (TMA) was established including HCC samples of 95 patients, corresponding tumorous liver tissues and normal liver samples as previously described [16]. Briefly, representative tissue blocks were selected as donor blocks for the TMA. Sections were cut from each block and stained with hematoxylin and eosin. Representative regions were chosen from each of the HCC and normal liver tissue samples. One cylindrical core tissue specimens per tumor block (diameter 0.6 mm) was punched from these regions and arrayed into the recipient paraffin block using a semiautomatic system (Beecher Instruments, Silver Spring, Maryland, USA). TMA slides were dewaxed and rehydrated using xylene and a series of graded alcohols, followed by heat-induced antigen retrieval using citrate buffer (pH 6). Staining was performed with a NovoLink Min Polymer Detection System (Leica Microsystems, Wetzlar, Germany) according to the manufacturer's instructions. For CYLD detection a polyclonal rabbit anti-CYLD antibody (Abcam, ab137524), for Ki67 staining a monoclonal rabbit anti–Ki67 antibody (Bethyl Laboratories, Inc, Montgomery, USA, IHC-00375) was used. Unspecific binding was excluded by omitting the primary antibody. For the immunohistochemical, semiquantitative assessment of CYLD expression, the product of the scores of staining intensity and quantity of immunoreactive tumor cells was calculated as previously described [17]. Briefly, the final immunohistochemical score (IHS; ranging from 0 to 12) was obtained by multiplication of the intensity and the quantity score. To investigate the relationship between CYLD expression and survival, patients were grouped into two categories. Patients with a CYLD expression under the median expression value were assigned to the low-expression group. Patients with an expression level larger than or equal to the median value were assigned to the high-expression group. This procedure, which results in size-balanced patient groups, was independently applied to cytoplasmic and nuclear CYLD expression. For ^{nuc}CYLD expression, levels $\geq$3, and for ^{cyto}CYLD expression, levels $\geq$6 were considered as high, respectively. Two pathologists independently assessed expression values. Sections were re-examined in case of disagreement.

All patients were treated at the University Hospital in Heidelberg, Germany, between 1998 and 2013. Decision for liver transplantation was made based on imaging findings in a multidisciplinary tumor board according to the national guidelines and the German Transplant Act, which are based on the Milan criteria and EASL guidelines [18]. The histological grade of tumor differentiation was assigned the Edmondson Grading System [19].

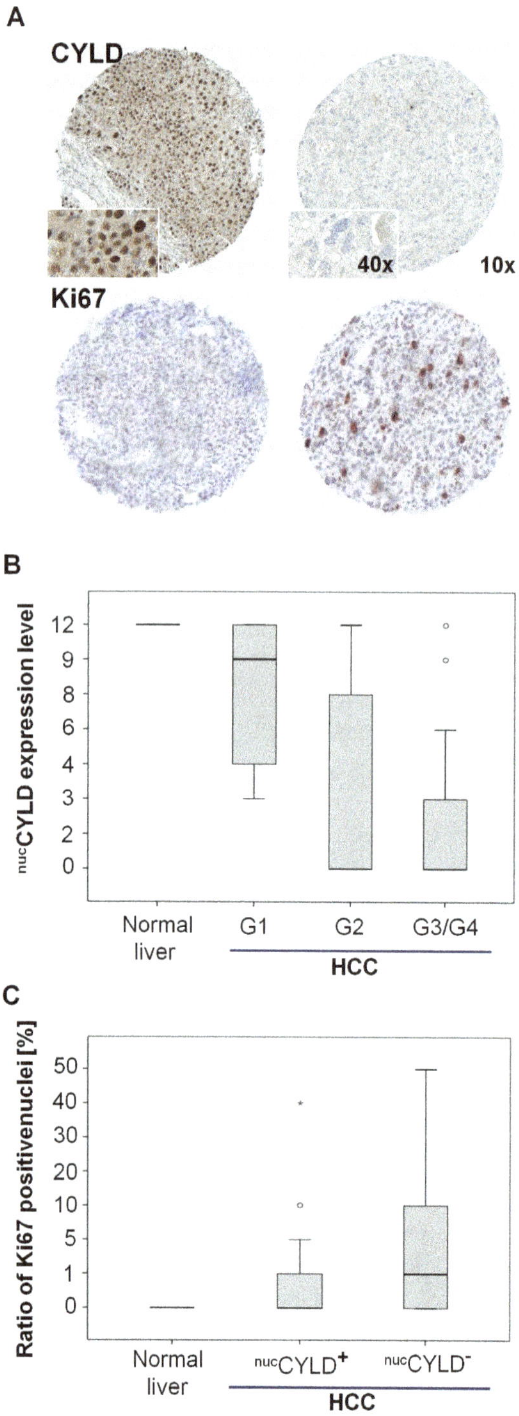

Figure 2. Nuclear CYLD expression in correlation to tumor grading in human HCC tissues. (**A**) Representative staining of positive and negative nuclear CYLD expression in HCC specimens. 10- and 40-fold magnification ($^{nuc}CYLD^{+}$; upper left and $^{nuc}CYLD^{-}$, upper right panel). Representative staining of corresponding Ki67 expression in HCC specimens. 10-fold magnification (lower panels). (**B**) Nuclear expression of CYLD (IHS score 0–12) in HCC (G1 = 13, G2 = 54, G4 = 25 G4 = 3) and normal liver tissues (N = 7) correlated to grading (Spearman correlation coefficient: −0.423, P<0.001). (C) Nuclear expression of CYLD related to the ratio of Ki67 positive nuclei in HCC ($^{nuc}CYLD^{+}$; N = 47; $^{nuc}CYLD^{-}$; N = 41) and normal liver tissues (N = 7) (Spearman correlation coefficient: −0.271, *P* = 0.006).

Cell culture experiments

The immortalized liver cell line THLE-2, the hepatoblastoma cell line HepG2 and the HCC cell lines Huh7 and Hep3B were purchased from ECACC. Cells were cultured in DMEM (Invitrogen, Karlsruhe, Germany), supplemented with 10% fetal calf serum (FCS, Biochrom, Berlin, Germany), 1% Pen/Strep (PAA Laboratories, Pasching, Austria), 1% HEPES and 1% L-Glutamine (Cambrex, Verviers, Belgium). Cells were cultivated at 37°C with 5% CO_2. Doxorubicin was purchased from Sigma-Aldrich (Hamburg, Germany).

For immunhistochemical staining 2.5×10^6 cells were seeded in 12-well plates on cover glasses (18 mm diameter). After treatment, cells were fixed with 4% PFA and stained for CYLD (same procedure used for the TMA staining, dilution 1:50, 1 h incubation). Hematoxylin and eosin (H&E) staining were performed according to standard procedures. Images were captured using an inverted microscope.

Western blotting

Protein extraction and preparation of total, nuclear and cytoplasmic extracts were performed as previously described [20,21]. Protein concentration was determined by Bradford protein assay (Bio-Rad, Munich, Germany). SDS-PAGE and Western blotting were performed according to standard procedures. Immunodetection was performed using the following primary antibodies: CYLD (E-4), IκB-α (C-21) (both Santa Cruz Biotechnology, Heidelberg, Germany), HDAC1 (Cell Signaling, Frankfurt, Germany) and α-Tubulin (Sigma-Aldrich, Munich, Germany).

Statistical Analysis

Overall survival was calculated from the date of surgery (OS, event = death by any cause). Survival time was "censored" for patients who did not experience an event. Those parameters not available for the analysis are depicted as "NA" (not available). Recurrence free survival (RFS) was not included in the study due to limited availability of recurrence data.

The relationship between staining index score and patient's age and gender, Edmonson grading, tumor size, vascular infiltration, viral hepatitis, bilirubin, serum AFP and Child-Pugh score was tested using a Chi-square test and quantified by the Spearman's rank correlation coefficient. Cox regression models were applied to assess the influence of explanatory variables on overall survival. For each endpoint, explanatory variables with univariate (Cox regression) probability only values <0.1 were included into a multiple Cox regression model. Hazard ratios were calculated to quantify prognostic effects. The Kaplan-Meier method was used to depict overall survival rates and differences assessed by log-rank test. All analyses were performed using SPSS 20 (IBM, NY, USA). *P* values <0.05 were considered statistically significant.

Results

CYLD expression in human HCC tissues

Downregulation of the deubiquitinase CYLD has been described as a frequent event in human HCC [10,11]. In addition, CYLD deletion led to HCC development in murine *knockout* models [13,14]. However, only little is known about subcellular CYLD localization and its association to the outcome of HCC patients. In order to assess CYLD expression, we analyzed 95 HCC tissue samples (N = 67 derived from liver resection, N = 28 from liver transplantation, respectively). Patients' characteristics concerning etiology, gender, and tumor stage are listed in Table 1. Subcellular CYLD expression was assessed (Fig. 1 and 2A, upper

Table 2. Univariate Cox analysis of different clinical, laboratory and histopathological parameters and CYLD expression for overall survival (OS).

Variables (N)		Univariate N*	HR (95% CI)	Global *P* value	Variables (N)		Univariate N*	HR (95% CI)	Global *P* value
sex					**CHILD**				
men	(69)	35	0.98 (0.47–2.04)	0.95	A	(64)	27	0.55 (0.29–1)	0.07
women	(19)	9	(Ref.)		B/C	(20)	14	(Ref.)	
grading					**alcohol**				
1–2	(67)	27	0.55 (0.296–1.0)	0.05	negativ	(65)	34	1.87 (0.86–4.09)	0.12
3–4	(28)	17	(Ref.)		positive	(21)	8	(Ref.)	
age					**viral hepatitis**				
<60	(35)	16	0.66 (0.35–1.25)	0.2	negative	(49)	28	1.43 (0.738–2.75)	0.29
>60	(53)	28	(Ref.)		B/C	(34)	13	(Ref.)	
tumor size					**bilirubin**				
<5 cm	(37)	10	0.37 (0.18–0.76)	0.007	normal	(55)	26	0.93 (0.49–1.8)	0.84
>5 cm	(46)	27	(Ref.)		increased	(28)	14	(Ref.)	
vascular invasion					**^{cyto}CYLD**				
negativ	(37)	13	0.54 (0.27–1.08)	0.08	negative	(33)	17	1.16 (0.63–2.15)	0.63
positive	(46)	25	(Ref.)		positive	(55)	27	(Ref.)	
serum AFP					**^{nuc}CYLD**				
<8 IU/ml	(42)	15	0.433 (0.22–0.85)	0.015	negative	(40)	27	2.14 (1.15–3.98)	0.02
>8 IU/ml	(35)	22	(Ref.)		positive	(48)	17	(Ref.)	

CI, confidence interval; HR, hazard ratio. N = 95; N*: Number of uncensored patients (patients who experienced the event).

Table 3. Multivariate Cox regression analysis of CLYD expression and clinical/laboratory/histopathological features for the prediction of overall survival (OS).

	Multivariate			
Variables	**(N)**	**N***	**HR (95% CI)**	**Global *P* value**
CHILD				
A	(53)	21	0.4 (0167–0.97)	0.04
B/C	(15)	9	(Ref.)	
grading				
1–2	(47)	17	0.7 (0.296–1.698)	0.44
3–4	(21)	13	(Ref.)	
^{nuc}CYLD				
negative	(27)	16	1.56 (0.71–3.41)	0.27
positive	(41)	14	(Ref.)	
tumor size				
<5 cm	(32)	8	0.34 (0.14–0.797)	0.01
>5 cm	(36)	22	(Ref.)	
vascular invasion				
negative	(29)	9	1 (0.392–2.68)	0.96
Positive	(39)	21	(Ref.)	
serum AFP				
<8 IU/ml	(38)	12	0.4 (0.17–1)	0.07
>8 IU/ml	(30)	18	(Ref.)	

CI, confidence interval; HR, hazard ratio. N = 95; N*: Number of uncensored patients (patients who experienced the event).

panels). 70 patients (74%) showed high nuclear and/or cytoplasmic CYLD expression, referred as ^{total}CYLD^{+}. In 25 patients (26%), only minor or absent CYLD expression was detected, both nuclear and cytoplasmic, referred as ^{total}CYLD^{-}. 52 patients (55%) showed positive nuclear staining for CYLD (^{nuc}CYLD^{+}). Among them, 39 (75%) were also positive for cytoplasmic expression (^{nuc}CYLD^{+}/^{cyto}CYLD^{+}, Fig. 1). There was a positive correlation between ^{nuc}CYLD^{+} and ^{cyto}CYLD^{+} ($P = 0.001$). To figure out differences in CYLD expression between patients treated with resection or transplantation, we compared subcellular CYLD expression in these two groups. CYLD expression levels for patients treated with resection or transplantation were similar (data not shown).

Correlation of CYLD with clinicopathological features

CYLD expression in HCC samples (both nuclear and cytoplasmic) was correlated with various clinicopathological features (Table 1). Median age of patients was 63 (±11.7) years (male:female ratio 3.5:1). 40% of patients had liver cirrhosis due to viral hepatitis B or C. Most patients had Child-Pugh score A (77%, B: 12%). No correlations between viral hepatitis or Child-Pugh score with $^{nuc/cyto}$CYLD expression were observed. ^{cyto}CYLD^{+} had a significant correlation with vascular invasion (Table 1, $P = 0.01$) and serum AFP (Table 1, $P = 0.02$). In contrary, ^{nuc}CYLD^{+} was not significantly associated with vascular invasion or serum AFP, but had a significant correlation with tumor grading (Table 1). Strikingly, the IHS for nuclear CYLD expression inversely correlated with both tumor grading (Spearman correlation coefficient −0.423, $P<0.001$, Fig. 2B) and Ki67-positivity (Spearman correlation coefficient −0.272, $P = 0.005$, Fig. 2C). In normal liver tissue (N = 7), median IHS for nuclear CYLD expression was 12. In HCC samples, the median score was 9 in G1 samples *vs.* 0 in G3/4 samples (Fig. 2B). 32% of the samples with a positive nuclear CYLD staining compared to 53% of negative samples showed a nuclear positivity of Ki67 defined as ≥1 Ki67-positive HCC cells per visual field, range 1–50 (data not shown).

Correlation of CYLD expression with outcome

N = 95 patients were eligible for survival analysis. For patients undergoing HCC resection or liver transplantation the 1-/3-/5-year survival rates were 79/68/50% for patients with ^{total}CYLD^{+}, and 77/50/30% and for those with ^{total}CYLD^{-}, respectively (log-rank: $P = 0.1$, HR 1.6, data not shown).

In total, 3 variables were found to be significantly associated with overall survival (OS) in univariate Cox regression analysis (Table 2): a) a tumor diameter less than 5 cm ($P = 0.007$, HR = 0.4), b) AFP under 8 IU/ml ($P = 0.015$, HR 0.4) and c) negative nuclear CYLD expression (^{nuc}CYLD^{-} = IHS≤3, $P = 0.02$, HR = 2.1). Strikingly, positive nuclear CYLD was a favourable prognostic factor for patients with HCC after surgery.

In the multiple Cox regression analysis, tumor size and CHILD score were independent prognostic factors ($P = 0.01$, HR = 0.34 and $P = 0.04$, HR = 0.4, Table 3). ^{nuc}CYLD^{+} did not prove to be an independent prognostic parameter ($P = 0.27$, Table 3). ^{cyto}CYLD^{-} patients showed non-significant differences for overall survival compared to the ^{cyto}CYLD^{+} group (IHS<6, $P = 0.6$, Fig. 3B, HR = 1.2, respectively) Importantly, ^{nuc}CYLD^{+} was significantly associated with improved OS in Kaplan-Meier analysis (^{nuc}CYLD^{+}: 1-/3-/5-year OS rates 81/73/63% *vs.* ^{nuc}CYLD^{-}: 75/50/26%, $P = 0.007$, Fig. 3A). The analysis was repeated with patients divided according to their surgical procedure (liver resection *vs.* liver transplantation). Patients in the ^{nuc}CYLD^{+} group after liver resection showed a non-significant

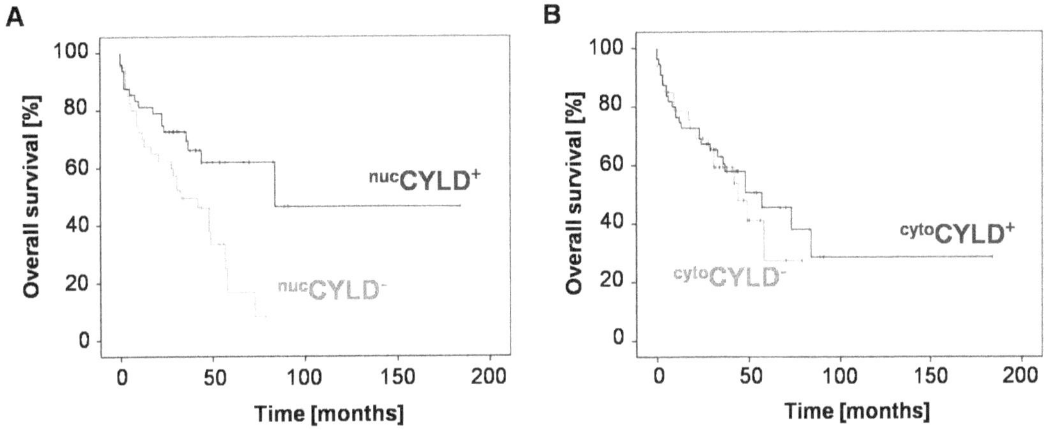

Figure 3. Overall survival of HCC patients with positive CYLD expression. (**A**) Overall Survival (OS) in patients with positive ($^{nuc}CYLD^+$; N = 48) and negative nuclear CYLD expression in HCC tissues ($^{nuc}CYLD^-$; N = 40; *P* = 0.007). (**B**) OS in patients with positive ($^{cyto}CYLD^+$, N = 55) and negative cytoplasmic CYLD expression ($^{cyto}CYLD^-$; N = 33; *P* = 0.6).

differences for OS, compared to the $^{nuc}CYLD^-$ group ($^{nuc}CYLD^+$: 1-/3-/5-year survival rates 77/64/59% *vs.* $^{nuc}CYLD^-$: 75/50/20%, *P* = 0.1, Fig. 4A). In patients after liver transplantation, $^{nuc}CYLD^+$ was associated with longer OS compared to $^{nuc}CYLD^-$, and a log-rank test confirmed significance ($^{nuc}CYLD^+$: 1-/3-/5-year survival rates 94/94/77% *vs.* ^{nuc}CYLD: 73/55/41%, *P* = 0.04, Fig. 4B). Analyzing CYLD expression in all subgroups ($^{nuc}CYLD^+$/$^{cyto}CYLD^-$, $^{nuc}CYLD^+$/$^{cyto}CYLD^+$, $^{nuc}CYLD^-$/$^{cyto}CYLD^+$ and $^{nuc}CYLD^-$/$^{cyto}CYLD^-$), no significant differences for overall survival were detected by the Kaplan-Meier approach. Among the subgroups, $^{nuc}CYLD^+$/$^{cyto}CYLD^-$ had the most favourable 5-year survival rate (*P* = 0.06; Fig.1).

Subcellular CYLD expression in HCC cell lines

To assess subcellular CYLD expression *in vitro*, total, cytoplasmic and nuclear CYLD expression levels in the non-malignant liver cell line THLE-2, the HCC cell lines Hep3B, Huh7 and in the hepatoblastoma cell line HepG2 were analyzed. Total and cytoplasmic CYLD expression was low in all 3 malignant cell lines compared to THLE-2 cells. Nuclear CYLD expression levels were hardly detectable, with no differences between the non-malignant liver cell line and liver cancer cells (Figure S1).

We have already shown that *knockdown* of CYLD increased the resistance towards chemotherapy [22]. Here, we observed induction of CYLD expression after chemotherapy with doxorubicin, which is frequently used for transarterial chemoembolization in HCC patients. The following analysis of subcellular CYLD expression 6 and 12 h after doxorubicin treatment revealed increased total, cytoplasmic and nuclear CYLD expression levels. This indicates a predominate role of increased CYLD protein translation rather than enhanced nuclear shuttling (Figure S2A, B). We additionally analyzed the TMA data and correlated cytoplasmic and nuclear CYLD expression. In cases with a cut-off value >3, ^{nuc}CYLD was also increased (Figure S2C). Immunohistological CYLD staining of HepG2 and Huh7 cells showed increased CYLD levels after doxorubicin treatment and additionally revealed induction of CYLD expression in nucleoli (Figure S3).

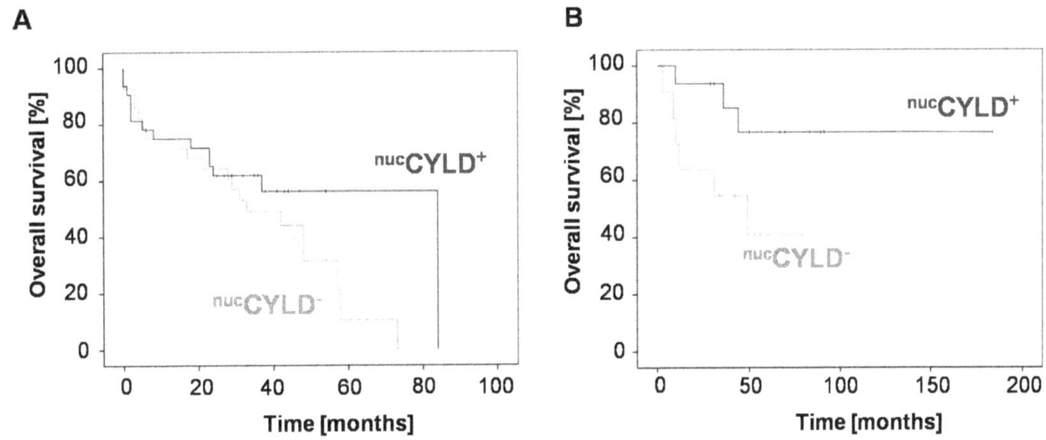

Figure 4. Correlation of CYLD expression with outcome after liver resection *vs.* liver transplantation. (**A**) Kaplan-Meier analysis for overall survival (OS) of patients receiving liver resection with positive ($^{nuc}CYLD^+$, N = 33) and negative nuclear CYLD expression ($^{nuc}CYLD^-$; N = 29; *P* = 0.1). (**B**) OS of patients receiving liver transplantation with positive ($^{nuc}CYLD^+$; N = 16) or negative nuclear CYLD expression ($^{nuc}CYLD^-$; N = 11; *P* = 0.04).

Discussion

In the present study, the clinicopathological relevance of the deubiquitinase CYLD was assessed in a series of 95 human hepatocellular carcinoma (HCC) samples, obtained from patients undergoing resection or liver transplantation as treatment of early stage HCC. Our key finding is a strong correlation of nuclear CYLD expression with overall survival of HCC patients. Importantly, nuclear CYLD inversely correlated with both tumor grading and Ki67 positivity in HCC patients.

Originally, CYLD has been described as a tumor suppressor gene in a rare tumor disease, called familial cylindromatosis (Brooke-Spiegler Syndrome) [4]. In recent studies, downregulation of CYLD has been described in various other malignancies, including HCC [10,11]. A reduced copy number of the CYLD gene was observed in more than 30% of human HCCs caused by chronic hepatitis C [23].

Suppression of CYLD is known to trigger oncogenic signaling, such as NF-κB, Wnt/ß-catenin and Bcl-3. However, the exact role of CYLD in cancer development is not fully understood. In murine *knockout* models, we and others revealed a central role of CYLD for hepatocarcinogenesis [12,13,14]. Activation of NF-κB signaling and chronic inflammation are discussed to trigger HCC development in mice lacking hepatic CYLD expression [9,10].

CYLD has been shown to be regulated at both transcriptional and post transcriptional level [24]. This opens up opportunities for targeting CYLD expression in human HCC. Constitutive activation of the Ras-Raf-MEK-ERK (MAPK; mitogen-activated protein kinase) signaling pathway is the major upstream signaling mechanism responsible for constitutive expression of the CYLD transcription inhibitor Snail1 [5]. We have already shown that CYLD expression in HCC cells can be triggered by the multikinase inhibitor sorafenib, by inhibition of Raf-1, as well as by blockage of the pro-survival kinases MEK and EGFR and identified the recovery of CYLD expression as an interesting approach for overcoming HCC resistance [22].

So far, the pathophysiological role of subcellular CYLD localization remains elusive. Various deubiqitinating enzymes are predominantly localized in the nucleus. Nuclear DUBs regulate major cellular processes such as gene expression, DNA repair and DNA replication. Deubiquitination of chromatin substrates impacts these processes at several levels, directly by altering protein stability (K-48) and localization (K-63-linked polyubiquitination) [6]. Nuclear USP7 has been shown to deubiquitinate forkhead box-containing transcription factor 4, provoking its nuclear export and hence its inactivation [25]. However, CYLD has been described to be mainly located in the cytoplasma and the perinuclear region [26,27]. Our study illustrates reduced nuclear CYLD expression in liver cancer cell lines. A correlation of CYLD mRNA and protein expression was described in previous studies [10]. Doxorubicin, which is a common agent used for transarterial chemoembolization procedures in HCC, induced CYLD expression in various subcellular compartments, including nucleoli. In addition, subcellular CYLD localization might be influenced by genetic alterations. In HEK293 cells, mutated, but not wildtype CYLD appeared in the nucleus. Overexpression of CYLD carrying a mutation of the small zinc-binding B box domain within the core of CYLDs USP domain led to nuclear accumulation of CYLD. Mutated CYLD showed equal DUB activity and specificity [8]. Our study showed that CYLD is able to locate in the nucleus. Further studies are required to elucidate the precise role of the b box domain and to uncover the molecular functions of nuclear CYLD. In HCC, it is still not known how subcellular CYLD localization is regulated.

This is the first study to present nuclear CYLD expression and its correlation with the outcome of HCC patients. Recently, it was reported that low CYLD mRNA and protein expression was paralleled by poor survival. In 76% of the HCC cases (N = 70, all patients undergoing resection) positive CYLD protein expression was described [28]. In our study, 74% out of 95 patients had positive nuclear and/or cytoplasmic expression. 41% out of 95 patients were positive for both nuclear and cytoplasmic CYLD expression ($^{cyto/nuc}$CYLD^{+}). We observed a significant association of ^{cyto}CYLD and ^{nuc}CYLD positivity. However, 25% of HCC tissues with positive nuclear CYLD expression were lacking cytoplasmic expression. Interestingly, a lack of nuclear CYLD expression correlated with poor differentiation (evaluated by Edmonson grading) and higher Ki67 positivity. It is well known that increased proliferation, indicated by high levels of Ki67 positive cells, is associated with earlier HCC recurrence after resection [29,30,31]. In addition, poor differentiation is associated with vascular invasion and unfavourable prognosis [32,33]. It is not known, however, whether increased proliferation or poor differentiation might influence nuclear CYLD expression or *vice versa*. An inverse correlation of CYLD protein expression with mitotic activity (as assessed by the MIB1-index), but not with tumor stage, has been reported by others in human HCC [12].

Resection of HCC remains the mainstay of treatment in patients with limited tumor size, normal bilirubin levels and the absence of portal hypertension [34]. However, liver transplantation is widely accepted as a curative therapeutic approach in well-selected patients with early stage HCC [35]. After liver transplantation, the 5-year survival rate was 63% in our study. Similar survival data after liver transplantation have been reported by other centers [36,37]. Following tumor resection 5-year survival rate was 31%. Other known well-defined factors, such as tumor size and Child-Pugh score, were confirmed as independent prognostic factors in patients after HCC resection or liver transplantation in our study [38]. The inferior survival rates after resection compared to transplantation, underline the clinical benefit of transplantation in selected patients [39].

Importantly, positive nuclear CYLD expression was significantly associated with improved OS in the cohort of resected and transplanted patients. So far, adjuvant treatment approaches are not established after curative surgery of HCC. Since the present retrospective study identifies a subgroup of patients with improved OS after curative resection and liver transplantation (^{nuc}CYLD^{+}), nuclear CYLD expression might be an interesting biomarker for prospective clinical trials in the adjuvant setting after HCC surgery.

So far, the functional role of nuclear CYLD remains unclear. We cannot exclude that nuclear expression of CYLD might be an early event in HCC development, which disappears upon tumor progression, or CYLD simply changes its subcellular location. Further insights into the regulation of subcellular CYLD expression would help to evaluate the pathophysiological contribution of CYLD localization to hepatocarcinogenesis and HCC progression.

In conclusion, we identified nuclear CYLD expression as a prognostic parameter for patients undergoing surgery in HCC patients. Thus, nuclear CYLD is a promising novel marker to predict outcome of HCC patients, and might help to identify patients with a reduced risk of recurrence after resection or transplantation.

Supporting Information

Figure S1 Low CYLD expression in HCC cell lines. Western blot analysis of basal CYLD expression levels in total, cytoplasmic and nuclear cell extracts derived from THLE-2 (non-malignant liver cell line), HepG2, Huh7 and Hep3B cells. Tubulin served as a loading control for total and cytoplasmic fractions, HDAC1 for nuclear fractions.

Figure S2 Subcellular CYLD expression in HCC cells after doxorubicin treatment and in TMA specimens. (A) HepG2 and (**B**) Huh7 cells were treated with doxorubicin for 6 and 12 h (1 μM). Western blot analysis of CYLD expression in total, cytoplasmic and nuclear cell extracts (upper panel). Analysis of CYLD expression in total, cytoplasmic and nuclear cell extracts from HCC cells 12 h after doxorubicin treatment on the same gel (lower panel). Tubulin served as loading control for total and cytoplasmic fractions, HDAC1 for nuclear fractions. (**C**) Boxplot summarizing nuclear expression of CYLD (IHS 0–12) within categories of cytoplasmic expression (IHS 0–12) in HCC patients.

Figure S3 Immunohistochemical CYLD staining of HCC cells. Representative pictures of H&E and CYLD staining of untreated and doxorubicin treated HepG2 (left panels) and Huh7 cells (right panels). Magnification 100x, scale bar 30 μm. Arrows indicate nucleoli.

Author Contributions

Conceived and designed the experiments: SW TU HSB. Performed the experiments: SW TU NW JL KB TL NK CE. Analyzed the data: SW TU NW JL KB TL FP. Contributed reagents/materials/analysis tools: HSB DJ KB PS NK CE. Wrote the paper: SW TU BCK JL KB PS KHW.

References

1. Venook AP, Papandreou C, Furuse J, de Guevara LL (2010) The incidence and epidemiology of hepatocellular carcinoma: a global and regional perspective. Oncologist 15 Suppl 4: 5–13.
2. Siegel R, Naishadham D, Jemal A (2012) Cancer statistics, 2012. CA Cancer J Clin 62: 10–29.
3. Breuhahn K, Gores G, Schirmacher P (2011) Strategies for hepatocellular carcinoma therapy and diagnostics: lessons learned from high throughput and profiling approaches. Hepatology 53: 2112–2121.
4. Bignell GR, Warren W, Seal S, Takahashi M, Rapley E, et al. (2000) Identification of the familial cylindromatosis tumour-suppressor gene. Nat Genet 25: 160–165.
5. Massoumi R, Kuphal S, Hellerbrand C, Haas B, Wild P, et al. (2009) Down-regulation of CYLD expression by Snail promotes tumor progression in malignant melanoma. J Exp Med 206: 221–232.
6. Atanassov BS, Koutelou E, Dent SY (2011) The role of deubiquitinating enzymes in chromatin regulation. FEBS Lett 585: 2016–2023.
7. Massoumi R, Chmielarska K, Hennecke K, Pfeifer A, Fassler R (2006) Cyld inhibits tumor cell proliferation by blocking Bcl-3-dependent NF-kappaB signaling. Cell 125: 665–677.
8. Komander D, Lord CJ, Scheel H, Swift S, Hofmann K, et al. (2008) The structure of the CYLD USP domain explains its specificity for Lys63-linked polyubiquitin and reveals a B box module. Mol Cell 29: 451–464.
9. Glittenberg M, Ligoxygakis P (2007) CYLD: a multifunctional deubiquitinase. Fly (Austin) 1: 330–332.
10. Hellerbrand C, Bumes E, Bataille F, Dietmaier W, Massoumi R, et al. (2007) Reduced expression of CYLD in human colon and hepatocellular carcinomas. Carcinogenesis 28: 21–27.
11. Urbanik T, Kohler BC, Boger RJ, Worns MA, Heeger S, et al. (2011) Down-regulation of CYLD as a trigger for NF-kappaB activation and a mechanism of apoptotic resistance in hepatocellular carcinoma cells. Int J Oncol 38: 121–131.
12. Pannem RR, Dorn C, Ahlqvist K, Bosserhoff AK, Hellerbrand C, et al. (2013) CYLD controls c-MYC expression through the JNK-dependent signaling pathway in hepatocellular carcinoma. Carcinogenesis.
13. Urbanik T, Boger RJ, Longerich T, Becker K, Ehrenberg KR, et al. (2012) Liver specific deletion of CYLDexon7/8 induces severe biliary damage, fibrosis and increases hepatocarcinogenesis in mice. J Hepatol 57: 995–1003.
14. Nikolaou K, Tsagaratou A, Eftychi C, Kollias G, Mosialos G, et al. (2012) Inactivation of the deubiquitinase CYLD in hepatocytes causes apoptosis, inflammation, fibrosis, and cancer. Cancer Cell 21: 738–750.
15. Carr BI (2004) Hepatocellular carcinoma: current management and future trends. Gastroenterology 127: S218–224.
16. Tschaharganeh DF, Chen X, Latzko P, Malz M, Gaida MM, et al. (2013) Yes-associated protein up-regulates Jagged-1 and activates the Notch pathway in human hepatocellular carcinoma. Gastroenterology 144: 1530–1542 e1512.
17. Macher-Goeppinger S, Bermejo JL, Wagener N, Hohenfellner M, Haferkamp A, et al. (2011) Expression and prognostic relevance of the death receptor CD95 (Fas/APO1) in renal cell carcinomas. Cancer Lett 301: 203–211.
18. European Association For The Study Of The L, European Organisation For Research And Treatment Of Cancer (2012) EASL-EORTC clinical practice guidelines: management of hepatocellular carcinoma. J Hepatol 56: 908–943.
19. Edmondson HA, Steiner PE (1954) Primary carcinoma of the liver: a study of 100 cases among 48,900 necropsies. Cancer 7: 462–503.
20. Vick B, Weber A, Urbanik T, Maass T, Teufel A, et al. (2009) Knockout of myeloid cell leukemia-1 induces liver damage and increases apoptosis susceptibility of murine hepatocytes. Hepatology 49: 627–636.
21. Urbanik T, Kohler BC, Boger RJ, Worns MA, Heeger S, et al. (2010) Down-regulation of CYLD as a trigger for NF-kappaB activation and a mechanism of apoptotic resistance in hepatocellular carcinoma cells. Int J Oncol 38: 121–131.
22. Urbanik T, Kohler BC, Boger RJ, Worns MA, Heeger S, et al. Down-regulation of CYLD as a trigger for NF-kappaB activation and a mechanism of apoptotic resistance in hepatocellular carcinoma cells. Int J Oncol 38: 121–131.
23. Hashimoto K, Mori N, Tamesa T, Okada T, Kawauchi S, et al. (2004) Analysis of DNA copy number aberrations in hepatitis C virus-associated hepatocellular carcinomas by conventional CGH and array CGH. Mod Pathol 17: 617–622.
24. Massoumi R Ubiquitin chain cleavage: CYLD at work. Trends Biochem Sci 35: 392–399.
25. van der Horst A, de Vries-Smits AM, Brenkman AB, van Triest MH, van den Broek N, et al. (2006) FOXO4 transcriptional activity is regulated by monoubiquitination and USP7/HAUSP. Nat Cell Biol 8: 1064–1073.
26. Garcia-Santisteban I, Zorroza K, Rodriguez JA (2012) Two nuclear localization signals in USP1 mediate nuclear import of the USP1/UAF1 complex. PLoS One 7: e38570.
27. Massoumi R, Podda M, Fassler R, Paus R (2006) Cylindroma as tumor of hair follicle origin. J Invest Dermatol 126: 1182–1184.
28. Hiroki Kinoshita HO, Toru Beppu, Akira Chikamoto, Hiromitsu Hayashi, Katsunori Imai, et al. (2013) CYLD downregulation is correlated with tumor development in patients with hepatocellular carcinoma. Molecular and Clinical Oncology.
29. D'Errico A, Grigioni WF, Fiorentino M, Baccarini P, Grazi GL, et al. (1994) Overexpression of p53 protein and Ki67 proliferative index in hepatocellular carcinoma: an immunohistochemical study on 109 Italian patients. Pathol Int 44: 682–687.
30. Watanabe J, Kushihata F, Honda K, Sugita A, Tateishi N, et al. (2004) Prognostic significance of Bcl-xL in human hepatocellular carcinoma. Surgery 135: 604–612.
31. Nakanishi K, Sakamoto M, Yamasaki S, Todo S, Hirohashi S (2005) Akt phosphorylation is a risk factor for early disease recurrence and poor prognosis in hepatocellular carcinoma. Cancer 103: 307–312.
32. Abdel-Wahab M, El-Husseiny TS, El Hanafy E, El Shobary M, Hamdy E (2010) Prognostic factors affecting survival and recurrence after hepatic resection for hepatocellular carcinoma in cirrhotic liver. Langenbecks Arch Surg 395: 625–632.
33. Nanashima A, Tobinaga S, Kunizaki M, Miuma S, Taura N, et al. (2010) Strategy of treatment for hepatocellular carcinomas with vascular infiltration in patients undergoing hepatectomy. J Surg Oncol 101: 557–563.
34. Llovet JM, Bru C, Bruix J (1999) Prognosis of hepatocellular carcinoma: the BCLC staging classification. Semin Liver Dis 19: 329–338.
35. Hoffmann K, Hinz U, Hillebrand N, Radeleff BA, Ganten TM, et al. (2011) Risk factors of survival after liver transplantation for HCC: a multivariate single-center analysis. Clin Transplant 25: E541–551.
36. Yao FY, Ferrell L, Bass NM, Watson JJ, Bacchetti P, et al. (2001) Liver transplantation for hepatocellular carcinoma: expansion of the tumor size limits does not adversely impact survival. Hepatology 33: 1394–1403.
37. Kornberg A, Kupper B, Tannapfel A, Buchler P, Krause B, et al. (2012) Patients with non-[18 F]fludeoxyglucose-avid advanced hepatocellular carcinoma on clinical staging may achieve long-term recurrence-free survival after liver transplantation. Liver Transpl 18: 53–61.
38. Kikuchi LO, Paranagua-Vezozzo DC, Chagas AL, Mello ES, Alves VA, et al. (2009) Nodules less than 20 mm and vascular invasion are predictors of survival in small hepatocellular carcinoma. J Clin Gastroenterol 43: 191–195.
39. Llovet JM (2004) Treatment of Hepatocellular Carcinoma. Curr Treat Options Gastroenterol 7: 431–441.

Comparison of Clinical Manifestations and Outcomes between Hepatitis B Virus- and Hepatitis C Virus-Related Hepatocellular Carcinoma: Analysis of a Nationwide Cohort

Dong Hyun Sinn[1], Geum-Youn Gwak[1]*, Juhee Cho[2,3], Seung Woon Paik[1], Byung Chul Yoo[1]

1 Department of Medicine, Samsung Medical Center, Sungkyunkwan University School of Medicine, Seoul, Korea, **2** Department of Health Science and Technology, Samsung Advanced Institute for Health Science and Technology, Sungkyunkwan University, Seoul, Korea, **3** Department of Health, Behavior and Society and Epidemiology, Johns Hopkins Bloomberg School of Public Health, Baltimore, United States of America

Abstract

Background: We analyzed whether difference exist in the clinical manifestations and outcomes of hepatocellular carcinoma (HCC) according to the two major etiologies of HCC from a nationwide, population-based, random HCC registry.

Methods: Of the 31,521 new HCC cases registered at the Korea Central Cancer Registry between 2003 and 2005, 4,630 (14.7%) were randomly abstracted, and followed up until December 2011. Of those, 2,785 hepatitis B virus (HBV)-related and 447 hepatitis C virus (HCV)-related HCC patients were compared.

Results: The mean annual incidence rates of HBV- and HCV-related HCC incidence per 100,000 persons were 20.8 and 4.9, respectively. The annual incidence rate of HBV-related HCC peaked at 50–59 age group (46.5 per 100,000 persons), while the annual incidence rate of HCV-related HCC increased gradually to the ≥70 year age group (13.2 per 100,000 persons). Large tumors (≥5 cm) and portal vein invasion at initial diagnosis were more frequent in HBV-related HCC, while multiple tumors were more frequent in HCV-related HCC. In outcome analysis, HBV-related HCC showed poorer survival than HCV-related HCC [median survival: 1.34 vs. 2.17 years, adjusted hazard ratio (95% confidence interval): 0.88 (0.78–0.98), $P = 0.03$, adjusted for age, gender, Child-Pugh class, AJCC/mUICC stage, and initial treatment modality]. However, when divided according to the AJCC/mUICC stage, survival difference was observed only for those with AJCC/mUICC stage IV tumor, but not for AJCC/mUICC stage I, II or III tumors. The treatment outcome of each modality (resection, ablation, and transarterial chemoembolization) was comparable between the two etiologies.

Conclusion: HBV-related and HCV-related HCC have clear differences in clinical manifestation, requiring different screening strategy according to etiology to optimize HCC surveillance in HBV-endemic area. However, etiology did not affect treatment outcomes and long-term survival within the same stage except for far advanced tumors.

Editor: Pierre Roques, CEA, France

Funding: The authors have no support or funding to report.

Competing Interests: The authors have declared that no competing interests exist.

* Email: gy.gwak@samsung.com

Introduction

Hepatocellular carcinoma (HCC) is the fifth most common cancer and the third leading cause of cancer-related deaths in the world [1]. HCC continues to increase progressively in incidence, being a major global health problem [2,3]. The two most important risk factors for HCC are the hepatitis B virus (HBV) and hepatitis C virus (HCV) infection [4]. Worldwide, approximately 54% of cases are attributed to HBV infection (which affects 400 million people globally), while 31% are attributed to HCV infection (170 million) [5]. HCC is a major cancer in Korea [6], with a high incidence rate [2]. High incidence rate of HCC closely reflects a high prevalence rate of HBV or HCV infection [2]. Korea is an endemic area of HBV infection [7], although the prevalence of HBV is rapidly decreasing due to a nationwide universal vaccination program [8]. HBV accounts for 68~78% of all HCC diagnosed in Korea [9]. Almost all Korean chronic hepatitis B patients are infected with HBV genotype C [10], which progresses more rapidly to HCC [8]. HCV accounts for 10~15% of HCC diagnosed in Korea [11], and >95% of Korean chronic hepatitis C patients are infected with HCV genotype 1b or 2 [12].

Despite the histological similarities in the resulting carcinomas, there are evidences suggesting two distinct oncogenic pathways and natural histories between these major etiologies of HCC. In

HBV infection, in addition to chronic inflammation, the integration of HBV DNA into the host hepatocyte DNA and the expression of viral proteins, which transactivate human oncogenes, may play a role in hepatocarcinogenesis, while in HCV infection, chronic inflammation seems to play a main role in oncogenesis [13–15]. Thus, cirrhosis almost always accompanies HCV-related HCC [16], but not in HBV-related HCC [17,18]. HBV infection usually occurs in the perinatal period in an endemic area, while the immune status of the host is still immature [8]. Meanwhile, HCV infection occurs in adults with a fully matured immune system [19]. A combination of virus-specific, host genetic, environmental, and immune-related factors will affect the HCC manifestations, thus these differences in hepatocarcinogenesis may affect clinical manifestations as well as patients outcome. Indeed, several previous studies have assessed the impact of viral etiology on clinical manifestation and long-term outcome [20–22]. However, still controversies exist whether different HCC surveillance and management strategies according to the viral etiologies are needed. This question has not been answered, in part, because most studies were performed on a single hospital base which inevitably has a selection bias, with limited sample size and limited follow-up period. The sample sizes were 205, 359 and 127 in reports by Shiratori et al.'s [20], Tanabe et al.'s [21], and Hiotis et al.'s [22], respectively. Therefore, in this study, we used data from population-based nationwide cancer registry which has less selection bias, with large study sample and long-term follow-up period, and assessed whether true differences exist in clinical manifestations and long-term outcomes of HCC patients between the two viral etiologies.

Methods

Data source

In Korea, the largest government-endorsed, population-based cancer registry, called the Korea Central Cancer Registry (KCCR), was established in 1980. Patients diagnosed with cancer receive additional economic assistance from the National Health Insurance Service when registered at the KCCR, hence, almost all incidences of cancer (>95%) occurring in the population are included in the registry [23]. Therefore, the KCCR has the advantage that it has high case completeness as a cancer registry. However, the KCCR do not collect detailed information, such as liver function, tumor characteristics, treatment modalities, etc. To fully collect detailed clinical, tumor characteristics as well as treatment information and long-term outcomes of Korean HCC patients, the Korean Liver Cancer Study Group (KLCSG) built a randomly selected, population based HCC cohort based on KCCR registry (KLCSG random cohort).

The KLCSG random cohort was built as follows: Between 2003 and 2005, a total of 31,521 new cases of HCC were registered at the KCCR from about 500 hospitals nationwide. First, 25–30 hospitals were randomly selected after being stratified by region and number of cases registered, then 16.5% of HCC cases from each year were randomly selected, this gave a total of 5,262 HCC cases. Three trained abstractors visited 32 hospitals throughout the country between May 2009 and May 2010, and obtained information of each case regarding the clinical and tumor characteristics and treatment modality. Among the 5,262 cases, abstraction was possible for 4,630 HCC cases (14.7%). The major reasons of abstraction failure included malignancy other than HCC (e.g., intrahepatic cholangiocarcinoma, hepatoblastoma, etc…), data duplication or unavailable data, etc. After excluding 110 cases, which the date of the diagnosis was not between 2003 and 2005, a total of 4,520 patients were enrolled in the KLCSG random cohort. The diagnosis of HCC was made clinically or histologically based on the guidelines proposed by the KLCSG and the National Cancer Center [6]. In brief, clinical diagnosis of HCC was defined by one imaging technique (spiral CT scan, dynamic MRI, or hepatic artery angiography) showing a compatible feature of HCC in patients with alpha-fetoprotein level of more than 400 ng/ml or two imaging techniques showing compatible feature of HCC in patients with alpha-fetoprotein level of less than 400 ng/ml [6].

Out of the 4,520 patients, we analyzed 3,232 patients with either HBV or HCV infection (HBV: 2,785, HCV: 447). HBV-related HCC was defined when the presence of hepatitis B surface antigen was documented with a history of chronic liver disease. HCV-related HCC was defined when the presence of HCV RNA or anti-HCV were documented with a history of chronic liver disease. Forty-one patients had dual HBV and HCV infection, and were excluded from the analysis. The study protocol was reviewed and approved by the Institutional Review Board at Samsung Medical Center. The requirement for the informed consent was exempted by the Institutional Review Board because the study was based on the retrospective analysis of existing administrative and clinical data. Patient records/information was anonymized and de-identified prior to analysis

Variables

The KLCSG random cohort registry collected information including age, gender, date of diagnosis, etiology, Child-Pugh class, tumor number, tumor size, presence of portal vein invasion and extrahepatic spread, American Joint Committee on Cancer (AJCC)/International Union Against Cancer (UICC) tumor-node-metastasis (TNM) stage, and applied treatment modality. At the time of data abstraction, Barcelona Clinic Liver Cancer (BCLC) staging and performance status was not collected. Hence, we re-coded the BCLC stage with Child-Pugh class, tumor size, tumor number and presence of portal vein invasion and extrahepatic spread, omitting performance status. Surgical resection, local ablation and transplantation were defined as curative therapies; and transarterial chemoembolization (TACE), transarterial chemoinfusion (TACI), systemic chemotherapy and radiation were regarded as palliative therapies. Survival data was collected from the National Statistics Service, and survival data of each patient were acquired up to December 2011.

Statistical analysis

Statistical analysis was performed using the chi-square test to compare discrete variables and the t-test for continuous variables between HBV and HCV-related HCC. The survival rate was calculated and plotted by using the Kaplan-Meier method. To assess whether etiology was associated with survival, the Cox proportional hazard model was used, and a P value of less than 0.05 was considered to be significant.

Results

Clinical characteristics

The baseline characteristics at diagnosis are compared in Table 1. Mean age at diagnosis was much younger in HBV than HCV-related HCC (53.9±9.7 vs. 65.4±8.8, $P<0.01$). In HBV-related HCC, a comparably significant proportion of patients were under 40 years old (7%). Sixty-five percent were age between 40 and 59, and 28% were over 60 years. While in HCV-related HCC, those diagnosed below the age of 40 years was rare (1%) and most patients (77%) were over 60 years. In HBV-related HCC, the mean age at diagnosis was much younger for men than

Table 1. Characteristics of study population.

Characteristics	HBV	HCV	*P*-value
Number	2,785	447	
Age (years, mean ± S.D)	53.9±9.7	65.4±8.8	<0.01
<40	193 (7%)	4 (1%)	
40–49	800 (29%)	22 (5%)	
50–59	1,010 (36%)	77 (17%)	
60–69	647 (23%)	197 (44%)	
≥70	135 (5%)	147 (33%)	
Male, n (%)	2,248 (81%)	339 (76%)	0.02
Laboratory values			
Albumin (g/dl)	3.5 (3.0–3.9)	3.4 (3.0–3.8)	<0.01
Total bilirubin (mg/dl)	1.1 (0.7–1.7)	1.0 (0.7–1.6)	0.33
Prothrombin time (INR)	1.15 (1.05–1.29)	1.15 (1.05–1.28)	0.67
Child-Pugh class			0.18
A	1,798 (65%)	299 (67%)	
B	734 (26%)	119 (27%)	
C	254 (9%)	29 (7%)	
Diagnostic methods			0.86
Histologic	458 (16%)	75 (17%)	
Clinical	2,327 (84%)	372 (83%)	
Tumor number			0.03
Single	1,972 (71%)	294 (66%)	
Multiple	813 (29%)	153 (34%)	
Maximal tumor size (cm)			<0.01
<2	387 (14%)	79 (18%)	
2–5	1,089 (39%)	217 (49%)	
≥5	1,309 (47%)	151 (34%)	
Portal vein invasion			<0.01
Yes	739 (27%)	73 (16%)	
Extrahepatic spread	316 (11%)	40 (9%)	0.13
AJCC/mUICC stage			0.08
I	294 (11%)	54 (12%)	
II	1,171 (42%)	206 (46%)	
III	776 (28%)	120 (27%)	
IV-A	299 (11%)	43 (10%)	
IV-B	245 (9%)	24 (5%)	
BCLC stage[†]			<0.01
O	202 (7%)	39 (9%)	
A	1,266 (46%)	233 (52%)	
B	255 (9%)	62 (14%)	
C	808 (29%)	84 (19%)	
D	254 (9%)	29 (7%)	
Milan criteria			
Within Milan (YES)	1,250 (45%)	239 (54%)	0.01
Treatment			0.53
Curative	516 (19%)	92 (21%)	
Palliative	1,597 (57%)	246 (55%)	
Experimental[*]	2 (0.1%)	1 (0.2%)	
None	670 (24%)	108 (24%)	
Specific modality			0.01
Resection	295 (14%)	34 (10%)	

Table 1. Cont.

Characteristics	HBV	HCV	P-value
Ablation	194 (9%)	54 (16%)	
Transplantation	27 (1%)	4 (1%)	
TACE	1,439 (68%)	231 (68%)	
TACI	100 (5%)	13 (4%)	
Systemic chemotherapy	30 (1%)	1 (0.3%)	
Radiation	28 (1%)	1 (0.3%)	

Abbreviation: HBV, hepatitis B virus; HCV, hepatitis C virus; S.D, standard deviation; INR, international normalized ratio; AJCC/mUICC, American Joint Committee on Cancer/International Union Against Cancer; BCLC, Barcelona Clinic Liver Cancer; TACE, transarterial chemoembolization; TACI, transarterial chemoinfusion.
*These 3 patients received ^{166}holmium injection therapy. Values are expressed as mean ± standard deviation, median (quartile), or no (%).
†BCLC stage and performance status was not collected at the time of data collection. Hence, BCLC stage was re-coded (staged) by authors with Child-Pugh class, tumor size, tumor number and presence of portal vein invasion and extrahepatic spread, without performance status.

women (53.2±9.3 vs. 57.2±10.7, $P<0.01$), while in HCV-related HCC, the mean age at diagnosis was marginally younger for men than women (64.9±8.6 vs. 66.9±9.4 for men vs. women, $P=0.05$).

We estimated the annual incidence rate of HCC using the mid-point-population of the study period (data not shown, available at National statistics service, http://kostat.go.kr). The mean annual incidence rates of HBV- and HCV-related HCC per 100,000 persons were 20.8 and 4.9, respectively. The mean annual incidence rates of men per 100,000 were 34.3 and 9.1 for HBV- and HCV-related HCC, respectively, and were 7.9 and 2.1 for HBV- and HCV-related HCC for women. The annual incidence rate of HBV-related HCC peaked at age group 50–59, while the annual incidence rates of HCV-related HCC gradually increased until age group over 70 (Fig. 1A). In HBV-related HCC, the annual incidence rate peaked at 50–59 (78.6 per 100,000) in men, while it was 60–69 (20.4 per 100,000) in women (Fig. 1B). In HCV-related HCC, the annual incidence rate gradually increased until age over 70 in both genders (Fig. 1C).

Male patients comprised significantly more proportion in HBV-related HCC than HCV-related HCC, the serum albumin level was significantly lower in HCV-related HCC, however, the Child-Pugh Class at diagnosis was similar in both groups (Table 1).

Tumor characteristics and treatment pattern

Large tumor (≥5 cm, 47% vs. 34%, $P<0.01$) and portal vein invasion (27% vs. 16%, $P<0.01$) were more frequent in HBV-related HCC, however, multiple tumor was more common in HCV-related HCC (34% vs. 29%, $P=0.03$). There was only a marginal difference according to AJCC/mUICC stage between HBV and HCV-related HCC (Table 1). When assessed according to the BCLC staging system (without performance status), the proportion of patients with BCLC stage C or D was higher in HBV-related HCC than in HCV-related HCC (29% vs. 19% and 9% vs. 7%), while the proportion of patients with stage 0, A or B was higher in HCV-related HCC than in HBV-related HCC (9% vs. 7%, 52% vs. 46% and 14% vs. 9%). The proportion of patients diagnosed at within the Milan criteria was significantly lower in HBV- than HCV-related HCC (45% vs. 54%, $P=0.01$, Table 1). In HBV-related HCC, the proportion of patients diagnosed outside the Milan criteria was highest in age <40 years group (67.4%, 58.0%, 51.3%, 53.3%, and 57.8% for age <40, 40 s, 50 s, 60 s and ≥70 years, respectively).

When stratified according to the treatment modality (curative, palliative vs. none), there was no difference of initial treatment modality between HBV- and HCV-related HCC. Of the specific treatment modality, resection was more common in HBV-related HCC (14% vs. 10%), while local ablation therapy was more common in HCV-related HCC (16% vs. 9%).

Outcomes

The 1, 3, and 5 year survival rate was 55%, 35%, and 27% for HBV-related HCC and was 68%, 40%, and 28% for HCV-related HCC. The median survival was significantly longer in HCV-related HCC (2.17 vs. 1.34 years, $P<0.01$, Fig. 2). The hazard ratio for survival was significantly lower in HCV-related HCC compared to HBV-related HCC in both un-adjusted and adjusted analysis (Table 2).

The independent factor for survival was similar for both HBV- and HCV-related HCC. Gender, Child-Pugh Class, AJCC/mUICC stage and treatment modality was independent factors associated with survival in both HBV- and HCV-related HCC (Table 3). Age (per year) was not an independent factor for survival in HBV-related HCC, while it was an independent factor for survival in HCV-related HCC (Table 3). However, when patients were grouped in 10-year intervals, the median survival was shortest in patients under 40 (0.83 years), followed by 40–49 (1.15 years), over 70 years (1.26 years), 60–69 (1.43 years), and longest in the 50–59 age group (1.58 years) in HBV-related HCC, showing poor survival in both extreme of age group. Patients under 40 showed shorter survival than the age 50–59 group in unadjusted analysis, but when adjusted, patients under 40 showed comparable survival (Table 3). Older age groups (60–69 and ≥70 years) showed significantly shorter survival than 50–59 age group in unadjusted and adjusted analysis. In HCV-related HCC, there were only a few patients in the 40 ($n=4$) and 40–49 ($n=22$), so those patients were grouped as under 50 years, 50–59, 60–69 and ≥70 years. Age per year was a significant factor associated with patient survival in HCV-related HCC (Table 3). Older age groups (60s, ≥70 years) showed poorer survival than the 50–59 age group in adjusted analysis (Table 3).

When stratified by tumor burden (AJCC/mUICC stage), survival was not different in AJCC/mUICC I, II, III tumors (Table 4). However, in AJCC/mUICC stage IV, long-term survival was significantly worse in HBV-related HCC than HCV-related HCC. When stratified by treatment, patients who received curative or palliative therapy, there was no significant difference in survival. However, survival was significantly worse for HBV-related HCC for patients who had not received therapy (Table 4). Even in AJCC/mUICC stage IV tumor, there was no

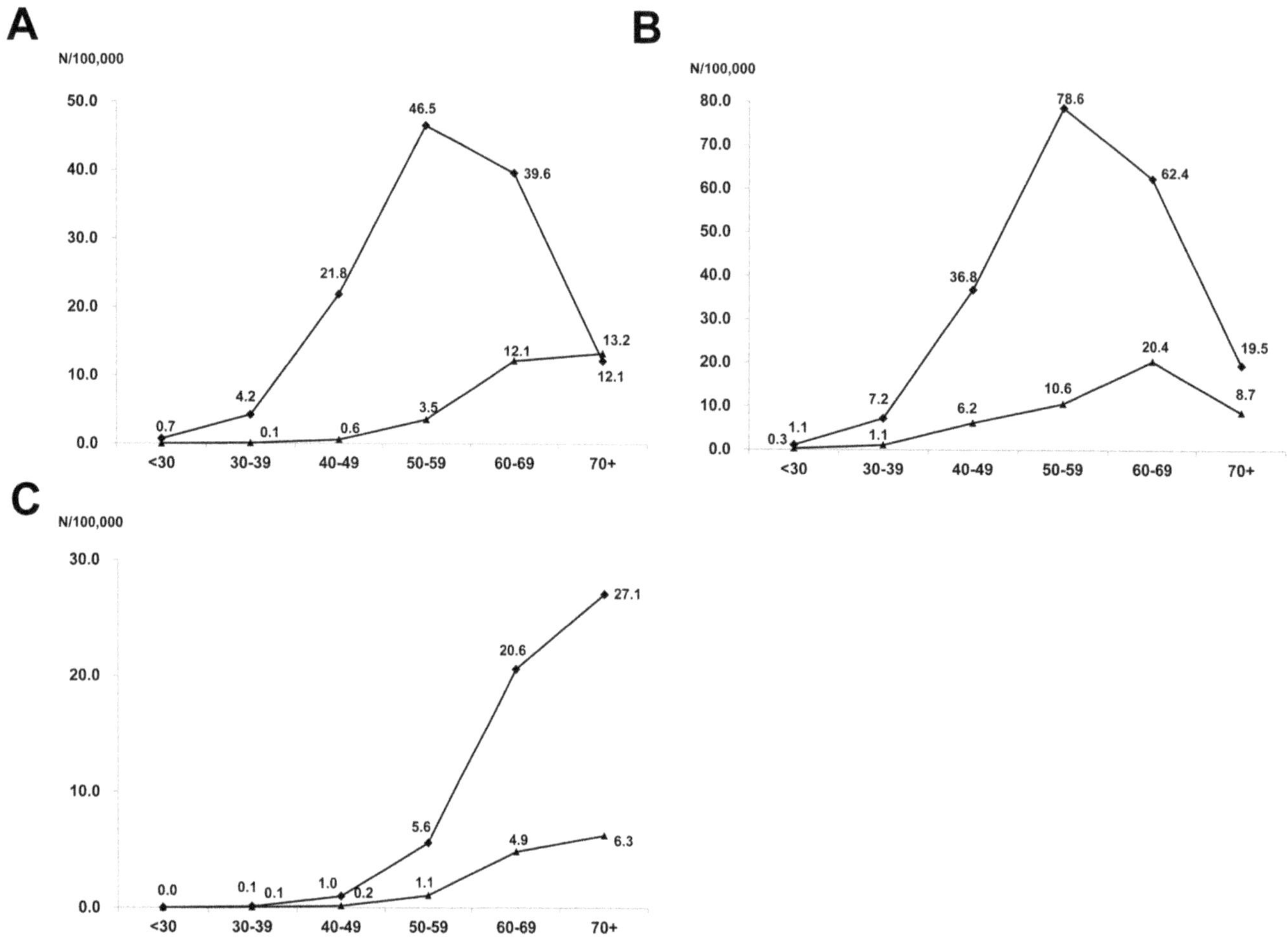

Figure 1. The age-specific incidence rates of hepatocellular carcinoma (HCC) by the etiology (A), by gender in HBV-related HCC (B) and by gender in HCV-related HCC (C). The annual incidence rates of HBV-related HCC peaked in the 50–59 age group, while the annual incidence rates of HCV-related HCC kept gradually increasing until age ≥70 s. Similar trend was observed after stratified by gender, although the peak mean annual incidence rates was observed in the 50–59 in men and in the 60–69 in women in HBV-related HCC (B). Diamonds (♦) and triangles (▲) represent for HBV and HCV-related HCC in (A), men and women in (B) and (C), respectively.

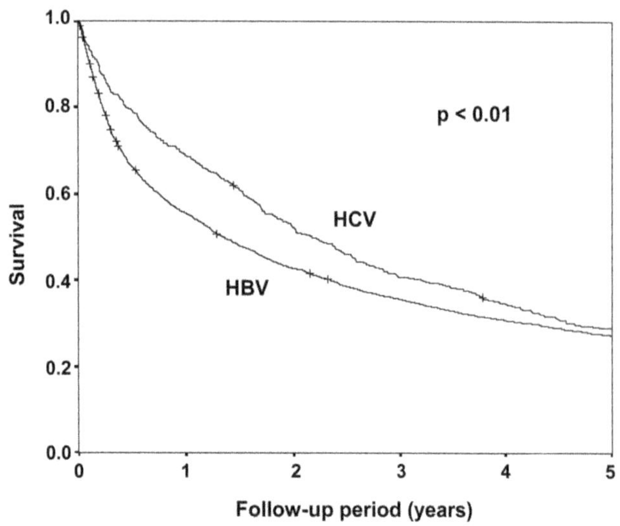

Figure 2. Long-term survival by etiology. The median survival was significantly longer in HCV-related HCC patients than in HBV-related HCC patients. (2.17 vs. 1.34 years, $P<0.01$).

significant different in survival for patients who received treatment, and the survival difference was significant for patients who had no therapy (Table 4).

Discussion

In this study, HCC patients clearly showed different clinical manifestation according to viral etiology (HBV vs. HCV). HBV-related HCC occurred at a younger age than HCV-related HCC. The annual incidence rate of HBV-related HCC peaked in the 50–59 year age group, while the annual incidence rate of HCV-related HCC gradually increased up to the over 70 year group. In HBV-related HCC, tumor was more likely to be single and larger, and accompanied by portal vein invasion. Overall, the long-term outcome was worse in HBV-related HCC than HCV-related HCC, however, the survival difference existed only for patients with advanced tumor (AJCC/mUICC stage IV). The outcome of each treatment modality (resection, ablation, and TACE) was also comparable between HBV- and HCV-related HCC.

In this study, we could estimate annual incidence rate of HCC by age groups and etiology for the first time in Korea, as the data was based on a nationwide population-based cohort, and could notice significant differences in the incidence rates of HCC by age

Table 2. Survival by etiology.

	Median survival (years)	Model 1		Model 2		Model 3		Model 4	
		HR (95% CI)	*P*-value	HR (95% CI)	*P*-value	HR (95% CI)	*P*-value	HR (95% CI)	*P*-value
HBV	1.34	Reference		Reference		Reference		Reference	
HCV	2.17	0.94 (0.84–1.05)	0.28	0.88 (0.78–0.99)	0.04	0.86 (0.77–0.98)	0.02	0.88 (0.78–0.98)	0.03

Abbreviation: HBV, hepatitis B virus; HCV, hepatitis C virus. HR, hazard ratio. Model 1 = crude hazard ratio, Model 2 = adjusted for age, gender, Model 3 = Model 2 + Child-Pugh class and AJCC/mUICC stage, Model 4 = Model 3 + initial treatment modality.

group and viral etiology. The highest age-specific incidence rates were observed in the 50–59 age group in HBV-related HCC, while the annual incidence rates of HCV-related HCC kept gradually increasing until the ≥70 group. This phenomenon may be explained by the fact that vertical transmission is the major route of HBV acquisition in Korea [24], while HCV is usually acquired in adulthood [19]. HCC rarely developed before the age of 50 years in HCV-related HCC, likewise in countries where HBV is not endemic [13]. However, in HBV-related HCC, the age-specific incidence rate was not low in patient age less than 50 years. A clear gender difference in the age-specific incidence rate of HBV-related HCC was also observed. In men, highest age-specific incidence rates were observed in the 50–59 age group (78.6 per 100,000), while it was highest in the 60–69 age group (20.4 per 100,000) in women. In HCV-related HCC, there was no significant difference in the peak age group between men and women.

Notably, there were significant differences in the tumor characteristic at diagnosis by viral etiology. HBV-related HCC were more likely to be single, large, and accompanied by portal vein invasion. Different oncogenic mechanism by different viruses may explain the observed differences in tumor characteristics. However, it might also be attributable to the currently recommended surveillance policy for HBV and HCV infected individuals in Korea. An HCC surveillance program has been included in National Cancer Screening Program in Korea since 2003 [9]. Patients over 40 year old with risk factors such as hepatitis B, hepatitis C and cirrhosis are recommended to undergo HCC surveillance by ultrasonography and alpha-fetoprotein levels at 6-month interval. Thus, early participation of HCV-infected patients in regular surveillance program before reaching the peak age of HCC development might have a positive influence on the characteristics of tumor at the time of diagnosis. HBV-related HCC patients were diagnosed at younger age, and the proportion of patients diagnosed outside the Milan criteria was also higher in young age group in HBV-related HCC patients. Several studies reported that most of HCC patients diagnosed at young age did not receive regular HCC surveillance, and presented at advanced stage [25,26]. As this study did not collect information regarding HCC surveillance before HCC diagnosis, careful interpretation is needed. Nevertheless, this data strongly suggest different surveillance strategy (e.g., different age cutoff for starting surveillance) according to the viral etiology is needed.

The decision to undergo HCC surveillance is determined by the level of risk for HCC, which is related to HCC incidence in a predefined at-risk population. Although we cannot provide the exact incidence rate of HCC according to each age group and etiology, we could roughly estimate the annual incidence rate of HCC based on population and prevalence rates of HBV and HCV infection in each age group. The estimated annual incidence rates of HCC in HBV infected patients were 0.02%, 0.09%, 0.5%, 0.8%, 1.2% and 1.1% for age 20–29, 30–39, 40–49, 50–59, 60–69 and ≥70 years, respectively. The estimated annual incidence rates of HCC in HCV infected patients were 0%, 0.02%, 0.1%, 0.4%, 0.8% and 0.6% for age 20–29, 30–39, 40–49, 50–59, 60–69 and ≥70 years, respectively. Similar annual incidence rates of HCC were observed in HBV infected patients who were about 10 years younger than in HCV infected patients. Thus, HBV-infected patients may require earlier participation in an HCC surveillance program compared to that of HCV infected patients.

In this study, we observed differences of overall survival according to the viral etiology. However, when stratified by tumor stage, patients who were diagnosed at AJCC/mUICC stage I, II and III, showed similar survival in HBV- and HCV-related HCC.

Table 3. Comparison of prognostic factors between hepatitis B virus- and hepatitis C virus-related hepatocellular carcinoma.

	HBV-related HCC				HCV-related HCC			
	Unadjusted		Adjusted		Unadjusted		Adjusted	
	HR (95% CI)	*P* value	HR (95% CI)	*P* value	HR (95% CI)	*P* value	HR (95% CI)	*P* value
Age (years)	1.00 (0.99–1.01)	0.16	1.00 (0.99–1.01)	0.13	1.01 (1.00–1.03)	0.01	1.01 (1.01–1.02)	0.03
<40	1.24 (1.04–1.48)	0.01	1.13 (0.95–1.35)	0.15	1.08 (0.64–1.81)	0.77	1.32 (0.78–2.23)	0.29
40–49	1.08 (0.97–1.21)	0.13	0.95 (0.85–1.06)	0.40				
50–59	Reference		Reference		Reference		Reference	
60–69	1.21 (1.08–1.35)	0.01	1.15 (1.03–1.29)	0.01	1.17 (0.87–1.59)	0.28	1.41 (1.04–1.91)	0.03
≥70	1.48 (1.21–1.78)	<0.01	1.22 (1.01–1.49)	0.04	1.53 (1.12–2.08)	0.01	1.46 (1.07–2.00)	0.01
Gender								
Female	Reference		Reference		Reference		Reference	
Male	1.27 (1.13–1.41)	<0.01	1.37 (1.22–1.54)	<0.01	1.06 (0.83–1.35)	0.63	1.37 (1.06–1.78)	0.01
Child-Pugh Class								
A	Reference		Reference		Reference		Reference	
B	2.20 (2.00–2.42)	<0.01	1.64 (1.48–1.81)	<0.01	2.03 (1.61–2.56)	<0.01	1.73 (1.36–2.20)	<0.01
C	2.82 (2.44–3.26)	<0.01	2.54 (2.19–2.95)	<0.01	2.89 (1.92–4.35)	<0.01	3.23 (2.08–5.00)	<0.01
AJCC/mUICC stage								
I	Reference		Reference		Reference		Reference	
II	1.68 (1.37–1.94)	<0.01	1.72 (1.45–2.05)	<0.01	1.43 (0.99–2.05)	0.05	1.16 (0.80–1.67)	0.42
III	3.32 (2.78–3.96)	<0.01	2.76 (2.31–3.33)	<0.01	2.29 (1.57–3.35)	<0.01	1.67 (1.13–2.45)	0.01
IV	6.07 (5.50–7.30)	<0.01	4.75 (3.94–5.72)	<0.01	4.16 (2.74–6.31)	<0.01	2.38 (1.54–3.68)	<0.01
Treatment								
Curative	Reference		Reference		Reference		Reference	
Palliative	2.83 (2.46–3.25)	<0.01	2.44 (2.11–2.81)	<0.01	2.63 (1.93–3.58)	<0.01	2.83 (2.04–3.91)	<0.01
None	7.78 (6.68–9.07)	<0.01	4.97 (4.24–5.83)	<0.01	5.36 (3.81–7.54)	<0.01	4.68 (3.26–6.71)	<0.01

Abbreviation: HBV, hepatitis B virus; HCC, hepatocellular carcinoma; HCV, hepatitis C virus; HR, hazard ratio.

Table 4. Adjusted difference in the survival between hepatitis B virus and hepatitis C virus related hepatocellular carcinoma by subgroup.

	Number of patients (HBV vs. HCV)	Median survival, year, (HBV vs. HCV)	Adjusted hazard ratio (95% CI)	*P*-value
AJCC/mUICC stage I	294 vs. 54	6.60 vs. 5.09	1.10 (0.73–1.66)	0.63
AJCC/mUICC stage II	1,172 vs. 206	2.95 vs. 3.19	0.86 (0.71–1.03)	0.10
AJCC/mUICC stage III	776 vs. 120	0.65 vs. 1.71	0.95 (0.76–1.19)	0.70
AJCC/mUICC stage IV	544 vs. 67	0.28 vs. 0.49	0.65 (0.49–0.88)	0.01
Stage IV and received treatment	311 vs. 33	0.48 vs. 0.95	0.69 (0.44–1.08)	0.11
Stage IV and received no treatment	233 vs. 34	0.12 vs. 0.24	0.64 (0.42–0.98)	0.04
Curative treatment	516 vs. 92	NR vs. 6.19	1.09 (0.78–1.53)	0.59
Resection	295 vs. 34	NR vs. NR	0.72 (0.39–1.35)	0.31
Ablation	194 vs. 54	7.06 vs. 4.47	1.13 (0.74–1.73)	0.55
Palliative treatment	1,597 vs. 246	1.48 vs. 2.12	0.95 (0.81–1.11)	0.53
TACE	1,439 vs. 231	1.72 vs. 2.23	0.97 (0.83–1.14)	0.76
None	672 vs. 109	0.18 vs. 0.33	0.75 (0.59–0.95)	0.02

Abbreviation: HBV, hepatitis B virus; HCV, hepatitis C virus; CI, confidence interval; NR, not reached. In each adjusted model, hepatitis B was used as reference for hepatitis C and following variables were adjusted: age, gender, Child-Pugh class, AJCC/mUICC stage, and initial treatment modality.

In AJCC/mUICC stage IV tumor, survival was significantly worse in HBV-related HCC. These findings are consistent with the study of Cantarini et al., which reported that HBV-related HCC is more aggressive than HCV-related HCC, especially for HCC diagnosed at an advanced stage [27]. Whether or not viral etiology should be considered in treatment decision is also an important issue. Indeed, several previous studies have tried to assess whether viral etiology is a significant factor determining treatment outcome, and found that viral etiology was not an independent factor for determining outcomes of HCC who underwent resection [28,29], ablation [30], or TACE [31]. In this study, we also found that viral etiology is not an independent factor associated with survival for patients who received therapy. Even in AJCC/mUICC stage IV tumor, survival was not significantly different when patients received treatment (Table 4). Therefore, although viral etiology should be considered in estimation of patient prognosis, it may have little impact on choosing therapeutic modality.

There are some limitations in this study. Information of some important prognostic factors (e.g., performance status, serum alpha-fetoprotein levels, and use of antiviral therapy, etc.) was not collected. The BCLC stage was not collected and could not be properly assessed. There are also some remained questions whether viral etiology would affect the treatment outcome of other types of treatment, such as transplantation or sorafenib. For liver transplantation, HBV-related HCC has been reported to be an independent factor associated with better survival than HCV-related HCC [32]. For sorafenib, the median survival in the Sorafenib HCC Assessment Randomized Protocol Trial (SHARP) trial (10.7 months) was longer than the median survival of same trial performed in the Asia-Pacific Study (6.5 months) [33,34]. Unfortunately, sorafenib had not been approved in Korea during period of the present study, so there were no patients who used sorafenib. Hence, it was impossible to assess the impact of viral etiology for the prognosis of patients treated with sorafenib. Lastly, this study only assessed first treatment modality. It is known that HCV-related tumors have higher recurrence rate after curative resection than HBV-related HCC [35], which may have affected long-term outcome.

Despite some limitations, this study provides highly reliable information from unselected nationwide cohort, which minimized selection bias, and large sample size with long term follow-up. HBV-related and HCV-related HCC have clear differences in clinical manifestation, requiring different screening strategy according to etiology to optimize HCC surveillance in HBV-endemic area. However, etiology does not affect treatment outcome and long-term survival within the same stage except for far advanced tumor.

Acknowledgments

This study was selected to use the KLCSG random cohort data in the 2012 KLCSG Research Contest. The authors thank all members of the KLCSG and the Korea Central Cancer Registry for their contribution to build the KLCSG random cohort.

Author Contributions

Conceived and designed the experiments: GYG. Performed the experiments: DHS GYG. Analyzed the data: DHS JC. Contributed reagents/materials/analysis tools: DHS JC. Wrote the paper: DHS GYG SWP BCY.

References

1. Ferlay J, Soerjomataram I, Dikshit R, Eser S, Mathers C, et al. (2014) Cancer incidence and mortality worldwide: Sources, methods and major patterns in GLOBOCAN 2012. Int J Cancer 13.doi: 10.1022/ijc.29210. [Epub ahead of print]
2. Yang JD, Roberts LR (2010) Hepatocellular carcinoma: A global view. Nat Rev Gastroenterol Hepatol 7: 448–458.
3. El-Serag HB (2011) Hepatocellular carcinoma. N Engl J Med 365: 1118–1127.
4. Forner A, Llovet JM, Bruix J (2012) Hepatocellular carcinoma. Lancet 379: 1245–1255.
5. Bruix J, Sherman M (2011) Management of hepatocellular carcinoma: an update. Hepatology 53: 1020–1022.
6. Korean Liver Cancer Study Group (2009) [Practice guidelines for management of hepatocellular carcinoma 2009]. Korean J Hepatol 15: 391–423.
7. Chae HB, Kim JH, Kim JK, Yim HJ (2009) Current status of liver diseases in Korea: hepatitis B. Korean J Hepatol 15 Suppl 6: S13–24.

8. Korean Association for the Study of the Liver (2012) KASL Clinical Practice Guidelines: Management of chronic hepatitis B. Clin Mol Hepatol 18: 109–162.
9. Song IH, Kim KS (2009) Current status of liver diseases in Korea: hepatocellular carcinoma. Korean J Hepatol 15 Suppl 6: S50–59.
10. Bae SH, Yoon SK, Jang JW, Kim CW, Nam SW, et al. (2005) Hepatitis B virus genotype C prevails among chronic carriers of the virus in Korea. J Korean Med Sci 20: 816–820.
11. Suh DJ, Jeong SH (2006) Current status of hepatitis C virus infection in Korea. Intervirology 49: 70–75.
12. Sinn DH, Paik SW, Kang P, Kil JS, Park SU, et al. (2008) Disease progression and the risk factor analysis for chronic hepatitis C. Liver Int 28: 1363–1369.
13. El-Serag HB, Rudolph KL (2007) Hepatocellular carcinoma: epidemiology and molecular carcinogenesis. Gastroenterology 132: 2557–2576.
14. Kim W, Oe Lim S, Kim JS, Ryu YH, Byeon JY, et al. (2003) Comparison of proteome between hepatitis B virus- and hepatitis C virus-associated hepatocellular carcinoma. Clin Cancer Res 9: 5493–5500.
15. Hai H, Tamori A, Kawada N (2014) Role of hepatitis B virus DNA integration in human hepatocarcinogenesis. World J Gastroenterol 20: 6236–6243.
16. Yeh MM, Daniel HD, Torbenson M (2010) Hepatitis C-associated hepatocellular carcinomas in non-cirrhotic livers. Mod Pathol 23: 276–283.
17. Zhou YM, Zhang XF, Li B, Sui CJ, Yang JM (2014) Prognosis after resection of hepatitis B virus-related hepatocellular carcinoma originating from non-cirrhotic liver. Ann Surg Oncol 21: 2406–2412.
18. Kalayci C, Johnson PJ, Davies SE, Williams R (1991) Hepatitis B virus related hepatocellular carcinoma in the non-cirrhotic liver. J Hepatol 12: 54–59.
19. The Korean Association for the Study of the Liver (2014) KASL clinical practice guidelines: Management of Hepatitis C. Clin Mol Hepatol 20: 89–136.
20. Shiratori Y, Shiina S, Imamura M, Kato N, Kanai F, et al. (1995) Characteristic difference of hepatocellular carcinoma between hepatitis B- and C- viral infection in Japan. Hepatology 22: 1027–1033.
21. Tanabe G, Nuruki K, Baba Y, Imamura Y, Miyazono N, et al. (1999) A comparison of hepatocellular carcinoma associated with HBV or HCV infection. Hepatogastroenterology 46: 2442–2446.
22. Hiotis SP, Rahbari NN, Villanueva GA, Klegar E, Luan W, et al. (2012) Hepatitis B vs. hepatitis C infection on viral hepatitis-associated hepatocellular carcinoma. BMC Gastroenterol 12: 64.
23. Ahn YO (2007) [Cancer registration in Korea: the present and furtherance]. J Prev Med Public Health 40: 265–272.
24. Choi MS, Sinn DH, Kim SA, Lee YS, Choi W, et al. (2012) The clinical and laboratory characteristics of patients with chronic hepatitis B using current or past antiviral therapy in Korea: a multi-center, nation-wide, cross-sectional epidemiologic study. Gut Liver 6: 241–248.
25. Kim JH, Choi MS, Lee H, Kim do Y, Lee JH, et al. (2006) Clinical features and prognosis of hepatocellular carcinoma in young patients from a hepatitis B-endemic area. J Gastroenterol Hepatol 21: 588–594.
26. Wang Q, Luan W, Villanueva GA, Rahbari NN, Yee HT, et al. (2012) Clinical prognostic variables in young patients (under 40 years) with hepatitis B virus-associated hepatocellular carcinoma. J Dig Dis 13: 214–218.
27. Cantarini MC, Trevisani F, Morselli-Labate AM, Rapaccini G, Farinati F, et al. (2006) Effect of the etiology of viral cirrhosis on the survival of patients with hepatocellular carcinoma. Am J Gastroenterol 101: 91–98.
28. Kao WY, Su CW, Chau GY, Lui WY, Wu CW, et al. (2011) A comparison of prognosis between patients with hepatitis B and C virus-related hepatocellular carcinoma undergoing resection surgery. World J Surg 35: 858–867.
29. Nishikawa H, Arimoto A, Wakasa T, Kita R, Kimura T, et al. (2013) Comparison of clinical characteristics and survival after surgery in patients with non-B and non-C hepatocellular carcinoma and hepatitis virus-related hepatocellular carcinoma. J Cancer 4: 502–513.
30. Chen PH, Kao WY, Chiou YY, Hung HH, Su CW, et al. (2013) Comparison of prognosis by viral etiology in patients with hepatocellular carcinoma after radiofrequency ablation. Ann Hepatol 12: 263–273.
31. Takayasu K, Arii S, Ikai I, Omata M, Okita K, et al. (2006) Prospective cohort study of transarterial chemoembolization for unresectable hepatocellular carcinoma in 8510 patients. Gastroenterology 131: 461–469.
32. Tandoi F, Ponte E, Saffioti MC, Patrono D, Mirabella S, et al. (2013) Liver transplantation for hepatocellular carcinoma within Milan Criteria in patients with Model for End-Stage Liver Disease score below 15: the impact of the etiology of cirrhosis on long-term survival. Transplant Proc 45: 2711–2714.
33. Llovet JM, Ricci S, Mazzaferro V, Hilgard P, Gane E, et al. (2008) Sorafenib in advanced hepatocellular carcinoma. N Engl J Med 359: 378–390.
34. Cheng AL, Kang YK, Chen Z, Tsao CJ, Qin S, et al. (2009) Efficacy and safety of sorafenib in patients in the Asia-Pacific region with advanced hepatocellular carcinoma: a phase III randomised, double-blind, placebo-controlled trial. Lancet Oncol 10: 25–34.
35. Huang YH, Wu JC, Chen CH, Chang TT, Lee PC, et al. (2005) Comparison of recurrence after hepatic resection in patients with hepatitis B vs. hepatitis C-related small hepatocellular carcinoma in hepatitis B virus endemic area. Liver Int 25: 236–241.

19

Risk of Deaths, AIDS-Defining and Non-AIDS Defining Events among Ghanaians on Long-Term Combination Antiretroviral Therapy

Fred Stephen Sarfo[1,2]*, Maame Anima Sarfo[1], Betty Norman[1], Richard Phillips[1,2], George Bedu-Addo[1,2], David Chadwick[3]

1 Komfo Anokye Teaching Hospital, Kumasi, Ghana, **2** Kwame Nkrumah University of Science and Technology, Kumasi, Ghana, **3** The James Cook University Hospital, Middlesbrough, United Kingdom

Abstract

Combination antiretroviral therapy (cART) has been widely available in Ghana since 2004. The aim of this cohort study was to assess the incidences of death, AIDS-defining events and non-AIDS defining events and associated risk factors amongst patients initiating cART in a large treatment centre. Clinical and laboratory data were extracted from clinic and hospital case notes for patients initiating cART between 2004 and 2010 and clinical events graded according to recognised definitions for AIDS, non-AIDS events (NADE) and death, with additional events not included in such definitions such as malaria also included. The cumulative incidence of events was calculated using Kaplan Meier analysis, and association of risk factors with events by Cox proportional hazards regression. Data were closed for analysis on 31st December, 2011 after a median follow-up of 30 months (range, 0–90 months). Amongst 4,039 patients starting cART at a median CD4 count of 133 cells/mm^3, there were 324 (8%) confirmed deaths, with an event rate of 28.83 (95% CI 25.78–32.15) deaths per 1000-person follow-up years; the commonest established causes were pulmonary TB and gastroenteritis. There were 681 AIDS-defining events (60.60 [56.14–65.33] per 1000 person years) with pulmonary TB and chronic diarrhoea being the most frequent causes. Forty-one NADEs were recorded (3.64 [2.61–4.95] per 1000 person years), of which hepatic and cardiovascular events were most common. Other common events recorded outside these definitions included malaria (746 events) and respiratory tract infections (666 events). Overall 24% of patients were lost-to-follow-up. Alongside expected risk factors, stavudine use was associated with AIDS [adjusted HR of 1.08 (0.90–1.30)] and death (adjusted HR of 1.60 [1.21–2.11]). Whilst frequency of AIDS and deaths in this cohort were similar to those described in other sub-Saharan African cohorts, rates of NADEs were lower and far exceeded by events such as malaria and respiratory tract infections.

Editor: Sarah L. Pett, Faculty of Medicine, Australia

Funding: Funding for setting up the database was provided by the HIV Research Trust, UK. The funder had no role in study design, data collection and analysis, decision to publish, or preparation of the manuscript.

Competing Interests: The authors have declared that no competing interests exist.

* Email: stephensarfo78@gmail.com

Introduction

Combination anti-retroviral therapy (cART) for the long-term management of HIV infection is administered to achieve long-term suppression of virological replication and to maintain CD4 cell counts at a level that reduces the risk of morbidity and mortality. It is encouraging that the effectiveness of cART in developing countries in sub-Saharan Africa has been reported to be similar, and often superior in clinical and immunologic outcomes when compared with those from the developed countries [1–8]. Evidence of the sustainability of these initially favourable immunological and clinical responses is beginning to emerge.

Deaths in the era of cART have largely been due to AIDS-defining clinical events in many such reports from developing countries. But the dynamics of mortality is believed to be changing in industrialised countries with non-AIDS defining clinical events assuming greater importance as causes of death as patients live longer on potent cART [9–11]. Non-AIDS defining events are classified as cardiovascular, renal, hepatic-related or non-AIDS-defining malignancies that are likely to have an impact on morbidity and mortality [12]. One report from Botswana indicated that the age-standardised incidence rates of non-AIDS defining events were comparable to those in the United States [13]. However, the spectra of disease entities included in this definition is debated [14,15] and does not capture infectious diseases such as malaria which is a common cause of morbidity among patients in sub-Saharan Africa.

Ghana like many other countries in sub-Saharan Africa started cART roll-out in 2004. We have recently published a comparative analysis of the effectiveness and tolerability of nevirapine and efavirenz based cART among a large cohort of Ghanaian HIV-infected patients [16]. The aim of this study is to present a comprehensive analysis of the incidence, causes and risk factors associated with AIDS, non-AIDS clinical events, immunological failure, immune reconstitution inflammatory syndrome, treatment-limiting toxicity, and mortality over the long-term in this Ghanaian cohort.

Methods

Ethical permission for this study was given by the Committee on Human Research Publications and Ethics of the Kwame Nkrumah University of Science and Technology and the Komfo Anokye Teaching Hospital, Kumasi, Ghana (ref: CHRPE/AP/073/13). Our institutional review board waived the need for a written informed consent since this was a retrospective, observational study and anonymised data were collected from patients' records. The study was conducted at the HIV clinic at the Komfo Anokye Teaching Hospital in Kumasi, Ghana, which provides HIV care to a large rural and urban population across central and northern Ghana. Antiretroviral therapy has been administered to patients meeting eligibility criteria since 2004 as has been previously described [16]. Data were extracted from the notes of patients starting ART between January 2004 and December 2010 and was closed for analysis by an intention-to-treat basis on 31st December 2011. For this analysis, AIDS-defining events, non-AIDS defining clinical events, immune reconstitution inflammatory syndrome, loss-to-follow up, death and adherence to therapy were defined as follows. An AIDS-defining clinical event was defined as the occurrence of any opportunistic infections or malignancy according the World Health Organisation (WHO) [17] criteria while the patient was on cART.

The diagnosis of a non-AIDS clinical event was adjudicated by consensus between FSS, BN and RP (BN and RP are Consultants in HIV Medicine at the Komfo Anokye Teaching Hospital). The conditions classified under NADEs included cerebrovascular accident (stroke), cerebral/sub-arachnoid hemorrhage, myocardial infarction, coronary artery disease, congestive cardiac failure, end-stage renal disease, renal failure, cirrhosis of the liver, esophageal varices, hepatic failure, hepatic coma, hepatic encephalopathy, intestinal adenocarcinoma/lymphoma, penile carcinoma, small cell lung carcinoma, malignant melanoma, hepatocellular carcinoma, squamous cell carcinoma, and squamous cell carcinoma of the anus as previously described [14,15]. Severity of specific NADEs in particular liver injury and renal failure were assessed using established Division of AIDS (DAIDS) tables for Grading Severity of Adult Adverse Experiences (NADEs).

Other medical diagnoses that did not fulfil the criteria for AIDS-defining events or serious NADEs were recorded and presented as "medical co-morbidities on cART". These included conditions such as malaria, urinary tract infections, new onset diabetes mellitus or hypertension.

In the present study immune reconstitution inflammatory syndrome (IRIS) was defined as the paradoxical worsening of a previously treated opportunistic infection [18] for which the clinician was able to demonstrate radiological evidence of exacerbation in the cases of tuberculosis or cerebral toxoplasmosis, and fundoscopic evidence of vitreous inflammation in the case of CMV retinitis. Cases of herpes zoster IRIS were defined clinically. Due to the inherent difficulty of differentiating an opportunistic infection with normal presentation and a disorder with presentation that is compatible with unmasking IRIS in our setting, the unmasking type of IRIS was not documented in charts in this cohort. Immunological failure was defined using WHO criteria as either the return of CD4 counts to pre-therapy baseline, or below and/or more than 50% fall from on-therapy CD4 peak-level (and/or more than 50% fall in CD4), or persistent low CD4 of less than 100 cells/μl after one year of therapy without other concomitant infection to explain the low CD4. Loss to follow up was defined as missing a clinic appointment by at least 3 months of the last scheduled visit to clinic. Death was defined as the demise of a patient from causes related to HIV/AIDS or from toxicity from antiretrovirals or other non-AIDS related causes if known. Confirmation of death was by death certification by medical doctors for patients who died on the wards or by patients' family for those who died outside the hospital. Patient adherence, assessed by pill count, was classified as excellent at each clinic visit if adherence level of ≥95% was achieved. Poor adherence was defined as any documented evidence of <95% of adherence during follow up.

Statistical analysis

Parametric and non-parametric methods were used to compare baseline characteristics of continuous data between patients started on either efavirenz, nevirapine or a protease inhibitor-based ART. A 1-way analysis of variance (ANOVA) or Kruskal-Wallis test was used to compare means or medians respectively. Comparisons of dichotomous data were performed using χ^2 or Fisher's exact test. Crude incidence rates of events were calculated in person-years of follow-up with 95% confidence intervals calculated using Normal approximation to the Poisson distribution. Risk factors associated with death and AIDS-defining events were assessed using multivariable Cox proportional hazards regression with factors attaining a significance level of <0.10 in univariate analyses included in the final model. For these survival analyses, the month in which patients started cART was set as month zero and one day of follow-up was added to patients who did not attend any follow-up visits after initiating therapy. Time to events of interest, namely AIDS-defining events, loss-to-follow up or mortality, was calculated by subtracting the date of the event from the date on which the patient was started on cART. Patients were censored at December 31, 2011 if there were no event of interest. Explanatory variables included in survival analyses were selected on the basis of their well-recognised impact on clinical outcomes such as AIDS-defining events, loss-to-follow up and deaths. The cumulative incidence of loss to follow up and deaths were calculated using the Kaplan Meier methodology. For all analysis, a 2-sided p-value <0.05 was set as the level of statistical significance. All data analyses were conducted using SPSS version 19.

Results

Baseline demographics and laboratory characteristics of study participants

Four thousand and thirty-nine (4,039) patients out of 10,500 (38.5%) patients registered between January 2004 and December 2010 initiated first line therapy. There was a female preponderance in a ratio of 2.1: 1.0 with a median age of patients of 38 years (range of 14–78). As shown in Table 1, 2,376 (58.8%) patients were started on efavirenz based cART compared with 1,623 (40.2%) on nevirapine based cART while 40 (1.0%) were initiated on protease inhibitor based cART because they had HIV-2 mono-infection or HIV-1/2 dual infection: 23 on ritonavir-boosted lopinavir and 17 on nelfinavir. 52.1% were started on an NRTI backbone of stavudine (d4T) and lamivudine (3TC) while 47.7%

Table 1. Baseline demographic, clinical and laboratory characteristics of patients initiating cART.

Characteristic	Efavirenz n = 2,376	Nevirapine n = 1,623	Protease inhibitors n = 40	Total n = 4,039	p-value
Male: female	1,028: 1,348	248: 1,375	11: 29	1,287: 2,752	<0.0001
Median (range) age	40 (14–77)	35 (15–75)	36 (25–65)	38 (14–77)	<0.0001
WHO clinical stage n (%)					0.09
1	165 (6.9)	106 (6.5)	2 (5.0)	273 (6.8)	
2	258 (10.9)	225 (13.9)	6 (15.0)	489 (12.1)	
3	1274 (53.6)	867 (53.4)	25 (62.5)	2166 (53.6)	
4	407 (17.1)	238 (14.7)	10 (10.0)	649 (16.1)	
No data	272 (11.4)	187 (11.5)	3 (7.5)	462 (11.4)	
Mean BMI ± SEM	20.1±0.09	20.5±0.10	21.0±0.62	20.3±0.07	0.0025
BMI categories					
<18.5 kg/m^2	868 (36.5)	543 (33.5)	11 (27.5)	1422 (35.2)	0.0047
18.5–24.5 kg/m^2	1145 (48.2)	804 (49.5)	20 (50.0)	1969 (48.8)	
>24.5 kg/m^2	291 (12.3)	246 (15.2)	6 (15.0)	543 (13.4)	
No data	72 (3.0)	30 (1.8)	3 (7.5)	105 (2.6)	
CD4 count Median (range)	127.5 (1–1085)	140.0 (0–676)	186.0 (1–1134)	134 (0–1134)	0.0006
CD4 categories					
<200 cells/ml	1684 (70.9)	1080 (66.5)	21 (52.5)	2785 (69.0)	<0.0001
200–350 cells/ml	611 (25.7)	495 (30.5)	12 (30.0)	1118 (27.7)	
>350 cells/ml	53 (2.2)	41 (2.5)	7 (17.5)	101 (2.5)	
No data	28 (1.2)	7 (0.5)	0 (0.0)	35 (0.9)	
Median (range) Hemoglobin (g/dl)	10.2 (2.6–19.4)	10.2 (3.2–19.8)	10.9 (6.8–16.3)	10.2 (2.6–19.8)	0.07
Mean ± SEM ALT (U/L)	40.5±0.87	32.0±0.75	39.3±6.64	37.1±0.60	<0.0001
Mean ± SEM AST (U/L)	53.6±0.93	45.2±0.95	51.0±11.6	50.2±0.68	<0.0001
eGFR (ml/min/1.73m^2) Median (IQR), n	64.0 (47.0–83.0) n = 1791	71.0 (54.0–89.0) n = 1240	66.5 (54.5–89.5) n = 32	66.0 (50.0–86.0) n = 3063	<0.0001
eGFR categories					
>60ml/min	1028 (57.4)	849 (68.5)	21 (65.6)	1898 (62.0)	<0.0001
30–59 ml/min	638 (35.6)	345 (27.8)	11 (34.4)	994 (32.5)	
15–29 ml/min	92 (5.1)	35 (2.8)	0 (0.0)	127 (4.1)	
<15ml/min	33 (1.8)	11 (0.9)	0 (0.0)	44 (1.4)	
HBV co-infection Positive/Negative (%)	143/761 15.8%	87/527 14.2%	3/13 18.8%	233/1301 15.2%	>0.05
NRTI backbone					
AZT +3TC	1083 (45.6)	819 (50.5)	23 (57.5)	1925 (47.7)	<0.0001
D4T +3TC	1286 (54.1)	804 (49.5)	13 (32.5)	2103 (52.1)	
Others	7 (0.3)		4 (10.0)	11 (0.2)	

BMI-Body Mass Index; ALT-Alanine transaminitis; AST- Aspartate transaminitis; eGFR- estimated glomerular filtration rate calculated using Cockroft Gault formula; AZT-zidovudine; 3TC- Lamivudine; d4T- stavudine.

were initiated on zidovudine (AZT) plus 3TC with 0.2% commencing other NRTIs.

The characteristics of patients enrolled in the clinic for care, proportion initiating cART, their WHO clinical stages, median CD4 counts and vital status for each calendar year from 2004 to 2010 are shown in Table 2. Overall, the median (IQR) follow-up time on cART for the cohort was 30 (12–54) months. There were 11,236.8 person years of follow up on cART with 2,748 patients (68%) still alive, 967 (24%) lost to follow up and 324 (8%) deaths at the time of closing data for the present analysis.

Immunological responses/events on cART

Changes in CD4 counts with cART. The median (IQR) CD4 count at baseline of 133 (50–218) increased to 314 (204–429) within 6 months of initiation of cART, $p<0.0001$. This initial increment was sustained at 12 months with a median (IQR) CD4 at 12 months of 355 (244–487), with further increases during follow up to month 90.

Immune reconstitution inflammatory disorders. There were 45 documented cases of IRIS with an overall incidence rate of 4.00 (2.92–5.36) events/1000 person years under follow up. Tuberculosis-associated IRIS was the commonest and manifested clinically as new pulmonary infiltrations (n = 16), lymphadenitis

Table 2. Enrolment, characteristics, follow-up and vital status of patients initiating cART according to calendar year of enrolment.

Year Characteristic	2004	2005	2006	2007	2008	2009	2010	TOTAL	p-value
No. enrolled for ART	1,700	2,020	1,819	1,782	1,738	636	705	10,400	
No. starting ART	769	695	819	658	590	272	236	4039	
% starting ART	45.2	34.4	45.0	36.9	33.9	42.8	33.5	38.8	
WHO Clinical stage, n (%)[§]									<0.0001
1	52 (7%)	33 (5%)	43 (5%)	47 (7%)	53 (9%)	28 (10%)	16 (7%)	273 (7%)	
2	109 (14%)	80 (12%)	113 (14%)	70 (11%)	63 (11%)	25 (9%)	29 (12%)	489 (12%)	
3	460 (60%)	402 (58%)	420 (51%)	355 (54%)	280 (47%)	134 (49%)	115 (49%)	2166 (54%)	
4	126 (16%)	121 (17%)	145 (18%)	98 (15%)	80 (14%)	38 (14%)	41 (17%)	649 (16%)	
No data	22 (3%)	59 (8%)	98 (12%)	88 (13%)	114 (19%)	47 (16%)	35 (15%)	452 (11%)	
Median (IQR) CD4 count	136 (51–213)	136 (65–211)	133 (51–212)	124 (33–220)	131 (48–228)	128 (41–251)	149 (57–231)	134 (51–218)	0.23
Vital status									<0.0001
Alive*	503 (65%)	426 (61%)	541 (66%)	467 (71%)	438 (74%)	186 (68%)	187 (79%)	2748 (68%)	
Dead	35 (5%)	40 (6%)	50 (6%)	104 (16%)	63 (11%)	14 (5%)	18 (8%)	324 (8%)	
Lost	231 (30%)	229 (33%)	228 (28%)	87 (13%)	89 (15%)	72 (27%)	31 (13%)	967 (24%)	
Person follow up years	3565.1	2531.8	2158.7	1393.8	936.4	455.2	195.8	11236.8	

* And accessing the clinic, [§] % of patients initiating cART.

Table 3. Frequencies and rates of Non-AIDS defining events (NADEs) and other medical disorders not meeting AIDS-defining or NADEs criteria.

NADEs events	Number of events	Proportion of patients in entire cohort with event (%), n = 4,039	Rate/1000 person years follow up (95% CI)
Hepatic disorders			
Chronic liver disease	13	0.3	1.16 (0.62–1.98)
Hepatitis B virus infection flares*	7	0.2	0.62 (0.25–1.28)
Cardiovascular events			
Stroke	8	0.2	0.71 (0.31–1.40)
Congestive cardiac failure	2	0.1	0.18 (0.02–0.64)
Renal disorders			
Stage 4 or 5 renal impairment	6	0.2	0.53 (0.19–1.16)
Non-AIDS malignancies			
Hepatocellular carcinoma	4	0.1	0.36 (0.10–0.91)
Oesophageal carcinoma	1	0.0	0.09 (0.00–0.05)
Total	41	1.0	3.64 (2.61–4.95)
Medical disorders not meeting NADEs Non-AIDS defining infectious disorders			
Malaria	746	18.5	66.39 (61.71–71.32)
Upper and lower respiratory infections	666	16.5	59.27 (54.85–63.95)
Dermatological infections	364	9.0	32.39 (29.15–35.90)
Gastroenteritis	314	7.7	27.94 (24.94–31.21)
Urinary tract infections	151	3.7	13.43 (11.38–15.76)
Ear nose and throat infections	102	2.5	9.08 (7.40–11.02)
Sepsis	29	0.7	2.58 (1.73–3.71)
Bacterial meningitis	5	0.1	0.45 (0.17–1.01)
Miscellaneous disorders			
Dyspeptic disorders	73	1.8	6.50 (5.09–8.17)
Post-herpetic neuralgia	52	1.3	4.63 (3.46–6.07)
Seizure disorders	24	0.6	2.14 (1.37–3.18)
Paraparesis (unknown cause)	10	0.3	0.88 (0.43–1.64)
Hemiparesis (unknown cause)	9	0.2	0.80 (0.37–1.52)
Monoparesis (unknown cause)	6	0.1	0.53 (0.19–1.16)
Proximal myopathy	3	0.1	0.27 (0.06–0.78)
New onset vascular risk factors			
Hypertension	94	2.3	8.36 (6.76–10.24)
Diabetes mellitus	9	0.2	0.80 (0.37–1.52)

* HBV flare was defined as an elevation of ALT >5X upper limit of normal in a patient with HBSAg sero-positivity.

(n = 2) and pleural effusions (n = 2) over a median of 2 months (range: 2 to 12 months). Others included herpes zoster (n = 13), cerebral toxoplasmosis (n = 9), CMV retinitis (n = 2) and cryptococcal meningitis (n = 1). The median age of patients experiencing IRIS was 38 years, 33 (73%) were females and the median CD4 count at initiation of cART was 73 (range, 2 to 314) cells/mm^3. At the close of data for analysis, 27 (60%) patients who developed IRIS were alive, 6 (13%) patients died and 12 (27%) were lost-to-follow up.

Incidence and risk factors for immunological failure. Although robust CD4 recovery was noted among most patients on cART, there were 407 immunological failures with a crude event rate of 3.62 (3.28–3.99) per 100 person years. The median (range) time to occurrence of immunological failure on first line cART was 24 (12–78) months. Factors significantly associated with the risk of immunological failure on multivariable Cox proportional hazards analysis were male sex with an adjusted HR of 1.85 (95% CI of 1.47–2.33), initiating cART below 40 years of age with an adjusted HR of 1.25 (1.01–1.55) and baseline CD4 strata below 200 cells/mm^3 with an adjusted HR of 3.62 (95% CI of 2.59–5.07).

Clinical events on cART

Non-AIDS defining clinical events. There were 41 NADEs with the commonest recorded events being hepatic disorders (n = 20), cardiovascular events (n = 10) and new onset severe renal impairment with eGFR below 30ml/min (n = 6); hepatocellular carcinoma (n = 4) and oesophageal carcinoma (n = 1) were the only non-AIDS defining malignancies. The hepatic disorders noted include liver cirrhosis, hepatitis B transaminitis flares and

Table 4. Frequencies and rates of AIDS-defining conditions.

Condition	Frequency of events n (%) n=681	Proportion of patients in entire cohort with event (%), n=4,039	Rate/1000 person years follow up (95% CI)
Pulmonary tuberculosis	179 (26.3)	4.4	15.93 (13.68–18.44)
Chronic diarrhoea	155 (22.8)	3.8	13.79 (11.71–16.14)
Esophageal candidiasis	75 (11.0)	1.9	6.67 (5.25–8.36)
Recurrent pneumonia	58 (8.5)	1.4	5.16 (3.92–6.67)
Oral candidiasis	45 (6.6)	1.1	4.00 (2.92–5.36)
Cerebral toxoplasmosis	38 (5.6)	0.9	3.38 (2.39–4.64)
Extrapulmonary tuberculosis	33 (4.8)	0.8	2.94 (2.02–4.12)
Kaposi sarcoma	31 (4.6)	0.8	2.76 (1.87–3.92)
CMV retinitis	17 (2.5)	0.4	1.51 (0.88–2.42)
HIV encephalopathy	16 (2.5)	0.4	1.42 (0.81–2.31)
Cryptococcal meningitis	12 (1.8)	0.3	1.07 (0.55–1.87)
Intracranial space occupying lesion*	9 (1.3)	0.2	0.80 (0.37–1.52)
Non-Hodgkin's disease	5 (0.7)	0.1	0.44 (0.14–1.04)
HIV wasting syndrome	3 (0.4)	0.1	0.27 (0.05–0.78)
Pneumocystis jirovercii pneumonia	2 (0.3)	0.0	0.18 (0.02–0.64)
CNS lymphoma	1 (0.1)	0.0	0.09 (0.00–0.50)
Herpes esophagitis	1 (0.1)	0.0	0.09 (0.00–0.50)
Invasive cervical carcinoma	1 (0.1)	0.0	0.09 (0.00–0.50)
Total	**681**		**60.60 (56.14–65.33)**

AIDS defining events were defined using WHO clinical criteria. * Causes of Intracranial space occupying lesion on CT scan were not documented but were presumed to be AIDS-defining events.

hepatocellular carcinoma which were all observed in patients with HBsAg sero-positivity. The overall crude NADE incidence rate (95% CI) was 3.64 (2.61–4.95) per 1000 person years as shown in Table 3.

By far, the commonest medical morbidity (not fulfilling AIDS nor NADEs criteria) was from infectious causes of which 2,377 events were documented (Table 3), with malaria being the commonest event. This is followed briefly by upper/lower respiratory tract infections (n = 666). Of the non-infectious medical comorbidities recorded, 94 patients developed hypertension and 9 Type 2 diabetes mellitus while on cART.

Causes and factors associated with AIDS-defining events on cART. Six hundred (600) patients (14.9%) experienced a total of 681 AIDS-defining events during follow up on cART with a crude (95% CI) event rate of 60.60 (56.14–65.33) per 1000 person years of follow up (Table 4). The median (range) time to development of first AIDS-defining event was 6 (2–90) months. Nine patients were documented to have had computed tomographic evidence of an intracranial space occupying lesions, but clinicians did not document the etiology of these mass lesions. For the purposes of the present study, they were judged to be AIDS-defining events. Factors significantly associated with the risk of developing an AIDS-defining event on cART on adjusted analyses were low body mass index below 16 kg/m^2, WHO clinical stages 3 or 4 at baseline and CD4 strata below 200 cells/mm^3 at initiation of therapy (Table 5).

Of the 600 patients who developed AIDS-defining events on cART, 317 (52.8%) were alive as at time of closure of data but 153 (25.5%) were subsequently lost-to-follow up and 130 (21.7%) died of AIDS. The median (range) duration between the first AIDS-defining diagnosis and death was 0.25 months (0 to 72 months) and that for loss-to-follow up was 4 months (0 to 76 months). Patients who developed an AIDS-defining event and were alive at the time of closure of data for analysis survived for a median of 34 months (range of 0 to 88 months).

The incidence, causes and risk factors associated with mortality

There were 324 (8.0%) deaths over the 11,263.8 person follow-up years giving a crude (95% CI) event rate of 28.83 (25.78–32.15) deaths per 1000-person follow up years. The median (range) time to death was 2 months (0–66) by Mann Whitney's U-test. 202 (62.3%) deaths occurred within the first 90-days of initiation of therapy, 88 (27.2%) from month 4 to month 12, 16 (4.9%) within the second year, 9 (2.8%) within the third year, 3 (0.9%) within the fourth year and 6 (1.9%) within the fifth year of follow up. The Kaplan Meier estimated cumulative incidence of mortality at 6, 12, 36, and 72 months were 6.8%, 7.9%, 9.0% and 9.8% respectively and of attrition (including 324 deaths and 958 loss-to-follow ups) from the programme were 17.3%, 20.7%, 27.8%, 34.5% and 36.5% respectively.

As shown in Table 6, significant factors associated with mortality in Cox proportional hazards model were male gender with an adjusted HR (95% CI) of 1.69 (1.29–2.21), advanced HIV disease – Stages 3 or 4 – with an adjusted HR (95% CI) of 2.20 (1.42–3.41), low CD4 strata below 200 cells/mm^3 with an adjusted HR (95% CI) of 2.39 (1.64–3.49), baseline BMI below 16 kg/m^2 with an adjusted HR (95% CI) of 2.60 (1.92–3.53) and starting on an NRTI backbone of d4T plus 3TC with an adjusted HR of 1.60 (1.21–2.11).

Table 5. Univariate and multivariate analysis of factors associated with risk of developing AIDS on cART.

Variable	Person follow-up time (yrs)	Number of events	Crude event rate (/1000 py), 95% CI	Unadjusted HR (95% CI)	p-value	Adjusted HR (95% CI)	p-value
Sex							
Male	3467	193	55.67 (48.09–64.10)	1.06 (0.89–1.25)	0.53	–	–
Female	7770	406	52.25 (47.29–57.59)	1.00			
Age							
≥40 years	5161	268	51.93 (45.90–58.53)	1.00 (0.94–1.07)	0.90	-	-
<40 years	6082	331	54.42 (48.72–60.61)	1.00			
WHO stage							
3 or 4	7803	477	61.13 (55.77–66.87)	1.73 (1.37–2.18)	<0.0001	1.45 (1.13–1.86)	0.0031
1 or 2	2370	84	35.44 (28.27–43.88)	1.00		1.00	
Baseline CD4 strata							
<200	7706	481	62.42 (56.96–68.25)	2.00 (1.64–2.45)	<0.0001	1.87 (1.49–2.35)	<0.0001
>200	3462	117	33.80 (27.95–40.50)	1.00		1.00	
Baseline BMI							
<16 kg/m^2	901	99	109.9 (89.3–133.8)	1.91 (1.54–2.38)	<0.0001	1.53 (1.20–1.94)	0.0005
≥16 kg/m^2	9189	483	52.56 (47.98–57.47)	1.00		1.00	
Baseline Hb							
<8g/dl	1176	87	73.98 (59.25–91.25)	0.92 (0.83–1.01)	0.06	1.01 (0.78–1.31)	0.94
≥8g/dl	8590	494	57.51 (52.55–62.81)	1.00		1.00	
NRTI backbone							
D4T plus 3TC	5276	322	61.03 (54.55–68.07)	1.18 (1.01–1.39)	0.04	1.08 (0.90–1.30)	0.09
AZT plus 3TC	5940	274	46.13 (40.83–51.93)	1.00		1.00	
NNRTI							
Efavirenz	6120	330	53.92 (48.26–60.06)	0.92 (0.78–1.08)	0.29	-	-
Nevirapine	5013	261	52.06 (45.94–58.78)	1.00			
Adherence							
Poor	3835	237	61.80 (54.18–70.18)	1.17 (0.99–1.38)	0.06	1.06 (0.89–1.27)	0.51
Excellent	6345	363	57.21 (51.48–63.41)	1.00		1.00	

Table 6. Univariate and multivariate analysis of factors associated with death on cART.

Variable	Patient follow-up time (years)	Number of events	Crude event rate (/1000 person years)	Unadjusted HR (95% CI)	p-value	Adjusted hazard ratio (95% CI)	p-value
Sex							
Male	3467	188	54.23 (46.75–62.56)	1.71 (1.37–2.14)	<0.0001	1.69 (1.29–2.21)	0.0001
Female	7770	136	17.50 (14.69–20.70)	1.00		1.00	
Age							
≥40 years	5161	143	27.71 (23.35–32.64)	0.94 (0.75–1.17)	0.55	–	–
<40 years	6082	180	29.60 (25.43–34.25)	1.00			
WHO stage							
3 or 4	7803	277	35.50 (31.44–39.94)	3.52 (2.34–5.30)	<0.0001	2.20 (1.42–3.41)	0.0004
1 or 2	2370	25	10.55 (6.82–15.57)	1.00		1.00	
Baseline CD4 strata							
<200	7706	276	35.81 (31.72–40.30)	3.13 (2.29–4.29)	<0.0001	2.39 (1.64–3.49)	<0.0001
>200	3462	45	13.00 (9.48–17.39)	1.00		1.00	
Baseline BMI							
<16 kg/m^2	901	88	97.67 (78.33–120.33)	3.79 (2.95–4.85)	<0.0001	2.60 (1.92–3.53)	<0.0001
≥16 kg/m^2	9189	214	23.29 (20.27–26.63)	1.00		1.00	
Baseline Hb							
<8g/dl	1176	76	64.63 (50.92–80.89)	2.43 (1.88–3.16)	<0.0001	1.28 (0.95–1.75)	0.11
≥8g/dl	8590	227	26.43 (23.10–30.10)	1.00		1.00	
NRTI backbone							
D4T plus 3TC	5276	216	40.94 (35.66–46.78)	2.04 (1.62–2.58)	<0.0001	1.60 (1.21–2.11)	0.001
AZT plus 3TC	5940	106	17.85 (14.61–21.58)	1.00		1.00	
NNRTI							
Efavirenz	6120	212	34.64 (30.13–39.63)	1.43 (1.14–1.81)	0.0024	1.15 (0.87–1.51)	0.32
Nevirapine	5013	108	21.54 (17.67–26.01)	1.00		1.00	
Adherence							
Poor	3835	147	38.33 (32.39–45.05)	1.52 (1.22–1.89)	0.0002	1.21 (0.95–1.56)	0.12
Excellent	6345	177	27.90 (23.94–32.32)	1.00		1.00	

Table 7. Causes of death among 188 patients who died in hospital while on first line cART.

Cause of death	Frequency
Pulmonary tuberculosis	37
Gastroenteritis with hypovolemic shock	30
Severe anemia	19
Pneumonia	18
Sepsis	16
Cerebral toxoplasmosis	12
HIV Encephalopathy	7
TB Immune reconstitution inflammatory syndrome	7
Disseminated Kaposi sarcoma	6
Enteric fever	4
End stage kidney failure	4
Lactic acidosis	4
Bacterial meningitis	4
Chronic liver disease	2
Cryptococcal meningitis	2
Steven's Johnsons syndrome due to nevirapine	2
Miscellaneous*	14
TOTAL	188

* Miscellaneous comprises of 1 case each of acute abdomen, amoebic liver abscess, CNS lymphoma, gluteal abscess, hepatocellular carcinoma, HBV flare, high grade non-Hodgkin's lymphoma, hyperglycemic hyperosmolar syndrome, strangulated umbilical hernia, otitis media, *Pneumocystis jirovercii* pneumonia, systemic candidiasis, tuberculous colitis, fulminant vasculitis with gangrene of toes and fingers.

Table 8. Frequencies of specific toxicities and treatment switches among Ghanaian cohort on long-term cART.

Toxicity	Frequency of toxicity among patients who developed any toxicity on ART n (%), n = 1,603	Proportion of patients who developed toxicity n (%)[§] n = 4,039	Frequency of treatment switches due to specific toxicity[#] n (%)	Proportion of patients with treatment switch due to toxicity, (%) n = 4,039
Anemia	675 (42.1)	527 (13.0)	62 (11.8)	1.5
Skin rash	295 (18.4)	281 (7.0)	44 (15.7)	1.1
Neuropsychiatric toxicity	235 (14.7)	218 (5.4)	39 (17.9)	1.1
Peripheral neuropathy	181 (11.3)	181 (4.5)	83 (45.9)	2.1
Severe hepatotoxicity	143 (8.9)	143 (3.5)	8 (5.6)	0.2
Lipoatrophy	40 (2.5)	40 (1.0)	34 (85.0)	0.8
Ptylism	14 (0.9)	14 (0.3)	0 (0.0)	0.0
Gastrointestinal disorders	12 (0.7)	12 (0.3)	0 (0.0)	0.0
Lactic acidosis	4 (0.2)	4 (0.1)	0 (0.0)	0.0
Myalgia	3 (0.2)	3 (0.1)	0 (0.0)	0.0
Hyperpigmentation	3 (0.2)	3 (0.1)	0 (0.0)	0.0
Pancreatitis	1 (0.1)	1 (0.0)	1 (100.0)	0.0
Column total	1,603	1,427 (35.3)	271	6.8

[#] This refers to the number of patients switching treatment due to specific toxicity specified on the row. % was determined by dividing the number of patients switching treatment due to a specific toxicity by the total number of patients with that particular toxicity in question.
[§] n(%) n refers to the number of patients who experienced specific toxicity and the % refers to number of patients with toxicity divided by the total number of patients starting ART which was 4,039. An individual patient may experience more than one toxicity during follow up and may experience a specific toxicity more than one episode during follow up.

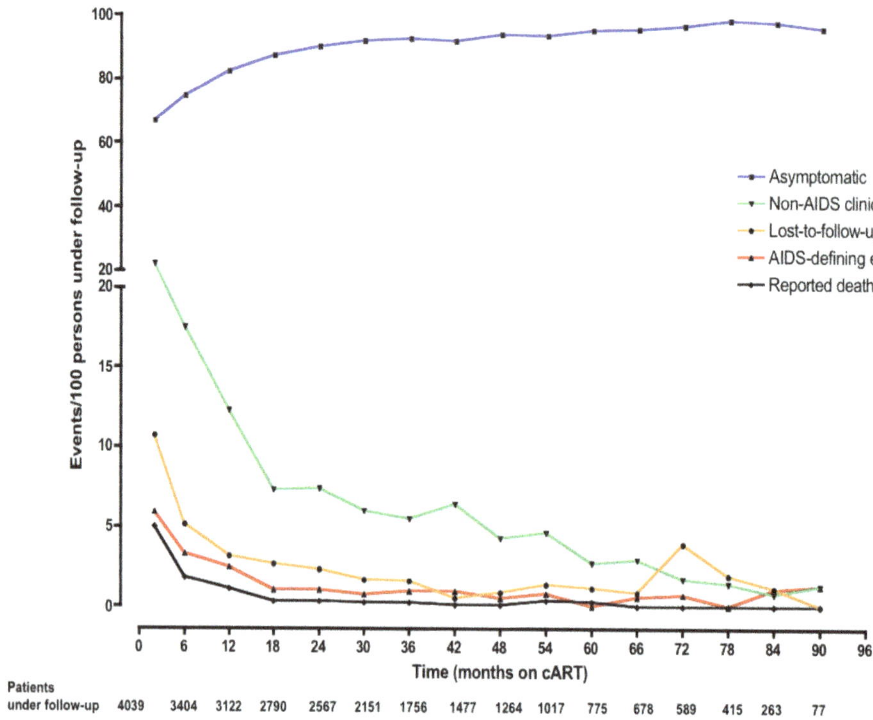

Figure 1. Six monthly incidence rates of Non-AIDS and AIDS events, deaths, loss to follow up and asymptomatic events among Ghanaian HIV-infected patients on long-term cART. Non-AIDS events comprised all medical conditions which are non-AIDS defining by WHO criteria.

In a series of 188 hospital-confirmed deaths, the causes of death are as shown in Table 7. The leading causes of death in this subset of patients were pulmonary tuberculosis, severe diarrhoea with hypovolaemic shock, severe anaemia, pneumonia and sepsis.

Treatment-limiting toxicities. Overall 35.3% (n = 4,039) of patients experienced toxicity during follow up. There were 1,603 documented episodes of cART-related toxicities among patients who started first line cART with an event rate of 14.3 events/100 person-years (95% CI, 13.6 to 15.0/100 person-years). As shown in Table 8, severe anemia, skin rash and neuropsychiatric toxicity were the commonest reported adverse events. 271 patients representing 6.8% of the entire cohort switched therapy due to toxicity.

Rates of major clinical events on cART. Figure 1 depicts the overall decline in the rates of AIDS-defining events, non-AIDS clinical events, mortality and loss to follow up over time on cART. The highest incidence rates of these events were observed within the first two months of initiating cART with rates of 22.1 non-AIDS clinical events per 100 patients, 10.7 lost-to-follow up per 100 patients, 5.9 AIDS defining events per 100 patients and 5.0 deaths per 100 patients under follow-up. One hundred and thirty-five (135) patients (3.3%) starting NNRTI-based first line cART were subsequently switched to a PI-based second line therapy on account of treatment failure at closure of data for analysis.

Discussion

This study is among the largest cohort studies documenting morbidity and mortality in an ART programme in sub-Saharan Africa. The data presented in this paper show that there is a sustained and robust immunological recovery on cART among this cohort of HIV-infected patients. This immune restoration accompanied improvements in morbidity as evidenced the steady decline in the incidence of deaths, losses to follow-up, AIDS-defining and non-AIDS defining clinical events. Attrition from the programme, due mainly to deaths and loss-to-follow up as well as AIDS-defining events, occurred predominantly within the first year of treatment and were predicted by clinical and laboratory indicators of advanced HIV disease at initiation of cART.

Several studies from both developed [19–23] and developing countries [1,24–29] have reported short-, medium- and recently long-term CD4 responses on cART. The findings from this study show that within a programme setting in sub-Saharan Africa, immunological responses to cART are sustainable over the long-term on a limited repertoire of first-line therapy. As expected, the median (IQR) CD4 counts at initiation of therapy of 133 (50–218) cells/mm^3 were low and comparable with those from several cohorts from developing countries [24–34] and serve as an indicator of the advanced stages of immunosuppression at which cART is initiated in these settings [35]. This notwithstanding, cART was associated with a near doubling in median CD4 counts within 6 months of therapy followed by more gradual and sustained increases throughout the period of observation for patients remaining under care. The vigorous restitution of CD4 cell counts within the first six months of therapy was accompanied by the occurrence of IRIS in some patients, of which tuberculosis was the commonest reported cause followed by herpes zoster and cerebral toxoplasmosis. Admittedly, compared with other cohorts where the reported frequency of IRIS has varied between 10% to 25% of all patients initiating cART [18,36–40], the overall frequency of 1.1% of IRIS reported among this cohort is low, and probably reflects the difficulties in the diagnosis of this clinical syndrome within settings of limited diagnostic support. Events were considered as IRIS when clinicians felt they had sufficient clinical and laboratory evidence to support the diagnosis.

For patients who stayed on cART for more than a year, 407 (10.1%) developed immunological failure according to WHO guidelines but only 135 (3.3%) patients in the cohort were switched to second line therapy. The spectra of clinical events classified as IRIS overlaps closely with those diagnosed as AIDS-defining events which occurred at a frequency of 17%. AIDS-defining events on cART occurred at a median time of 6 months, were predicted by low CD4 cell counts, prior AIDS and low BMI at initiation of therapy and were associated with an increased risk of subsequent attrition from the programme. These show that the occurrence of AIDS-defining events in the proximal phases of cART is an indicator of early treatment failure and is representative of progression of HIV disease which cART may be incapable of halting, even when appropriate treatment for opportunistic infections is concurrently commenced. The implication is that cART should be started much earlier, requiring patients to be diagnosed earlier, as has been suggested by others [35,41].

The crude incidence rates of Non-AIDS-defining events of 3.64/1000 person-years is lower compared to that of cohorts from Botswana [13] and the United States [13] of 10.0 py, and 12.4 py, respectively, that of a multicentre Latin American cohort [42] of 8.4/1000 person-years and that of the Eurosida cohort [11] of 17.7 (95% CI of 16.6 to 18.7/1000 py, n = 12,844). The median follow up for the cohorts from Botswana [13], the USA [13], and Latin America [42] were 36 months, 18 months and 30 months respectively which is comparable with the 30 months of follow up of this cohort. However, the retrospective nature of the present study and the relatively short median follow-up in this cohort could have accounted for the lower incidence rates of NADEs. Of the 41 NADEs in this cohort, hepatic disorders (n = 20) were the commonest NADE followed by cardiovascular events (n = 10), end-stage renal disease (n = 6) and non-AIDS malignancies of which hepatocellular carcinoma (n = 4) and one case of oesophageal carcinoma were reported. Overall, 24 of the 41 documented NADEs were associated with HBSAg seropositivity making HBV co-infection an important determinant of NADEs in this cohort. The order of events were different from those in the cohort from Botswana where out of 18 NADEs, 9 were cardiovascular, 4 were renal, five were malignancies and none were of hepatic in etiology [13]. As a composite outcome measure, non-AIDS events are a heterogeneous collection of several end-points with multifactorial aetiologies and risk factors, and also dependent on the presence of chronic hepatitis B co-infection and chronic vascular inflammation due to persistence of HIV viral replication [43–52]. The multi-dimensional composition of risk factors for NADEs together with the relatively limited observation of events and some missing data restricted analysis of risk factors for these events in this cohort.

Malaria was the leading cause of non-AIDS-defining infectious morbidity on cART and was often treated with artemisinin-based antimalarial therapy. The fact that within this HIV cohort, tuberculosis and malaria were the leading causes of AIDS and non-AIDS infectious morbidity respectively underscores their importance among the most important public health challenges Sub-Saharan Africa is attempting to overcome. Unlike in developed countries where AIDS-related mortality on cART is being superseded by Non-AIDS-related mortality [52], causes of death in this cohort were predominantly driven by AIDS-related events of which tuberculosis was the leading cause followed by gastroenteritis with hypovolemic shock, severe anaemia and pneumonia, as in other cohorts from developing countries. Of the NADEs, end-stage kidney disease and liver-related disease were among the common causes of mortality. It is also noteworthy that 6 deaths were attributed directly to cART-related toxicity: two cases of Stevens Johnson's syndrome from nevirapine and four cases of clinically suspected lactic acidosis from stavudine. cART toxicity is a cardinal factor influencing the durability and therefore the effectiveness of cART and 35.3% of patients experienced one form of toxicity or the other with 6.8% discontinuing therapy on account of toxicity. Use of a stavudine was independently associated with increased risk of death, hence the withdrawal of this antiretroviral from the Ghanaian ART programme is justified. Given the high prevalence of renal impairment among this cohort (38.8%) [53], replacement of stavudine by tenofovir should however be approached with caution due to the well-known association between tenofovir and risk for renal tubular toxicity. It is encouraging that the DART study has provided some reassuring data on the safety of tenofovir among Africans [54]. Furthermore given the high prevalence of hepatitis B co-infection in this cohort, the benefits of tenofovir in slowing the progression of liver disease may outweigh possible renal toxicity.

The analyses presented in this study have limitations worth noting. As over 60% of patients presenting to the clinic did not start cART, and many with advanced HIV/AIDS were lost to follow-up, it is likely there were many deaths in this group. Hence the population studied was skewed towards those patients who survived long enough to start cART, who may have had different causes of death to those not starting cART. The trajectories of CD4 over time reflect those of patients who remained on cART and thus are influenced by survivor bias. Furthermore the sources of ascertainment of causes of deaths in a significant proportion of patients were by verbal autopsy by relatives whose accuracy may be limited. In spite of these the specific causes of death could be verified by medical certification in 188 (58%) out of 324 events. Similarly, the classification of AIDS-defining events, IRIS and NADEs were influenced by availability of data and arrived at by consensus between the authors and local experts.

In summary, cART is effective over the long-term for a substantial proportion of this Ghanaian cohort of HIV-infected patients. Within the constraints of limited resources as it pertains to the ART programme in Ghana, cART was associated with a sustained and durable immunological recovery in most patients, an improvement in morbidity from HIV-infection and trend towards reduction in mortality over the long-term among patients remaining on therapy and in care.

Author Contributions

Conceived and designed the experiments: FSS DC. Performed the experiments: FSS DC. Analyzed the data: FSS MAS. Contributed reagents/materials/analysis tools: FSS BN GBA RP. Wrote the paper: FSS DC.

References

1. Laurent C, Ngom Gueye NF, Ndour CT, Gueye PM, Diouf M, et al. for the ANRS 1215/1290 Study Group (2005) Long-term benefits of highly active antiretroviral therapy in Senegalese HIV-1 infected adults. J Acquir Immune Defic Syndr. 38: 14–17.
2. Desclaux A, Ciss M, Taverne B, Sow PS, Egrot M, et al. (2003) Access to antiretroviral drugs and AIDS management in Senegal. AIDS. 17 (Suppl): S95–S101.
3. Akileswaran C, Lurie MN, Flanigan TP, Mayer KH (2005) Lessons learned from use of highly active antiretroviral therapy in Africa. Clin Infect Dis. 4: 376–385.
4. Braitstein P, Brinkhof MW, Dabis F, Schechter M, Boulle A, et al. (2006) Antiretroviral Therapy in Lower Income Countries (ART-LINC) Collaboration; Antiretroviral Therapy Cohort Collaboration (ART-CC) groups. Mortality of

HIV-1-infected patients in the first year of antiretroviral therapy: comparison between low-income and high-income countries. Lancet. 367: 817–824.
5. Coetzee D, Hilderbrand K, Boulle A, Maartens G, Louis F, et al. (2004) Outcomes after two years of providing antiretroviral treatment in Khayelitsha, South Africa. AIDS. 18: 887–895.
6. Severe P, Leger P, Charles M, Noel F, Bonhomme G, et al. (2005) Antiretroviral therapy in a thousand patients with AIDS in Haiti. N Engl J Med. 353: 2325–2334.
7. Wester CW, Kim S, Bussmann H, Avalos A, Ndwapi N, et al. (2005) Initial response to highly active antiretroviral therapy in HIV-1C-infected adults in a public sector treatment program in Botswana. J Acquir Immune Defic Syndr. 40: 336–343.
8. Hawkins C, Achenbach C, Fryda W, Ngare D, Murphy R (2007) Antiretroviral durability and tolerability in HIV-infected adults living in urban Kenya. J Acquir Immune Defic Syndr. 45(3): 304–310.
9. Deeks SG, Phillips AN (2009) HIV infection, antiretroviral treatment, ageing and non-AIDS related morbidity. BMJ. 338: a3172.
10. Phillips AN, Neaton J, Lundgren JD (2008) The role of HIV in serious diseases other than AIDS. AIDS. 22: 2409–2418.
11. Mocroft A, Reiss P, Gasiorowski J, Ledergerber B, Kowalska J, et al. (2010) Serious fatal and nonfatal Non-AIDS-defining illnesses in Europe. J Acquir Immune Defic Syndr. 55: 262–270.
12. Centers for Disease Control (1992) 1993 revised classification system for HIV infection and expanded surveillance case definition for AIDS among adolescents and adults. MMWR Recomm Rep. 41: 1–19.
13. Wester CW, Koethe JR, Shepherd BE, Stinnette SE, Rebeiro F, et al. (2011) Non-AIDS-defining events among HIV-1-infected adults receiving combination antiretroviral therapy in resource-replete versus resource-limited urban setting. AIDS. 25 (12): 1471–1479.
14. Division of AIDS, NIAID (1994) Division of AIDS Table for Grading Severity of Adult Adverse Experiences. Rockville, MD: National Institute of Allery and Infectious Diseases.
15. Division of AIDS, NIAID (2004) Division of AIDS Table for Grading Severity of Adult Adverse Experiences. Rockville, MD: National Institute of Allery and Infectious Diseases; December.
16. Sarfo FS, Sarfo MA, Kasim A, Phillips R, Booth M, et al. (2014) Long-term effectiveness of first-line non-nucleoside reverse transcriptase inhibitor (NNRTI)-based antiretroviral therapy in Ghana. J Antimicrob Chemother. 69(1): 254–261.
17. WHO (2010) Antiretroviral therapy for HIV infection in adults and adolescents, recommendations for a public health approach 2010 revision. Available: http:/www.int/entity/hiv/pub/arv/adult2010/en/index.html. Accessed 2012 July 25.
18. Müller M, Wandel S, Colebunders R, Attia S, Furrer H, IeDEA South and Central Africa, et al. (2010) Immune reconstitution inflammatory syndrome in patients starting antiretroviral therapy for HIV infection: a systematic review and meta-analysis. Lancet Infect Dis. 10: 251–261.
19. Wolbers M, Battegay M, Hirschel B, Furrer H, Cavassini M, et al. (2007) CD4+ T-cell count increase in HIV-1-infected patients with suppressed viral load within 1 year after start of antiretroviral therapy. Antivir Ther. 12: 889–897.
20. Moore RD, Keruly JC (2007) CD4+ cell count 6 years after commencement of highly active antiretroviral therapy in persons with sustained virologic suppression. Clin Infect Dis. 44: 441–446.
21. Mocroft A, Phillips AN, Gatell J, Ledergerber B, Fisher M, et al. (2007) Normalisation of CD4 counts in patients with HIV-1 infection and maximum virological suppression who are taking combination antiretroviral therapy: an observational cohort study. Lancet. 370(9585): 407–413.
22. Smith CJ, Sabin CA, Youle MS, Kinloch-de Loes S, Lampe FC, et al. (2004) Factors influencing increases in CD4 cell counts of HIV-positive persons receiving long-term highly active antiretroviral therapy. J Infect Dis. 190: 1860–1868.
23. Gras L, Kesselring AM, Griffin JT, van Sighem AI, Fraser C, et al. (2007) CD4 cell counts of 800 cells/mm^3 or greater after 7 years of highly active antiretroviral therapy are feasible in most patients starting with 350 cells/mm^3 or greater. J Acquir Immune Defic Syndr. 45: 183–192.
24. Sow PS, Otieno LF, Bissagnene E, Kityo C, Bennink R, et al. (2007) Implementation of an antiretroviral access program for HIV-1-infected individuals in resource-limited settings: clinical results from 4 African countries. J Acquir Immune Defic Syndr. 44: 262–267.
25. Charalambous S, Innes C, Muirhead D, Kumaranayake L, Fielding K, et al. (2007) Evaluation of a workplace HIV treatment programme in South Africa. AIDS. 21: S73–8.
26. Stringer JS, Zulu I, Levy J, Stringer EM, Mwango A, et al. (2006) Rapid scale-up of antiretroviral therapy at primary care sited in Zambia: feasibility and early outcomes. JAMA. 296: 782–93.
27. Lawn SD, Myer L, Bekker LG, Wood R (2006) CD4 cell count recovery among HIV-infected patients with very advanced immunodeficiency commencing antiretroviral treatment in Sub-Saharan Africa. BMC Infect Dis 6: 59.
28. Erhabor O, Ejele OA, Nwauche CA (2006) The effects of highly active antiretroviral therapy (HAART) of Stavudine, Lamivudine and nevirapine on the CD4 lymphocyte count of HIV-infected African: the Nigerian experience. Niger J Clin Pract. 9: 128–133.
29. Ferradini L, Jeannin A, Pinoges L, Izopet J, Odhiambo D, et al. (2006) Scaling up of highly active antiretroviral in a rural district of Malawi: an effectiveness assessment. Lancet. 367: 1335–1342.
30. Kilaru KR, Kumar A, Sippy N, Carter AO, Roach TC (2006) Immunological and virological responses to highly active antiretroviral therapy in a non-clinical trial setting in a developing Caribbean country. HIV Med. 7: 99–104.
31. Tuboi SH, Harrison LH, Sprinz E, Albernaz RK, Schechter M (2005) Predictors of virologic failure in HIV-1-infected patients starting highly active antiretroviral therapy in Porto Alegre, Brazil. J Acquir Immune Defic Syndr. 40: 324–328.
32. Marins JR, Jamal LF, Chen SY, Barros MB, Hudes ES, et al. (2003) Dramatic improvement in survival among adult Brazilian AIDS patients. AIDS. 17: 1675–1682.
33. Dai Y, Qiu ZF, Li TS, Han Y, Zuo LY, et al. (2006) Clinical outcomes and immune reconstitution in 103 advanced AIDS patients undergoing 12-month highly active antiretroviral therapy. Chin Med J (Engl). 119: 1677–1682.
34. Srasuebkul P, Ungsedhapand C, Ruxrungtham K, Boyd MA, Phanuphak P, et al. (2007) Predictive factors for immunological and virological endpoints in Thai patients receiving combination antiretroviral treatment. HIV Med. 8: 46–54.
35. Nash D, Katyal M, Brinkhof MWG, Keiser O, May Margaret, et al. (2008) Long-term immunologic response to antiretroviral therapy in low-income countries: Collaborative analysis of prospective studies: The Antiretroviral Therapy in Lower Income Countries (ART-LINC) Collaboration of the International epidemiological Databases to Evaluate AIDS. AIDS. 22(17): 2291–2302.
36. Novak RM, Richardson JT, Buchacz K, Chmiel JS, Durham MD, et al. (2012) Immune reconstitution inflammatory syndrome (IRIS) in the HIV outpatient study (HOPS): incidence and implications. AIDS. 26(6): 721–730.
37. Ratman I, Chiu C, Kandala NB, Easterbrook PJ (2006) Incidence and risk factors for immune reconstitution inflammatory syndrome in an ethnically diverse HIV type-1-infected cohort. Clin Infect Dis. 42: 418–27.
38. French MA, Price P, Stone SF (2004) Immune restoration disease after antiretroviral therapy. AIDS. 18: 1615–1627.
39. Cooney EL (2002) Clinical indicators of immune restoration following highly active antiretroviral therapy. Clin Infect Dis. 34: 224–233.
40. Shelburne SA, Hamill RJ, Rodriguez-Barradas MC, Greenberg SB, Atmar RL, et al. (2002) Immune reconstitution inflammatory syndrome: emergence of a unique syndrome during highly active antiretroviral therapy. Medicine (Baltimore). 81: 213–227.
41. Lawden C, Chene G, Morlat P, Raffi F, Dupon M, et al. (2007) HIV-infected adults with a CD4 cell count greater than 500 cells/mm^3 on long-term combination antiretroviral therapy reach same mortality rates as the general population. J Acquir Immune Defic Syndr. 44: 262–267.
42. Belloso WH, Orellana LC, Grinsztejn B, Madero JS, La Rosa A, et al. (2010) Analysis of serious non-AIDS events among HIV-infected adults at Latin American sites. HIV MED. 11: 554–564.
43. Calza L, Manfredi R, Verucchi G (2010) Myocardial infarction risk in HIV-infected patients: epidemiology, pathogenesis, and clinical management. AIDS. 24(6): 789–802.
44. Kuller LH, Tracy R, Belloso W, deWit S, Drummond F, et al. (2008) Inflammatory and coagulation biomarkers and mortality in patients with HIV infection. PLoS Med. 5: e203.10.1371/journal.pmed.0050203.
45. Lau B, Sharret AR, Kingsley LA, Post W, Palella FJ, et al. (2006) C-reactive protein is a marker for human immunodeficiency virus disease progression. Arch Intern Med. 166: 64–70.
46. Torriani FJ, Komarow L, Parker RA, Cotter BR, Currier JS, et al. (2008) Endothelial dysfunction in human immunodeficiency virus-infected antiretroviral-naïve sujects before and after starting potent antiretroviral therapy. J Am Coll Cardiol. 52: 569–576.
47. Friis-Moller N, Reiss P, Sabin CA, Weber R, Monteforte A, et al. (2007) DAD Study group. Class of antiretroviral drugs and the risk of myocardial infarction. N Engl J Med. 356: 1723–1735.
48. Obel N, Thomsen HF, Kronborg G, Larsen CS, Hilderbrandt PR, et al. (2007) Ischaemic heart disease in HIV-infected and HIV-uninfected individuals: a population-based cohort study. Clin Infect Dis. 44: 1625–1631.
49. Triant VA, Lee H, Hadigan C, Grinspoon SK (2007) Increased acute myocardial infarction rates and cardiovascular risk factors among patients with human immunodeficiency disease. J Clin Endocrinol Metal. 92: 2506–2512.
50. Currier JS (2002) Cardiovascular risk associated with HIV therapy. J Acquir Immune Defic Syndr.(Suppl 1): 31 S16–23. Discussion S4–5.
51. Crum-Cianflone N, Hullsiek KH, Marconi V, Weintrob A, Ganesan A, et al. (2009) Trends in the incidence of cancers among HIV-infected persons and the impact of antiretroviral therapy: a 20-year cohort study. AIDS.23: 41–50.
52. Neuhaus J, Angus B, Kowalska JD, La Rosa A, Sampson J, et al. for the INSIGHT SMART and ESPRIT study groups (2010) Risk of all-cause mortality associated with non-fatal AIDS and serious non-AIDS events among adults infected with HIV. AIDS. 24: 697–706.
53. Sarfo FS, Keegan R, Appiah L, Shakoor S, Phillips R, et al. (2013) High prevalence of renal dysfunction and association with risk of death amongst HIV-infected Ghanaians. J Infect. 67(1): 43–50.
54. Reid A, Stöhr W, Sarah Walker A, Williams IG, Kityo C, et al. (2008) Severe renal dysfunction and risk factors associated with renal impairment in HIV-infected adults in Africa initiating antiretroviral therapy. Clin Infect Dis. 46: 1271–1281.

Association of HLA-DP/DQ and STAT4 Polymorphisms with HBV Infection Outcomes

Yun Liao[9], Bei Cai[9], Yi Li, Jie Chen, Chuanmin Tao, Hengjian Huang, Lanlan Wang*

Department of Laboratory Medicine, West China Hospital, Sichuan University, Chengdu, Sichuan Province, China

Abstract

Background: Though HLA-DP/DQ is regarded to associate with HBV susceptibility and HBV natural clearance, its role in hepatocellular carcinoma (HCC) development is obscure. And the role of STAT4 in HBV susceptibility and clearance as well as HCC development is still contentious. Therefore, we conducted this study, aiming to clarify these obscure relationships.

Methods: We recruited 1312 Chinese Han subjects including healthy controls, HBV carriers and HCC patients in the experiment stage. The meta-analysis included 3467 HCC patients and 5821 HBV carriers to appraise the association with HCC development.

Results: Consistent with previous studies, HLA-DP/DQ associated with HBV susceptibility and HBV natural clearance ($p < 0.05$). However, the experiment showed that HLA-DP rs3077, rs9277535 and rs7453920 did not associate with HCC development (dominant model, rs3077, OR = 0.86, 95%CI = 0.62–1.18; rs9277535, OR = 0.94, 95%CI = 0.68–1.30; rs7453920, OR = 0.75, 95%CI = 0.44–1.27). Meta-analysis again consolidated this conclusion (allele model, rs3077, OR = 0.94, 95%CI = 0.87–1.02; rs9277535, OR = 1.04, 95%CI = 0.97–1.11; rs7453920, OR = 0.89, 95%CI = 0.76–1.02). As for STAT4 rs7574865, we did not find any significant association with HBV susceptibility (OR = 0.91, 95%CI = 0.66–1.26) or HBV natural clearance (OR = 1.13, 95%CI = 0.86–1.49). Moreover, current data failed to acquire positive connection of rs7574865 with HCC development (experiment, OR = 0.86, 95%CI = 0.62–1.19; meta-analysis, OR = 0.87, 95%CI = 0.74–1.03), which may be due to the small sample size.

Conclusions: HLA-DP/DQ polymorphisms (rs3077, rs9277535, rs7453920) did not associate with HCC development, but did correlate with HBV susceptibility and HBV natural clearance. STAT4 rs7574865 seemed not to correlate with HBV susceptibility or natural clearance. And it seemed rather ambiguous in its role on HCC development at present.

Editor: Ferruccio Bonino, University of Pisa, Italy

Funding: This study was funded in full by grants from Natural Science Foundation of China (grant numbers 81072443, 81100536, and 81273256). The funders had no role in study design, data collection and analysis, decision to publish, or preparation of the manuscript.

Competing Interests: The authors have declared that no competing interests exist.

* Email: wangll_wch@163.com

[9] These authors contributed equally to this work.

Introduction

Hepatitis B virus (HBV) infection is one of the major causes of chronic hepatitis and the main risk factor for liver cirrhosis and hepatocellular carcinoma (HCC) [1]. Approximately 350 to 400 million people are HBV carriers worldwide and 1 million deaths from HBV-related diseases, including cirrhosis, liver failure and HCC [2].

Most HBV infections which occurred in adults are often self-limited, with spontaneous clearance of HBV from blood and liver. However, some of the infections in adults do not resolve but develop into persistent infection (though less than 5%) [3]. After HBV persistent infection, about 20% patients would progress to cirrhosis and 5–10% would develop HCC. As for the reason why some adults could achieve spontaneous clearance, and some would develop into chronic hepatitis and even HCC, still remains to be further illustrated. Recent Genome-Wide Association studies (GWAS) revealed that HLA-DP/DQ polymorphisms (HLA-DP rs3077, rs9277535, HLA-DQ rs2856718, rs7453920) associated with HBV clearance [4,5], from a genetic perspective to investigate the etiology of chronic hepatitis B. Subsequently, these findings were validated by many a study [6–10], especially in Asians, like Chinese Han, Japanese, Korean and so on. Hu and his colleagues [7] first pointed out that HLA-DP/DQ not only associated with HBV clearance, but also correlated with HCC development, with HLA-DQ rs2856718 significantly decreasing HCC risk and rs3077 an approaching significant effect on HCC development. Moreover, in their further research [11], they found additional HLA-DQ single nucleotide polymorphism (SNP) rs9272105 correlated with HCC development, however, when they validated the previous SNPs, they only found rs9277535 pertained to HCC development, which was regarded as insignificant in their previous study [7], vice versa, the previous proved-to-be significant SNPs (rs3077, rs2856718) did not reach statistical significance again. Additionally, several other studies including GWAS studies did not acquire that these SNPs correlated with HCC development [8,11–13]. Therefore, up to now, no confirmative conclusion could be drawn on which SNPs of HLA-DP/DQ would play the decisive role in the development of HCC.

Still, one GWAS study [12] described above also revealed Signal Transducer and Activator of Transcription 4 (STAT4) rs7574865 significantly correlated with HBV-related HCC except for HLA-DQ polymorphism. However, when they examined whether this SNP associated with chronic HBV (CHB) infection, they found results little more than a trend of higher frequency for G allele in chronic HBV carriers compared with those who did not carry HBV. Clark et al [14] recruited Vietnamese as the investigated subjects to explore the relationship between STAT4 rs7574865 and HCC development, only to find a trivial role contributing to HCC development ($P = 0.047$). And Chen's study [15] did not find any significant association at all ($P = 0.57$). These seemingly conflicting results sparked our great interest. Whether STAT4 did exert influence on HCC development as well as HBV seroclearance still remains obscure.

Therefore, in this study, we mainly aimed to investigate the association of HLA-DP rs3077, rs9277535, HLA-DQ rs7453920 and STAT4 rs7574865 with HCC development, chronicity of HBV infection in Han population dwelling in West China, both from experiment and meta-analysis perspective to clarify the currently ambiguous role of these SNPs with HCC development, and to validate their correlations with HBV susceptibility and clearance from the experiment.

Materials and Methods

Patients

The present study recruited 1312 Chinese Han subjects, including 450 chronic HBV carriers, 227 hepatocellular carcinoma patients and 635 healthy controls, from March to July in 2013 in West China Hospital. Chronic HBV carriers were defined as those who had histories of at least 6 months HBsAg positivity (HBsAg+) as well as no HBsAb (anti-HBs negative) existed in the serum, with no evidence supporting cirrhosis or HCC. The diagnosis of HCC was confirmed by a pathological examination and/or alpha-fetoprotein elevation (>400 ng/ml) plus imaging examination (i.e. magnetic resonance imaging and/or computerized tomography). The controls comprised two groups: 398 subjects with HBV natural clearance (NC subjects) and 237 subjects who were negative for all the serum biomarkers of HBV (HBsAg, anti-HBs, HBeAg, anti-HBe, anti-HBc) (healthy control, HC). Subjects with natural clearance (NC subjects) were those who were negative for HBsAg, but positive for both anti-HBs and anti-HBc. All the control subjects had normal liver functions. And those who were coinfected with hepatitis A, C, D virus or human immunodeficiency virus (HIV) were excluded from this study. All patients consented to sample collection for this study and written informed consent was obtained for each participant. This study was approved by the Institutional Review Board of West China Hospital of Sichuan University. The procedures are in accordance with the Helsinki Declaration.

Serological testing

Serology markers of HBV including HBsAg, HBeAg, anti-HBs, anti-HBe and anti-HBc were analyzed using Elecsys Modular E170 immunoassay (Roche Diagnostics, GmbH, Mannheim, Germany) or I2000 immunoassay (Abbott co., USA) in accordance with manufacturers' instruction. Clinical biochemistry analysis on ALT, AST, TB, DB, ALP, ALB and GGT were conducted on Cobas c702 assay with photocolorimetric method (Roche Diagnostic, GmbH, Mannheim, Germany). HBV DNA from 200 μl serum was extracted by NucliSENS easyMAG system (Biomerieux Company, Paris, France), the viral load was measured using Roche Light Cycler 480α (Roche Diagnostics, Basel, Switzerland).

HLA-DP/DQ and STAT4 polymorphism genotyping

All the four SNPs (HLA-DP rs3077, rs9277535; HLA-DQ rs7453920; STAT4 rs7574865) were genotyped using polymerase chain reaction-high resolution melting (HRM) analysis performed on Light Cycler 480 (Roche Diagnostics, Penzberg, Bavaria, Germany). Genomic DNA kit (Biotake Corporation, Beijing, China) was used to extract the free circulating DNA from the blood sample and the concentration was measured by Nanodrop 2000c spectrophometer (Thermo Scientific, DE). SNP genotyping was performed in a 20 μL reaction system contained 10 μL Roche Master Mix (Roche Applied Science) which comprises FastStart Taq DNA Polymerase and the High Resolution Melting Dye in a reaction buffer, 2.4 μL 25 mM $MgCl_2$, 0.2 μL 10 μmol/L Forward Primer and 0.2 μL 10 μmol/L Reverse Primer, 6.2 μL deionized water and finally 1 μL DNA sample as recommended by the manufacturer. The whole genotyping process encompasses four programmes, namely, pre-denaturation, amplification, high resolution melting and cooling. When finished, the results were analyzed by the corresponding Gene Scanning Software v1.2 (Roche Diagnostic) primarily based on the shape of the melting curve. Primers used in this study were shown in Table S1.

Meta-analysis on association of HLA-DP/DQ and STAT4 with HCC development

We searched Pubmed, Embase to screen the eligible studies. Such words were used in the search strategy: "HLA-DP" or "HLA-DQ" or "rs3077" or "rs9277535" or "rs7453920" or "STAT4" or "rs7574865" and "liver cancer" or "hepatocellular carcinoma" or "HCC". The detailed screening process is shown in Figure 1. Data were collected by two investigators (Yun Liao and Bei Cai). The inclusion criteria are listed as follows: 1) the article assessed the genotype frequencies of HLA-DP/DQ or STAT4 between HBV and HCC; 2) study design was a case-control study; 3) the diagnosis of each stage of liver disease conforms to the American Association for the Study of Liver Disease [16,17]; 4) odds ratio with the 95% confidence interval [95%CI] was reported or could be figured out through the available data. The studies which did not meet above principles were not included. We mainly extracted the odds ratio and the 95%CI from each study so as to fully take advantage of every related study.

Quality of each study included in this study was assessed using the Newcastle-Ottawa Scale (NOS), which has in total 3 categories: 4 stars for selection, up to 2 stars for comparability and 3 stars for exposure/outcome. Nine stars were regarded as the highest quality and studies with more than 6 stars were deemed as the high quality study [18].

Statistical analysis

Hardy-Weinberg equilibrium (HWE) was independently appraised for each polymorphism. Continuous variables with skewed distribution were described with median and interquartile and the Kruskal-Wallis H test was used for these data. Pearson's chi-square test or Fisher's exact test were used to analyze the allele case-control comparisons. Association of SNPs with development as well as susceptibility of HBV infection was estimated by figuring out the odds ratio (OR) and 95% Confidence Interval (CI). When

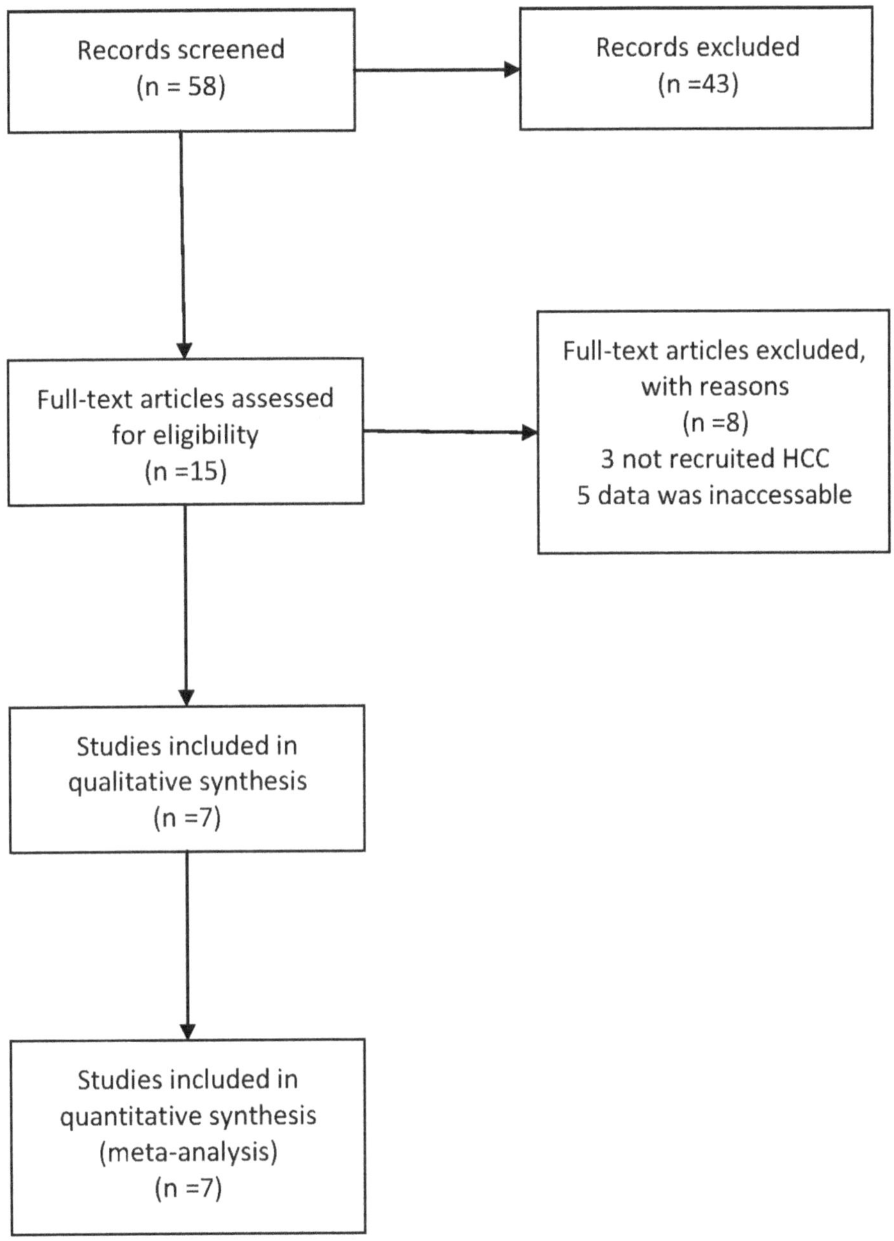

Figure 1. Flow diagram for article screening.

comparing the two group of subjects (case and control), several analytic methods were used: allele frequency distribution of the two groups (allele A versus allele B, A as the major allele, B as the minor allele, this applied to the following methods); genotypic distribution (AA versus AB versus BB); dominant model (AB+BB versus AA). Haplotype analysis was performed to explore whether HLA-DP/DQ polymorphisms were in strong linkage disequilibrium (LD) or they independently contribute to the susceptibility of HBV infection, and can capture additional significant variants since it's more sensitive than the single SNP analysis. Haplotypes with frequencies of more than 0.03 were analyzed. Pearson's chi-squared test was used for case–control comparisons.

Meta-analysis was adopted to comprehensively evaluate the correlation of genetic factors with HCC development. The heterogeneity for the included articles was evaluated using Cochran's Q test, I^2 statistics (the heterogeneity could be accepted if $P>0.1$ and $I^2 \leq 50\%$). If the value is less than 50%, we could think that no heterogeneity existed among the included studies, and then fixed-effects model was used to evaluate the odds ratios. While if I^2 value is more than 50%, random-effects model was used. Additionally, if all the studies were from one ethnicity, we did not perform subgroup analysis. Sensitivity analysis was performed to evaluate the reliability of the results.

All the analyses were performed using SPSS 13.0 (SPSS Inc., Chicago, IL, USA), STATA 12.0 (version 12.0), comprehensive meta-analysis (version 2.0, Englewood, NJ, USA) and SHEsis online software (http://analysis.bio-x.cn/myAnalysis.php) [19]. A two-sided P value<0.05 was deemed as statistically significant.

Results

Clinical characteristics of included subjects

The median age for HC patients was 42 (range: 29–53) years, for NC patients was 49 (range: 41–59) years, for HBV patients was 46 (range: 36–57) years and for HCC patients was 49 (42–59) years. HCC group has a higher proportion of male patients (80.2%), in comparison with HBV group (63.8%), SC group (51.2%) or NC group (38.0%). All the polymorphisms in the four groups were in Hardy-Weinberg equilibrium (P>0.05). The detailed clinical characteristics of the four groups were shown in Table 1.

We next analyzed the association of HLA-DP/DQ and STAT4 genotypes with clinical indicators in each group. Data showed that rs3077 genotype AA tended to associate with a higher aspartate amino transferase (AST), especially in HCC patients (P = 0.05). But no other polymorphisms were found to correlate with these indicators (HLA-DQ rs7453920 was excluded due to its too skewed distribution of genotypes) (Table S2).

Association analysis of HLA-DP/DQ, STAT4 polymorphisms with HBV clearance and susceptibility

To identify genetic variations associated with HBV susceptibility, we first compared genotype frequencies of HLA-DP/DQ, STAT4 between HBV group and NC group respectively. The minor allele frequencies of HLA-DP/DQ in both the two groups (HBV vs. NC) were as follows: rs3077, 0.271 vs. 0.324; rs9277535, 0.276 vs. 0.378; rs7453920, 0.067 vs. 0.116; rs7574865, 0.336 vs. 0.336). After adjusting age and sex to control for potential confounders, we observed that rs3077 non-GG genotype, rs9277535 non-GG genotype and rs7453920 non-GG genotype favored HBV seroclearance respectively (adjusted dominant model, rs3077, OR = 0.70, 95%CI = 0.53–0.93; rs9277535, OR = 0.54, 95%CI = 0.40–0.72; rs7453920, OR = 0.48, 95%CI = 0.33–0.70) (Table 2). Allele model further confirmed that rs3077 allele A, rs9277535 allele A and rs7453920 allele A, all had protective effect on HBV seroclearance (rs3077, OR = 0.77, 95%CI = 0.63–0.96; rs9277535, OR = 0.63, 95%CI = 0.51–0.77; rs7453920, OR = 0.55, 95%CI = 0.39–0.77). But STAT4 rs7574865 seemed not to correlate with HBV clearance (dominant model, OR = 0.91, 95%CI = 0.66–1.26, p = 0.571) (Table 2).

Next, we appraised the correlation between HBV and HC subjects. HLA-DP rs3077 and rs9277535 still correlated with HBV susceptibility (adjusted dominant model, rs3077, OR = 0.60, 95%CI = 0.43–0.84; rs9277535, OR = 0.51, 95%CI = 0.36–0.72). But we did not find significant association between rs7453920 and HBV susceptibility this time (OR = 0.74, 95%CI = 0.46–1.18) (Table 2). However, since the minor allele frequency of rs7453920 in HBV carriers resembles HCC patients, we combined the two groups and reappraised the correlation of rs7453920 with HBV susceptibility. Univariate analysis showed that rs7453920 tended to associate with HBV susceptibility in dominant model (OR = 0.66, 95%CI = 0.43–1.01, p = 0.053). Additionally, we made a comparison between the control subjects (NC+HC) and virus-carrying group (HBV+HCC). Results showed that HLA-DP rs3077, rs9277535 and even HLA-DQ rs7453920 were significantly pertinent to HBV susceptibility. However, we still did not find significant association existed between STAT4 rs7574865 and HBV susceptibility (P>0.05).

Association analysis of HLA-DP/DQ, STAT4 polymorphisms with HCC development and the meta-analysis

To identify the correlation of these genetic factors with HBV progression, we compared the genotype frequency between HCC group and HBV group. The minor allele frequencies in the two groups were shown as follows (HCC vs. HBV): rs3077, 0.254 vs. 0.271; rs9277535, 0.276 vs. 0.276; rs7453920, 0.047 vs. 0.067; rs7574865, 0.322 vs. 0.336). Univariate analysis showed that none of the gene polymorphisms associated with HCC development

Table 1. Clinical characteristics of subjects recruited in this study.

Group	HC	NC	HBV	HCC
number of subjects	237	398	450	227
age (years)*	42 (29–53)	49 (41–59)	46 (36–57)	49 (42–59)
Gender (male/female)*	90/147 (38.0)	204/194 (51.2)	287/163 (63.8)	191/47 (80.2)
HBsAg+	0	0	450	227
HBsAb+	0	398	0	0
HBeAg+	0	0	65	56
HBeAb+	0	0	369	183
HBcAb+	0	398	450	221
ALT(IU/L)*	16 (11.5–22.5)	20 (14–26)	24 (17–38)	40 (27–64)
AST(IU/L)*	18 (15–22)	21 (17–25)	25 (20–32)	44 (31–66)
TP(g/L)	69.3 (65.3–73.9)	71.4 (67.9–74.7)	71.8(67.6–75.3)	70.4 (66.2–73.6)
ALB(g/L)	43.8 (40.9–46.3)	45.3 (42.9–47.6)	44.9 (42.0–47.3)	40.9 (37.7–43.8)
TB (μmol/L)	11.1 (8.2–14.75)	11.7 (9.5–15.5)	13.8 (10.5–17.8)	15.1 (11.5–20.3)
GGT(IU/L)*	16 (11–26)	18.0 (12.0–28.5)	21 (13–36)	78.0 (43.7–172.7)
PLT*	168 (126.5–211)	178 (139.75–212.25)	152 (114.5–191.0)	116 (75–169)

*Significant difference existed among all the four groups; HC, healthy control; NC, natural clearance subjects; HBV, hepatitis B virus patients; HCC, hepatocellular carcinoma patients; ALT, alanine aminotransferase; AST: aspartate aminotransferase; ALB, albumin; TB, total bilirubin; TP, total protein; GGT, gamma-glutamyl transpeptidase.

Continuous variables were described as median and interquatile range.

Table 2. Association of HLA-DP/DQ and STAT4 polymorphisms with HBV susceptibility, HBV natural clearance and HCC development.

Genotype	HC	percentage	NC	percentage	HBV	percentage	HCC	percentage	HBV vs. HC		HBV vs. NC		HCC vs. HBV	
									OR (95%CI)	P	OR (95%CI)	P	OR (95%CI)	P
rs3077														
GG	100	42.2%	175	44.2%	233	53.3%	128	57.1%	1		1		1	-
AG	115	48.5%	185	46.7%	171	39.1%	78	34.8%	**0.64 (0.46–0.89)**	**0.008**	**0.69 (0.52–0.92)**	**0.012**	0.83 (0.59–1.17)	0.289
AA	22	9.3%	36	9.1%	33	7.6%	18	8.0%	0.64 (0.36–1.16)	0.14	0.69 (0.41–1.15)	0.151	0.99 (0.54–1.83)	0.982
Dominant									**0.64 (0.46–0.88)**	**0.006**	**0.69 (0.53–0.91)**	**0.009**	0.86 (0.62–1.18)	0.35
Adjusted*									**0.60 (0.43–0.84)**	**0.003**	**0.70 (0.53–0.93)**	**0.012**	-	-
G	315	66.5%	535	67.6%	637	72.9%	334	74.6%	1		1		1	-
A	159	33.5%	257	32.4%	237	27.1%	114	25.4%	**0.74 (0.58–0.94)**	**0.013**	**0.77 (0.63–0.96)**	**0.017**	0.92 (0.71–1.19)	0.515
rs9277535														
GG	83	35.6%	136	36.8%	226	51.8%	118	53.4%	1		1		1	-
AG	110	47.2%	188	50.8%	179	41.1%	84	37.5%	**0.60 (0.42–0.84)**	**0.003**	**0.57 (0.43–0.77)**	**<0.001**	0.90 (0.64–1.26)	0.54
AA	40	17.2%	46	12.4%	31	7.1%	19	8.5%	**0.28 (0.17–0.48)**	**<0.001**	**0.41 (0.24–0.67)**	**<0.001**	1.17 (0.64–2.17)	0.608
Dominant									**0.51 (0.37–0.71)**	**<0.001**	**0.54 (0.41–0.72)**	**<0.001**	0.94 (0.68–1.30)	0.705
Adjusted*									**0.51 (0.36–0.72)**	**<0.001**	**0.54 (0.40–0.72)**	**<0.001**	-	-
G	276	59.2%	460	62.2%	631	72.4%	320	72.4%	**1**		**1**		1	-
A	190	40.8%	280	37.8%	241	27.6%	122	27.6%	**0.55 (0.44–0.70)**	**<0.001**	**0.63 (0.51–0.77)**	**<0.001**	0.99 (0.77–1.29)	0.989
rs7453920														
GG	199	84.0%	302	77.2%	391	87.9%	203	90.6%	1		1		1	-
AG	33	13.9%	87	22.3%	48	10.8%	21	9.4%	0.74 (0.46–1.19)	0.213	**0.43 (0.29–0.62)**	**<0.001**	0.84 (0.49–1.45)	0.534
AA	5	2.1%	2	0.5%	6	1.3%	0	0.0%	0.61 (0.18–2.03)	0.416	2.32 (0.46–11.56)	0.292		
Dominant									0.72 (0.46–1.13)	0.156	**0.47 (0.32–0.68)**	**<0.001**	0.75 (0.44–1.27)	0.286
Adjusted*									-	-	**0.48 (0.33–0.70)**	**<0.001**	-	-
G	431	90.9%	691	88.4%	830	93.3%	427	95.3%	1		1		1	-
A	43	9.1%	91	11.6%	60	6.7%	21	4.7%	0.72 (0.48–1.09)	0.121	**0.55 (0.39–0.77)**	**<0.001**	0.68 (0.41–1.13)	0.137
rs7574865														
GG	97	40.9%	181	46.3%	190	43.2%	104	46.8%	1		1		1	-
GT	113	47.7%	157	40.2%	204	46.4%	93	41.5%	0.92 (0.66–1.29)	0.634	1.24 (0.92–1.66)	0.151	0.83 (0.59–1.17)	0.295
TT	27	11.4%	53	13.6%	46	10.5%	25	11.2%	0.87 (0.51–1.48)	0.609	0.83 (0.53–1.29)	0.401	0.99 (0.58–1.71)	0.979
dominant	140		210		250		118		0.91 (0.66–1.26)	0.571	1.13 (0.86–1.49)	0.368	0.86 (0.62–1.19)	0.37
G	307	64.8%	519	66.4%	584	66.4%	301	67.8%	1		1		1	-
T	167	35.2%	263	33.6%	296	33.6%	143	32.2%	0.93 (0.74–1.78)	0.555	1.0 (0.82–1.23)	0.998	0.94 (0.73–1.19)	0.602

*Logistic regression analysis adjusted for age and sex. For those insignificant results in univariate analysis, we did not adjust the results; HC, healthy control; NC, natural clearance; HBV, hepatitis B virus patients; HCC, hepatocellular carcinoma.

(dominant model, rs3077, OR = 0.86, 95%CI = 0.62–1.18; rs9277535, OR = 0.94, 95%CI = 0.68–1.30; rs7453920, OR = 0.75, 95%CI = 0.44–1.27; rs7574865, 95%CI = 0.86, 95%CI = 0.62–1.19) (Table 2).

Then, based on current study, we adopted meta-analysis, from a more powerful way, to illuminate the correlation between these host genetic factors and HBV progression. In total, fifty-eight articles were searched, but only data from seven studies can be extracted, including five studies [7,8,12,20,21] focused on HLA-DP/DQ, two studies [14,15] researched STAT4 rs7574865. Quality assessment of all the included studies showed that only study conducted by Al-Qahtani et al. [21] scored less than 6 points and thus was regarded as study of low quality. All the other studies were of high quality. The clinical characteristics as well as the quality scores of the enrolled studies were shown in Table S3 and Table S4. Plus our data, in total, 3467 HCC patients and 5821 HBV carriers were included in this meta-analysis. We extracted the effect size and its 95% confidence interval to appraise the correlation for HLA-DP/DQ and genotype frequencies for STAT4 rs7574865. Meta-analysis based on data from three studies [7,8,12] plus our present data, including 2997 HCC patients and 3738 HBV patients, showed that HLA-DP rs3077 did not correlate with HCC development (allele model, OR = 0.94, 95%CI = 0.87–1.02) using fixed model effects (Table 3, Figure 2A). Since moderate heterogeneity existed among all the studies ($I^2 = 46.7\%$), we adopted random effects model to reappraise the correlation and results also indicated its insignificant association with HCC development (OR = 0.95, 95%CI = 0.84–1.06) (Table 3, Figure 2B). When it came to HLA-DP rs9277535 and HLA-DQ rs7453920, consistent with all the studies [7,8,20,21], the two polymorphisms (rs9277535: 3386 HCC patients and 5621 HBV patients; rs7453920: 2813 HCC patients and 3347 HBV patients) showed no connection with HCC development (allele model, rs9277535, OR = 1.04, 95%CI = 0.97–1.11; rs7453920, OR = 0.89, 95%CI = 0.76–1.02) (Table 3, Figure 2C, 2D). Two studies [14,15] investigated STAT4 rs7574865 with HCC development, combined with our present data (in total, 962 HCC patients and 1418 HBV patients), we failed to find any significant association with HCC development (dominant model, OR = 0.87, 95%CI = 0.74–1.03, p = 0.113) (Table 3, Figure S1). Sensitivity analysis was performed through omitting studies with rather small sample size. And results were not significantly influenced (data now shown) and our conclusions were credible. Egger's test showed that no publication bias existed among all the polymorphisms (Figure S2).

Haplotype analysis

Haplotype was constructed based on the 3 HLA-DP/DQ polymorphisms and were analyzed for their associations with HBV susceptibility, HBV seroclearance and HCC development. Based on rs3077 (minor allele A), rs9277535 (minor allele A) and rs7453920 (minor allele A), when comparing the target haplotype with remaining haplotype combinations, haplotype block GGG was significantly associated with HBV seroclearance (OR = 1.60, 95%CI = 1.31–1.96), block GAG favored virus clearance (OR = 0.56, 95%CI = 0.40–0.70). When comparison was made between HBV and HC subjects, haplotype block GGG still associated with increased risk of HBV infection (OR = 1.69, 95%CI = 1.34–2.14), while GAG and AAG connected with reduced risk of HBV infection (GAG, OR = 0.53, 95%CI = 0.37–0.77; AAG, OR = 0.70, 95%CI = 0.52–0.94). Moreover, we analyzed haplotype in HCC and HBV groups to acquire haplotype that was linked to HCC development.

Table 3. Meta-analysis results of HLA-DP/DQ and STAT4 polymorphisms with HCC development.

SNPs	Gene	case/control	OR	95%CI	I^2	Effects model
rs3077	HLA-DP	2997/3738	0.94	0.87–1.02	46.7%	F
rs3077	HLA-DP	2997/3738	0.95	0.84–1.06	46.7%	R
rs9277535	HLA-DP	3386/5621	1.04	0.97–1.11	5.7%	F
rs7453920	HLA-DQ	2813/3347	0.89	0.76–1.02	28.0%	F
rs7574865	STAT4	962/1418	0.87	0.74–1.03	0.0%	F

Note: OR, odds ratio; F, fixed-effects model; R, random-effects model.

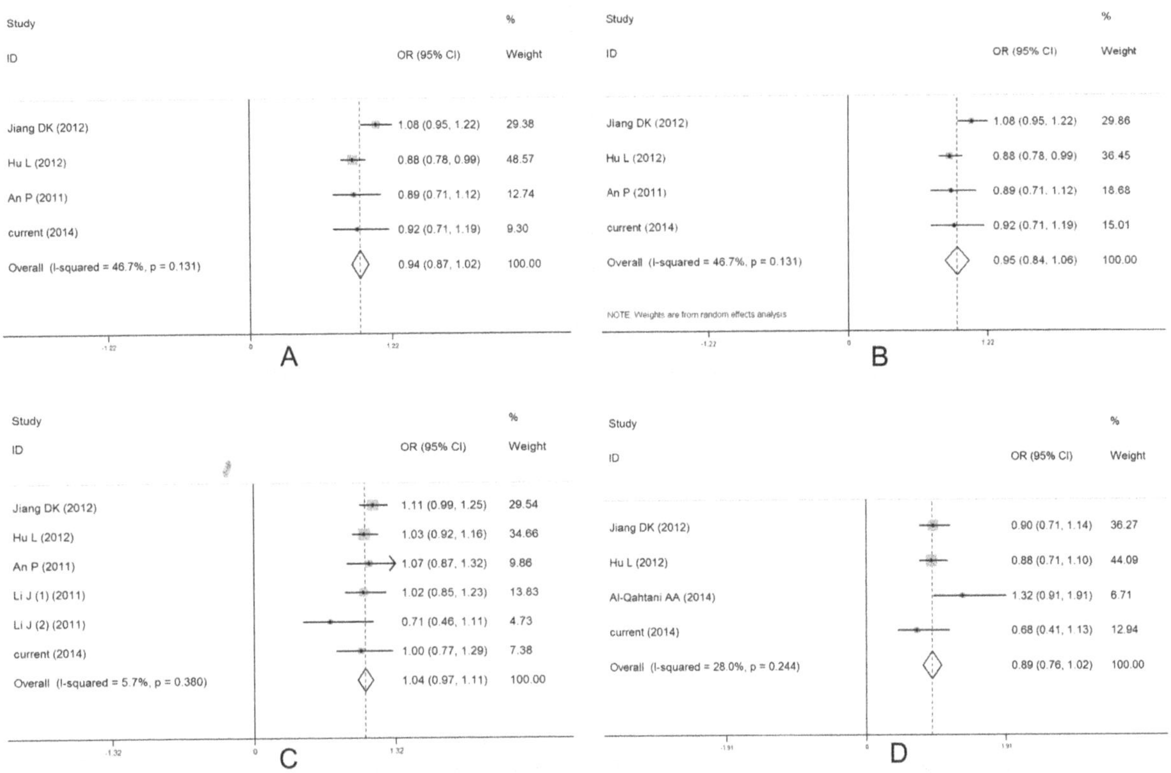

Figure 2. Forest plot for association of rs3077, rs9277535 and rs7453920 with HCC development. (A) Meta-analysis for rs3077 calculated in Fixed-effects model; (B) Meta-analysis for rs3077 calculated in Random-effects model; (C) Forest plot for rs9277535 with HCC development, Li J (1) represents southern Han Chinese, while (2) represents northern Han Chinese; (D) Forest plot for rs7453920 with HCC development.

However, no haplotype presented significant association with HCC development ($p>0.05$) (Table 4).

Discussion

In this study, we investigated HLA-DP/DQ and STAT4 polymorphisms with HBV susceptibility, viral clearance and HCC development in Han population residing in the Southwest of China. And our study first pointed out that currently hot spots (HLA-DP rs3077, rs9277535, HLA-DQ rs7453920, rs2856718) did not correlate with HCC development, either from experiment data or meta-analysis results, but they did associate with HBV susceptibility as well as HBV natural clearance. As for STAT4 rs7574865, it has no impact on HBV susceptibility and seroclearance, but its role in HCC development remains contentious.

Consistent with previous findings, HLA-DP rs3077, rs9277535, HLA-DQ rs7453920 still correlated with HBV seroclearance ($p<0.05$), and rs3077 allele A, rs9277535 allele A as well as rs7453920 allele A served as the protective role in HBV clearance. When analyzing HBV susceptibility between HBV patients and HC subjects, rs3077 and rs9277535 still associate with HBV susceptibility, but rs7453920 presented an insignificant result. This might be due to the limitation of sample size in HC group. Since the MAFs in HC and NC, HBV and HCC resemble, we divided all the patients into two groups: control (NC+SC) and HBV carrier (HBV+HCC). Next, we reappraised the correlation of rs7453920 with HBV susceptibility, and significant correlation existed. But the phenomenon implied that rs7453920 had weaker effect on HBV susceptibility compared with HLA-DP rs3077 and rs9277535.

As is listed before, only several studies [7,8,13–15,20,21] investigated the correlation of HLA-DP/DQ with HCC development, but quite conflicting results were acquired. In order to clarify this obscure correlation, we recruited HCC patients and replicated the experiments to further give an explanation on the conflicting results. But based on our experimental data and the haplotype analysis on HCC development, only negative results were achieved. Due to the limitation of our sample size, we subsequently performed meta-analysis to circumvent these confounding factors such as the sample size and the inherent heterogeneity in the study subjects. However, meta-analysis results again contradicted that HLA-DP rs3077, rs9277535 and HLA-DQ rs7453920 are not pertinent to HCC development. Besides, based on the weak or even insignificant connection of these SNPs with liver function indicators (Table S2), they would not be predictors for liver damage after HBV infection, and further implied that they could not predict the development of liver diseases, which, from another perspective, supported the conclusion both achieved from the experiment and meta-analysis. However, HLA-DQ rs2856718 seemed to significantly correlated with HCC development [7], and from meta-analysis, its role in HCC development seemed to be definite ($OR = 0.88$, $95\%CI = 0.81–0.95$) (Figure S3) and therefore we did not include it in this study.

Previous study has demonstrated that the risk alleles of HLA-DP polymorphisms (rs3077 G, rs9277535 G) associated with a decreased expression level of HLA-DP mRNA [22]. HLA-DP is

Table 4. Haplotype analysis of rs3077, rs9277535 and rs7453920 with HBV susceptibility, seroclearance and HCC development.

Haplotype	case(freq)	control(freq)	OR	95%CI	p value
(A)					
AAA	24 (0.029)	20 (0.042)	0.66	0.36–1.22	0.183
AAG	132 (0.158)	97 (0.208)	0.7	0.52–0.94	0.016
AGG	71 (0.085)	37 (0.080)	1.05	0.69–1.59	0.811
GAG	67 (0.080)	65 (0.139)	0.53	0.37–0.77	0.0006
GGG	511 (0.661)	224 (0.481)	1.69	1.34–2.14	1.10E-05
(B)					
AAG	132 (0.158)	129 (0.178)	0.83	0.64–1.08	0.174
AGG	71 (0.085)	69 (0.096)	0.85	0.60–1.20	0.346
GAG	67 (0.080)	95 (0.131)	0.56	0.40–0.77	0.0004
GGA	25 (0.029)	22 (0.031)	0.92	0.51–1.64	0.769
GGG	511 (0.611)	348 (0.480)	1.6	1.31–1.96	5.91E-06
(C)					
AAG	77 (0.175)	132 (0.158)	1.1	0.81–1.50	0.55
AGG	28 (0.063)	71 (0.085)	0.71	0.45–1.12	0.136
GAG	37 (0.083)	67 (0.080)	1.02	0.67–1.55	0.942
GGG	280 (0.634)	511 (0.611)	1.04	0.81–1.34	0.732

(A) Haplotype analysis on HBV susceptibility; (B) Haplotype analysis on HBV seroclearance; (C) Haplotype analysis on HCC development.

expressed on the surface of antigen-presenting cells and belong to HLA-αmolecules, which can bind and present antigen epitopes to CD4+ T helper cell [23]. The decreased HLA-DP expression attributed to carrying risk alleles of HLA-DP rs3077 and rs9277535 might thus influence the antigen presentation, incurring immune evasion of the virus. One recent study [24] indicated HLA-DP polymorphisms might interact with HBV genome mutations to determine the outcomes of HBV infection, with HLA-DP protective genotypes relating to decreased prevalence of viral mutations which contributed to HCC development. Given the seemingly irrelevant role of HLA-DP/DQ in HCC development, the role of the association of HLA-DP/DQ polymorphisms with HBV viral mutations in HBV outcomes have dimmed. However in this study, we only validated those hot spots, which might lead to some missing causative polymorphisms. Considering the population heterogeneity, it would be better to sequence HLA-DP/DQ to unveil the polymorphisms that would play decisive role in HCC development.

STAT4 is a transcription factor which regulated immune response, transmitted signals from interleukin-12 (IL-12) and typeinterferon (IFN) to induce IFN-γ production [25–27]. Few studies had ever linked STAT4 with HBV diseases and HCC development before the GWAS studies came into being [12]. In light of current conflicting conclusions [12,14,15], we performed this validation study. Our present data doubted the discovery by the GWAS study that rs7574865 associated with HCC development [12]. Considering the limit of relatively small sample size, we performed this meta-analysis. Meta-analysis combined the two studies plus our current data including in total 962 HCC patients and 1418 HBV patients, and still failed to determine any significant association but only a trend with HCC development (OR = 0.87, 95% = 0.74–1.03). However, based on the sample size, the detection power of current meta-analysis still cannot challenge the conclusion drew by the GWAS study [12]. Therefore, in regard to STAT4 rs7574865 with HCC development, large cohort studies with high quality are warranted to validate this conclusion, particularly from multiple ethnicities to eliminate the race heterogeneity. Besides, we did not find any significant association of STAT4 rs7574865 with HBV seroclearance as well as the susceptibility when comparing HBV patients with seroclearance subjects and negative controls respectively. Accordingly, all these mentioned above suggested an irrelevant role of STAT4 rs7584865 in HBV susceptibility, at least in Chinese Han population, but seemingly a rather obscure association with HCC development awaiting more high-quality studies to corroborate.

Apart from what mentioned above, our study has several limitations. Firstly, we only replicated those currently hot SNPs but with conflicting relationship with HCC development, and the selected SNPs might not fully represent the related genes. In this way, we may have missed some representative and decisive gene polymorphisms. Secondly, when appraising the relationship of these gene polymorphisms with HCC development, we lacked virus genotype information, since Zhang et al. [24] suggested that different genotypes would have distinct outcomes stratified by HLA-DP polymorphism. Meanwhile, we lacked detailed information on the fibrosis stage and the presence of cirrhosis or not, so further studies are needed to comprehensively analyze the genotype frequencies of these gene polymorphisms in each stage of HBV related liver disease. Thirdly, the rather small number size limited the detection power in HCC group, though this has been remedied by the subsequent meta-analysis. And when analyzing the relationship of STAT4 rs7574865 with HCC using meta-analysis, we did not include the GWAS study, since all the other three studies held points similar to negative conclusion. If included, the positive relationship is definite, but this conclusion still warrants more studies in different ethnicities to substantiate. Moreover, since too few studies investigated each SNP and were included in the meta-analysis, we did not further conduct subgroup analysis stratified by quality of the studies, ethnicities etc., due to the probably insufficient statistical power. Fourthly, since the role of HLA-DP/DQ in HBV susceptibility as well as natural clearance is rather certain now, we did not take meta-analysis to summarize the associations.

These limitations notwithstanding, our study first summarized that current hot SNPs (rs3077, rs9277535, rs7453920) selected from HLA-DP/DQ did not associate with HCC development, from perspective of both experiment and meta-analysis. And consistent with previous studies, HLA-DP/DQ associated with HBV susceptibility and virus seroclearance. As for the recently emerged STAT4 rs7574865, experimental data contradicted its association with HBV susceptibility and HCC development. But given the rather limited sample size and the insignificant but tended-to-be significant meta-analysis results, the correlation of rs7574865 with HCC development still awaits large cohort studies to validate. Anyway, this study further corroborated the association of HLA-DP/DQ polymorphisms (rs3077, rs9277535 and rs7453920) with HBV seroclearance and first pinpointed their irrelevant role in HCC development. Future study could sequence HLA-DP/DQ genes to unveil the decisive polymorphisms associating with HCC development in multiple races and further explore how these polymorphisms impact on HBV clearance and HCC development and another study with large sample size to validate the correlation of rs7574865 with HCC development.

Supporting Information

Figure S1 Forest plot for association of STAT4 rs7574865 with HCC development.

Figure S2 Publication bias of the four polymorphisms discussed in this study. (A) Publication bias for rs3077; (B) Publication bias for rs9277535; (C) Publication bias for rs7574865; (D) Publication bias for rs7453920.

Figure S3 Forest plot for association of HLA-DQ rs2856718 with HCC development.

Table S1 Information of primers used in this study.

Table S2 Association of HLA-DP/DQ and STAT4 polymorphisms with clinical indicators.

Table S3 Clinical characteristics of the enrolled studies in the meta-analysis.

Table S4 Quality assessment for all included studies using the Newcastle-Ottawa Scale.

Checklist S1 Prisma checklist for the meta-analysis.

Author Contributions

Conceived and designed the experiments: Y. Liao BC LW. Performed the experiments: Y. Liao BC. Analyzed the data: Y. Liao Y. Li JC. Contributed reagents/materials/analysis tools: CT HH. Contributed to the writing of the manuscript: Y. Liao LW.

References

1. Lai CL, Ratziu V, Yuen MF, Poynard T (2003) Viral hepatitis B. Lancet 362: 2089–2094.
2. Dienstag JL (2008) Hepatitis B virus infection. N Engl J Med 359: 1486–1500.
3. Ganem D, Prince AM (2004) Hepatitis B virus infection–natural history and clinical consequences. N Engl J Med 350: 1118–1129.
4. Kamatani Y, Wattanapokayakit S, Ochi H, Kawaguchi T, Takahashi A, et al. (2009) A genome-wide association study identifies variants in the HLA-DP locus associated with chronic hepatitis B in Asians. Nat Genet 41: 591–595.
5. Mbarek H, Ochi H, Urabe Y, Kumar V, Kubo M, et al. (2011) A genome-wide association study of chronic hepatitis B identified novel risk locus in a Japanese population. Hum Mol Genet 20: 3884–3892.
6. Guo X, Zhang Y, Li J, Ma J, Wei Z, et al. (2011) Strong influence of human leukocyte antigen (HLA)-DP gene variants on development of persistent chronic hepatitis B virus carriers in the Han Chinese population. Hepatology 53: 422–428.
7. Hu L, Zhai X, Liu J, Chu M, Pan S, et al. (2012) Genetic variants in human leukocyte antigen/DP-DQ influence both hepatitis B virus clearance and hepatocellular carcinoma development. Hepatology 55: 1426–1431.
8. An P, Winkler C, Guan L, O'Brien SJ, Zeng Z (2011) A common HLA-DPA1 variant is a major determinant of hepatitis B virus clearance in Han Chinese. J Infect Dis 203: 943–947.
9. Cheng HR, Liu CJ, Tseng TC, Su TH, Yang HI, et al. (2013) Host genetic factors affecting spontaneous HBsAg seroclearance in chronic hepatitis B patients. PLoS One 8: e53008.
10. Seto WK, Wong DK, Kopaniszen M, Proitsi P, Sham PC, et al. (2013) HLA-DP and IL28B polymorphisms: influence of host genome on hepatitis B surface antigen seroclearance in chronic hepatitis B. Clin Infect Dis 56: 1695–1703.
11. Li S, Qian J, Yang Y, Zhao W, Dai J, et al. (2012) GWAS identifies novel susceptibility loci on 6p21.32 and 21q21.3 for hepatocellular carcinoma in chronic hepatitis B virus carriers. PLoS Genet 8: e1002791.
12. Jiang DK, Sun J, Cao G, Liu Y, Lin D, et al. (2013) Genetic variants in STAT4 and HLA-DQ genes confer risk of hepatitis B virus-related hepatocellular carcinoma. Nat Genet 45: 72–75.
13. Zhang H, Zhai Y, Hu Z, Wu C, Qian J, et al. (2010) Genome-wide association study identifies 1p36.22 as a new susceptibility locus for hepatocellular carcinoma in chronic hepatitis B virus carriers. Nat Genet 42: 755–758.
14. Clark A, Gerlach F, Tong H, Hoan NX, Song le H, et al. (2013) A trivial role of STAT4 variant in chronic hepatitis B induced hepatocellular carcinoma. Infect Genet Evol 18: 257–261.
15. Chen K, Shi W, Xin Z, Wang H, Zhu X, et al. (2013) Replication of genome wide association studies on hepatocellular carcinoma susceptibility loci in a Chinese population. PLoS One 8: e77315.
16. Bruix J, Sherman M (2005) Management of hepatocellular carcinoma. Hepatology 42: 1208–1236.
17. Lok ASF, McMahon BJ (2007) Chronic hepatitis B. Hepatology 45: 507–539.
18. Stang A (2010) Critical evaluation of the Newcastle-Ottawa scale for the assessment of the quality of nonrandomized studies in meta-analyses. Eur J Epidemiol 25: 603–605.
19. Shi YY, He L (2005) SHEsis, a powerful software platform for analyses of linkage disequilibrium, haplotype construction, and genetic association at polymorphism loci. Cell Res 15: 97–98.
20. Li J, Yang D, He Y, Wang M, Wen Z, et al. (2011) Associations of HLA-DP variants with hepatitis B virus infection in southern and northern Han Chinese populations: a multicenter case-control study. PLoS One 6: e24221.
21. Al-Qahtani AA, Al-Anazi MR, Abdo AA, Sanai FM, Al-Hamoudi W, et al. (2014) Association between HLA Variations and Chronic Hepatitis B Virus Infection in Saudi Arabian Patients. PLoS One 9: e80445.
22. O'Brien TR, Kohaar I, Pfeiffer RM, Maeder D, Yeager M, et al. (2011) Risk alleles for chronic hepatitis B are associated with decreased mRNA expression of HLA-DPA1 and HLA-DPB1 in normal human liver. Genes Immun 12: 428–433.
23. Diaz G, Amicosante M, Jaraquemada D, Butler RH, Guillen MV, et al. (2003) Functional analysis of HLA-DP polymorphism: a crucial role for DPbeta residues 9, 11, 35, 55, 56, 69 and 84-87 in T cell allorecognition and peptide binding. Int Immunol 15: 565–576.
24. Zhang Q, Yin J, Zhang Y, Deng Y, Ji X, et al. (2013) HLA-DP polymorphisms affect the outcomes of chronic hepatitis B virus infections, possibly through interacting with viral mutations. J Virol 87: 12176–12186.
25. Thierfelder WE, van Deursen JM, Yamamoto K, Tripp RA, Sarawar SR, et al. (1996) Requirement for Stat4 in interleukin-12-mediated responses of natural killer and T cells. Nature 382: 171–174.
26. Nguyen KB, Watford WT, Salomon R, Hofmann SR, Pien GC, et al. (2002) Critical role for STAT4 activation by type 1 interferons in the interferon-gamma response to viral infection. Science 297: 2063–2066.
27. Yu H, Pardoll D, Jove R (2009) STATs in cancer inflammation and immunity: a leading role for STAT3. Nat Rev Cancer 9: 798–809.

Increased Expression of Cathepsin L: A Novel Independent Prognostic Marker of Worse Outcome in Hepatocellular Carcinoma Patients

Jian Ruan[1*§], Hang Zheng[1§], Wenguang Fu[2], Peng Zhao[3], Ning Su[4], Rongcheng Luo[1*]

1 Cancer Center, Traditional Chinese Medicine-Integrated Hospital, Southern medical University, Guangzhou, Guangdong, People's Republic of China, 2 Department of Hepatobiliary Surgery, The Affiliated Hospital of Luzhou Medical College, Luzhou, Sichuan, People's Republic of China, 3 Department of Medical Oncology, The First Affiliated Hospital, School of Medicine, Zhejiang University, Hangzhou, Zhejiang, People's Republic of China, 4 Department of Oncology, Guangzhou Chest Hospital, Guangzhou, Guangdong, People's Republic of China

Abstract

Objectives: To investigate the expression and role of Cathepsin L (CTSL) in Hepatocellular carcinoma (HCC) tissue and cell line (MHCC-97H), and to evaluate the clinical and prognostic significance of CTSL protein in patients with HCC.

Methods: The expression of CTSL was examined in HCC tissue and MHCC-97H cells by Western-blotting, Real-time PCR and immunohistochemical staining. Cell growth curve assay and colony formation assay were used to verify the effect of CTSL on the proliferation and tumor progression ability of MHCC-97H cells. Tumor formation assay in nude mice was used to analyze the effect of CTSL on the tumorigenicity of MHCC-97H cells.

Results: The status of CTSL protein in carcinoma tissues is much higher than that in paracarcinoma tissues. The overall survival of the patients with high CTSL expression was significantly shorter than the low CTSL expression group. high CTSL expression was significantly correlated with advanced clinical staging, histological grade and tumor recurrence. In vitro experiments demonstrated that over-expression of CTSL in MHCC-97H cells promoted cell proliferation and tumor progression ability. Down-regulation of CTSL showed the opposite effects. Over-expression of CTSL increase the tumorigenicity of MHCC-97H cells by in vivo experiments. Moreover, multivariate analysis suggested that CTSL expression might be an independent prognostic indicator for the survival of HCC patients after curative surgery.

Conclusions: CTSL might involve in the development and progression of HCC as a oncogene, and thereby may be a valuable prognostic marker for HCC patients.

Editor: William B. Coleman, University of North Carolina School of Medicine, United States of America

Funding: This project is supported by the National Natural Science Foundation of China (Grant No. 81001212), The Science and Technology Foundation of Zhejiang Province (Grant No. 2012C33011), Foundation of State Key Laboratory of Oncology in South China (Grant No. HN2011-03), Zhejiang Provincial Chinese Medicine Research Foundation (Grant No. 2010ZB062, 2011ZQ012), Foundation of Zhejiang Provincial Educational Committee (Grant No. Y201019175), and Natural Science Foundation of Guangdong (Grant No. s2012010008209). The funders had no role in the study design, data collection and analysis, decision to publish, or preparation of the manuscript.

Competing Interests: The authors have declared that no competing interests exist.

* Email: software23@163.com (JR); luorc0001@126.com (RCL)

§ These authors contributed equally to this work.

Introduction

Hepatocellular carcinoma (HCC) is a highly lethal cancer whose prognosis is poor. It ranks the third cause for cancer deaths in East Asia and sub-Saharan Africa, and the second for male cancer deaths in China [1]. Now, the incidence of HCC is also increasing in the United States and Europe [2]. Surgical resection remains to be the standard choice of treatment for patients in the early stage of HCC. However, even with radical resection, 60–70% of patients develop metastasis and recurrence within five years after surgery. Although several clinicopathological features including a poorly differentiated phenotype, large-sized tumor, and portal venous invasion have been found to contribute to the poor prognosis in HCC patients before operation, the underlying molecular mechanisms of the development of HCC remain unclear. Thus, it is urgent to study the pathogenesis of HCC.

CTSL, a lysosomal endopeptidase expressed in most eukaryotic cells, is a member of the papain-like family of cysteine proteinases [3]. Although commonly recognized as a lysosomal protease, CTSL is also secreted. This broad-spectrum protease is potent in degrading several extracellular proteins (laminins, fibronectin, collagens I and IV, elastin, and other structural proteins of basement membranes) as well as serum proteins and cytoplasmic and nuclear proteins [4]. CTSL plays a major role in antigen processing, tumor invasion and metastasis, bone resorption, and turnover of intracellular and secreted proteins involved in growth regulation [5,6,7,8,9,10,11,12]. Increased CTSL level was found in multiple tumor types and associated with short survival of several cancers [13,14,15,16,17,18,19].

However, no research on CTSL has been done in HCC so far. To explore the exact role of CTSL in HCC, we investigated whether the expression of CTSL protein is different between tumor tissues and normal tissues, whether CTSL has any role in the development and progression of HCC, and whether CTSL is a prognostic factor in HCC after curative surgical treatment.

Materials and Methods

Patients and Specimens

Fresh tumor tissue samples with paired non-cancerous liver tissue samples of 26 HCC patients were obtained in operation from the Nanfang hospital. A total of 82 paraffin-embedded HCC samples, which were histologically and clinically diagnosed in patients with radical surgery in Nan Fang hospital, between 2000 and 2003, were also included in this study. Resected specimens, fixed in 10% formalin solution and then embedded in paraffin, were longitudinally sliced into 4-mm-thick sections. Representative sections were prepared and stained with hematoxylin and eosin for histologic examination. Western-blot was used to confirm the specificity of CTSL staining in fresh HCC tissues with paired non-cancerous liver tissues and MHCC-97H cell line. None of these patients had received radiotherapy or chemotherapy prior to surgical treatment. Clinical and pathological data of the 82 patients with HCC were collected, such as age, tumor size, stage, differentiation grade and recurrence. The tumor stages were classified according to the 2002 TNM staging system of Union for International Cancer Control (UICC). Tumor differentiation was classified using the Edmondson grading system. Clinical follow-up information was obtained by telephone or from the outpatient records.

Written Ethics Approval and Patient Consent from the Nanfang Hospital Research Ethics Committee were obtained. Participants were recruited and human experimentation was conducted in Nanfang Hospital. We have obtained written informed consent from all participants involved in the study.

Cell Culture

The HCC cell lines MHCC-97H, MHCC-97L, Huh-7, HepG2, SMMC-7721, Bel-7404 and human colorectal carcinoma cell lines (CaCO2 and LoVo) were obtained from The Cell Bank of Type Culture Collection of Chinese Academy of Sciences. MHCC-97H cells were established from the cell line MHCC97. Spontaneous pulmonary metastasis occurred in 100% of recipient

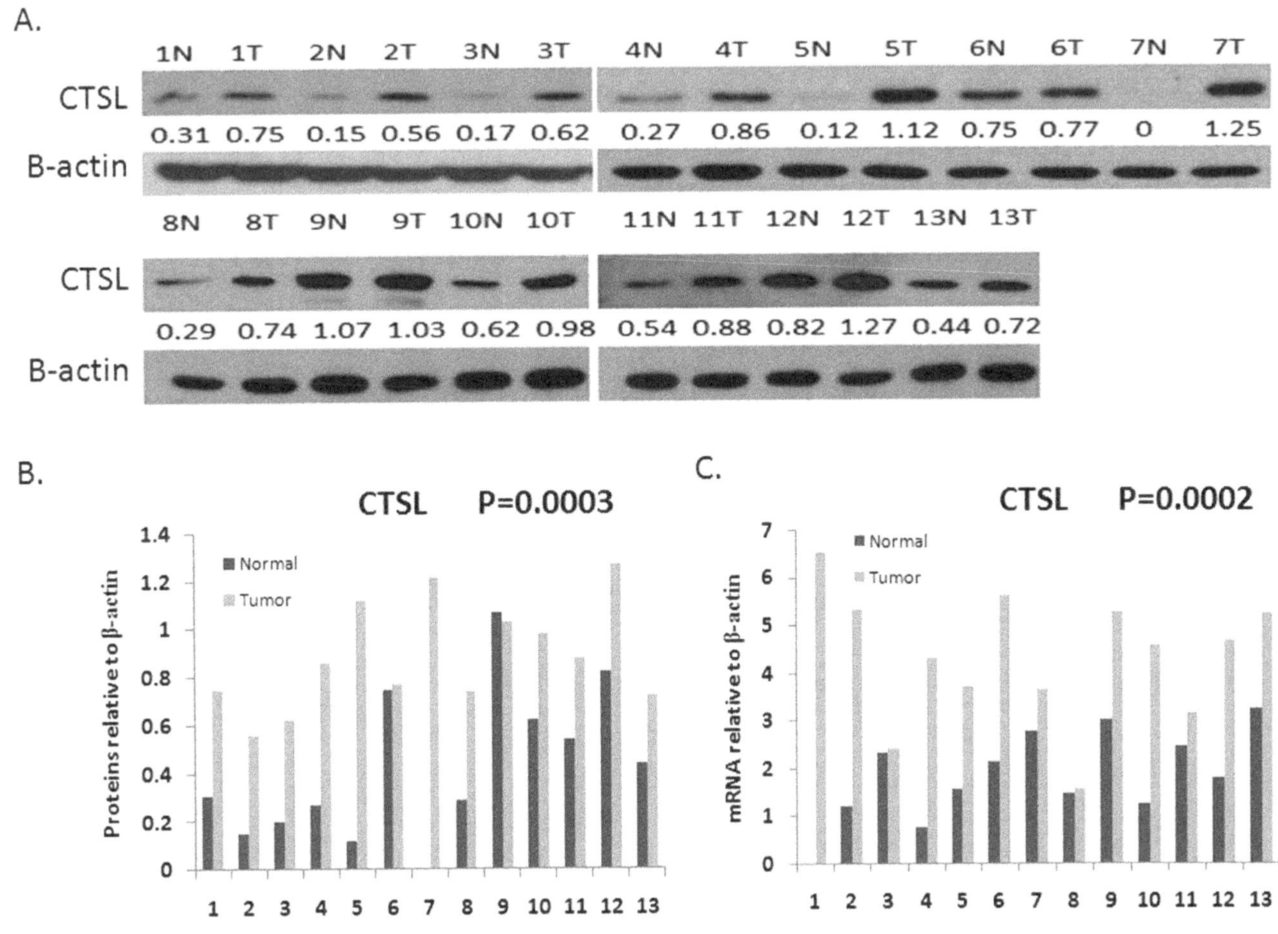

Figure 1. Expression levels of CTSL in HCC tissues. A. Expression levels of CTSL protein in 13 paired HCC tissues by Western blotting. N, paracarcinoma (normal) liver tissues. T, HCC tissues. B. Quantitative analysis of CTSL protein in 13 paired HCC tissues. C. mRNA levels of CTSL in 13 paired HCC tissues by real-time PCR.

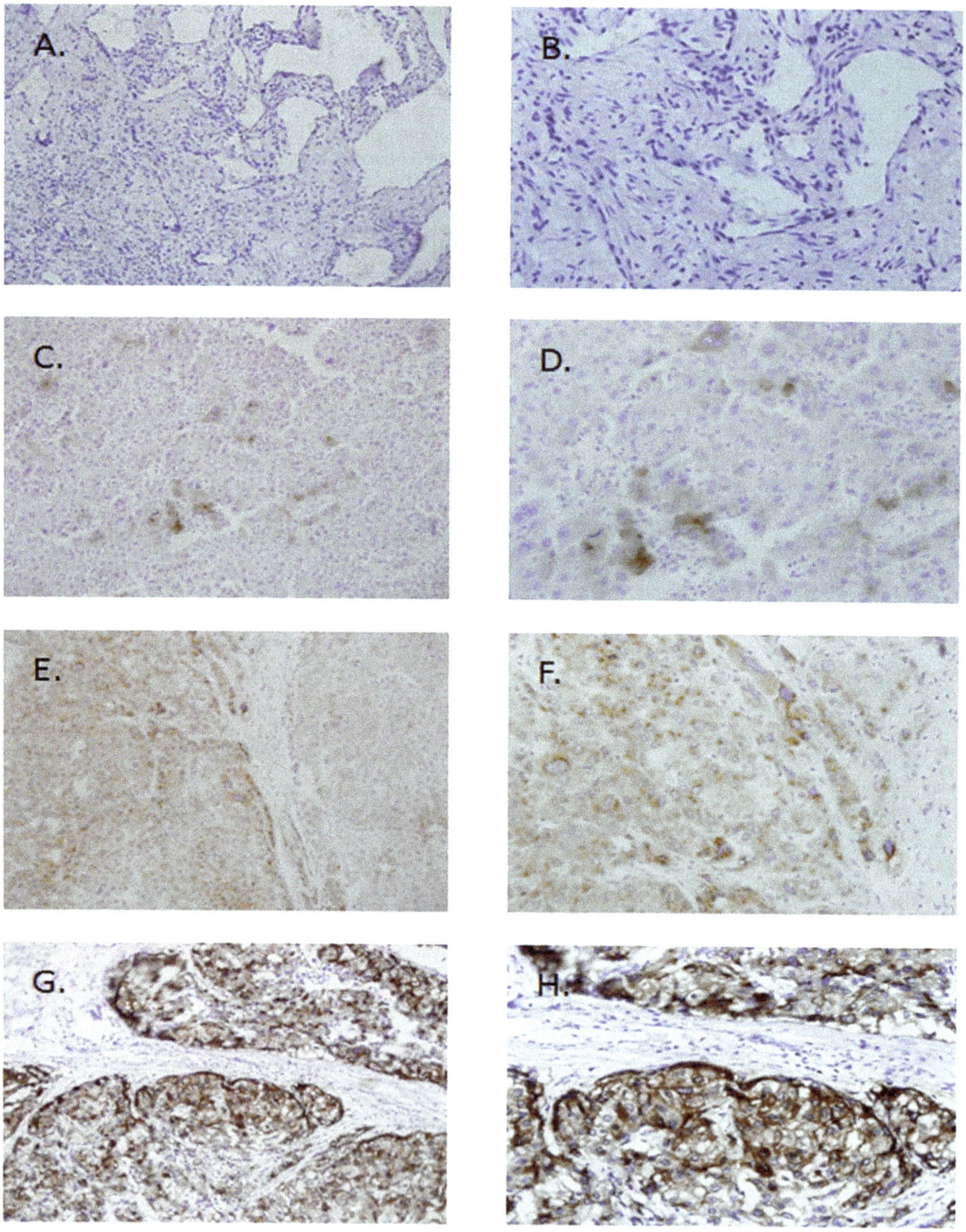

Figure 2. Analysis of CTSL protein in tissues by immunohistochemistry. A and B, CTSL expression is negative in normal liver cells. C and D, CTSL expression is weak in well-differentiated HCC cells. E and F, CTSL expression is moderate in moderately differentiated HCC cells. G and H, CTSL expression is strong in poorly differentiated HCC cells. (A, C, E, G ×200; B, D, F, H ×400).

nude mice after orthotopic inoculation of MHCC-97H. Cells were maintained in RPMI 1640 medium (Gibco, Invitrogen, Carlsbad, CA) supplemented with 10% fetal bovine serum (FBS; Hyclone, Logan, UT), penicillin (100 units/ml), and streptomycin (100 units/ml) at 37°C in humidified 5% CO_2 incubator.

Western Blotting Analysis

Cell and tissue samples were solubilized in SDS lysis buffer, and the protein concentrations were detected by the BCA protein assay kit (PIERCE, Rockford, IL). Equal amounts of protein samples (30 μg/lane) were separated by electrophoresis through 9.0% resolving SDS–polyacrylamide gel, and then transferred to PVDF membranes (Amersham Pharmacia Biotech Inc in Piscataway, NJ). Block the non-specific binding sites by immersing the

Table 1. Relationship between CTSL expression and clinicopathologic features of HCC patients.

Clinicopathologic parameters	n	CTSL expression		P value
		Positive (%)	Negative (%)	
All cases	82	47(57.3%)	35(42.7%)	
Gender				0.652
Male	61	32(52.5%)	29(47.5%)	
Female	21	15(71.4%)	6(28.6%)	
Age(years)				0.583
<50	58	30(51.7%)	28(48.3%)	
≥50	24	17(70.8%)	7(29.2%)	
Tumor size(cm)$^{\Delta}$				0.706
<5	47	26(55.3%)	21(44.7%)	
≥5	35	21(60.0%)	14(40.0%)	
Serum HBsAg				0.342
Positive	66	35(53.0%)	31(47.0%)	
Negative	16	12(75.0%)	4(25.0%)	
Serum AFP(ng/ml)				0.256
<25	30	14(46.7%)	16(53.3%)	
≥25	52	33(63.5%)	19(36.5%)	
Cirrhosis				0.019
Presence	64	40(62.5%)	24(37.5%)	
Absence	18	7(26.7%)	11(72.3%)	
UICC stage				0.026
I+II	59	35(59.3%)	24(40.7%)	
III+IV	23	12(52.2%)	11 (47.8%)	
Metastasis/Recurrence				0.001
Yes	58	40(69.0%)	18(31.0%)	
No	24	7(29.2%)	17(70.8%)	
Edmondson grade				0.007
Low (I/II)	62	32(51.6%)	30(48.4%)	
High (III/IV)	20	15(75.0%)	5(25.0%)	

Δ: The largest dimension of the tumor specimen.

membrane into 5% non-fat milk in TBST solution for 1 hr, and then incubate the membrane with a primary monoclonal antibody to CTSL (Santa Cruz Biotechnology) for 2 hr at room temperature (RT). After washing 3 times in with TBST (TBS+0.5% Tween-20), the membranes were incubated with a secondary antibody (diluted 1:1000 in TBS-T) for 1 hr at RT. The membranes were washed and proteins were detected by enhanced chemiluminescence system (Amersham Pharmacia Biotech) following manufacturer's instructions. Anti-GAPDH mouse monoclonal antibody was used to confirm equal loading of lysates (1:1000; Santa Cruz Biotechnology). Image J software was used to analyze the gray value.

Real-time RT-PCR Analysis

Total RNA from human tissues was extracted using Trizol reagent (Invitrogen) according to the manufacturer's instructions. cDNA was synthesized from 1 μg of total RNA by use of the SuperScript III First-Strand Synthesis System (Invitrogen). Real-time PCR was carried out using CFX96 Real-Time System (BIO-RAD). SYBR green 2× master mixture (Invitrogen) was used in a total volume of 10 μL. The primer sequences were as follows: CTSL sense 5′- CTGGTGGTTGGCTACGGATT-3′, antisense 5′-CTCCGGTCTTTGGCCATCTT-3′, GAPDH sense 5′-TGTTGCCATCAATGACCCCTT-3′, antisense 5′-CTCCACGACGTACTCAGCG-3′, GAPDH was used as an internal control. All reactions were run in triplicate in three independent experiments.

Immunohistochemical Analysis

Immunohistochemical (IHC) staining was performed using Dako Envision system (Dako, Carpinteria, CA) according to the manufacturer's instructions. The paraffin-embedded specimens were cut into 4 mm sections and baked 1 h at 65°C. All sections were deparaffined with xylenes and rehydrated through graded ethanol series to distilled water. Then, the sections were submerged into EDTA antigenic retrieval buffer (pH 8.0) and microwaved for antigenic retrieval. The sections were treated with 0.3% H_2O_2 for 15 min to block the endogenous peroxidase at RT, and then were treated with normal goat serum for 30 min to reduce the nonspecific binding. Consequently, the sections were incubated with rabbit polyclonal anti-CTSL antibody (1:50; Santa Cruz Biotechnology) overnight at 4°C. After washing, the sections

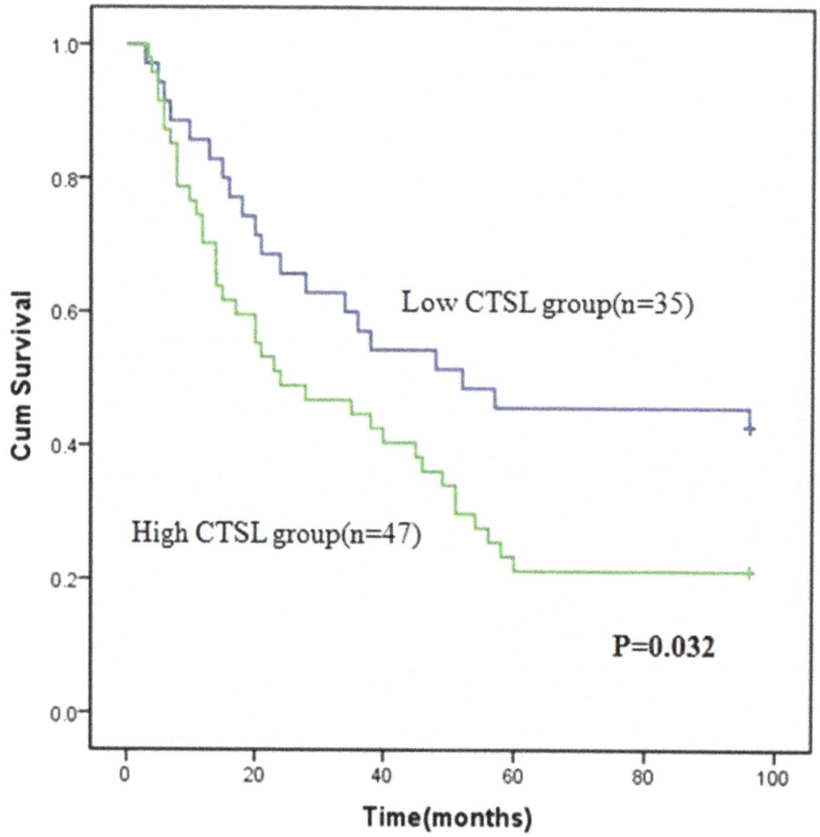

Figure 3. Survival curves for patients with high CTSL expression versus low CTSL-expressing carcinoma. The 5-year overall survival rate was 22.7% in the high CTSL protein expression group (green line), but it was only 41.4% in the low expression group (blue line), P = 0.032.

were incubated with biotinylated anti-goat secondary antibody (Zymed) followed by further incubation with streptavidin-horse-radish peroxidase (Zymed) at 37°C for 30 min. Diaminobenzidine (DAB) was used for color reaction, and the antibody was replaced by normal goat serum for negative controls.

The immunohistochemically stained tissue sections were scored independently by two pathologists blinded to the clinical parameters, and the final score was the average of the scores by two observers. We used the intensity and extent of the staining to evaluate the expression of CTSL. The staining intensity was scored as 0 (no staining), 1 (weak staining exhibited as light yellow), 2 (moderate staining exhibited as yellow brown), 3 (strong staining exhibited as brown). Extent of staining was scored as 0 (0%), 1 (1to 25%), 2 (26 to 50%), 3 (51 to 75%), and 4 (76 to 100%), according to the percentages of the positive staining areas relative to the whole carcinoma area or entire section for the normal samples. The sum of intensity and extent score was used as the final staining scores (0 to 7) for CTSL. For the purpose of statistical evaluation, tumors having a final staining score of <3 classified tumors with low CTSL expression and score >3 classified as high CTSL expression.

Vector construction and transfection

The pcDNA3.0 vector was used to generate pcDNA-CTSL. The CTSL shRNA Plasmid was purchased from Santa Cruz Biotechnology (Cat. No: sc-29939-SH). Vector transfection was performed according to the instructions, MHCC97H cells and CaCO2 cells were transfected with pcDNA expressing CTSL or empty vector and MHCC97H were also used to knock-down the expression of CTSL. MHCC97H cells and CaCO2 cells expressing CTSL or empty vector were selected for 14 days with G418 after infection. MHCC97H transfected with CTSL-shRNA was selected for 14 days with puromycin after infection.

Colony Formation Assay

For colony formation assay, cells were seeded evenly in 6-well plates (2×10^2 cells per well) and cultured for 14 days. Then the cells were fixed with methanol for 10 min, stained with 1% crystal violet for 1 min. Each group of cells was performed in triplicate.

3-(4, 5-dimethylthiazol-2-yl)-2, 5-diphenyltetrazolium Bromide Reduction (MTT) Assay

Cells were seeded into 96-well plates at 2000 cells/well. Each sample had four replicates. The cells were incubated with 0.2% MTT for 4 h at 37°C, 100 μl DMSO/well was added to the culture cells to dissolve the crystals, and cells were counted every day by reading the absorbance at 490 nm.

Tumor Formation in an Animal Model

Equivalent amounts of MHCC97H-CTSL cells and MHCC97H-Con cells (5×10^5 cells) were injected subcutaneously into the right flank of female BALB/c nude mice (Shanghai Slac Laboratory Animal Co. Ltd, Shanghai, China) at 5 weeks of age (15–17.5 g). Tumorigenesis procedure was observed by measuring solid tumors in 3 dimensions with a caliper for 21 days. Animals

Table 2. Univariate survival analysis of 82 patients with HCC.

Variable	n	Overall survival		*P* value
		2-year	5-year	
CTSL expression				0.032
Positive	47	50.3%	22.7%	
Negative	35	64.3%	41.4%	
Gender				0.421
Male	61	62.2%	38.6%	
Female	21	64.1%	40.0%	
Age(years)				0.022
<50	58	67.6%	48.5%	
≥50	24	53.2%	30.3%	
Tumor size(cm)$^{\Delta}$				0.015
<5	47	65.7%	42.1%	
≥5	35	52.6%	31.7%	
Serum HBsAg				0.103
Positive	66	62.3%	33.9%	
Negative	16	65.1%	37.1%	
Serum AFP(ng/ml)				0.001
<25	30	72.2%	42.3%	
≥25	52	54.1%	21.8%	
Cirrhosis				0.093
Presence	64	63.4%	32.5%	
Absence	18	69.8%	37.2%	
UICC stage				0.001
I+II	59	72.4%	40.1%	
III+IV	23	54.6%	22.5%	
Metastasis/Recurrence				0.000
Yes	58	50.4%	22.1%	
No	24	65.2%	34.6%	
Edmondson grade				0.017
Low (I/II)	62	70.3%	43.1%	
High (III/IV)	20	60.4%	36.8%	

Δ: The largest dimension of the tumor specimen.

Table 3. Cox regression analysis of patients with HCC.

Variables	Univariate		*P* value
	HR	CI(95%)	
CTSL expression(1 = down, 2 = over)	3.025	2.297~4.067	0.002
Gender(1 = male, 2 = female)	0.342	0.113~1.146	0.091
Age(1<50, 2≥50)	0.676	0.412~1.412	0.352
Serum HBsAg(1 = negative, 2 = positive)	1.466	0.523~3.736	0.401
Serum AFP(1<25 ng/ml, 2≥25 ng/ml)	2.012	1.152~3.712	0.017
Tumor size(1<5 cm, 2≥5 cm)	1.756	1.218~3.321	0.039
Cirrhosis(1 = Absence, 2 = Presence)	1.365	0.643~2.789	0.302
Metastasis/Recurrence(1 = no, 2 = yes)	3.345	1.730~6.125	0.000
UICC stage(1 = I+II, 2 = III+IV)	2.141	1.121~3.568	0.031
Edmondson grade(1 = High (III/IV), 2 = Low (I/II))	0.739	0.361~1.536	0.563

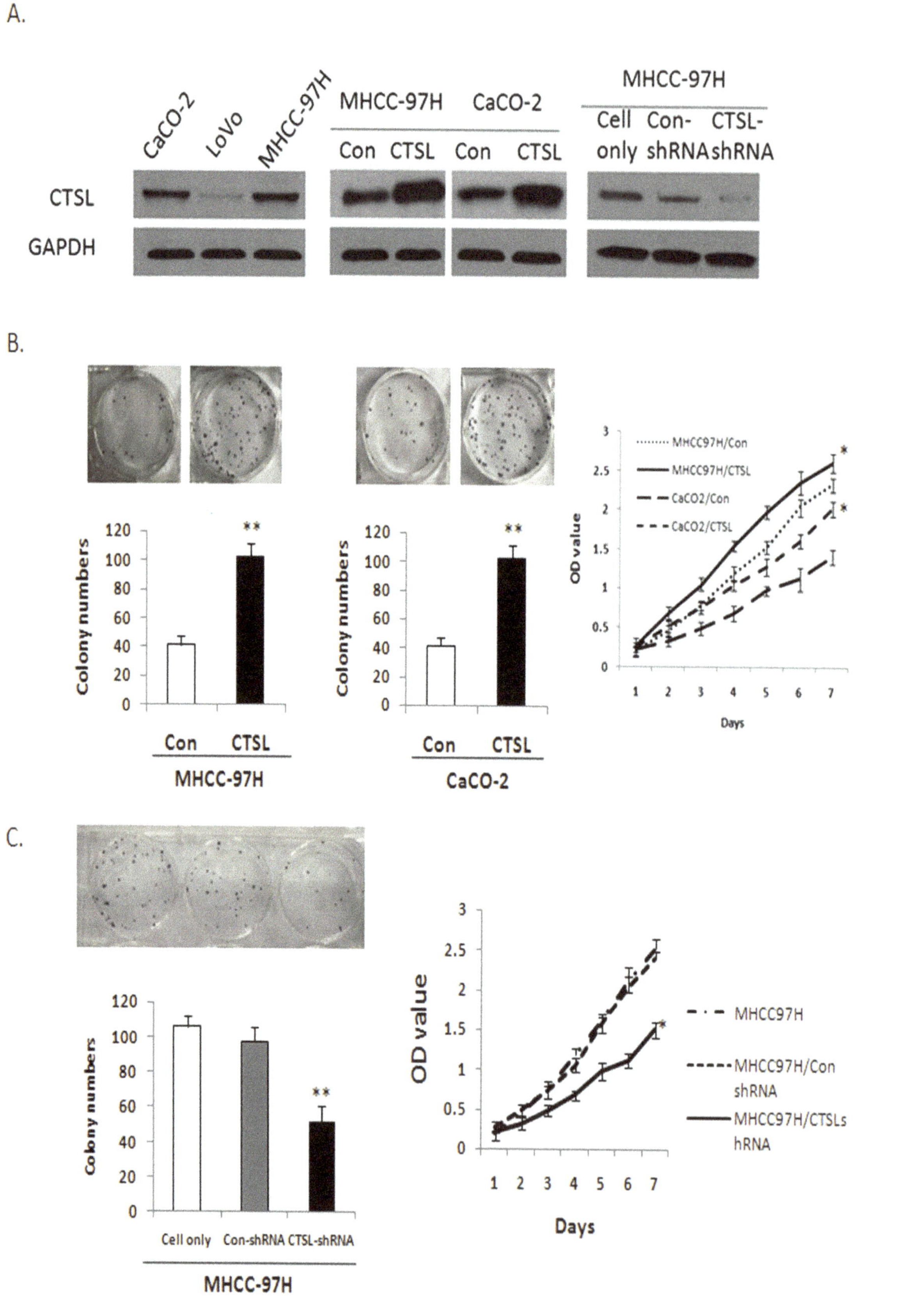

Figure 4. The effect of CTSL on the proliferation and tumor progression ability of MHCC-97H cells. A. Western blotting analysis of CTSL protein expression in HCC cell line (MHCC-97H), colorectal carcinoma cell lines (CaCO2 and LoVo), stably CTSL-expressed MHCC-97H cell line, stably CTSL-expressed CaCO2 cell line, empty vector stable cell lines (MHCC-97H-Con or CaCO2-Con), and MHCC-97H cell line transfected by CTSL-shRNA or Con-shRNA. B. Colony formation assay and MTT assay of MHCC-97H cells and CaCO2 cells with over-expression of CTSL. (Colony formation assay:

MHCC-97H-Con (vector) vs MHCC-97H-CTSL, P = 0.0042; CaCO2-Con (vector) vs CaCO2-CTSL, P = 0.0072. MTT: MHCC-97H-Con (vector) vs MHCC-97H-CTSL, P = 0.012; CaCO2-Con (vector) vs CaCO2-CTSL, P = 0.035). C. Colony formation assay and MTT assay of MHCC-97H cells with down-regulated CTSL. (Colony formation assay: MHCC-97H-Con-shRNA vs MHCC-97H-CTSL-shRNA, P = 0.003; MTT: MHCC-97H-Con-shRNA vs MHCC-97H-CTSL-shRNA, P = 0.001. (**P<0.01 as compared to parental groups, *P<0.05 as compared to parental groups).

were sacrificed 21 days after injection. The experiments on mice had been approved by the ethics committee at Nanfang hospital.

Statistical Analysis

Statistical analyses were performed using a statistical software package (SPSS13.0, Chicago, IL). The significance of CTSL mRNA levels was determined by t-test. The chi-square test was used to analyze the relationship between CTSL expression and clinicopathological characteristics. Survival times were evaluated using the Kaplan and Meier survival curves, and compared by the log-rank test. The significance of various variables for survival was analyzed by multivariate survival analysis using Cox's regression model. P-value less than or equal to 5 percent were considered to be statistically significant.

Results

The Expression of CTSL in HCC Tissues

To determine the expression of CTSL protein in HCC tissues, Western blotting was performed in 13 HCC tissues with paired non-cancerous tissues. Among 11 of 13 HCC tissues with paired normal tissues, clearly increased levels of CTSL expression was detected in all the tumors tissues in comparison to the paired non-cancerous tissues (Figure 1A and 1B). However, the levels of CTSL expression were similar in both tumors tissues and non-cancerous tissues in the rest 2 paired HCC tissues (Figure 1A, patient samples No. 6 and No. 9). We then determined whether the increased expression of CTSL occurred at mRNA level. We obtained an extra 13 paired HCC samples for real-time RT-PCR analysis. As shown in Figure 1C, the expression level of CTSL mRNA is significantly higher in tumor tissues. These data suggested that CTSL might serve as a oncogene in HCC.

To verify this observation, we further examined the expression of CTSL protein in 82 paraffin-embedded HCC samples and 16 normal liver (non-cancerous) samples by immunohistochemical analysis. As shown by immunohistochemical analysis, 35 of 82 (42.7%) paraffin-embedded HCC tissues showed weak or negative staining of CTSL protein, while 30 of 82 (36.6%) HCC tissues showed mainly moderate CTSL staining (in the membrane and cytoplasm of cancer cell) and 17 of 82 (20.7%) showed strong staining in tumor cells. Thirteen of the 16 non-cancerous tissues indicated negative staining of CTSL and the rest two non-cancerous tissues showed weak expression (Figure 2).

Additionally, the incidence of CTSL protein expression in well-differentiated carcinoma was significantly lower than that in poor-differentiated tumors, and CTSL expression was significantly related with tumor differentiation (P = 0.007) (Table 1).

Correlation of CTSL Expression with Clinicopathological Features and Outcomes

The association between CTSL expression and the clinicopathological outcomes is shown in Table 1. CTSL expression was significantly correlated with liver cirrhosis, stage, Recurrence and tumor differentiation. There was no significant correlation between CTSL expression and age, gender, Tumor size, Serum HBsAg or Serum AFP (Table 1).

Correlation of CTSL Expression with Overall Survival

The median follow-up time for overall survival was 78 months for all patients. The 2-year and 5-year overall rates for all patients were 65.6% and 33.6%, respectively. Among these patients, the overall survival of the patients with low CTSL expression (5-year overall rate, 41.4%) was significantly higher than the high CTSL expression group (5-year overall rate, 22.7%) (P = 0.032, Figure 3). Besides CTSL expression level, age, tumor size, serum AFP, stage, tumor recurrence and tumor differentiation were also significantly correlated with overall survival in univariate analysis (Table 2). Furthermore, overall survival was possibly correlated with liver Cirrhosis (P = 0.093).

The Cox proportional hazards mode was employed to evaluate the effects of the independent factors on overall survival. These factors include CTSL expression, gender, age, tumor size, Serum HBsAg, serum AFP, tumor size, liver cirrhosis, stage, tumor recurrence and tumor differentiation. The results showed that CTSL expression, serum AFP, tumor size, tumor recurrence and stage were recognized as independent prognostic factors of survival (Table 3). Therefore, Multivariate analysis indicated that CTSL protein expression has a significant correlation with poor prognosis of HCC patients as an independent factor.

CTSL Might Affect the Proliferation and Tumor Progression Ability of MHCC-97H Cells

The protein levels of CTSL of six HCC cell lines were shown in Fig. S1. The data showed that MHCC-97H expressed highest level of CTSL protein and thus was chosen for further study on the biological function of CTSL. In addition, as shown in Figure 4A, the expression level of CTSL was high in MHCC-97H and CaCO2 cells compared to LoVo cells. To further investigate whether CTSL could enhance the proliferation and tumor progression ability of HCC cells (MHCC-97H) and colorectal cancer cell lines (CaCO2), we established stable MHCC-97H cell line and CaCO2 cell line that expressed CTSL (MHCC-97H-CTSL or CaCO2-CTSL) or empty vector (MHCC-97H-Con or CaCO2-Con). Over-expression of CTSL promoted cell proliferation and malignant transforming ability of MHCC-97H cells and CaCO2 cells by colony formation assay and MTT assay (Figure 4B). To further investigate the effect of CTSL in the proliferation and malignant transforming ability of HCC cells (MHCC-97H), we established stable MHCC-97H cell lines with down-regulation of CTSL by shRNA sequences against CTSL (MHCC-97H-CTSL-shRNA). As shown in Figure 4A, the expression level of CTSL was significantly decreased in MHCC-97H-CTSL-shRNA cells compared to control cells (MHCC-97H-Con-shRNA). Knocking-down of CTSL in MHCC-97H cells decreased malignant transforming ability and cell proliferation (Figure 4C), suggesting that over-expression of CTSL might involve in the development of HCC.

Over-expression of CTSL promoted the Tumor Growth in Nude Mice

In vivo experiment was performed to evaluate the effect of CTSL over-expression in nude mice. As shown in Figure 5A and 5B, the growth rate and tumor weight of CTSL tumors were found to be much higher than those with control (MHCC-97H-Con). As

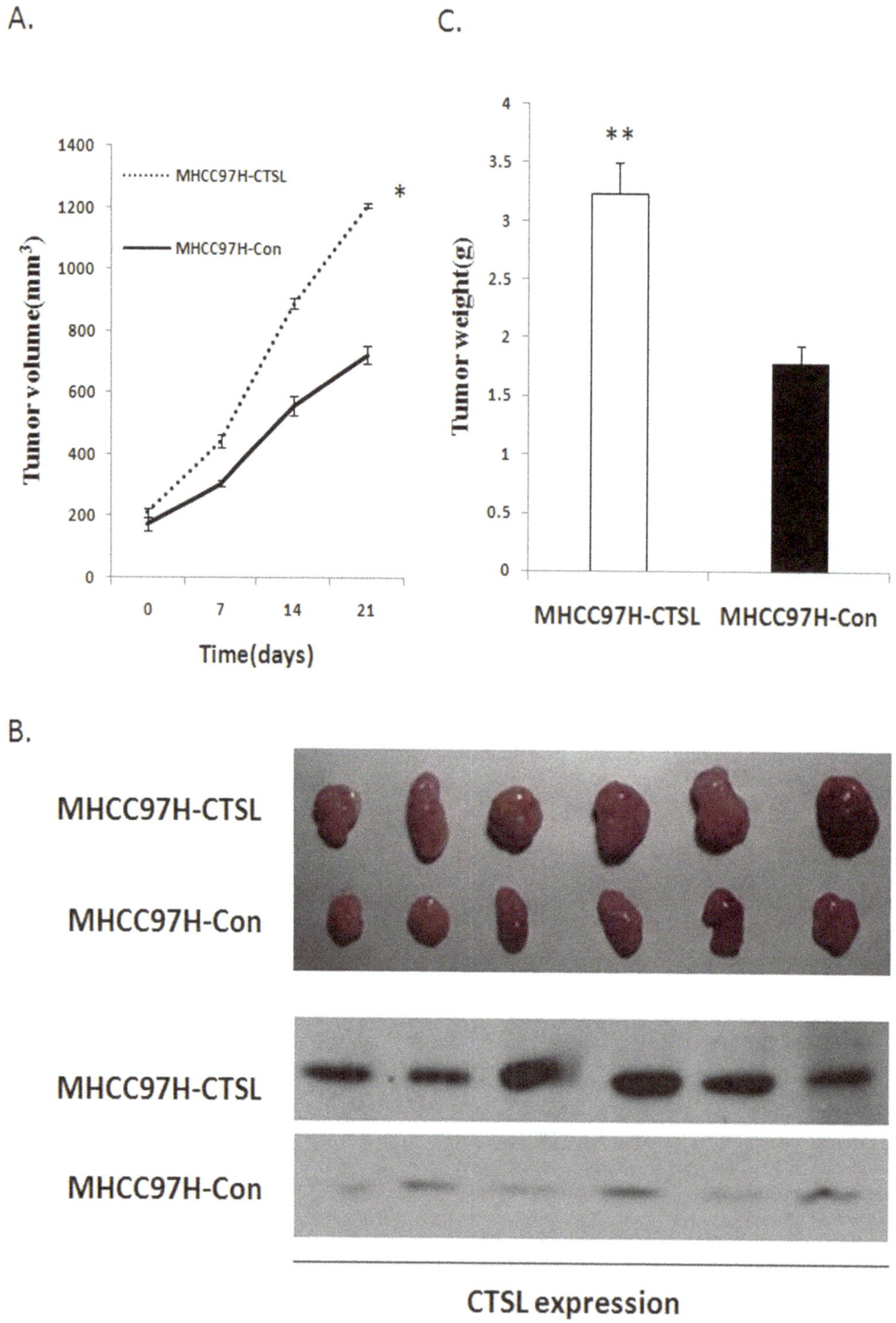

Figure 5. Effect of CTSL knockdown on subcutaneous tumorigencity of MHCC-97H. A. Tumor growth curve of after injection of nude mice with CTSL or control vector expressing MHCC-97H cells. ($P<0.001$) B. The picture of tumors from nude mice with CTSL or control vector expressing MHCC-97H cells. C. The weight of tumors from nude mice with CTSL or control vector expressing MHCC-97H cells ($P=0.005$). (**$P<0.01$ as compared to control groups, *$P<0.05$ as compared to control groups).

shown in Figure.5C, a remarkable increase of tumor size of groups MHCC-97H-CTSL was observed as compared with that of the control group. The result suggested that over-expression of CTSL promoted tumorigenicity of MHCC-97H cells in vivo.

Discussion

The occurrence and development of HCC are a comprehensive pathologic process involving complex alterations in oncogenes and tumor suppressor genes, which play roles in cell proliferation, cell-cycle control and cell apoptosis through regulation of multiple signal transduction pathways.

The first observed function of CTSL in cancer progression was its ability to promote cancer metastasis [20]. Early experimental studies revealed that the metastatic capability of tumor cells was correlated with CTSL activity. For example, subpopulations of high metastatic potential of murine B16 melanoma cell lines were found to express higher levels of CTSL when compared to their low-metastatic counterparts [21]. The invasive ability of brain tumor cells was markedly reduced by full-length antisense cDNA of CTSL [12]. Moreover, the finding that CTSL contribute to anti-apoptosis is also a well accepted observation experimentally. Enhanced susceptibility of CTSL-deficient A549 lung cells to spontaneous and anti-Fas-induced apoptosis was reported, with a possible mechanism involving altered Cathepsin D processing by CTSL [22]. However, Up to now, little has been known about whether CTSL is involved in HCC progression. Thus, in this study, we tried to investigate the role of CTSL on the development of HCC.

As shown by immunohistochemical analysis in our study, 20.7% paraffin-embedded HCC cancer tissues showed strong membrane and cytoplasm staining of CTSL, 36.6% HCC tissues showed moderate CTSL staining and 42.7% showed negative staining in tumor cells, while the non-cancerous tissues presented mainly negative expression of CTSL, indicating that CTSL might play an important role in the development and progression of HCC. In addition, as determined by immunohistochemistry, the incidence of CTSL protein expression in poor-differentiated carcinoma was significantly higher than that in well-differentiated tumors, suggesting that high level of CTSL expression was related to poor tumor differentiation. Additionally, we have shown that CTSL expression was correlated with liver cirrhosis, stage, Recurrence and tumor differentiation. There was no significant correlation between CTSL expression and age, gender, Tumor size, Serum HBsAg or Serum AFP. Our study suggests that high level of CTSL expression might be positively correlated with worse tumor biological features, such as rapid tumor progression and metastases, and that CTSL plays an important role in the development and progression of HCC. Furthermore, we have shown by multivariate analyses that patients with CTSL protein expression in carcinoma had a poor prognosis than those without CTSL expression, and that serum AFP, tumor size, tumor recurrence and stage and the status of CTSL protein were independent factors influencing overall survival, indicating that CTSL is a powerful prognostic index of survival in HCC. These findings also suggested that clinicopathological features together with detection of CTSL in HCC tissue could be valuable in evaluating prognosis or designing individual therapeutic policy for HCC.

In spite of the potential significance of CTSL in HCC, functional role of CTSL in HCC have not been clearly defined. Demonstration of its oncogenic activity in HCC is still lacking. To understand the functions of CTSL, the endogenous CTSL expression in an HCC cell line (MHCC-97H) was silenced by shRNA. Cell properties of the CTSL-depleted cells were then analyzed and compared with the control cells in various functional assays. The results showed that CTSL knockdown stable clones displayed suppressed cell proliferation ability. Additionally, over-expression of CTSL promoted the aggressive behaviors of MHCC-97H cells. Our study has also provided the first validation about the oncogenic capacity of CTSL expression in vivo. MHCC-97H with high level of CTSL expression displayed increased ability to form tumors in nude mice. All these studies affirmed our findings that CTSL exerts oncogenic effect on MHCC-97H cells.

CTSL expression status, combined with clinicopathological features and other biomarkers of HCC, may be useful to stratify patients for individual treatment, such as those of chemotherapy or TACE(Transcatheter Arterial Chemoembolization). Further investigation in other patient population or group is required to verify these hypotheses. Since the number of the cases in this study was not too big, the relationship between CTSL expression and metastases still requires to be evaluated. A recent study showed that CTSL might promote chemoresistance by their ability to resist various apoptotic stimuli in glioblastoma Cells, however the study was about brain cancer and the case scale was small [8]. Therefore, further studies are needed to clarify the mechanisms by which CTSL is involved in the development and progression of HCC.

Altogether, this study show that the first evidences of the expression and clinical significance of CTSL in HCC, suggesting that CTSL might involve in the development of HCC as a tumor promoter, and thereby may serve as a valuable prognostic marker for HCC patients.

Acknowledgments

We gratefully thank Chengwei Lv from the cancer biotherapy center for the collection and maintenance of the cell lines used in this research.

Author Contributions

Conceived and designed the experiments: JR HZ PZ NS. Performed the experiments: JR HZ PZ NS. Analyzed the data: JR HZ PZ NS WF. Contributed reagents/materials/analysis tools: JR HZ PZ NS. Contributed to the writing of the manuscript: JR HZ RCL.

References

1. Tung-Ping PR, Fan ST, Wong J (2000) Risk factors, prevention, and management of postoperative recurrence after resection of hepatocellular carcinoma. Ann Surg 232: 10–24.
2. Capocaccia R, Sant M, Berrino F, Simonetti A, Santi V, et al. (2007) Hepatocellular carcinoma: trends of incidence and survival in Europe and the United States at the end of the 20th century. Am J Gastroenterol 102: 1661–1670, 1660, 1671.
3. Kirschke H, Langner J, Wiederanders B, Ansorge S, Bohley P (1977) Cathepsin L. A new proteinase from rat-liver lysosomes. Eur J Biochem 74: 293–301.
4. Reiser J, Adair B, Reinheckel T (2010) Specialized roles for cysteine cathepsins in health and disease. J Clin Invest 120: 3421–3431.
5. Kane SE, Gottesman MM (1990) The role of cathepsin L in malignant transformation. Semin Cancer Biol 1: 127–136.
6. Kenig S, Frangez R, Pucer A, Lah T (2011) Inhibition of cathepsin L lowers the apoptotic threshold of glioblastoma cells by up-regulating p53 and transcription of caspases 3 and 7. Apoptosis 16: 671–682.
7. Zheng X, Chu F, Chou PM, Gallati C, Dier U, et al. (2009) Cathepsin L inhibition suppresses drug resistance in vitro and in vivo: a putative mechanism. Am J Physiol Cell Physiol 296: C65–C74.
8. Zajc I, Hreljac I, Lah T (2006) Cathepsin L affects apoptosis of glioblastoma cells: a potential implication in the design of cancer therapeutics. Anticancer Res 26: 3357–3364.

9. Jean D, Rousselet N, Frade R (2006) Expression of cathepsin L in human tumor cells is under the control of distinct regulatory mechanisms. Oncogene 25: 1474–1484.
10. Strojnik T, Kavalar R, Trinkaus M, Lah TT (2005) Cathepsin L in glioma progression: comparison with cathepsin B. Cancer Detect Prev 29: 448–455.
11. Colella R, Casey SF (2003) Decreased activity of cathepsins L+B and decreased invasive ability of PC3 prostate cancer cells. Biotech Histochem 78: 101–108.
12. Levicar N, Dewey RA, Daley E, Bates TE, Davies D, et al. (2003) Selective suppression of cathepsin L by antisense cDNA impairs human brain tumor cell invasion in vitro and promotes apoptosis. Cancer Gene Ther 10: 141–151.
13. Jagodic M, Vrhovec I, Borstnar S, Cufer T (2005) Prognostic and predictive value of cathepsins D and L in operable breast cancer patients. Neoplasma 52: 1–9.
14. Sullivan S, Tosetto M, Kevans D, Coss A, Wang L, et al. (2009) Localization of nuclear cathepsin L and its association with disease progression and poor outcome in colorectal cancer. Int J Cancer 125: 54–61.
15. Xu X, Yuan G, Liu W, Zhang Y, Chen W (2009) Expression of cathepsin L in nasopharyngeal carcinoma and its clinical significance. Exp Oncol 31: 102–105.
16. Macabeo-Ong M, Shiboski CH, Silverman S, Ginzinger DG, Dekker N, et al. (2003) Quantitative analysis of cathepsin L mRNA and protein expression during oral cancer progression. Oral Oncol 39: 638–647.
17. Miyamoto K, Iwadate M, Yanagisawa Y, Ito E, Imai J, et al. (2011) Cathepsin L is highly expressed in gastrointestinal stromal tumors. Int J Oncol 39: 1109–1115.
18. Yan JA, Xiao H, Ji HX, Shen WH, Zhou ZS, et al. (2010) Cathepsin L is associated with proliferation and clinical outcome of urothelial carcinoma of the bladder. J Int Med Res 38: 1913–1922.
19. Niedergethmann M, Wostbrock B, Sturm JW, Willeke F, Post S, et al. (2004) Prognostic impact of cysteine proteases cathepsin B and cathepsin L in pancreatic adenocarcinoma. Pancreas 29: 204–211.
20. Chauhan SS, Goldstein LJ, Gottesman MM (1991) Expression of cathepsin L in human tumors. Cancer Res 51: 1478–1481.
21. Yang Z, Cox JL (2007) Cathepsin L increases invasion and migration of B16 melanoma. Cancer Cell Int 7: 8.
22. Wille A, Gerber A, Heimburg A, Reisenauer A, Peters C, et al. (2004) Cathepsin L is involved in cathepsin D processing and regulation of apoptosis in A549 human lung epithelial cells. Biol Chem 385: 665–670.

Permissions

All chapters in this book were first published in PLOS ONE, by The Public Library of Science; hereby published with permission under the Creative Commons Attribution License or equivalent. Every chapter published in this book has been scrutinized by our experts. Their significance has been extensively debated. The topics covered herein carry significant findings which will fuel the growth of the discipline. They may even be implemented as practical applications or may be referred to as a beginning point for another development.

The contributors of this book come from diverse backgrounds, making this book a truly international effort. This book will bring forth new frontiers with its revolutionizing research information and detailed analysis of the nascent developments around the world.

We would like to thank all the contributing authors for lending their expertise to make the book truly unique. They have played a crucial role in the development of this book. Without their invaluable contributions this book wouldn't have been possible. They have made vital efforts to compile up to date information on the varied aspects of this subject to make this book a valuable addition to the collection of many professionals and students.

This book was conceptualized with the vision of imparting up-to-date information and advanced data in this field. To ensure the same, a matchless editorial board was set up. Every individual on the board went through rigorous rounds of assessment to prove their worth. After which they invested a large part of their time researching and compiling the most relevant data for our readers.

The editorial board has been involved in producing this book since its inception. They have spent rigorous hours researching and exploring the diverse topics which have resulted in the successful publishing of this book. They have passed on their knowledge of decades through this book. To expedite this challenging task, the publisher supported the team at every step. A small team of assistant editors was also appointed to further simplify the editing procedure and attain best results for the readers.

Apart from the editorial board, the designing team has also invested a significant amount of their time in understanding the subject and creating the most relevant covers. They scrutinized every image to scout for the most suitable representation of the subject and create an appropriate cover for the book.

The publishing team has been an ardent support to the editorial, designing and production team. Their endless efforts to recruit the best for this project, has resulted in the accomplishment of this book. They are a veteran in the field of academics and their pool of knowledge is as vast as their experience in printing. Their expertise and guidance has proved useful at every step. Their uncompromising quality standards have made this book an exceptional effort. Their encouragement from time to time has been an inspiration for everyone.

The publisher and the editorial board hope that this book will prove to be a valuable piece of knowledge for researchers, students, practitioners and scholars across the globe.

List of Contributors

Guoliang Qiao, Jun Li and Feng Shen
Department of Hepatic Surgery, Eastern Hepatobiliary Surgery Hospital, Second Military Medical University, Shanghai, China

Yuan Le and Lianghuan Wang
Department of Biochemistry and Molecular Biology, Second Military Medical University, Shanghai, China

Qi Zhao, Juan Liu and Chengyong Qin
Department of Gastroenterology, Provincial Hospital Affiliated to Shandong University, Jinan, China

Tao Li
Department of Infectious Diseases, Provincial Hospital Affiliated to Shandong University, Jinan, China

Jianni Qi
Central Laboratory, Shandong Provincial Hospital affiliated to Shandong University, Jinan, China

Sandhya V. G. Nair, Ziaullah and H. P. Vasantha Rupasinghe
Department of Environmental Sciences, Faculty of Agriculture, Dalhousie University, Truro, Nova Scotia, Canada

Zhihua Ren, Wenhong Jiang and Yongping Jiang
Biopharmagen Corp., Suzhou, China

Yanan Wang
Department of Laboratory Diagnosis, Suzhou Municipal Hospital Affiliated Nanjing Medical University, Suzhou, China

Zhihua Ren, Wei Dai and Yongping Jiang
Biopharmaceutical R&D Center, Chinese Academy of Medical Sciences & Peking Union Medical College, Suzhou, China

Wei Dai
Department of Environmental Medicine, New York University Langone Medical Center, Tuxedo, New York, United States of America

Jian-Hong Zhong, Yang Ke, Yan-Yan Wang, Liang Ma, Jie Chen, Xue-Mei You, Zhi-Yuan Zhang, Shi-Dong Lu and Le-Qun Li
Hepatobiliary Surgery Department, Affiliated Tumor Hospital of Guangxi Medical University, Nanning, PR China

Hang Li
Ultrasound Department, Affiliated Tumor Hospital of Guangxi Medical University, Nanning, PR China

Nan Xiao
Department of General Surgery Education, Guangxi Medical University, Nanning, PR China

Xin-Ping Ye
Hepatobiliary Surgery Department, the First Affiliated Hospital of Guangxi Medical University, Nanning, PR China

Yoshiki Murakami, Masaru Enomoto, Akihiro Tamori and Norifumi Kawada
Department of Hepatology, Osaka City University Graduate School of Medicine, Osaka, Japan

Toshihito Tanahashi
Department of Medical Pharmaceutics, Kobe Pharmaceutical University, Kobe, Japan

Toshihito Tanahashi, Rina Okada and Takeshi Azuma
Division of Gastroenterology, Department of Internal Medicine, Kobe University Graduate School of Medicine, Kobe, Japan

Hidenori Toyoda and Takashi Kumada
Department of Gastroenterology, Ogaki Municipal Hospital, Ogaki, Japan

Y-h Taguchi
Department of Physics, Chuo University, Tokyo, Japan

Somenath Datta, Alip Ghosh, Debanjali Dasgupta, Amit Ghosh, Shrabasti Roychoudhury, Soumyojit Das, Kausik Das, Keya Basu, Simanti Datta, Abhijit Chowdhury and Soma Banerjee
Centre for Liver Research, Institute of Post Graduate Medical Education & Research, Kolkata, India

Gaurav Roy
Molecular Virology Laboratory, Department of Biotechnology, Jamia Millia Islamia, New Delhi, India

Subash Gupta
Centre for Liver & Biliary Surgery, Indraprastha Apollo Hospital, New Delhi, India

Analabha Basu
National Institute of Biomedical Genomics, Kalyani, India

Youwen Tan, Guohong Ge, Tengli Pan, Danfeng Wen, Li Chen, Xuejun Yu and Xinbei Zhou
Department of Hepatosis, The Third Hospital of Zhenjiang Affiliated Jiangsu University, Zhenjiang, China

Youwen Tan and Jianhe Gan
Department of Infectious Diseases, The First Affiliated Hospital of Soochow University, Suzhou, China

Boyoung Park, Kyu-Won Jung, Chang-Mo Oh, Kui Son Choi, Mina Suh and Jae Kwan Jun
National Cancer Control Institute, National Cancer Center, Goyang-si, Korea

Zhiping Huang
Department of hepatopancreatobiliary Surgery, Yongchuan Hospital, Chongqing Medical University, Yongchuan, Chongqing, China

Peng Zhang, Haiqing Wang, Lunan Yan and Wentao Wang
Department of Liver Surgery, Liver Transplantation Center, West China Hospital of Sichuan University, Chengdu, Sichuan Province, China

Darren M. Hutt and Daniela Martino Roth
Department of Cell and Molecular Biology, The Scripps Research Institute, La Jolla, California, United States of America

Hélène Vignaud, Christophe Cullin and Marion Bouchecareilh
Institut de Biochimie et Génétique Cellulaires, CNRS UMR 5095, Université de Bordeaux, Bordeaux, France

Hyunsoo Kim, Jiyoung Park and Youngsoo Kim
Department of Biomedical Sciences, Seoul National University College of Medicine, Seoul, Republic of Korea

Kyunggon Kim, Jonghwa Jin and Youngsoo Kim
Department of Biomedical Engineering, Seoul National University College of Medicine, Seoul, Republic of Korea

Su Jong Yu and Jung-Hwan Yoon
Department of Internal Medicine, Seoul National University College of Medicine, Seoul, Republic of Korea

Ji-Gang Zhang, Xiao-Yu Li, Yu-Zhu Wang, Sheng-Ying Gu, Xin Wu, Guan-Hua Zhu, Qin Li and Gao-Lin Liu
Department of Pharmacy, Shanghai First People's Hospital, School of medicine, Shanghai Jiao Tong University, Shanghai, P. R. China

Qi-Di Zhang
Department of Gastroenterology, Shanghai First People's Hospital, School of medicine, Shanghai Jiao Tong University, Shanghai, P.R. China

Eun-Jung Lee, Ik-Jae Lee, Won Woo Kim, Yang-Gun Suh and Jinsil Seong
Department of Radiation Oncology, Yonsei University College of Medicine, Seoul, Korea

Hyo Jin Park and Sang-Jun Ha
Department of Biochemistry, Yonsei University, Seoul, Korea

Shen-Chih Chang, Po-Yin Chang, Brendan Butler, Binh Y. Goldstein, Nai-Chieh Y. You, Aileen Baecker, Sander Greenland and Zuo-Feng Zhang
Department of Epidemiology, University of California Los Angeles Fielding School of Public Health, Los Angeles, CA, United States of America

Lina Mu
Department of Social and Preventive Medicine, State University of New York at Buffalo, Buffalo, NY, United States of America

Lin Cai
Department of Epidemiology, Fujian Medical University, Fuzhou, Fujian, China

Shun-Zhang Yu
Department of Epidemiology, Fudan University School of Public Health, Shanghai, China

David Heber and Qing-Yi Lu
Center for Human Nutrition, University of California Los Angeles David Geffen School of Medicine, Los Angeles, CA, United States of America

Liming Li
Department of Epidemiology, Peking University School of Public Health, Beijing, China

Sander Greenland
Department of Statistics, University of California Los Angeles College of Letters and Science, Los Angeles, CA, United States of America

Gaétan Bour, Marc Aprahamian, Jacques Marescaux and Jean-Marc Egly
Institut de Recherche contre les Cancers de l9Appareil Digestif (IRCAD), Strasbourg, France

Fernand Martel and Jean-Marc Egly
IGBMC, Department of Functional Genomics and Cancer, CNRS/INSERM/Université de Strasbourg, BP 163, Illkirch, C. U. Strasbourg, Strasbourg, France

Laurent Goffin, Bernard Bayle and Jacques Gangloff
ICube laboratory UMR, CNRS 7357, University of Strasbourg, Strasbourg, France

Stefan Welte, Toni Urbanik, Christin Elßner, Nicole Kautz, Bruno Christian Koehler, Dirk Jaeger and Henning Schulze-Bergkamen
National Center for Tumor Diseases, Department of Medical Oncology, Internal Medicine VI, Heidelberg University Hospital, Heidelberg, Germany

Nina Waldburger, Federico Pinna, Thomas Longerich and Kai Breuhahn
Institute of Pathology, Heidelberg University Hospital, Heidelberg, Germany

Justo Lorenzo Bermejo
Institute of Medical Biometry and Informatics, Heidelberg University Hospital, Heidelberg, Germany

Karl-Heinz Weiss
Department of Gastroenterology, Toxicology, and Infectious Diseases, Heidelberg University Hospital, Internal Medicine IV, Heidelberg, Germany

Peter Schemmer
Department of General and Transplant Surgery, Heidelberg University Hospital, Heidelberg, Germany

Henning Schulze-Bergkamen
Department of Gastroenterology, Diabetology and Rheumatology, Internal Medicine II, Marien-Hospital, Wesel, Germany

Dong Hyun Sinn, Geum-Youn Gwak, Seung Woon Paik and Byung Chul Yoo
Department of Medicine, Samsung Medical Center, Sungkyunkwan University School of Medicine, Seoul, Korea

Juhee Cho
Department of Health Science and Technology, Samsung Advanced Institute for Health Science and Technology, Sungkyunkwan University, Seoul, Korea
Department of Health, Behavior and Society and Epidemiology, Johns Hopkins Bloomberg School of Public Health, Baltimore, United States of America

Fred Stephen Sarfo, Maame Anima Sarfo, Betty Norman, Richard Phillips and George Bedu-Addo
Komfo Anokye Teaching Hospital, Kumasi, Ghana

Fred Stephen Sarfo, Richard Phillips and George Bedu-Addo
Kwame Nkrumah University of Science and Technology, Kumasi, Ghana

David Chadwick
The James Cook University Hospital, Middlesbrough, United Kingdom

Yun Liao, Bei Cai, Yi Li, Jie Chen, Chuanmin Tao, Hengjian Huang and Lanlan Wang
Department of Laboratory Medicine, West China Hospital, Sichuan University, Chengdu, Sichuan Province, China

Jian Ruan, Hang Zheng and Rongcheng Luo
Cancer Center, Traditional Chinese Medicine-Integrated Hospital, Southern medical University, Guangzhou, Guangdong, People's Republic of China

Wenguang Fu
Department of Hepatobiliary Surgery, The Affiliated Hospital of Luzhou Medical College, Luzhou, Sichuan, People's Republic of China

Peng Zhao
Department of Medical Oncology, The First Affiliated Hospital, School of Medicine, Zhejiang University, Hangzhou, Zhejiang, People's Republic of China

Ning Su
Department of Oncology, Guangzhou Chest Hospital, Guangzhou, Guangdong, People's Republic of China

Index

www.ingramcontent.com/pod-product-compliance
Lightning Source LLC
LaVergne TN
LVHW060557210926
848485LV00005B/1327
* 9 7 8 1 6 3 2 4 2 8 9 5 0 *